CLINICAL MEDICINE IN OPTOMETRIC PRACTICE

CLINICAL MEDICINE
IN
OPTOMETRIC
PRACTICE

Bruce G. Muchnick, O.D.
Assistant Professor of Optometry
Pennsylvania College of Optometry
Philadelphia, Pennsylvania

with 300 illustrations

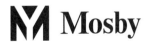 Mosby

St. Louis Baltimore Boston Chicago London Madrid Philadelphia Sydney Toronto

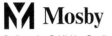

Mosby

Dedicated to Publishing Excellence

Editor: Martha Sasser
Associate Developmental Editor: Kellie F. White
Project Manager: Linda Clarke
Production Editor: Vicki Hoenigke
Designer: Renée Duenow

Printed in the United States of America
Composition by the Clarinda Company
Printing/binding by Maple Vail

Mosby–Year Book, Inc.
11830 Westline Industrial Drive
St. Louis, Missouri 63146

Library of Congress Cataloging-in-Publication Data
Clinical medicine in optometric practice / [edited by] Bruce G.
  Muchnick. — 1st ed.
      p.   cm.
    Includes bibliographical references and index.
    ISBN 0-8016-6306-7
    1. Ocular manifestations of general diseases.   2. Eye—Diseases.
  3. Optometry.   I. Muchnick, Bruce G.
    [DNLM: 1. Optometry—methods.   2. Vision Disorders—diagnosis.
  3. Vision Disorders—therapy.   WW 704 C641 1994]
  RE65.C56   1994
  617.7′5—dc20
  DNLM/DLC
  for Library of Congress   93-46868
                                                                    CIP

94 95 96 97 98 CL/MY 9 8 7 6 5 4 3 2 1

Contributors

Angelo M. Anaclerio, M.D., S.C.
Private Practice
Danville Eye Clinic and Cataract Center
Danville, Illinois

Martin Jan Bergman, M.D.
Clinical Assistant Professor of Medicine
Medical College of Pennsylvania
Philadelphia, Pennylvania;
Chief of Rheumatology
Taylor Hospital
Ridley Park, Pennsylvania

David C. Bright, O.D.
Assistant Chief, Optometry Service
Department of Veteran Affairs
West Los Angeles, California;
Associate Professor
Southern California College of Optometry
Fullerton, California

Jerry Cavallerano, O.D., Ph.D.
Staff Optometrist
Beetham Eye Institute
Joslin Diabetes Center
Boston, Massachusetts;
Associate Professor
New England College of Optometry
Boston, Massachusetts

Connie L. Chronister, O.D., F.A.A.O.
Associate Professor
Pennsylvania College of Optometry
Philadelphia, Pennsylvania

Philip Gilman, M.D.
Clinical Assistant Professor of Medicine
The Medical College of Pennsylvania
Department of Medicine, Gastroenterology
    Division
Episcopal Hospital
Philadelphia, Pennsylvania

Janice L. Glass, R.N.
Post-Anesthesia Care Unit Nurse
Anesthesia Department
Montgomery Hospital Medical Center
Norristown, Pennsylvania

Barry B. Goldberg, M.D.
Professor of Radiology
Director, Division of Ultrasound
Department of Radiology
Thomas Jefferson University Hospital and
    Medical School
Philadelphia, Pennsylvania

**Andrew S. Gurwood, B.S., O.D.,
    F.A.A.O.**
Assistant Professor of Clinical Sciences
Clinical Sciences
The Eye Institute of the Pennsylvania College of
    Optometry
Philadelphia, Pennsylvania

David S. Kountz, M.D.
Assistant Professor of Medicine
Director of Ambulatory Care
Division of Internal Medicine
Department of Medicine
Hahnemann University
Philadelphia, Pennsylvania

Allan T. Luskin, M.D.
Associate Professor of Immunology/
    Microbiology
Associate Professor of Medicine
Rush Medical Center
Chicago, Illinois;
Associate Professor of Immunology
Illinois College of Optometry
Chicago, Illinois

John F. Maher, M.D., F.A.C.S.
Instructor
Southern California College of Optometry
Fullerton, California

Brian P. Mahoney, O.D.
Chief, Optometry Section
Veteran's Administration Hospital
Wilmington, Delaware
Adjunct Instructor
Pennsylvania College of Optometry
S.U.N.Y. College of Optometry

Lawrence A. May, M.D., F.A.C.P.
Assistant Clinical Professor of Medicine
University of California-Los Angeles School of
    Medicine
Los Angeles, California

John McGreal, O.D.
Center Director of Missouri Eye Institute
St. Louis, Missouri

Daniel A. Merton, B.S., R.D.M.S.
Research Sonographer
Radiology, Division of Diagnostic Ultrasound
Thomas Jefferson University Hospital
Philadelphia, Pennsylvania

Leonard V. Messner, O.D.
Associate Professor
Director—Center for Advanced Ophthalmic
    Care
Illinois Eye Institute
Illinois College of Optometry
Chicago, Illinois

John H. Nishimoto, O.D.
Assistant Professor
Director of Residency Programs
Southern California College of Optometry
Fullerton, California

Al Philips, M.D., O.D.
Veteran's Administration Hospital
East Orange, New Jersey

Elois G. Rogers-Philips, M.D.
Co-Principal Investigator
Newark Inner City Minority–Based Community
    Clinical Oncology Program
University of Medicine and Dentistry of
    New Jersey
Newark, New Jersey

David P. Sendrowski, O.D., F.A.A.O.
Assistant Professor
Chief, Ocular Disease and Special Testing
    Service
Ocular Disease/Pathology Service
Southern California College of Optometry
Fullerton, California

Ronald E. Serfoss, O.D.
Private Practice
Danville Eye Clinic and Cataract Center
Danville, Illinois

Michael R. Silver, M.D.
Associate Professor
Director of Clinical Services
Pulmonary and Critical Care Medicine
Director Respiratory Care Unit
Department of Medicine
Rush-Presbyterian-St. Luke's Medical Center
Chicago, Illinois

George E. White, O.D.
Associate Professor
Department of Internal Clinical Education
Pennsylvania College of Optometry/The Eye
  Institute;
Director of Eye Services
John F. Kennedy Memorial Hospital
Department of Ophthalmology
Philadelphia, Pennsylvania

Alexander S. Zwil, M.D.
Assistant Professor, Psychiatry and Human
  Behavior
Director, Comprehensive Neuropsychiatry
  Program
Psychiatry and Human Behavior
Jefferson Medical College
Philadelphia, Pennsylvania

To my parents
MIRIAM AND IRVING MUCHNICK

Preface

The idea for this book grew out of a need for a text devoted to exploring the ways that clinical medicine can be integrated into the optometric practice. The goal of this book is to answer the most relevant of questions posed to me during my clinical medicine lectures to students and doctors of optometry: "How do I integrate this information into my office routine?"

The reader will note that the book has been divided into three parts. Part one discusses the medical diagnostic armamentarium available to the optometrist, from physical diagnosis to laboratory testing and radiology. It emphasizes the integration of these strategies into the optometric work-up.

Part two concentrates on the medical specialties that impact on eyecare. Here are presented the pathogenesis and evolution of systemic disorders, which sensitize the optometrist to the myriad of symptomologies indicative of underlying disease. I wanted this section of the book to help an optometrist faced with a patient who is, by virtue of their history and symptomology, suspicious for systemic disease. In addition, by examining the most recent diagnostic and therapeutic regimens available, this section serves as a quick reference guide for eyecare practioners and helps them gain familiarity with the medical conditions of their patients. In summary, Part two shows how the wide range of medical conditions and their therapeutic strategies impact on the delivery of eyecare.

Part three addresses the most likely scenario for the eyecare practitioner: the patient who presents with an ocular disorder that itself is suspicious for systemic disease. This section examines the possibility that your patient's anterior or posterior segment pathology is related to a systemic disease. By identifying the eye pathology, these chapters will guide the optometrist back to the appropriate chapters in Part two that describe the possible associated systemic disorders.

Since the fundamental philosophy guiding *Clinical Medicine in Optometric Practice* is an attempt to unify primary eyecare with clinical medicine, I felt strongly that as many chapters as possible be written by teams of optometrists and medical specialists. I sincerely hope that the team approach taken in the writing of this book symbolically forshadows an age of enlightened eyecare delivery. May all our patients benefit from the hard work of these dedicated authors.

Bruce G. Muchnick, O.D.

Acknowledgments

The completion of this text is due in no small part to a great number of people who helped in its production. I wish to acknowledge my editors at Mosby–Year Book, among them Mr. David Marshall, Ms. Kellie White, Ms. Martha Sasser, and Ms. Vicki Hoenigke, all of whom were a joy to work with.

Throughout this text are the many fine photographs of Mrs. Jane Stein, Ophthalmic Photographer of the Eye Institute of the Pennsylvania College of Optometry. Chapter Two photographs were taken by Mr. Scott Rowan and some photographs in Chapter Six are from Celeste Mruk, M.D.

Many thanks go to Dr. Sarah Foster and Dr. John Godfrey for their assistance in producing Chapter One, and to Ms. JoEllen Ritz and Ms. Beth L. Schultz for their assistance in producing Appendix B. Many, many thanks go to Ms. Beatrice Nunnally and Ms. Ruby Washington, who word processed almost all of the manuscript for publication. A special acknowledgement goes to Dr. Christopher Rinehart and Dr. Pierrette Dayhaw-Barker for suggesting me for this text.

For their inspiration throughout my optometric career, I wish to acknowledge some of the finest educators in our profession: Dr. Lorraine Lombardi, Drs. Gilda and the late George Crozier, Dr. Thomas Lewis, Dr. Louis Catania, Dr. Larry Gray, Dr. Linda Casser, and the entire faculty of the Pennsylvania College of Optometry. Also, thanks go to Dr. Samuel Cutler, Dr. Nibondh Vacharat, Dr. Bernard Blaustein, and Dr. Richard Sowby, who taught me much about the history and practical aspects of Optometry and Medicine.

And finally, for her love and support during this often difficult four-year project, a special thanks to my wife, Dr. Margaret Muchnick.

Contents

CLINICAL MEDICINE IN OPTOMETRIC PRACTICE

PART I

Diagnostic Procedures

1

The Physical Examination

LAWRENCE A. MAY

KEY TERMS

Observation	*Macules*	*Vertigo*
Palpation	*Papules*	*Otalgia*
Percussion	*Nodules*	*Tinnitis*
Auscultation	*Xanthelasma*	*Goiter*
Bruit	*Vesicle*	*Hemoptysis*
Transient Ischemic Attack	*Bullae*	*Ascites*
Stethoscope	*Pustule*	*Dysuria*
Sphygmomanometer	*Dysphonia*	*Hematuria*
Dyspnea	*Dysphagia*	*Dysmenorrhea*
Pruritus	*Otorrhea*	

---

*T*his chapter focuses on the art and science of the physical examination. It is impossible to appreciate clinical medicine without a sensitive understanding of the history, techniques, utility, and limitations of physical diagnosis.

To detect disease, the earliest clinicians relied entirely on observations that they made of their patients. Physical diagnosis advanced with refinements in the techniques of palpation and percussion. Finally, the introduction of instrumentation for auscultation permitted evaluation of sounds produced by the internal organs (Fig. 1-1).

The techniques of observation, palpation, percussion, and auscultation provide the framework necessary to achieve the primary goals of the physical examination. The first goal is to provide the initial basis for making decisions regarding laboratory and radiologic testing. The second goal is

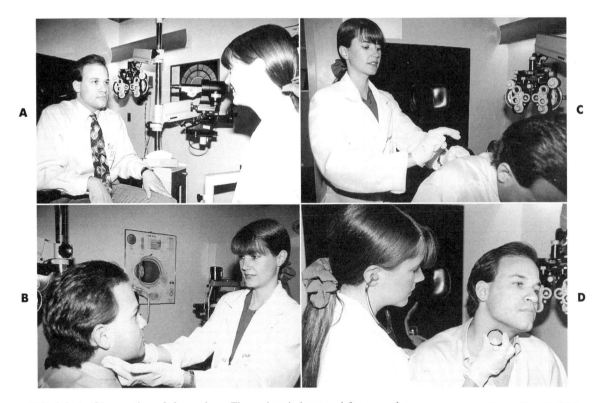

FIG. 1-1 **A, Observation of the patient:** The patient is inspected for general appearance, any asymmetry, posture, gait, and speech problems, and nutritional state. **B, Palpation of the patient:** The tactile sense is used to feel for masses, underlying abnormalities, and abnormal heart impulses. **C, Percussion of the patient:** A sound is produced by underlying structures when a sharp blow is delivered to an overlying site on the skin. This sound is evaluated to identify various problems in the underlying structures. **D, Auscultation of the patient:** Sounds produced by underlying organ systems are heard with the aid of the stethoscope.

to facilitate the doctor-patient relationship. The third goal is to detect any disease at an early stage. Finally, the examination provides important baseline information.

To master those aspects of the physical examination that are integral to the optometric practice, the student must learn and perform the techniques in the clinical setting. Only through repeated exposure to its methods and instrumentation can physical diagnosis as an art and discipline be appreciated and applied.

As science and medicine progress in complexity, it is all too easy for the examination to become depersonalized. The physical examination encompasses the patient's physical and emotional pain.

It embodies the sensitivity that the clinician develops in responding to a fellow human being.

BASIC PROCEDURES

Four primary skills are essential in performing an appropriate physical examination. These skills are observation, palpation, percussion, and auscultation.

The physical examination requires detailed *observation* by the practitioner from the moment the patient is first greeted. The examiner should evaluate the general appearance of the patient with regard to wellness, alertness, nutritional state, and posture. Any asymmetry of the body should be

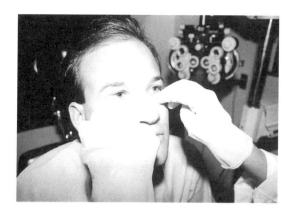

FIG. 1-2 Palpation: Small areas of skin or underlying masses may be palpated by use of one or two fingers moved in a circular pattern. Large masses are palpated with all the fingers or with the palm.

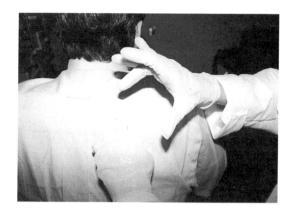

FIG. 1-3 Percussion: The examiner's left middle finger is placed over the site to be examined and pressed firmly on the skin.

noted, inspected, and evaluated. In addition, observations should be made about the patient's gait and speech pattern. Finally, the mental status of the patient should be evaluated.

Observation is followed by touching the patient's skin, a procedure known as *palpation*. Palpation of the body permits assessment of any irregularity, enlargement, hardness, or heat associated with inflammation. To perform palpation, the clinician uses touch to evaluate the characteristics of an internal organ system. Most often the fingers and the palms of the hand are used because these are exquisitely sensitive detectors of underlying pressure and contour gradients. Palpation involves an intimacy that is critical for the development of the complex doctor/patient relationship (Fig. 1-2).

The technique of *percussion* is performed by striking an area of the body to produce and evaluate the resulting sound. Percussion provides information about the size of an underlying organ, the presence of fluid in a normally air-filled cavity, and the presence of excessive dilatation due to trapped air. To perform percussion, the clinician's left middle finger is placed firmly against the patient's body. The tip of the right middle finger is then struck against the left middle finger to produce the resulting sound (Figs. 1-3 and 1-4).

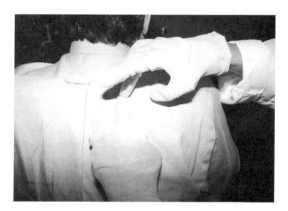

FIG. 1-4 Percussion: The examiner's right middle finger sharply strikes the left middle finger. The resulting sound is evaluated by the examiner.

Each organ produces a characteristic sound that results from the shock wave of the percussion as it passes through various tissues. Changes in the organ's size, density, or tissue composition result in characteristic changes in the sound produced. As the clinician gains experience with this skill, valuable predictions can be made concerning the health of an organ system.

With the addition of simple yet refined instruments, such as the stethoscope, *auscultation* has become an essential part of the physical examination. Listening with the stethoscope allows detec-

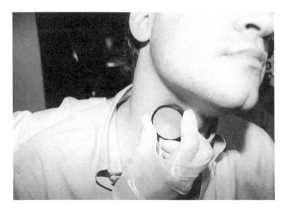

FIG. 1-5 Auscultation of the carotid artery: The diaphragm of the stethoscope is used on the patient, who is sitting or supine. The patient's head is turned away from the stethoscope and the patient holds his breath. The examiner listens to the carotid artery just above the clavicle, on the center of the neck, and just under the angle of the jaw.

tion of adventitious lung sounds that suggest pneumonia or heart failure (see Chapter 10). Auscultation is also used to evaluate the heart for murmurs that suggest valvular dysfunction. Of particular interest to the optometrist is the use of auscultation to detect the presence of *bruits* due to narrowing of blood vessels secondary to atherosclerosis. The carotid bruit is a significant finding in a patient experiencing the visual symptoms associated with a *transient ischemic attack* (TIA) (Fig. 1-5).

THE INSTRUMENTS

The four cardinal skills of the physical examination are enhanced by the use of other medical instruments. The instruments used to examine the ears, nose, throat, larynx, esophagus, stomach, rectum, colon and joints fall under the category of endoscopes. These scopes enable the examiner to look within the body through natural or surgically created holes. Simpler equipment is also used to help perform various tests. Refinements in these instruments have accelerated as each decade passes, but the decision to employ this technology is costly, and the diagnosis ultimately depends on

the human skills of history taking and physical examination.

The mandatory equipment for the routine physical examination includes the *stethoscope* for auscultation, the penlight for specific illumination and pupil testing, the otoscope for the ear examination, the ophthalmoscope for the eye examination, safety pins for sensory testing, a 128-Hz tuning fork for audition, and a reflex hammer for deep tendon reflex testing. Other equipment includes a nasal speculum and illuminator, *sphygmomanometer* for blood pressure measurement, tongue depressors, and cotton-tipped applicators. Barrier protection for the clinician and patient includes gloves, mask, and eye protection (Fig. 1-6).

THE LANGUAGE OF THE PHYSICAL EXAMINATION

Language is an important element of the physical examination; although language is a means of communication, it can also be a source of confusion. Clinicians communicating with patients during the physical examination must be aware of the need to interpret medical terminology so that the patient understands it (Table 1-1). The language of the physical examination includes eponyms and colorful descriptives that can both frighten and confuse patients. Although eponyms bestow honor on clinicians who made observations and disseminated them to their peers, they have no value in terms of description. In general, description is preferable to use of eponyms.

The sheer number of fascinating eponyms associated with the eye indicates how central the eye has been in the development of the physical examination. A few of the ocular signs of systemic disease that are denoted by eponyms include Adie's tonic pupil, Brushfield's spots of the iris, the Kayser-Fleischer corneal ring, Hollenhorst plaques of the retinal vasculature, and Horner's syndrome.

A myriad of eponyms denote lid abnormalities associated with hyperthyroidism (see Chapter 14), such as von Graefe lid lag, the infrequent blinking known as Stellwag's sign, the tremor of the

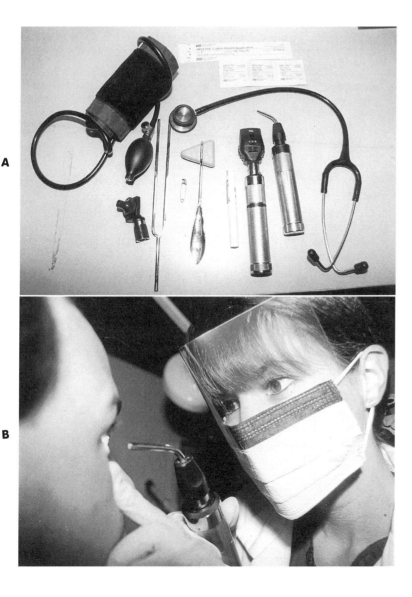

A

B

FIG. 1-6 A, The instruments of the physical examination: Included here are the stethoscope, penlight, otoscope, ophthalmoscope, safety pins, tuning fork, reflex hammer, nasal illuminator, sphygmomanometer, tongue depressor, and cotton-tipped applicators. **B, Barrier protection for doctor and patient:** Included here are mask, gloves, and eye protection.

closed lids known as Rosenbach's sign, and the lag of the lower lid during globe elevation known as Griffith's sign. A similar litany of famous names is attached to other important signs in the physical examination.

The physical examination sometimes uses colorful language to help describe a clinical observation. Numerous examples are associated with the eye. The copper-wiring associated with arteriosclerotic change in the retina, the nerve infarctions known as *cotton-wool spots,* and the mutton fat precipitates of the cornea seen in granulomatous uveitis all illustrate colorful and descriptive language.

Similarly, sputum has been described with such terms as "rusty," "currant jelly," or "prune juice." Each description indicates a certain type of infectious organism. The characteristic skin rash of chickenpox or its reactivation as herpes zoster is referred to as "dew drops on a petal." In patients

TABLE I-I *System-by-System Useful Vocabulary*		
Organ or System	*Medical Term*	*Definition*
Ear	Audiometer	A device that measures hearing
	Presbycusis	Hearing loss with age
	Otitis	Inflammation of the ear
	Phonasthesia	Voice weakness
Mouth	Stomatitis	Inflammation of the mouth
Chest	Bronchitis	Inflammation of the bronchus
	Dyspnea	Shortness of breath or difficulty breathing
	Hemoptysis	Coughing up blood
	Apnea	Temporary cessation of respiration
Heart	Bradycardia	Slow heart rate
	Tachycardia	Fast heart rate
	Cardiomegaly	Heart enlargement
Breast	Gynecomastia	Excessive male breast development
	Lactation	Milk secretion
	Mammogram	X-ray of breast
	Mastitis	Inflammation of the breast
Abdomen	Colitis	Inflammation of intestine
	Cholecystitis	Inflammation of gallbladder
Urogenital system	Nephropathy	Kidney disease
	Pyelogram	X-ray of kidney
	Metrorrhagia	Uterine bleeding
	Hematuria	Red blood cells in urine
	Pyuria	White blood cells in urine
Musculoskeletal system	Arthritis	Inflammation of joint
	Myopathy	Muscle disease
	Scoliosis	Lateral deviation of the spine
Nervous system	Dysesthesia	Abnormal sensation
	Agnosia	Loss of recognition of sensory stimuli
	Paresis	Weakness
	Neuropathy	Nerve damage
	Aphasia	Inability to speak

with cirrhosis of the liver, dilated veins may form around the umbilicus which have been called the caput Medusa, named for the mythologic goddess who had snakes in place of hair. These poetic descriptions all help visualize the abnormalities being described.

THE HISTORY

While taking the patient's history, the clinician establishes a rapport with the patient and makes critical observations. The history begins with a detailing of the chief complaint (the reason the patient has come to the clinician), a history of previous illnesses, current medications, family medical history, social situation, and all other pertinent information that helps to explain a symptom or diagnose a disease (Table 1-2).

The chief complaint is best described as a brief statement by the patient of the reason for seeking medical attention. A chronologic history of present symptoms allows the clinician to understand the

TABLE 1-2 *A Format for the Physical Examination and History*

Major Section	Goal	Detailed Questioning or Explanation
Chief complaint	Learn why patient is seeking medical attention.	Quote the patient's words exactly as stated.
History of present illness	Ascertain recent changes in the health of the patient pertaining to the chief complaint.	Ascertain earliest symptom; follow chronology and evolution of symptoms to present day.
Past medical history	Assess patient's general health prior to present illness.	Ascertain prior health, past illness, injuries, hospitalizations, surgery, allergies, immunizations, diet, current medications, and sleep habits.
Occupational history	Ascertain the risk the patient faces at work of exposure to disease-producing substances or environments.	List occupations, protective devices, and duration of exposure to noxious substances.
Family history	Ascertain health of parents, siblings, and other blood relatives.	List genetic and environmental causes of all family deaths and illnesses.
Social history	Ascertain life style, sexual, and biographical information.	Ascertain substance abuse; alcohol use (how much and when); cigarette or tobacco; drugs (cocaine, marijuana, etc.)
Review of systems	Compile a summary of common complaints of each body system.	Determine major symptoms of each of the following organs and systems: general, skin, head, eyes, ears, nose, mouth, throat, breasts, chest, and vascular, gastrointestinal, urinary, genital, musculoskeletal, and neurologic systems.

evolution of a developing disease. The medical history should include answers to questions concerning the state of the patient's general health, past medical conditions, trauma, previous surgeries, allergies, alcohol or drug abuse, and current medications. A family history may reveal a relevant genetic pattern. This medical history provides an excellent format for the optometric patient with systemic disease.

VITAL SIGNS

The vital signs include measurements of the patient's temperature, pulse, blood pressure, respiratory rate, height, and weight. Normal temperature is considered 98.6° F, but a temperature may be slightly higher or lower. A temperature eleva-

tion may be a sign of disease, indicating a reaction of the body to infection. Circadian variation sometimes causes people who are ill, to have a normal temperature in the morning and an elevated temperature later in the day. Fevers tend to be highest at night (Fig. 1-7). Any patient coming to the optometrist's office with signs of systemic inflammation should have an oral temperature reading.

The pulse is assessed for rate and regularity. A normal rate is 50 to 70 pulses per minute but may be lower in a young athlete or in an elderly heart patient with a disease of the conduction system. Elevated pulse rate occurs with increased respiration; this is known as normal sinus arrhythmia. Premature beats may be perceived as early, extra, or skipped beats because a long pause follows the

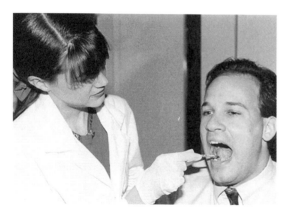

FIG. 1-7 **Measuring the patient's temperature:** Use of an oral thermometer can determine a patient's temperature. A sterile thermometer is shaken so that its initial reading is well below 98.6° F. It is placed beneath the tongue of a patient and read in one minute.

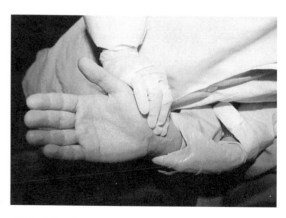

FIG. 1-8 **Measuring the patient's pulse:** The index finger, middle finger, and fourth finger are placed over the radial artery (wrist pulse) below the base of the patient's thumb. The pulse is counted for 30 seconds and multiplied by two to get a pulse rate for one minute.

early beat. The pulse may be rapidly irregularly irregular, as with atrial fibrillation (Fig. 1-8). All optometric patients can be evaluated for pulse rate; any finding of bradycardia (slow rate) or an irregular heart beat in a glaucoma patient warrants a call to the family physician before beginning a beta-blocker for glaucoma treatment.

Blood pressure is measured with a sphygmomanometer and stethoscope by auscultating and evaluating changes in the pulse as pressure is released from the cuff (Fig. 1-9). The first heart sound heard as pressure is released represents the systolic pressure, or the pressure that is maximally achieved when the heart pumps. Continued auscultation reveals disappearance of the pulse, which represents the diastolic pressure, or the pressure during the filling phase of the heart. Blood pressure is arbitrarily judged to be high based on an accepted normal reading of 140/90 mm Hg or less, but blood pressure must be interpreted in the context of age, the relative excitement of the patient, and measurement limitations. For example, a very thick arm may produce an artificially elevated blood pressure, and the clinician must use a wide thigh cuff to determine pressure accurately. Blood pressure readings are mandatory for any optometric patient who is to be dilated with phenylephrine

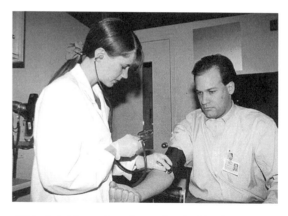

FIG. 1-9 **Measuring the patient's blood pressure:** The sphygmomanometer provides an indirect measurement of blood pressure by detecting the appearance and disappearance of the Korotkoff sounds over an artery compressed by an air-filled bladder. Evaluation of both arms may be necessary.

because this sympathomimetic can raise systemic blood pressure temporarily.

Respiratory rate can be a clue to underlying breathing difficulties. In very ill patients, various types of respiratory patterns may indicate metabolic abnormalities or levels of coma. *Dyspnea* (difficulty in breathing) in a glaucoma patient may preclude the use of beta-blockers because of their tendency to exacerbate asthma.

Height and weight are important measurements. Changes in weight must be measured and ultimately explained. Significant weight gain is associated with pseudotumor cerebri, which causes elevated intracranial pressure. Headache and reduced visual acuity can accompany the papilledema that is secondary to elevated intracranial pressure. A significant finding in these patients is often a history of recent weight gain. Height and weight can easily be measured in the optometrist's office or recent readings can be obtained with the patient's permission from the family physician.

EXAMINATION OF THE SKIN

The skin, or integument, is the outer aspect or covering of the body and is the first system to be examined. The medical examination should be performed with the patient completely naked, so that every area of the skin can be evaluated. The optometric evaluation of the skin is usually limited to the head, neck, arms, and hands. The detection of possible skin cancers is a critical element of this part of the physical examination. Skin cancers are detected by observation and confirmed by removal of tissue and subsequent examination under the microscope (biopsy). The patient may present with symptoms of skin disease, including *pruritus* (itching), a rash, and changes in skin, hair, or nails.

Examination of the facial skin can be useful in determining significant disease. Pigmented lesions such as seborrheic keratoses must be differentiated from melanoma. The characteristics of melanoma include irregular borders and surface details and changes in color. The inflamed tissue is red but may become white from necrosis or turn blue from deep invasion of the melanoma. Pigmented lesions should always be observed, measured, described, documented with drawings or photographs.

Many clinical diagnoses derive from observing the facial skin. Skin coloring may be a risk factor in the development of skin cancer. The clinician should therefore caution a fair-skinned patient about the importance of sun screens. Areas of red-

ness and roughness, known as actinic keratoses, or sun damage, should be treated for cosmetic reasons and for their tendency to become malignant.

Thinning of the skin with visible vessels, called telangiectasias, may be a normal variation or the result of sun damage. Telangiectasias may also be spider angiomas, which when compressed seem to fill from the center with spider-like tentacles. Spider angiomas may indicate estrogen excess or may be related to a specific skin disease like acne rosacea.

Small papules or pimples may be normal variations or may require a referral to another physician for the treatment of acne. Blackheads around the eyes in older patients can be treated for cosmetic purposes.

The color of the facial skin is changed by the presence of some diseases. For example, pallor of the skin may indicate anemia, and a yellowing complexion may suggest underlying jaundice or liver disease.

Skin Terminology

It is important to become familiar with the terminology used to describe skin lesions. Localized changes in the color of usually flat red lesions of 1 cm or less in size are called *macules* (for example, freckles). Elevated areas less than 1 cm in diameter are called *papules* (for example, acne). Rashes that have a flat, red area are called maculopapular. A patch is a macule greater than 1 cm in diameter (for example, vitiligo).

Raised areas greater than 1 cm are referred to as *nodules*. Plaques have a large surface area in relation to their height. For example, the skin lesion present in psoriasis is a scaling plaque. Plaques that are yellow are often called xanthomas, or they may be small seborrheic cysts. Xanthomas on the eyelid are known as *xanthelasma* and may be a sign of elevated cholesterol.

An elevation of the skin with a clear fluid accumulation of less than 1 cm just beneath the upper layer is called a *vesicle*. A cold sore is a type of vesicle. Accumulations of clear fluid larger than 1 cm are called *bullae*. Vesicles and bullae are clear because their fluid is not infected. An accumulation of fluid that is thicker, more opaque, and yellow, green or orange is called a pustule and may indicate active infection.

In summary, the skin examination is divided into two parts. The first part consists of detection of pruritus or changes in skin color, hair, and nails. The second part consists of inspection and palpation of the hair, nails, and skin of the neck, face, back, chest, abdomen, arms, and legs. All lesions should be described and documented and clinico-pathologic correlations made (see Chapter 8). Any suspicious skin lesion found on the optometric examination should be documented and the patient monitored or referred to the family physician or a dermatologist.

EXAMINATION OF THE EYE

Following the skin evaluation, the eyes are examined. Significant eye symptoms include loss of visual acuity, field loss, eye pain, redness, diplopia, tearing, discharge, or trauma. This examination includes a visual acuity measurement, confrontational visual field testing, pupil testing, extraocular muscle motility assessment, and fundus evaluation with an ophthalmoscope. The skin around the eyes is checked carefully for any lesions, such as basal cell carcinoma. Basal cell lesions can appear as small, red, or bleeding sores found especially around the eyes and bridge of the nose. Lastly, the cornea is evaluated for pterygium, and the lid is everted to look for conjunctival cysts, lumps, or changes in color. We omit an in-depth discussion of the ocular portion of the physical examination in deference to the reader's expertise.

EXAMINATION OF THE NOSE

Significant nasal symptoms include frequent nose bleeds, nasal discharge, nasal obstruction, sinus infection, and hay fever. Frequent nose bleeds, or epistaxis, are usually due to nose picking, but malignancy must be considered. Examination of the nose requires inspection of its outer detail as well as its internal structures, which are viewed with the assistance of a nasal illuminator (Fig. 1-10). Examination of the nasal mucosa indicates whether

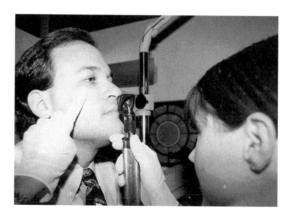

FIG. 1-10 The nasal illuminator: The nasal illuminator aids in the evaluation of the nose.

it is swollen and pale (as in allergic rhinitis), swollen and red (as in a viral rhinitis), and dry and cracking (from environmental changes such as dryness). By obtaining a nasal illuminator head for the ophthalmoscope, the optometrist can easily perform this examination. A practitioner can often discover clues to illicit drug use, such as punctate ulcerations from cocaine or actual perforation of the nasal septum from a vasoconstricting illicit drug. Nasal tumors can be detected through careful observation.

EXAMINATION OF THE MOUTH

Significant complaints of oral cavity problems include bleeding gums, frequent sore throats, *dysphonia* (hoarseness, voice changes), and postnasal drip. *Dysphagia,* or difficulty swallowing, is a significant symptom of obstruction or neurologic problems. The oral cavity is examined with a light and a tongue depressor to allow visualization of all structures (Fig. 1-11). The posterior pharynx and tonsils are examined for inflammation, infection, enlargement, and abnormal lesions that might be cancerous.

The underside of the tongue and the area between the teeth and the lips, should be examined to identify premalignant or potentially malignant conditions. Normal variations, such as torus palatinus, a bony structure emanating from the hard pal-

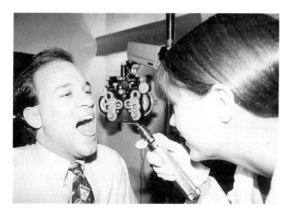

FIG. 1-11 Examination of the mouth: A penlight and optional tongue depressor are used to evaluate the teeth, gums, buccal mucosa, tongue, tonsils, uvula, and lips.

ate, must be differentiated from more serious conditions. When anything abnormal is visualized — whether a white plaque known as leukoplakia, a red plaque known as erythroplakia, a lump, or a bony prominence — it should be palpated to provide a more complete description. Any abnormalities noted on the oral examination warrant a referral to the family physician or dentist.

EXAMINATION OF THE EAR

Significant ear complaints include hearing loss, *otorrhea* (ear discharge), *vertigo* (dizziness), *otalgia* (pain), *tinnitis* (ringing in the ears) and ear infection. Examination of the ear requires observation of its external structures for abnormalities such as squamous cell carcinoma. The ear canal and drum are then inspected with the assistance of an otoscope. Significant signs of inflammation include redness or swelling of the canal and drum and a loss of the drum light reflex, suggestive of fluid behind the drum. An excessive accumulation of cerumen (ear wax) can block the canal or press against the tympanic membrane and produce hearing loss.

Two hearing tests can easily be performed by the optometrist in the office. Both tests make use of a 512-Hz tuning fork. The Rinne test involves placement of a vibrating tuning fork on the mas-

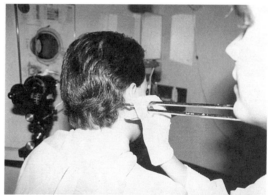

A

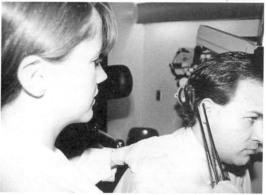

B

FIG. 1-12 The Rinne auditory test: A, A vibrating tuning fork is placed on the mastoid process. **B,** When the patient no longer hears a sound, the tuning fork is removed and brought to the ear opening. The sound should continue to be audible to the patient.

toid sinus of the patient (Fig. 1-12). The patient hears the sound by bone conduction. When the sound dies off, the patient signals the examiner, who then removes the fork and brings it to the opening of the patient's ear. The sound should still be audible because air conduction is superior to bone conduction. If the patient has a conductive hearing loss, then bone conduction, which bypasses the obstruction, will be superior to air conduction.

A second method, the Weber test, also makes use of a vibrating 512-Hz tuning fork. This time the tuning fork is placed on the center of the patient's forehead. The Weber test evaluates bone conduction between the ears. Normally, the patient

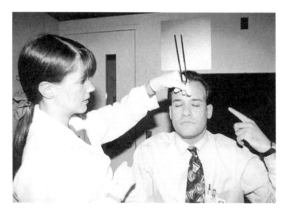

FIG. 1-13 The Weber test: A vibrating tuning fork is placed in the center of the patient's forehead. Normally the vibration sounds are equally loud to both ears. A conduction deficit lateralizes the sound to the affected side. A sensorineural deficit lateralize the sound to the unaffected side.

hears a sound in both ears. If the sound is louder in one ear, that ear may have a conduction deficit. To prove this principle, plug one ear with a finger to produce a conduction deficit and hum softly. The sound seems louder in the occluded ear. Of course, if there is a sensorineural deficit to one ear, the sound is lateralized to the unaffected side (Fig. 1-13).

EXAMINATION OF THE NECK

Following the examination of the head, eyes, ears, nose, and mouth, which all require primarily observational skills with the assistance of instruments, the clinician should focus on the neck. Significant presenting symptoms of neck problems include anomalous lumps, goiter, pain, tenderness, and neck stiffness. The multiple structures in the neck should be observed and carefully palpated.

First, the midline position of the trachea is confirmed by observation. Then the neck is inspected for any asymmetry or visible abnormal lumps. An enlarged central lump is suggestive of an enlarged thyroid, or *goiter*. Lumps along the sides of the neck are suggestive of enlarged lymph nodes. Enlarged salivary glands can be observed and pal-

pated under the chin. Dilation of the veins of the neck may suggest congestive heart failure.

Palpation of the neck is the most critical part of the examination. The thyroid should be palpated; and if there is a suggestion of an enlarged thyroid, the patient is asked to swallow a sip of water. The act of swallowing allows the thyroid to move up and down, making it easier to palpate (Fig. 1-14). The symmetry, size, and consistency of the thyroid should be described. The optometrist should palpate the thyroid of any patient exhibiting signs of Graves' disease (see Chapter 14).

The lymph nodes should be described in the entire neck and head area. Whenever inflammation of the eye is present, the optometrist should examine the preauricular lymph nodes, which are the major area of lymph drainage (Fig. 1-15). There are lymph nodes along the jugular vein in the neck, across the back (the posterior cervical lymph nodes), behind the ear, under the jaw bone (the submandibular lymph nodes), and under the chin (the submental lymph nodes).

Any lymph node enlargement must be explained because it is a key sign in many diseases. Such enlargement is usually due to inflammation or infection, but lymph nodes that grow and become firm, hard, or irregular may be indicative of a lymph node tumor known as lymphoma. In other situations, a tumor arising elsewhere in the body can metastasize and cause enlarged and hardened lymph nodes.

Lymph nodes must be palpated in the supraclavicular area just above the clavicle, in the axilla (armpit), and in the inguinal (groin) area. Although painful lymph nodes are often associated with inflammation or infection, painless lymph nodes can be associated with malignant change.

The carotid artery should be palpated to gain information regarding poor blood flow and changes in the heart valves. An important examination is auscultation of the carotid arteries. This involves listening for abnormal sounds suggestive of narrowing of the artery. Detection of these sounds, called bruits, sometimes requires a carotid work-up (Fig. 1-16). Causes of carotid bruits include excessive blood flow (in a young person),

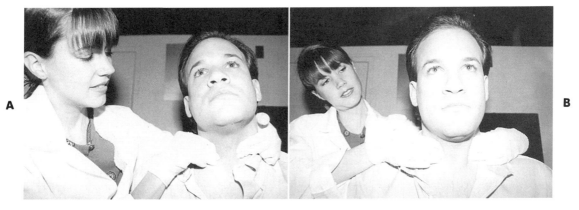

FIG. 1-14 Palpation of the thyroid: A, Anterior approach: The patient tilts his chin slightly to the right as the examiner grasps the right sternocleidomastoid muscle and displaces the larynx to the patient's right side by use of the examiner's left hand. The patient swallows and the right lobe of the thyroid is felt moving up and down against the examiner's right thumb and fingers. The process is reversed for the left lobe. **B,** Posterior approach: The examiner places both hands on the patient's sternocleidomastoid muscles. The left hand pushes the trachea to the right while the patient swallows. The right lobe is felt against the sternocleidomastoid muscle with the right hand. The process is reversed for the left lobe.

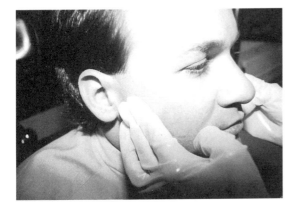

FIG. 1-15 Palpation of preauricular lymph node: The preauricular lymph node is found just in front of the ear where the jaw articulates with the cranium. This node may become enlarged and painful with viral conjunctivitis.

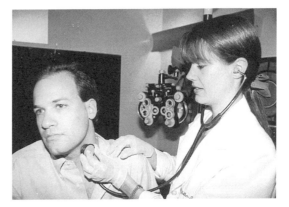

FIG. 1-16 Auscultation for carotid bruit: Thrombus development in the carotid artery causes the normally smooth and laminar blood flow to become disturbed and produce a "whooshing" sound heard between the two quick beats of the carotid pulse. Instead of the normal "blub-dup, blub-dup" the sound becomes "blub-woosh-dup, blub-woosh-dup."

transmission of a murmur from the heart, or narrowing of the carotid arteries. Any patient presenting with the ocular symptoms of a transient ischemic attack warrants a carotid auscultation because carotid plaques may occlude the ocular blood flow, causing sudden loss of vision. Usually these changes are monocular when they originate in the carotid artery. Whether the optometrist hears a bruit or not, the patient requires a carotid work-up by a vascular specialist as long as all other causes of the transient attack have been eliminated (see Chapter 9).

EXAMINATION OF THE LUNGS

Patients with lung problems (see Chapter 11) may present with complaints of cough, chest pain, dyspnea (difficulty breathing or shortness of breath), sputum production, *hemoptysis* (coughing up blood), or a history of lung disease, such as asthma, emphysema, tuberculosis, or sarcoidosis. The lungs should be examined by inspecting for abnormalities in symmetry, scoliosis (lateral curvature of the spine), and audible wheezes during inspiration or expiration.

Following this evaluation, the lung is percussed by pressing on the chest or the back with the middle finger of one hand and striking it with the middle finger of the other hand. A resonant note is indicative of hollowness produced by the presence of air. A dull note suggests fluid, which can accumulate in a patient with pneumonia or heart failure. An abnormal accumulation of fluid in the pleural sac is known as pleural effusion.

The stethoscope is then used to listen for abnormal lung sounds. In the healthy patient, the practitioner should be able to hear air coming into the lungs on inspiration and going out on expiration. If there is spasm of the bronchial tubes, the clinician may hear a wheeze suggestive of asthma. Fluid in the lungs produces a crackle, or rale, which is sometimes likened to the sound made by rubbing hair between two fingers. Louder variations of that sound are known as wheezes, or rhonchi. Rales and rhonchi suggest fluid, which may be caused by congestive heart failure or infection such as pneumonia. Sometimes sounds are heard that can be cleared by asking the patient to cough. The disappearance of adventitious sounds with coughing probably indicates a benign condition.

Monitoring the length of inspiration versus expiration can be helpful. Normal vesicular breathing produces a long inspiration and shorter expiration. Bronchial breathing has a prolonged expiration indicative of early obstructive changes.

The optometrist should be reminded that beta-blockers used for the topical treatment of glaucoma can exacerbate asthma. Some patients may be unaware that they have asthma. It is therefore recommended that the optometrist contact the patient's physician before prescribing a beta-blocker in order to determine whether a pulmonary problem has been diagnosed.

EXAMINATION OF THE HEART

The most frequent cardiac complaints include chest pain, coughing, dyspnea while lying flat or asleep, high blood pressure, palpitations, syncope, fatigue, peripheral edema (fluid in the legs), and a history of heart attack or abnormal electrocardiograms (see Chapter 9). Before the advent of echocardiography, the clinical examination of the heart was the most elegant and most challenging in internal medicine. It was incumbent on the clinician to determine by clinical means whether a patient had a narrowing of the aortic valve, known as aortic stenosis, or a leaking valve causing aortic insufficiency or aortic regurgitation.

The clinician can hear systolic ejection sounds suggestive of an atrial septal defect, which is a hole in the superior aspect of the heart. The clinician might hear a click and a late systolic murmur associated with the most common valve abnormality, known as mitral valve prolapse.

The heart is examined in the context of its sounds, their radiation into the axilla or the neck, and the effect they have on the carotid pulse. Palpation is used to detect a displaced primary impulse, suggesting a change in the heart's size. Palpation can also detect abnormal movement of the blood through the heart, known as a thrill. The heart is percussed to determine whether it is enlarged.

Auscultation is carefully performed by listening for murmurs indicative of heart valve dysfunction. These murmurs are described in terms of their intensity, duration, location, and transmission. Many murmurs, if not most, are physiologic or functional. A murmur is a sound indicative of a relative increase in blood flow through the valve opening, and it suggests either a narrowing, a leak, or simply a normal variant. Other heart sounds that indicate malfunction, such as S_4 gallops, precede the first heart sound and are indicative of a non-compliant ventricle. An S_3 gallop follows the second heart sound and indicates a dilated or poorly functioning heart muscle.

The echocardiogram uses sound waves to measure the heart sound, as well as the function of the valve. It establishes whether a disease is present.

It is important for the optometrist to realize that beta-blockers may exacerbate bradycardia and other significant heart conditions. Before the optometrist treats glaucoma with topical beta-blockers, the patient's family physician should be consulted to verify that the drug will not exacerbate an underlying heart condition. Some heart conditions are treated with beta-blockers, and the patient may already be on such oral medications. Topical application of an additional beta-blocker may cause overdosage. To reduce the chance of systemic absorption of a topical beta-blocker, the patient must be taught the technique of punctal occlusion when an eye drop is being applied.

EXAMINATION OF THE BREAST

Patients may present with breast complaints, including lumps, discharge from the nipple, pain and tenderness, and abnormal findings from a self-examination. Breasts in both men and women should be examined in the routine medical examination. In men, palpation is used to detect the abnormal accumulation of breast tissue, known as gynecomastia, or the rare case of male breast cancer.

Examination of the female breasts entails visual inspection, followed by palpation. The skin of the breast is inspected for changes, lumps, retractions, and asymmetries. Palpation can determine whether dominant masses are present. Radiographs of the breasts, known as mammograms, are recommended to supplement the physical examination.

The breasts should be examined regularly, and a good physical examination should include teaching and encouraging monthly self-examination on the part of the patient. Breast examination is not part of the routine optometric examination, and any patient with a breast complaint should be referred to a family physician or surgeon. A patient with a history of breast carcinoma requires a dilated fundus examination to rule out metastasis to the retina.

EXAMINATION OF THE ABDOMEN

Abdominal complaints include pain, nausea, vomiting, rectal bleeding, jaundice, and pruritus. Examination of the abdomen begins with inspection for the obvious signs of obesity or muscular laxity. Scars, engorged veins, abdominal contours, and visible masses should be noted. The abdomen is then percussed to detect any enlargement of the liver or spleen, and any dullness suggestive of an underlying mass. The abdomen is then palpated, feeling for the liver's edge on the right side of the body and the spleen's edge on the left. Sometimes abdominal palpation requires that the patient be placed in a left lateral position to ascertain enlargement. The mid-abdomen is palpated carefully, particularly in older patients, looking for signs of dilatation of the aorta, known as an aortic aneurysm.

The abdomen is then auscultated for bruits, which can indicate narrowing of the renal artery or the presence of atherosclerosis in the abdominal aorta. Auscultation is particularly important in assessing patients with unusual blood pressure elevations because those elevations can be due to narrowing, or stenosis, of the renal artery.

When abdominal distension is present, the clinician needs to look for the signs of *ascites,* which is fluid in the abdomen. Ascites can occur as a result of a generalized accumulation of fluid secondary to heart failure, liver failure, or tumors. Because fluid produces a change in the percussion sound, one clinical sign of ascites is a change in the distribution of dullness. Shifting of the dullness may be induced by placing a hand in the middle and taping the side of the abdomen while turning the patient. In this way a fluid wave can be produced.

In addition to these physical signs, the clinician can use an ultrasound examination to confirm a clinical suspicion of ascites. The patient who presents to the optometrist with symptoms of nausea, vomiting, and intestinal cramps, along with the ocular signs of uveitis, must be evaluated for inflammatory bowel disease (see Chapter 12).

EXAMINATION OF THE GENITOURINARY TRACT AND PELVIS

Typical pelvic complaints include pain, *dysuria* (pain on urination), incontinence, *hematuria* (blood in the urine), discharge, lesions, impotence or dyspareunia (painful intercourse), infertility, and *dysmenorrhea* (painful menstruation).

A pelvic examination of the female patient begins with an inspection of the external structures for signs of abnormalities. The pelvic examination involves all of the physical examination skills and also a scraping of cells from the cervix, known as a Pap smear. Abnormal cervical cells may be the first sign of an underlying cervical or uterine malignancy. Next, a speculum is inserted into the vaginal canal to visualize the vaginal wall and cervix. The speculum is kept in place while a sample of the cervical and uterine cells are obtained for the Pap smear. The speculum is then removed.

Palpation is used to evaluate the size of the uterus, uterine irregularities, enlargement of the ovaries, or abnormal masses in the area surrounding the uterus. Uterine palpation takes place by inserting one finger into the vaginal canal while another finger deeply palpates the surface of the abdomen. A rectovaginal examination takes place to ascertain whether a fullness that is felt in the patient's side is due to the bowel or to the pelvic organs. Performing a pelvic examination is critical in the early detection of cervical, uterine, or ovarian cancer.

The male genitals are inspected for changes in size of the external genitalia, particularly the testicles, and for lesions on the scrotum or penis. Palpation of the testicles is essential for determining symmetry, changes in abnormal lumps or bumps, and the presence of hardness. Testicular tumors are common tumors occurring in men under the age of 30. Although female breast examination and

screening have achieved considerable media attention, the need to instruct men in routine genital self-examination is often overlooked.

Another common abnormality of the male genitalia is the varicocele, which is an abnormal dilatation of the vein of the spermatic cord. Varicoceles are usually asymptomatic, but they are sometimes implicated in cases of subfertility. Enlargements of the epididymis, known as spermatoceles, also may be noted and may require corroboration by a urologic specialist.

Coughing or straining is necessary to elicit hernias, which result from breaks or discontinuities in the abdominal wall, allowing herniation of bowel. This condition requires surgical repair.

EXAMINATION OF THE RECTUM

Constipation, diarrhea, and abdominal pain are complaints necessitating a detailed rectal exam. In male patients, the rectal examination includes observation and palpation to determine the size and consistency of the prostate and to detect any signs of prostate cancer, early polyps, or tumors of the rectal area.

Examination of the rectum is improved by the use of a scope. A small anoscope is used to look for rectal abnormalities. Rigid sigmoidoscopes allow examination of 25 cm of the bowel. A flexible sigmoidoscope may go up to 60 cm.

The detail with which one approaches the examination depends on the age of the patient. Significant risk factors for colon cancer includes the age of the patient and a family history of colon cancer (see Chapter 12).

EXAMINATION OF THE MUSCULOSKELETAL SYSTEM

Musculoskeletal complaints include paresis (weakness) or paralysis, muscle stiffness, joint pain, limited movement, and a history of gout, arthritis, or deformity. The orthopedic examination must be done in a disciplined fashion, looking at every joint and assessing the integrity of the joint for both disease and function. Inspect for signs of inflammation, swelling, warmth, and redness, and examine each joint through its full range of motion. Whether it be the shoulder, the elbow, the knee, or the hip, each joint has a specific range of functional capabilities. Restrictions in function and elicitation of pain are important findings to record. They may be indicative of disease intrinsic to the joint, such as degenerative change or rheumatoid arthritis, or extrinsic to the joint, involving the tendons, muscles, or ligaments that surround it. The term arthritis is often used to describe musculoskeletal pain, but that diagnosis is appropriate only when inflammation of a joint is involved (see Chapter 7).

The examination begins with the small joints of the hands and feet and then extends to the shoulders, elbows, wrists, hips, knees, and ankles. Following this is an examination of the neck, mid-back, and lower back. The neck has a prescribed range of motion, which includes flexion forward, extension backward, lateral rotation to the right and left, and flexion to each side. The measurement of each movement should be recorded in degrees, and any limitation, pain, or spasm should be noted.

The mid-back is inspected for lateral curvature, known as scoliosis, palpated for pain, and guided through a routine set of movements that indicate whether function is normal.

The same examination is performed on the lower back. Lower back evaluation is complex because the most common back afflictions involve irritation to the nerves that emanate from the spine and continue down the leg. For example, patients with knee pain may have an intrinsic disease of the knee, such as arthritis, bursitis, tendinitis, or torn cartilage. Alternatively, the pain may reflect irritation of the nerves that supply the knee from the level of the back.

The spinal examination also involves palpation of the sacroiliac joint and the sciatic notch to rule out irritation of the sciatic nerve at the level of the back. Even the examination of the legs is directed at determining dysfunction in the back. This examination includes maneuvers such as straight-leg raising, reflex examination, and determination of

strength and sensation in the independently innervated areas of the foot.

The dorsal web of the foot is supplied by the nerves of the L5-S1 spinal disc and the medial aspect of the foot by those of the L4-L5 disc. Examination of these is more appropriately part of the neurologic examination, but they are essential in examination of the back as well.

The optometrist must rule out significant collagen-vascular disease in all cases of anterior uveitis. Ankylosing spondylitis usually presents in a male uveitis patient aged 20 to 40 with chronic lower back pain. A male patient in the same age group with arthritic joint pain and dysuria may have Reiter's syndrome. Young children who present with uveitis, particularly in a white, quiet eye, and who have posterior synechiae, cataract, and corneal edema or keratopathy, should be referred to a pediatric rheumatologist to rule out juvenile rheumatoid arthritis (see Chapters 7 and 18).

EXAMINATION OF THE LOWER EXTREMITY

Following the neurologic examination (see Chapter 2), the lower extremities are examined. The feet and legs are inspected for changes in color. A lack of hair growth may be indicative of poor arterial supply.

The pulses in the legs are assessed, starting with the femoral pulse in the groin, the popliteal pulse behind the knees, the posterior tibial pulse behind the ankle, and the dorsalis pedis pulse on the dorsum of the foot (approximately between the first and second toes).

Evaluation of arterial insufficiency in the legs is extremely important. To test the feet for swelling, place pressure on the skin and note whether a residual indentation remains, indicating peripheral edema. Palpate the calf for any abnormalities that might suggest deep vein thrombophlebitis.

In diabetics the skin of the feet should be inspected with special care, looking particularly between the toes for signs of cracking or fungal infection. The skin is also assessed for lesions, especially for evidence of dryness.

THE PHILOSOPHY OF THE PHYSICAL EXAMINATION

There are three categories of the physical examination. The first is the general physical, which provides an overall assessment of the patient. The second is the focused examination, in which one particular area of the body is inspected in great detail, and the entire examination is directed at that organ system or the related areas that might produce the patient's chief symptom. This is true, for example, in the assessment of the common problem of back pain. In that case, the back is inspected in greater detail, and a careful neurologic examination is made of the lower extremity to determine possible nerve dysfunction emanating from the back.

SPECIAL EXAMINATIONS: THE HEADACHE PHYSICAL

A third category is the examination focused on the evaluation of a specific medical problem, such as headache (see Chapter 16). In a patient complaining of headache, greater attention must be focused on the head and neck areas, where dysfunction does give rise to the symptom. To the optometrist, this means a precise ophthalmoscopic examination with attention to venous pulsations of the nerve head, the absence of which indicates a possible in-

crease of intracranial pressure. Visual field defects suggest intracranial tumor. Even refractive error may cause headache. All these possibilities must be differentiated from temporal arteritis, an inflammation of the temporal artery. In this case palpation of the temporal artery should be performed to detect swelling or pain.

Palpation of the sinuses for tenderness and transillumination of the sinuses (Fig. 1-17) for fluid that might indicate sinusitis are part of the comprehensive examination for headache. Examination of the temporomandibular joint for tenderness, clicking, and spasm or the muscles in that area might be helpful in eliciting temporomandibular joint dysfunction as the cause of headache. The neck is examined by assessing its range of motion in flexion and extension, as well as lateral flexion and rotation, and the presence or absence of spasm in the trapezius muscle is noted.

SUMMARY

Medical technology has overshadowed the physical examination for many physicians. The care and detail once given to the cardiac examination are sometimes dismissed and the patient is simply referred for an expensive echocardiogram. The painstaking detail of a neurologic assessment is replaced by an MR scan. The importance of palpat-

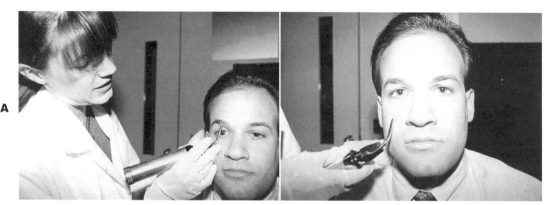

FIG. 1-17 A, Transillumination of the frontal sinus: A transilluminator is placed against the upper brow of a patient just under the superciliary ridge. In a completely dark room the sinus is illuminated. Dark structures interrupting the transilluminated appearance may represent tumors within the sinus. **B, Transillumination of the maxillary sinus:** A transilluminator is placed against the lower maxillary sinus to illuminate the sinus in a completely dark room.

ing the prostate to detect early prostatic carcinoma has at times been supplanted by a screening blood test known as a prostate specific antigen (PSA).

It is the physical examination that suggests whether or not medical technology should be applied. The careful physical examination is the essence of the doctor's contribution to the patient's medical care and the basis for subsequent treatment.

It is hoped that this chapter provides a useful introduction and guide, a basis for continued learning, and a new attitude of respect for and interest in the elegance and significance of the physical examination.

BIBLIOGRAPHY

Bates B: *A guide to physical examination and history taking,* ed 5, Philadelphia, 1991, JB Lippincott.

Braunwald E: *Heart disease: a textbook of cardiovascular medicine,* ed 4, Philadelphia, 1992, WB Saunders Co.

Burnside JW and McGlynn TJ: *Physical diagnosis,* ed 17, Baltimore, 1987, Williams & Wilkins.

Cassel EJ: *Talking with patients: clinical technique,* Cambridge, MA, MIT Press, 1985.

Cattau EL Jr and others: The accuracy of the physical examination in the diagnosis of suspected ascites, *JAMA* 247:1164, 1982.

D'Ambrosia RD: *Musculoskeletal disorders: regional examination and differential diagnosis,* ed 2, Philadelphia, 1986, JB Lippincott.

DeGowin R: *DeGowin and DeGowin's bedside diagnostic examination,* ed 6, New York, 1994, MacMillan.

DeWeese DD: *Otolaryngology: head and neck surgery,* ed 8, St. Louis, 1993, Mosby-Year Book.

Fitzpatrick TB and Freeberg, IM: *Dermatology in general medicine,* New York, 1987, McGraw-Hill.

Fletcher RH and Fletcher SW: Has medicine outgrown physical diagnosis? (editorial), *Ann Intern Med* 117:786, 1992.

Gorrol, May L, and Mulley AG: *Primary care medicine,* Philadelphia, 1994, JB Lippincott.

Gorlin R and Zucker HD: Physician's reaction to patients: a key to teaching humanistic medicine, *N Engl J Med* 308:1057, 1983.

Lookingbill DP and Marks JG Jr: *Principles of dermatology,* Philadelphia, 1986, WB Saunders Co.

Sackett DL: The science of the art of the clinical examination, *JAMA* 267:2650, 1992.

Schwartz MH: *Textbook of physical diagnosis— history and examination,* Philadelphia, 1989, WB Saunders Co.

Weinberger SE: *Principles of pulmonary medicine,* Philadelphia, 1992, WB Saunders Co.

Werner SC and Ingbar SCH, editors: *The thyroid: a fundamental and clinical text,* New York, 1991, Harper and Row.

Wilson JD and Foster DW: *Williams' textbook of endocrinology,* Philadelphia, 1992, WB Saunders Co.

2

The Neurologic Examination

BRUCE G. MUCHNICK

*T*he visual pathway from the retina to the occipital lobe is so lengthy that intracranial lesions are likely to affect some part of the functional visual system. The key to diagnosing the location and nature of such a lesion lies in the determination of its effect on the visual system and on other neurologic structures. The site of the lesion can be inferred from neurologic deficits identified by the practitioner. Confirmation of the lesion's location is made by radiography, computed tomography (CT scan), or magnetic resonance (MR) imaging (see Chapter 4). Finally, the nature of the lesion is tentatively deduced from the radiographic results along with the patient's history, symptoms, and clinical signs.

This chapter describes a basic neurologic evaluation for the optometrist. The chapter first describes the evaluation of the patient's mental status, reflexes, sensory and motor functions, and cerebellar functions. The remainder of the chapter is devoted to evaluation of the cranial nerves.

THE PRINCIPLES OF NEUROLOGIC DIAGNOSIS

Patients may present to the optometrist with no complaints at all or with ocular or neurologic symptoms. Neurologic symptoms are clues that help to establish the presence of a lesion and must be differentiated from a psychogenic problem or malingering.

The eye examination may reveal the presence of a visual pathway disturbance as evidenced by a decrease in visual acuity, pupillary defects, visual field changes on perimetry testing, color vision distortions, or optic nerve head problems.

Whether or not a defect is discovered in the visual pathway, a neurologic screening should be performed on every patient. If no ocular or neurologic deficits are discovered, the optometrist must determine the cause of any symptoms. If no symptoms or signs are present, the patient is followed routinely. (Fig. 2-1 is a flow chart for the neurologic evaluation of the eye care patient.)

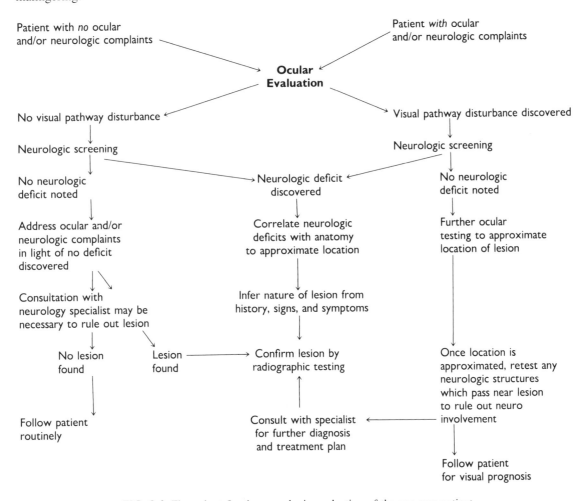

FIG. 2-1 Flow chart for the neurologic evaluation of the eye care patient.

Symptoms Without Clinical Signs

If no clinical signs are present in a symptomatic patient (see the box below), it is necessary to rule out the presence of disease. This is done by consultation with the family physician, neurologist, ophthalmologist, neuro-eye specialist, internist, or endocrinologist. For example, if a patient complains of headache and the ocular examination and neurology screening reveal no significant findings, one must decide whether to refer the patient for further evaluation or monitor the patient oneself.

Radiographic studies and laboratory work may be necessary to establish a diagnosis. Psychogenic symptoms and malingering can be ruled out in this way.

Visual Defects with No Obvious Neurologic Problems

If a visual pathway deficit is discovered but no neurologic problem is found, further neurologic testing is warranted to rule out the effects of a lesion on neurologic structures passing near the suspected site.

First, the location of the lesion is determined by its effect on the patient's visual field. With an intimate understanding of neuroanatomy, one can identify nearby neurologic structures and infer what neurologic deficits would occur if these nearby nerves were damaged. Finally, perform the neurologic evaluation, paying particular attention to any deficits that would occur given the lesion's suspected location. Be careful to elicit only findings that are truly present.

Ocular and Neurologic Defects

You may examine a patient with both ocular and neurologic defects. Whether the patient is symptomatic or asymptomatic, these findings must be correlated with the relevant neuroanatomy to localize the lesion. The nature of the lesion may be tentatively inferred at this point based on the patient's history, symptoms, and signs and the approximate location of the lesion.

The differential diagnosis can be narrowed down by radiographic findings. Conventional radiography, CT scan, MR imaging, and color Doppler ultrasonography all help in determining the diagnosis (see Chapter 4).

In most cases you will want to consult with a specialist, who will oversee the advanced diagnostic and treatment options available to the patient. Referral to a neurology specialist helps in pinpointing a more generalized problem. Treatment is based on the cause of the lesion. Surgery or other forms of treatment may be recommended by vascular specialists or neurosurgeons. Eventually, low vision adaptations may be necessary.

THE NEUROLOGIC SCREENING

For practical purposes, the neurologic examination is divided into six areas that impact on optometric practice: evaluation of the patient's mental status, motor and sensory functions, cerebellar functions, reflexes, and cranial nerve functions (see the box below).

Evaluation of Mental Status

Table 2-1 and the box on p. 25 discuss the evaluation of mental status.

SIGNIFICANT NEUROLOGIC SYMPTOMS

Headache
Confusion
Unsteadiness
Visual problems
Speech problems
Tremors
Numbness
Weakness

THE NEUROLOGIC SCREENING

Mental status
Motor function
Sensory function
Cerebellar function
Reflex function
Cranial nerve function

As you talk with the patient, judge from his responses whether he seems alert and aware. Does he seem confused? Is he acting in a rational manner? Is he oriented to time and place? If he is disoriented, does he have short-term or long-term memory loss?

You can test memory loss by presenting a set of three common words to the patient and asking him to repeat them to you minutes later. A memory loss may be due to a temporal lobe lesion.

Is the patient speaking clearly and using vocabulary appropriately? A dysfunction in speech can help localize a lesion. A patient who vocalizes meaningless words has *dysphasia,* which may indicate a brain lesion of the left hemisphere.

If a patient talks sensibly but has difficulty in producing sound, there is a disruption in the motor function that produces speech. This problem can occur anywhere along the pathway from the brain to the mouth.

Is the patient exhibiting inappropriate emotions,

such as sudden laughter or crying? This type of emotional display may be due to bilateral cerebral damage.

Can the patient recognize common objects? Inability to do so is called *agnosia.* If the patient closes his eyes and cannot identify an object by touching it, he may have a lesion in the nondominant parietal lobe.

Can the patient carry out simple instructions? Inability to do so is called *dyspraxia* and may be due to a deep frontal lobe lesion.

Finally, can the patient copy a simple drawn figure? Inability to do so may be caused by a posterior parietal lobe lesion.

Evaluation of Motor Functions

Muscle weakness is a fairly nonlocalizing finding because it can be caused by disturbances in the cerebrum, brainstem, spinal cord, nerves, neuromuscular junction, or muscles. To screen for muscle weakness, have the patient flex and extend both arms and legs against resistance (Fig. 2-2). Note any weakness of one limb when comparing the two.

Evaluation of Sensory Functions

Neurologic evaluation should include tests for the senses of touch, pain, and vibration. Loss of these senses may indicate a spinal cord lesion. The following tests are performed with the patient's eyes closed. To test for the sense of touch, stroke the patient's fingers with a tissue after asking him to

---

EVALUATION OF MENTAL STATUS

Consciousness
Orientation
Memory
Speech
Appropriate affect
Object recognition
Praxis

TABLE 2-1 *Localizing Value of Mental Status Evaluation*

Medical Condition	Description of Problem	Neurologic Structures Affected
Coma	Decreased level of consciousness	Nonlocalizing
Disorientation	Lack of orientation to time and place	Temporal lobe
Amnesia	Memory loss	Temporal lobe
Aphasia	Speech problem	Frontal, temporoparietal lobe
Inappropriate affect	Inappropriate emotional display	Bilateral cerebral damage
Agnosia	Inability to recognize objects	Nondominant parietal lobe
Apraxia	Inability to follow orders	Frontal lobe

FIG. 2-2 Evaluation of motor function: The forearms are tested for flexion and extension by exerting a force against the examiner, who holds the patient by the wrist. This tests roots C5-C6 (flexion) and C6-C8 (extension).

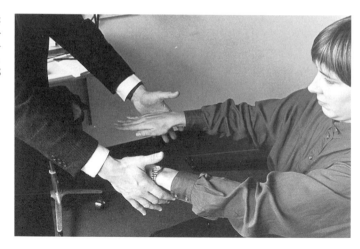

FIG. 2-3 Evaluation of tactile sense: The patient is asked to close her eyes. Her fingers and toes are lightly touched with a tissue. A significant finding is a marked decrease in sensitivity.

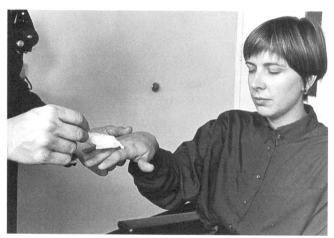

tell you when he feels the stroke of the tissue (Fig. 2-3). Repeat the test on the patient's toes.

To test for pain sensation, touch your patient on the fingers and hand with the point of a safety pin. Begin touching the fingers and hand, alternating the sharp tip with the blunt end, and determine whether the patient can discern the difference between sharp and dull sensations (Figs. 2-4 and 2-5). Repeat this test on the patient's toes.

Finally, test vibration sense using a 128-Hz tuning fork. Strike the tuning fork with your hand and place it over the base of the nail bed on the patient's index finger. Place your index finger under the patient's finger tip so you can feel the vibration also (Fig. 2-6). Ask the patient to report when he no longer feels the vibration.

Evaluation of Cerebellar Functions

To test for cerebellar disorders, perform a "finger-to-nose" test. Hold your finger at arm's length from the patient. Ask the patient to touch his nose with his index finger and then touch your index finger. Repeat this several times with the patient's eyes open and then closed (Fig. 2-7). A patient with a disorder of the cerebellum tends to overshoot the target. This response is called *past pointing.*

Another convenient test for cerebellar function is the *Romberg test.* Have the patient stand in front of you with heels and toes together. Ask the patient to close his eyes and attempt to balance himself. Be prepared to catch him if he falls off balance. This test assesses the posterior columns.

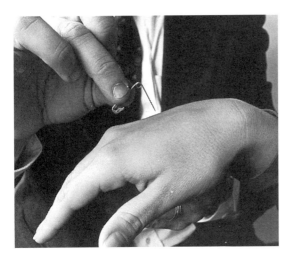

FIG. 2-4 Evaluation of pain sense: The patient is asked to close her eyes. With the sharp end of a safety pin the fingers and toes are lightly pricked.

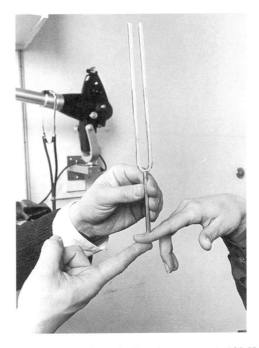

FIG. 2-6 Evaluation of vibration sense: A 128-Hz tuning fork is tapped to produce a vibration. The base of the fork is placed on the base of the patient's fingernail. The patient closes her eyes and reports when she can no longer feel the vibration. A significant finding is a reduced vibration sense.

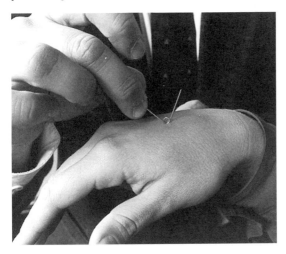

FIG. 2-5 Evaluation of pain sense: The procedure described in Fig. 2-4 is repeated with the dull end of the pin. The examiner alternates the sharp and dull ends of the pin and the patient is asked to compare sharp and dull sensation as the examiner moves proximally.

You may also ask the patient to raise his arms palms up while balancing with eyes shut (Fig. 2-8). Patients with a hemiparesis drops one arm and the fingers flex. This is called *pronator drift*.

The most important cerebellar function test is examination of gait (Fig. 2-9). First, observe the patient as he walks away from you. Then have him walk toward you on his toes. Finally, have him walk away from you putting heel to toe. Loss of this ability can occur in cerebellar dysfunction due to such diseases as syphilis.

Watch for normal posture and proper arm movement. Cerebellar *ataxia* is heightened by gait testing. Lower extremity muscle weakness may also be evaluated in this way.

Evaluation of Reflexes

The neurology tests should include an evaluation of deep tendon reflexes. A loss of these reflexes may occur in some cerebellar disorders. Of the many reflex tests to choose from, the patellar tendon reflex test is most important.

Have the patient sit on the edge of a table or chair and dangle his feet. Place your hand on the quadriceps muscle of one leg and strike the patellar tendon with a reflex hammer. You should feel the quadriceps contract and see the knee extend (Fig. 2-10).

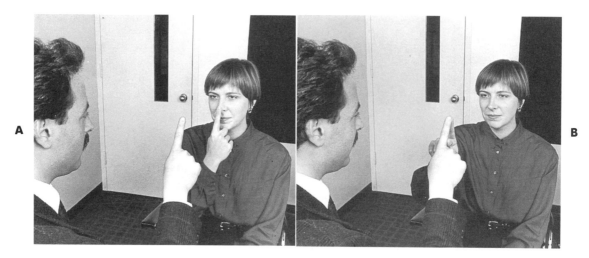

FIG. 2-7 (**A** and **B**) **Evaluation of cerebellar function** ("finger-to-nose" test): The examiner holds his finger outstretched at arm's length from the patient. With eyes open the patient first touches her nose and then touches the examiner's finger. This sequence is repeated several times. Then it is repeated with the patient's eyes shut. Cerebellar disease causes overshooting of the target and digital tremor.

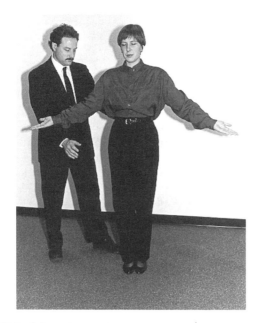

FIG. 2-8 Variation of the Romberg test for pronator drift.

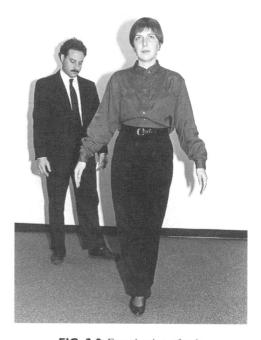

FIG. 2-9 Examination of gait.

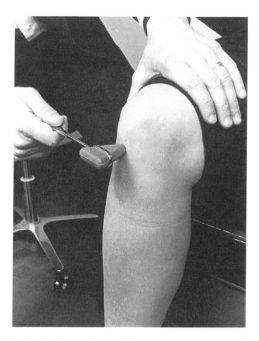

FIG. 2-10 Evaluation of deep tendon reflexes: The patellar tendon reflex is tested by positioning the patient on the edge of the examination chair or table so that her legs dangle freely with no obstruction. The examiner lightly places one hand on the quadriceps muscle. The patellar tendon is struck firmly by the base of the hammer. Extension of the knee should occur, and contraction of the quadriceps should be felt. This tests the nerves at roots L2 to L4.

Loss of deep tendon reflexes occurs in some cases of Adie's tonic pupil. In any patient presenting with a light near dissociation pupil, deep tendon reflex evaluation is mandatory, because a significant number of cases of bilateral Adie's tonic pupil in men are caused by syphilis.

CRANIAL NERVE TESTING

The cranial nerves control the five senses, allowing the patient to interact with the environment—to feel it, move through it, experience it, and alter it. These twelve pairs of nerves, which extend from the brain to vital organs throughout the body, are necessary for the patient's everyday activities.

The cranial nerves may be affected by a wide range of conditions, including trauma, demyelination from multiple sclerosis, development of space-occupying lesions (such as tumors or aneurysms), intracranial inflammation from meningitis, cerebrovascular ischemia from stroke, and infection.

The cranial nerves receive sensory (afferent) input from internal organs and from the skin, as well as special sensory input from the eyes, ears, and nose. The motor (efferent) innervation is supplied via the cranial nerves to voluntary and involuntary muscles throughout the body.

Each cranial nerve should be tested and evaluated in terms of its ability to function. All of the following tests can be performed in the optometrist's office (Table 2-2).

First Cranial Nerve—Olfactory Nerve

The olfactory nerve is a special afferent cranial nerve composed of sensory fibers only. It serves the sole function of olfaction, the ability to discern smells. To test the olfactory nerve, the patient shuts his eyes and one nostril is occluded. The patient's open nostril is presented with a variety of vials, each containing a concentrated extract such as coffee, peppermint, or vanilla. The patient is asked to sniff and identify each smell (Fig. 2-11). The loss of olfactory ability is called *anosmia* and can be caused by trauma to the skull, frontal lobe masses or seizures or viral infection. Olfactory nerve testing is rarely performed because it is an unreliable test of cranial disease.

Second Cranial Nerve—Optic Nerve

Like the olfactory nerve, the optic nerve contains only special sensory afferent fibers. The optic nerve functions to convey visual information from the retina to the occipital lobe via the visual pathway. The optic nerve is tested in the office by visual acuity measurement, color testing, pupil testing, visual fields testing, and optic nerve head evaluation via ophthalmoscope or stereo biomicroscopy.

Visual fields testing has great localizing value when an intracranial lesion affects the visual path-

TABLE 2-2 *The Cranial Nerves*

Cranial Nerve	No.	Innervation	Primary Function	Test
Olfactory	I	Sensory	Smell	Identify odors
Optic	II	Sensory	Vision	Visual acuity, visual fields, color, nerve head
Oculomotor	III	Motor	Upper lid elevation Extraocular eye movement Pupil constriction Accommodation	Physiologic "H" and near point response
Trochlear	IV	Motor	Superior oblique muscle	Physiologic "H"
Trigeminal	V	Motor Sensory	Muscles of mastication Scalp, conjunctiva, teeth	Corneal reflex Clench jaw/palpate Light touch comparison
Abducens	VI	Motor	Lateral rectus muscle	Abduction/physiologic "H"
Facial	VII	Motor Sensory	Muscles of facial expression Taste—anterior two thirds of tongue	Smile, puff cheeks, wrinkle forehead, pry open closed lids
Vestibulocochlear	VIII	Sensory	Hearing Balance	Rinne test Weber test
Glossopharyngeal	IX	Motor Sensory	Tongue and pharynx Taste—posterior one third of tongue	Gag reflex
Vagus	X	Motor Sensory	Pharynx, tongue, larynx, thoracic and abdominal viscera Larynx, trachea, esophagus	Gag reflex
Accessory	XI	Motor	Sternomastoid and trapezius muscles	Shrug, head turn against resistance
Hypoglossal	XII	Motor	Muscles of tongue	Tongue deviation

way. Prechiasmal lesions usually cause monocular field defects. Chiasmal lesions produce heteronymous hemianopsias, and postchiasmal lesions produce homonymous hemianopsias. The further posterior the lesion, the more congruous (alike) the two fields appear.

Third Cranial Nerve—Oculomotor Nerve

The oculomotor nerve contains only motor fibers. These fibers include (1) somatic efferent fibers innervating the levator palpebral superioris, superior rectus, medial rectus, inferior rectus, and inferior oblique muscles of the eye, and (2) visceral efferent motor fibers innervating the constrictor pupillae and ciliary muscles with parasympathetic fibers via the ciliary ganglion.

Because the third nerve innervates four of the six extraocular muscles, it is tested by having the patient's eyes follow a near target as you draw out a physiologic "H" pattern, causing adduction (medial rectus), depression while abducting (inferior rectus), and elevation (superior rectus and inferior oblique). Pupillary constriction is tested by the light reflex, and accommodation can be tested on

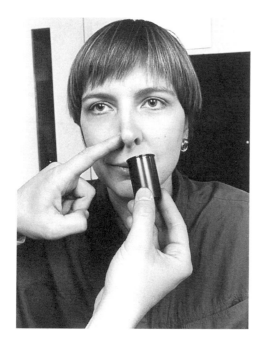

FIG. 2-11 Testing the olfactory nerve: One nostril is occluded by the examiner. The patient is asked to sniff extracts of peppermint, vanilla, and coffee and attempts to identify each of them.

a near target. Loss of third nerve function may cause diplopia, and an eye that is "down-and-out" with ptosis and mydriasis.

Fourth Cranial Nerve—Trochlear Nerve

The trochlear nerve supplies only somatic efferent motor fibers to the superior oblique muscle of the eye. The superior oblique is tested, as previously described, by having the patient's eyes follow a near target as you trace an "H" pattern. The trochlear nerve causes superior oblique contraction, which rotates the eye inward, downward, and outward. This nerve is best isolated by having the patient adduct and look down toward the nose.

The trochlear nerve is the only cranial nerve to exit from the dorsal aspect of the brain, and it has the longest intracranial course of any cranial nerves. Lesions affecting the fourth nerve include injury, inflammatory disease, compression from an aneurysm of the posterior cerebral and superior cerebellar arteries, and cavernous sinus entities. A lesion affecting the trochlear nerve causes diplopia and *torticollis* (twisted neck).

Fifth Cranial Nerve—Trigeminal Nerve

The trigeminal nerve supplies both sensory and motor fibers to the face and periorbital area. The afferent sensory fibers supply sensation to the face, scalp, conjunctiva, tongue, teeth, tympanic membrane, and mucous membranes of the paranasal sinuses. Motor efferent fibers function to innervate several facial muscles, including the muscles of mastication.

Three tests are used to evaluate the trigeminal nerve: the corneal reflex test, the sensory division test, and the motor division test. The corneal reflex is evaluated by gently touching the temporal side of the cornea with a thin sterile braid of cotton as the patient looks down and toward his nose. Normally, the patient immediately shuts his eyes. This tests both the sensory fifth nerve and the motor portion of the seventh, or facial, nerve, which is responsible for lid closure (Fig. 2-12**A**).

To test the sensory division of the fifth nerve, the patient is asked to close his eyes. Lightly touch one side of his forehead with a tissue. Then touch the other side and ask the patient to compare sensations. A reduced sensation of touch on one side may indicate a *hemiparesthesia*. The test is repeated on the cheeks to test the second division of the trigeminal and on the chin to test the third division (Fig. 2-12**B**).

The motor component of the trigeminal nerve is tested by having the patient clench his teeth to produce a prominence of the masseter muscle. Palpate both masseters and compare the muscle tone of both (Fig. 2-12**C**).

One of the most common causes of sensory loss of the fifth nerve is fracture of a facial bone, especially a blow-out fracture of the orbital floor. This trauma may cause ipsilateral reduction or loss of feeling on the cheek. Vascular damage, tumors of the pons, and trauma may cause damage to the motor neuron or its axons.

Sixth Cranial Nerve—Abducens Nerve

The abducens nerve supplies only somatic efferent motor fibers to the lateral rectus muscle of the

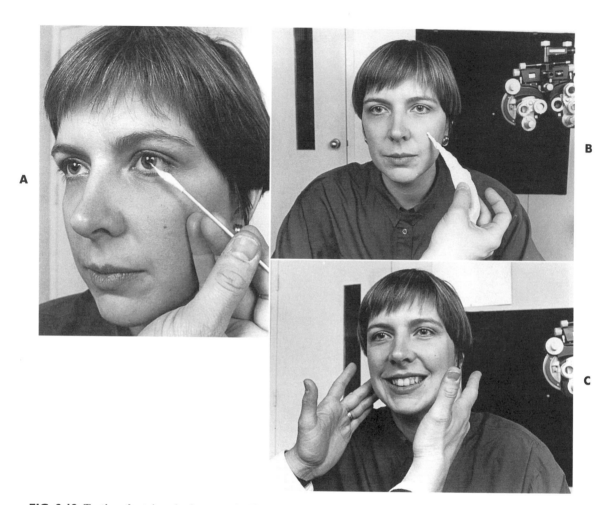

FIG. 2-12 Testing the trigeminal nerve: A, The corneal reflex: The patient is asked to look downward and inward while the examiner touches the temporal cornea with a small bit of cotton. Immediate closure of both eyelids should occur. **B,** The sensory distribution of the trigeminal nerve is tested by asking the patient to compare the sensation of light touch on both sides of the forehead, cheek, and chin. **C,** The motor component of the trigeminal nerve is tested by palpating the masseter muscles of a patient who is clenching her teeth and comparing the muscle tone of both sides.

eye. This muscle functions to abduct the eye.

To test the abducens nerve, have the patient's eyes follow a near target through the physiologic "H" pattern. An inability to abduct the eye indicates a possible abducens deficit. Patients with abduction deficit may complain of diplopia and may appear esotropic. Causes of abducens deficit include aneurysms of the posterior cerebellar or basilar arteries or internal carotid arteries, cerebellar tumors, meningitis, trauma, increased intracranial pressure, and cavernous sinus pathology.

Seventh Cranial Nerve—Facial Nerve

The facial nerve supplies (1) efferent motor innervation to the muscles of facial expression and lacrimal gland (and others), and (2) sensory afferent fibers from the anterior two thirds of the tongue for taste. Testing of the facial nerve involves examination of the muscles it innervates. Four tests easily evaluate the seventh nerve. First, have the patient smile or bare his teeth without laughing. Look for any asymmetry of the cheeks which might indicate a hemiparesis of the nerve (Fig.

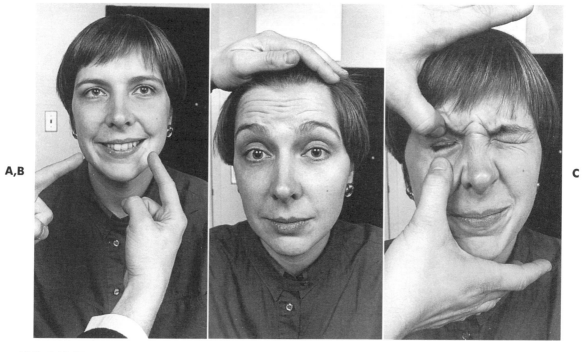

A,B **C**

FIG. 2-13 Testing the facial nerve: A, The patient bares her teeth and the nasolabial folds on either side of the face are compared. **B,** The patient wrinkles her forehead and the wrinkling of the two sides is compared. **C,** The examiner attempts to pry open the patient's tightly shut eyelids.

2-13**A**). Next, push in on the patient's cheeks with your fingers while the patient attempts to puff out both cheeks. Then have the patient attempt to wrinkle his forehead. A weakness of one side of the forehead causes a diminution in the wrinkling on the affected side (Fig. 2-13**B**). Finally, have the patient tightly shut his eyes while you attempt to pry the eyelids open. A weakness of the facial nerve allows relatively easy parting of the lids (Fig. 2-13**C**).

Bell's palsy is a common lower motor neuron lesion of the facial nucleus or its axon. All voluntary and reflex muscles ipsilateral to the lesion are affected. The result is facial asymmetry with drooping of the eyebrow, a smooth nasolabial fold, drooping of the corner of the mouth, and a reduced blink reflex on the affected side. All patients presenting with a new case of Bell's palsy should have a Lyme titer determination because Lyme disease can produce hemifacial palsy (see Chapter 6).

Eighth Cranial Nerve—Vestibulocochlear Nerve

The eighth cranial nerve carries two special sensory afferent fibers—one for vestibular function, or balance, and one for audition, or hearing. Evaluation of the eighth cranial nerve for audition is covered in Chapter 1. The *Rinne* and *Weber tests* are easy to perform in the examination room and can help differentiate conductive deficits from neurosensory lesions (Fig. 2-14) (see Chapter 1). At present there is no useful screening test to evaluate balance or vestibular function. Damage to the hearing apparatus or eighth cranial nerve can be caused by injury, tumors, or infection. Damage to the vestibular apparatus is most often caused by a tumor called an acoustic neuroma, which leads to dizziness, hearing loss, nausea, loss of balance, tinnitus, deafness, and Bell's palsy. These symptoms occur because the eighth and seventh nerves run together along part of their paths.

FIG. 2-14 Testing the vestibulocochlear nerve: A, The Rinne test for audition: A tuning fork is held against the mastoid process until it can no longer be heard. The still-vibrating fork is then brought to the ear. **B,** The Weber test for audition: A tuning fork is struck and placed in the center of the forehead, and the patient compares the loudness on both sides.

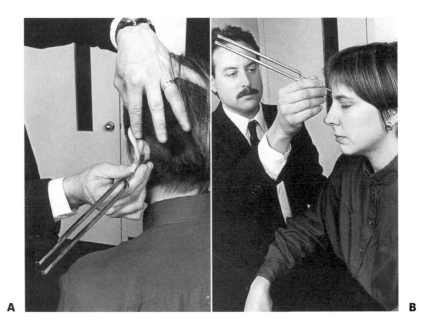

A B

Ninth Cranial Nerve—Glossopharyngeal Nerve

The ninth cranial nerve supplies motor fibers to the parotid gland and the pharynx. It also supplies sensory fibers from the carotid body (to monitor oxygen tension in the blood) and from the posterior third of the tongue, mediating the taste sensation in the posterior tongue. Because the ninth cranial nerve innervates the pharynx, testing the gag reflex evaluates the integrity of the nerve. Lightly stroking the wall of the pharynx should cause the patient to gag. A damaged nerve results in an absence of this reflex. The tenth and eleventh cranial nerve pathways are so close to those of the ninth that one rarely sees an isolated lesion of one of these nerves.

Another test to evaluate the integrity of the ninth and tenth nerves is to ask the patient to open his mouth and say, "ahh." This raises the soft palate high up in the back of the oral cavity. The uvula, a small, cone-shaped piece of tissue suspended from the back of the throat, should elevate without lateral deviation (Fig. 2-15). Paralysis of the ninth nerve causes a pulling of the uvula to the unaffected side.

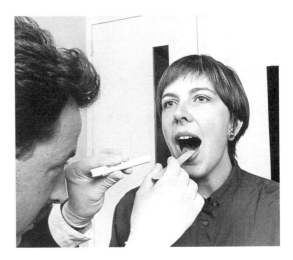

FIG. 2-15 Testing the glossopharyngeal nerve and vagus nerve: The patient sticks out her tongue and says, "ahhh." This elevates the soft palate. The uvula should elevate without lateral deviation.

Tenth Cranial Nerve—Vagus Nerve

The tenth cranial nerve has both sensory and motor components. It receives sensory afferent fibers from the larynx, trachea, esophagus, pharynx, and abdominal viscera and sends efferent motor fibers

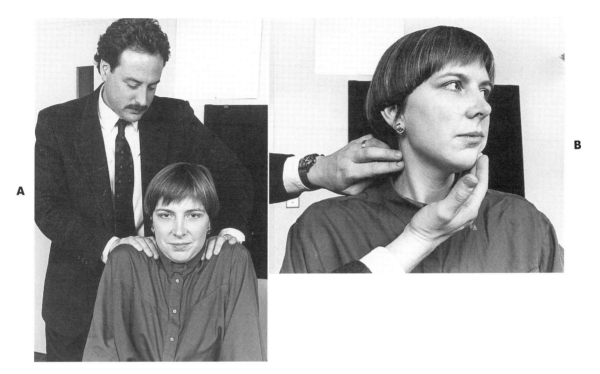

FIG. 2-16 Testing the accessory nerve: A, The examiner pushes down on the shoulders of the patient, who tries to shrug against the resistance. **B,** The patient turns her head against the examiner's hand while the sternomastoid muscle is palpated for tone. The patient then turns to the other side. The muscle tone on both sides is compared.

to the pharynx, tongue, larynx, and thoracic and abdominal viscera.

A unilateral lesion affecting the vagus nerve causes a loss of laryngeal function, producing hoarseness and difficulty in swallowing. To evaluate the vagus (and the ninth cranial nerve), perform the "ahhh" test described in the preceding section on the ninth cranial nerve (Fig. 2-15). Causes of unilateral vagus lesions include trauma from surgical procedures of the neck (such as carotid endarterectomy or thyroidectomy), aortic aneurysm, and metastatic carcinoma, in which enlarged paratracheal lymph nodes can compress the vagus nerve.

Eleventh Cranial Nerve—Accessory Nerve

The accessory nerve carries only efferent motor fibers to supply innervation to the sternomastoid and trapezius muscles. Damage to this nerve causes a drooping of the ipsilateral shoulder and loss of trapezius function on the affected side. The patient may have difficulty turning his head to the side opposite the lesion.

To test the eleventh nerve, place your hands on the patient's shoulders and press downward as the patient attempts to shrug the shoulders against your resistance (Fig. 2-16,**A**). Another test involves having the patient attempt to turn his head against resistance. Place your hand on the left side of the patient's face and push against the patient's left cheek as he tries to turn his head to his left. Palpate the patient's right sternomastoid muscle and feel it tighten as the patient attempts to turn his head to the left. Repeat the process with the patient attempting to turn his head to the right against resistance (Fig. 2-16**B**). Damage to the eleventh

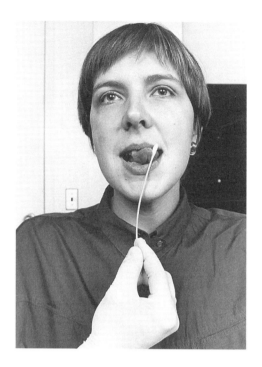

FIG. 2-17 Testing the hypoglossal nerve: The patient sticks out his tongue and moves it laterally against resistance from a cotton-tipped applicator.

cranial nerve can occur as a result of radical nerve surgery or trauma.

Twelfth Cranial Nerve—Hypoglossal Nerve

The twelfth cranial nerve supplies efferent motor fibers to all intrinsic and extrinsic muscles of the tongue (except the palatoglossus). Damage to the nerve results in paralysis of the tongue on the affected side. Therefore, when the patient sticks out his tongue, it deviates to the side of the lesion (Fig. 2-17).

To test the hypoglossal nerve, ask the patient to stick out his tongue and move it right and left against resistance offered by the examiner, who holds a cotton-tipped applicator on the lateral aspect of the tongue.

Bibliography

Brazio PW, Masdeu JC, and Biller J: *Localization in clinical neurology,* Boston, 1985, Little, Brown, & Co.

Dejong RN and others: *Essentials of the neurological examination, Essentials booklet,* pp 1-53 Smith Kline & Co.

Pelligrino TR: A faster, focused neurologic exam, *Emerg Med,* p 71, Sept. 30, 1990.

Prior JA, Silberstein JS, and Stang JM: Chapter 18. In *Physical diagnosis—the history and examination of the patient,* ed 6, St. Louis, 1981, Mosby–Year Book.

Swartz Mark H: Chapter 18. In *Textbook of physical diagnosis,* Philadelphia, 1989, WB Saunders Co.

Weiner WJ, Goetz CG, editors: *Neurology for the non-neurologist,* Philadelphia, 1981, Harper and Row.

Wilson-Pauwels L and others: *Cranial nerves: anatomy and clinical comments,* Toronto, 1988, BC Decker.

3

Laboratory Medicine

BRUCE G. MUCHNICK

INTRODUCTION TO LABORATORY TESTING

Laboratory testing impacts heavily on modern eye care. Routine blood testing and urinalysis are or- dered for the preoperative medical evaluation of patients awaiting ocular surgery. The eye care practitioner can use portable and relatively inex- pensive instruments to monitor serum and urine glucose levels in patients with or suspected of hav- ing diabetes mellitus (see Chapter 13). Patients who present with hypertensive retinopathy, arte- riolar sclerotic changes, and retinal vascular plaques can have their serum cholesterol and tri- glyceride levels determined by in-office tabletop instruments. A battery of special hematology, chemistry, and immunology laboratory tests is used to evaluate systemic disorders underlying re- current uveitis (see Chapter 18). The patient who presents with early signs of Graves' thyroidopathy should have laboratory testing to evaluate endo- crine function (see Chapter 14). Infections such as cytomegalovirus retinopathy, gonorrhea, and tox- oplasmosis are detected by serology testing (see Chapter 6). For the most part, eye disease can be diagnosed from a careful history, symptoms, clin- ical signs, and in-office procedures. The diagnosis of systemic disease with ocular manifestations, however, mandates the use of laboratory medicine.

THE LOCAL LABORATORY

To gain familiarity with laboratory testing, meet with the laboratory manager of the local medical laboratory and tour the facilities. Observe how the tests are actually performed. The laboratory will instruct you on how to order specific tests, what instructions the patient needs to follow (such as fasting), what forms need to be filled out, where the patient is to report or where the sample needs to be sent, and the cost of the test. Be sure to get a "Lab User's Guide" from the laboratory. This guide lists all the tests available, as well as information concerning each test, how the sample is collected, patient preparation, interpretation of results, and methodology. This guide and the laboratory manager are invaluable sources of information when laboratory testing is indicated.

THE LABORATORY STRUCTURE

The medical laboratory is divided into several sections. These include anatomic pathology to examine tissue biopsy and acid-fast stains; blood bank for transfusions; the chemistry section to analyze myriad blood compounds; hematology to study the cells and plasma of the blood; immunology to detect infections and inflammation; microbiology to identify infectious agents; nuclear medicine to scan tissues and organs using injected radiopharmaceuticals; and urinalysis. The individual laboratory tests ordered on a given patient fall under one of these sections.

BLOOD ANALYSIS

The chemicals, solids, and plasma of the blood may be analyzed by a wide variety of laboratory techniques. The study of the formed elements of the blood and the blood-forming tissues is known as hematology. The biochemical make-up of the blood, which can reflect the presence of systemic disease, is analyzed in chemistry. Immunology serum testing analyzes diseases characterized by antibody-antigen reactions. Blood cultures to detect, isolate, and identify potentially pathogenic organisms causing bacteremia are studied by mi-

crobiology. Nuclear medicine makes use of radionuclides in the diagnosis and management of disorders, and in some cases blood must be sampled and analyzed.

Blood Appropriation

Blood may be obtained from capillaries, veins, or bone marrow for laboratory analysis.

Fingerstick (Finger Puncture) (Fig. 3-1). Blood sampled from a finger capillary is of a small volume and is used when a larger amount of venous blood is not needed or cannot be obtained. It is most useful for single chemical tests, such as glucose or cholesterol levels, and has the advantage of being an easy technique for patients to learn when personal sampling is necessary. It may not be as accurate as venous blood sampling, however, and may not provide enough volume to perform a blood chemistry profile.

The fingertip to be sampled is swabbed with alcohol and allowed to air dry. A small lancet or steel scalpel blade is used to puncture the skin. It should be deep enough for blood to flow freely when pressure is applied to the area just adjacent to the wound. Never squeeze the fingertip to gain more blood, as this dilutes the sample with interstitial fluid. Micropipets are used to collect the sample, and, if necessary, diluting agents may be

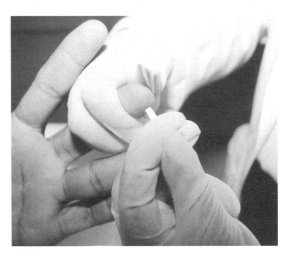

FIG. 3-1 Fingerstick (finger puncture): Blood is sampled from a finger capillary.

added. Other potential puncture sites include the heel in infants and the earlobe in adults.

Venipuncture (Fig. 3-2). Large samples of blood may be obtained from the superficial veins of the midarm, wrist, and back of the hand. These sample sizes are appropriate for blood chemistry profiles and special blood testing.

To obtain venous blood from the midarm, a tourniquet is applied above the site of needle insertion, allowing for better visibility of distended veins due to blockage of venous drainage. The area is then cleansed. A needle is inserted into the vein and an evacuated container is connected to the needle for the blood collection. The tourniquet is then removed, the needle is withdrawn, and a gauze pad is placed over the site. Pressure is applied for a few minutes to halt any blood flow. Anticoagulating agents can be added to the blood sample; these preserve blood cell morphology yet prevent blood coagulation.

Hematology

Complete Blood Count (CBC). In general, the CBC provides an overview of hematologic abnormalities reflecting systemic disease states (Table 3-1). It is particularly useful in the evaluation of anemia and leukemia, although hematologic changes may occur in infection and inflammation. Any patient presenting with clinical signs of anemia, such as dilated retinal veins, retinal hemorrhaging, retinal edema, and exudates, or leukemia, with infiltration and hemorrhages of the lids and conjunctiva, needs a hematologic evaluation including a CBC.

The CBC includes the red blood count, indices and morphology, white blood cell count and *dif-*

TABLE 3-1 *Complete Blood Count: Normal Values*

Test	Normal Range	
	Male	*Female*
RBC ($\times 10^6/\mu L$)	4.6-6.2	4.2-5.4
WBC ($\times 10^6/\mu L$)	4.8-10.8	4.8-10.8
Hgb (g/dl)	14.0-18.0	12.0-16.0
Hct (%)	42-52	37-47
MCV (fl)	83-101	
MCH (pg)	27-37	
MCHC (%)	32-37	
MCV (fl)	80-94	81-91
Platelet ($\times 10^3/\mu L$)	150-400	

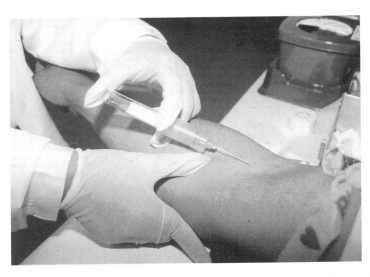

FIG. 3-2 Venipuncture: A large sample of blood is obtained from the superficial view of the midarm.

ferential, hematocrit and *hemoglobin* ("H and H"), platelet count, and other hematologic tests. It is ordered from the laboratory on a hematology order form and costs about $30.00. The blood is obtained by venipuncture or fingerstick, and results are available within a few hours.

Red Blood Cell (RBC) Count. The red blood cell, or erythrocyte, transports oxygen and carbon dioxide and helps control the pH of the blood. Erythropoietic dysfunction or blood loss is indicated by results outside the normal range of 4.6 to 6.2 million/mm^3. A decrease in the RBC occurs in hemorrhaging and anemia (see Chapter 15). Polycythemia presents as an increase in the RBC and may cause markedly dilated and tortuous retinal veins as well as disc edema.

The RBC is ordered on a hematology form supplied by the laboratory and, if not part of a CBC, costs about $10.00. Blood is obtained by venipuncture or fingerstick, and results are available within a few hours.

Red Blood Cell Indices. These erythrocyte parameters help diagnose specific anemias and are based on the hemoglobin concentration, the hematocrit, or the packed cell volume, and the RBC count. They are usually provided as part of the CBC.

Red Blood Cell Morphology. A blood smear is stained with Wright's stain, and the erythrocyte appearance is examined microscopically. The cell membrane, biconcavity, central area of pallor, size, shape, and inclusions are all evaluated. It is part of the CBC, and samples may be obtained by fingerstick or venipuncture. It is useful in the evaluation of red cell disorders and is ordered through hematology. The cost of this test is around $11.00.

White Blood Cell (WBC) Count. This is a count of the total number of leukocytes, or white blood cells, in 1 μl of whole blood. The normal WBC count is between 4,500 and 11,000 cells/mm^3. An elevation in the number of white blood cells is known as leukocytosis and, in most cases, indicates an infectious process, usually involving a bacterial cause. A decrease in the WBC count is called leukopenia and may arise from acute viral infections, starvation, drugs, and stress. In gen-

eral, the WBC count is useful in the detection of leukemias and infections.

The WBC count gives only the total number of leukocytes and is of limited value in diagnosis. Significant additional information is provided when a differential count of the various leukocyte types is performed. Collection for a WBC count is by venipuncture or fingerstick and is ordered through hematology, usually as part of a CBC.

Differential. The differential identifies the various types of leukocytes. Because the WBC yields only the total number of white blood cells, it may have limited value in the differential diagnosis of anemias, leukemias, infections, and inflammations. To this end, the various types of leukocytes are differentiated and counted. These include the neutrophils, lymphocytes, monocytes, eosinophils, and basophils (Table 3-2). Changes in each of these leukocytes may indicate certain disease states and are of great value in the differential diagnosis. The test is ordered through hematology and costs about $21.25. The sample is collected by fingerstick or venipuncture.

Neutrophils. These leukocytes comprise 56% of the total WBC and are the most abundant of all the cells seen. Reduction in the number of neutrophils can occur in acute viral infections and starvation. Elevations in the number of neutrophils can be due to bacterial infection, inflammation, tumors, and drugs.

Eosinophils. Comprising up to 8% of the total WBCs, the eosinophil number may be elevated as a result of allergic reactions or parasitic disease. Reduction in eosinophils may be due to stress.

TABLE 3-2 *Differential (Adult Range): Normal Values*

Cell Type	Normal Range
Neutrophil	40%-74%
Lymphocytes	19%-48%
Monocytes	3.4%-9.0%
Eosinophils	0%-8.0%
Basophils	0%-1.5%

Basophils. Up to 1.5% of the WBCs are basophils, which contain heparin. A rapidly falling basophil count may indicate an anaphylactic reaction.

Lymphocytes. Comprising 19% to 48% of the WBCs, the lymphocytes are formed in the lymph nodes and thymus gland. Elevations may occur in chronic lymphocytic leukemia and in viral infections, such as mononucleosis, measles, and chickenpox.

Monocytes. These leukocytes are formed in the bone marrow and are increased in response to chronic inflammatory disorders.

Platelet Count. Because the platelets are necessary for blood coagulation, the platelet count helps in the evaluation of bleeding disorders. The test determines the number of platelets per cubic millimeter of blood. The normal platelet count is 150,000 to 400,000/mm^3. A low platelet count is referred to as thrombocytopenia. The test is ordered through hematology, and blood is collected by fingerstick or venipuncture. Cost of a platelet count is about $16.00.

Thrombocytopenia may be due to an immunologic response, drugs, transfusion, or infection. A rise in thrombocytes (thrombocytosis) may be due to myeloproliferative syndromes, iron deficiency, or malignant disease.

The Red Blood Cell Indices. It is important to establish the relationship between the size, number, and hemoglobin content of the erythrocytes in order to correctly diagnose the various types of anemias. To this end, an examination of the stained peripheral blood smear (collected by venipuncture or fingerstick method) reveals the red blood cell characteristics. The hematocrit (Hct), hemoglobin (Hgb), mean cell volume (MCV), mean cell hemoglobin concentration (MCHC), and mean cell hemoglobin (MCH) help in the specific diagnosis of the various types of anemia.

Hematocrit (Hct). Hematocrit is defined as the volume of packed red blood cells found in 100 ml of blood and is expressed as a percentage. The normal hematocrit is 42% to 52% in males and 37% to 47% in females. Increased levels may occur in heart failure or chronic anoxia. It is useful in evaluating anemias. Hematocrit is ordered through hematology and costs about $17.25.

Hemoglobin (Hgb). When ordered with the hematocrit, hemoglobin is known as the "H + H." Hemoglobin is the oxygen-carrying pigment of the erythrocyte, and its level is reported as grams per

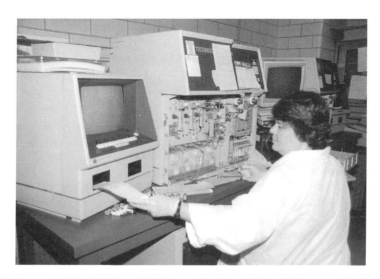

FIG. 3-3 CBC instrument: The Technicon H-1 System in a hospital-based laboratory for hematology studies.

100 ml (dl) of blood. The normal hemoglobin level in men is 14 to 18 g/dl and in women is 12 to 16 g/dl. Increased hemoglobin level may occur in chronic heart failure or anoxia. It is useful in evaluating anemias. It is ordered through hematology and costs about $17.75.

Mean cell volume (MCV). This is the average volume of an erythrocyte, expressed as cubic microns per red cell. The normal value is 83 to 101 fl.

Mean cell hemoglobin concentration (MCHC). This is the amount of hemoglobin per 100 ml (dl) of erythrocytes. The normal MCHC is 32 to 37 g/dl.

Mean cell hemoglobin (MCH). This is the average hemoglobin content of an individual erythrocyte. The normal is 27 to 37 pg. The cost of the test is about $17.75.

CBC Instrumentation. The CBC is performed in hospital-based and private laboratories by large, automated analyzers. The use of computers has reduced the time necessary to analyze multiple blood samples (Fig. 3-3).

CBC Procedure, Ordering, and Results. The CBC is ordered through a hematology request form available from the laboratory. The blood sample is obtained by a venipuncture or fingerstick technique. Any abnormal results in a routine CBC should be reviewed by a pathologist or the patient's family medical doctor or internist. The cost of the complete CBC is about $30.00 (Fig. 3-4).

Blood Chemistry

Biochemical Profile. Any variety of blood chemicals may be analyzed in order to help in the diagnosis and management of disease states. Twelve of the most common and meaningful of these chemistry tests can be performed by ordering a chemistry panel, also known as the simultaneous multiple analysis (SMA-12). With the advent of sophisticated instrumentation, the physician is encouraged to order the most appropriate tests necessary to profile the patient. The SMA-12, on the other hand, is useful as a multiple organ system survey. The test may include the following blood chemicals: total protein, albumin,

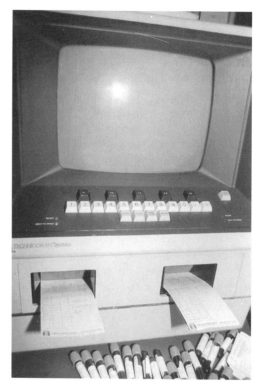

FIG. 3-4 Results of a CBC are displayed both on the computer screen and on a hard-copy report.

calcium, phosphorus, cholesterol, glucose, bilirubin, blood urea nitrogen, creatinine, uric acid, alkaline phosphatase, lactic acid dehydrogenase, and serum glutamic-oxaloacetic transaminase (Table 3-3).

The biochemical profile, or SMA-12 test, is ordered on the chemistry request form available from the laboratory. The blood sample is obtained via the venipuncture technique. It is intended primarily as a screening, and follow-up of abnormal chemical findings should include selective testing. The SMA-12 test is also performed as a routine blood test before ocular surgery. The cost of a chemistry profile is about $58.25.

Total serum protein. Proteins are used as cotransporters and buffers in the blood. The protein level, together with the albumin level, is used to evaluate a patient's nutritional status, liver function, and nephrotic syndromes. The normal serum

TABLE 3-3 *Biochemical Profile: Normal Ranges*

Protein	6.0-8.5 g/dl
Albumin	3.2-5.2 g/dl
Calcium	8.5-10.6 mg/dl
Phosphorus	2.5-4.5 mg/dl
Cholesterol	150-239 mg/dl
Glucose (fasting)	70-115 mg/dl
Bilirubin	0.1-1.2 mg/dl
Creatinine	0.6-1.4 mg/dl
Uric Acid	3.8-8.5 mg/dl (male)
	2.2-7.7 mg/dl (female)
Blood urea nitrogen	8-20 mg/dl
Alkaline phosphatase	38-126 U/L
Lactic acid dehydrogenase	297-618 U/L
Serum glutamic-oxaloacetic transaminase	5-35 U/L

value of protein is 6.0 to 8.5 g/dl. Patients who present with nutritional-type amblyopia, alcoholism, or anorexia warrant a protein level determination (see Chapter 12). The cost of the total serum protein test is about $20.00.

Serum albumin. Albumin is a specific protein whose level is a good indicator of nutritional status. It is also useful in the evaluation of liver disease, chronic alcoholism, kidney disease, Crohn's disease, burns, and heart disease. The normal value for albumin is 3.2 to 5.2 g/dl. The cost of the albumin test is about $20.00.

Calcium. Calcium is essential for heart, muscle, and nerve function, as well as blood coagulation. The normal calcium level in adults is 8.5 to 10.6 mg/dl. Elevated calcium levels occur in carcinoma, alcoholic dehydration, sarcoidosis, tuberculosis, histoplasmosis, leukemia, and hyperthyroidism. Low calcium levels are seen in malnutrition and low protein levels, because calcium is bound to serum albumin. Eye patients who present with corneal band keratopathy, lithiasis of the conjunctiva, and corneal arcus juvenilis may have abnor-

mal calcium levels and deserve a serum test. Cost is about $25.00.

Phosphorus. Elevated levels of phosphorus, an inorganic blood compound, may be found in some patients with sarcoidosis and diabetic ketosis. Decreased levels are found in acute alcoholism and malabsorption syndrome. The normal value in adults is 2.5 to 4.5 mg/dl. The phosphorus level is often evaluated relative to the calcium level. The cost of the phosphorus test is about $20.00.

Cholesterol. No longer considered an adequate evaluation of serum lipid levels, elevated total cholesterol levels are, however, associated with increased risk of coronary artery disease in middle-aged men. For appropriate determination of relevant cholesterol levels, it is recommended that low density and high density lipoprotein cholesterol also be determined as part of a lipid profile. Eye patients with pronounced arcus juvenilis and retinal Hollenhorst plaques should have cholesterol levels determined. Cholesterol is both ingested and synthesized in the liver. It is used for fat transport and hormone formation. Desirable level is less than 200 mg/dl, and 200 to 239 mg/dl is considered "borderline-high." The test costs about $13.25.

Glucose. For the fasting blood glucose level, the patient should be instructed to fast for an 8-hour period before the test. Serum glucose is useful in the diagnosis of diabetes mellitus. The normal adult value is 70 to 115 mg/dl, and borderline hyperglycemia is considered 115 to 140 mg/dl. A fasting glucose of over 200 mg/dl establishes the diagnosis of diabetes mellitus. Readings of 140 to 200 mg/dl necessitate an oral glucose tolerance test. Cost of a glucose test is about $16.00. Patients with no significant medical history who present with possible diabetic retinopathy or neuropathy should have serum glucose level determined.

Bilirubin. This is a test of liver function. Bilirubin is a bile pigment, the breakdown product of erythrocyte hemoglobin. It circulates in the plasma bound to albumin. It is a waste product and must be eliminated. Elevated bilirubin can occur in hepatitis, cirrhosis, alcoholism, and some anemias.

Patients who present with jaundice, with possible yellowing of the conjunctiva, have high concentrations of bilirubin. The normal bilirubin level is 0.1 to 1.2 mg/dl. Cost of this single test is about $35.00.

Blood urea nitrogen (BUN). The BUN is a renal function test. The formation of urea, the end product of protein metabolism, accounts for most of nitrogen excretion. Urea is excreted in the urine. An elevated BUN indicates renal insufficiency, shock, or heart failure. Low BUN may be due to malnutrition, protein deficiency, or liver disease. A normal value for BUN in the adult is 8 to 20 mg/dl. The cost of this test is about $12.00.

Creatinine. This is a renal function test that is more specific for renal function than is the BUN. Creatinine is a nitrogenous waste product. Normal levels are 0.6 to 1.4 mg/dl. Creatinine is elevated in kidney disease with nephron destruction and is a fairly specific renal test. Cost of the test is about $27.00.

Uric acid. Uric acid is a major product of metabolism. It is cleared from the plasma in the kidney. Normal levels are 3.8 to 8.5 mg/dl in men and 2.2 to 7.7 mg/dl in women. Elevated levels occur in gout, diabetes mellitus, hypertension, atherosclerosis, and myocardial infarction. Low levels of uric acid are seen in Wilson's disease. Cost of the test is $25.00.

Alkaline phosphatase (AP). Alkaline phosphatase is an enzyme found in the serum, bone, kidney, spleen, lung, and other organs, where it catalyzes biochemical reactions. AP acts to help mediate bone formation. The normal value in adults is 38 to 126 IU/L. Elevated levels of AP may be due to liver problems such as jaundice or space-occupying lesions. If there is no liver disease, elevated AP levels may be due to bone pathology, such as carcinoma or fracture. Elevated AP levels may be found following ocular trauma, that causes a blow-out fracture of the orbital floor. The AP is normally elevated during pregnancy and in childhood and adolescence. Average cost of the test is $32.00.

Lactic acid dehydrogenase (LDH). An enzyme widespread throughout body tissues, such as the

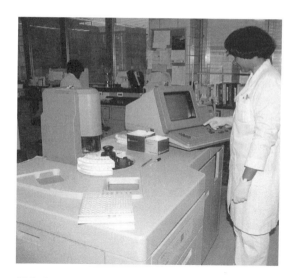

FIG. 3-5 The Ektachem 700 for simultaneous multiple blood analysis when performing a blood chemistry profile.

heart, brain, liver, kidney, and skeletal muscles, LDH is elevated when one of these tissues is damaged. Elevated LDH occurs in myocardial infarction. The normal value is 300 to 610 U/L. Average cost of the test is $25.00.

Serum glutamic-oxaloacetic transaminase (SGOT). An enzyme originating in the bone, kidney, heart, spleen, liver, and lung, SGOT is most useful as a liver function test. The normal value is 8 to 40 U/L. Elevation occurs in cirrhosis, congestive heart failure, alcoholism, and shock. Cost of the SGOT is about $27.00.

The Instruments of Chemistry. Three levels of instruments are available to perform biochemical analysis. At the laboratory, large, computerized instruments perform simultaneous analysis of multiple samples. Such instruments as the Ektachem 700 and the Ektachem 400 streamline the evaluation of many serum samples (Figs. 3-5 and 3-6).

Results are produced on a hard-copy printout and normal values are given following each test. Any abnormal findings are flagged with an asterisk or indicator of some sort, helping to speed the reading of the results.

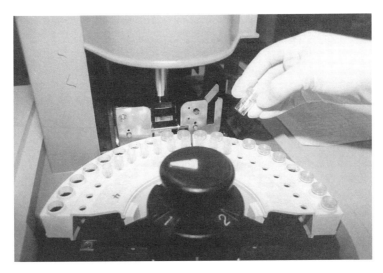

FIG. 3-6 Several samples of blood are prepared for the Ektachem 700. The sampling probe automatically "sips" each container of blood, delivers the sample to the analyzer, and self-cleans between samplings.

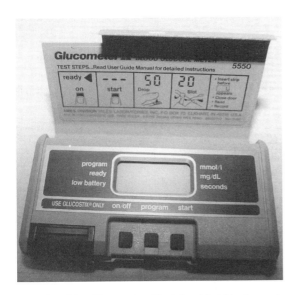

FIG. 3-7 The Glucometer II: A hand-held instrument used by diabetics to monitor blood glucose levels.

At the other end of the spectrum are hand-held instruments. These portable devices are used to evaluate single chemistry tests. Most often these are used by insulin-dependent diabetics to monitor

serum glucose. Blood is sampled by a fingerstick, and the sample is introduced into the instrument. Within minutes a single reading is shown on an LED screen. The portability of these devices is a great help to the diabetic who wishes to maintain an active life style (Fig. 3-7).

A compromise between the large-sized instruments of the laboratory and the hand-held devices are the portable, mid-sized analyzers. These instruments can handle a multitude of chemistry tests but are limited to a one-at-a-time approach. Therefore, the tests are more useful in the office than the laboratory. They have the advantage of offering a plethora of chemistry tests in one portable instrument. Blood is sampled by a fingerstick, and each test takes about two minutes. An example of this instrument is the Reflotron (Fig. 3-8).

URINALYSIS

The normal patient excretes about 1 L of urine daily. Waste products of metabolism are carried away by the urine, as well as a multitude of dissolved substances. Changes in the chemical constituents of the urine may yield important informa-

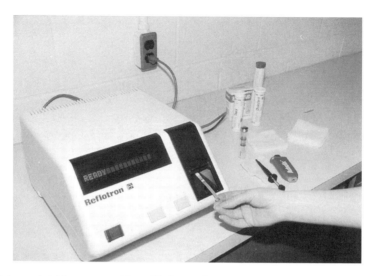

FIG. 3-8 The Reflotron: A table-top, portable, mid-size analyzer, useful for glucose, cholesterol, and other blood chemistry tests.

tion related to the presence of disease. To this end, urinalysis provides a technique of examining the urine to help in the evaluation and management of disorders.

Urinalysis actually encompasses several tests that can be performed in the laboratory, office, or home. Urinalysis is divided into macroscopic testing and microscopic testing. Macroscopic testing includes an evaluation of the sample's appearance, specific gravity, color, and pH. Also included are tests to detect the presence of protein, glucose, ketone bodies, bilirubin, nitrite, occult blood, leukocyte esterase, and urobilinogen (Table 3-4). Microscopic studies include tests of the urine sediment following centrifugation of the sample to look for red or white blood cells, bacterial colonies, casts, and crystals (Table 3-5).

Macroscopic Evaluation

Appearance. The macroscopic evaluation begins with the visual appearance of the urine. Because there are a wide range of urine constituent concentrations, urine specimens present with a wide variety of characteristic colors, from pale yellow to dark amber. The normal color of urine is a result of metabolic breakdown products such as

TABLE 3-4 *Urinalysis: Normal Ranges Macroscopic (Dipstick)*

Color	Yellow
Appearance	Clear
Specific gravity	1.003-1.035
pH	5-8.5
Protein	Negative
Glucose	Negative
Ketones	Negative
Bilirubin	Negative
Occult blood	Negative
Nitrate	Negative
Urobilinogen	Negative
Leukocyte esterase	Negative

bile, as well as pigments found in the patient's diet. Evaluation of the appearance of urine includes not only color but also an inspection for stringy mucus, which may be due to infection.

Blood in the urine is called hematuria and is a significant finding necessitating a medical evaluation. Dark brown urine may occur in jaundice, indicating possible liver disease.

Specific Gravity. The specific gravity of the urine sample may reflect the degree of hydration present. It is an indicator of renal function and is dependent on the urine volume and presence of excreted solids. Normal urine specific gravity is about 1.020.

Urine Volume. The volume of urine typically increases in uncontrolled diabetes mellitus. Patients with a complaint of polyuria should be evaluated for diabetes.

Dipstick Testing. Urine must be collected in clean, usually disposable, containers. The patient is asked to void into the container after following any specific instructions, such as fasting or 24-hour collection.

The use of dipsticks containing a number of tests on each stick expedites macroscopic urinalysis. These tests include glucose, protein, ketones, blood, pH, bile, bilirubin, nitrite, leukocyte esterase, and urobilinogen (Fig. 3-9).

Glucose. Normal urine does not contain enough glucose to cause a positive result on a dipstick. Therefore, a positive urine glucose finding should be treated as an abnormality, and an evaluation to rule out diabetes mellitus is mandatory. Because a positive urine glucose test does not confirm the presence of the disease, serum glucose remains a more meaningful test than urine glucose testing alone. This is significant when considering in-office glucose testing of patients with diabetic retinopathy or neuropathy.

Protein. Protein found in the urine (proteinuria) is an important indicator of renal disease. The protein, when found in urine, is usually albumin. The list of disorders causing proteinuria includes glomerulonephritis, renal failure, systemic lupus erythematosus, and many others. Proteinuria appears early in renal disease and may be the only clinical sign of the abnormality.

Ketone Bodies. Ketone bodies are intermediates of fat metabolism formed in the liver. It is an important screening test in diabetics, children, pregnancy, all hospital admissions, and presurgical evaluations. Large amounts occur in diabetic ketoacidosis. They occur when fat instead of carbo-

TABLE 3-5 *Urinalysis: Microscopic*

RBC	0-5 cells
WBC	0-2 cells
Casts	0-1 cast (hyaline)
Crystals	Variable
Bacteria	Negative

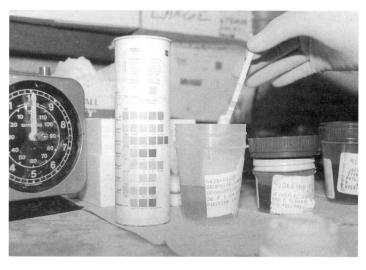

FIG. 3-9 Dipstick testing: Each stick contains a number of tests, expediting macroscopic urinalysis.

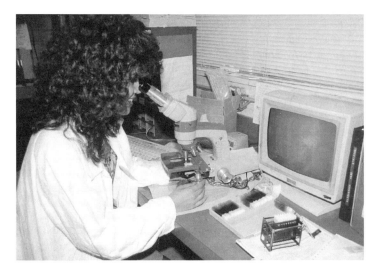

FIG. 3-10 Microscopic evaluation of urine: Microscopic evaluation of the urine sample is necessary if the dipstick test is abnormal.

hydrate is used for energy. The presence of ketone bodies in the urine of a diabetic indicates that the patient is not adequately controlled.

Blood. Blood in the urine (hematuria) may be detected visually as a smoky brown–appearing sample, chemically by a dipstick, or microscopically. Hematuria is usually due to some urinary tract disease, whereas occult (hidden) blood may be due to any number of renal disorders.

pH. Although it can vary widely, the normal pH of urine is usually between 5.0 and 8.5. Changes in the pH value may be due, for example, to a urinary tract infection, which can cause an alkaline shift (e.g., 9.0).

Bile. Bilirubin is formed from hemoglobin, bound to serum protein, and carried to the liver for processing. Bile is then produced and excreted into the intestine. An increase in bilirubin occurs when chemicals or viruses interfere with liver function.

Urine Urobilinogen and Bilirubin. Urobilinogen and bilirubin form from hemoglobin metabolism and are both considered bile pigments. Both are tested by dipstick. Bilirubin can appear in the urine in hepatitis, bile duct obstruction, and chem-

ical injury to the liver. Elevated urobilinogen occurs in jaundice and cirrhosis.

Microscopic Evaluation

Urine can be centrifuged and the sediment examined for casts, cells, crystals, and bacteria. Casts usually indicate renal disease. Red and white blood cells indicate hematuria or infection. Crystals are usually a normal finding.

Casts. These bits of concealed protein form as a plug within the kidney tubule and then are washed into the urine. Casts can be seen only microscopically. Casts of red blood cells usually indicate glomerular inflammation or a renal vascular disorder.

Cells. The finding of red cells in the urine may indicate kidney trauma, exercise, passage of stones, tumors, and renal calculi (such as may occur when patients are taking certain carbonic anhydrase inhibitors). White blood cells indicate infection within the urinary tract.

Ordering Urinalysis

To order a urinalysis, use the laboratory's urinalysis order form. Either collect the specimen from the patient and deliver to the laboratory within two hours, or have the laboratory collect the sample. The average cost of a full urinalysis is about $12.00.

Urinalysis in Eye Care

Urinalysis is an effective screening test for renal and hepatobiliary function, as well as for glucose. Macroscopic evaluation of the urine is easily performed in the private office setting by use of the dipstick. Have your local laboratory demonstrate to you the proper dipstick technique and resulting interpretation.

The dipstick technique uses any number of chemical strips containing reagent tests which are sensitive to compounds present in the urine. These strips are dipped into the urine sample, and a certain amount of time is allowed for color transformation of the reagents. These colors are then compared with a normal standard color chart. Dipsticks may be purchased from a local laboratory or medical supply house.

Microscopic evaluation of the urine is performed if the dipstick is positive for occult blood, protein, or other factors. Microscopic evaluation requires a trained laboratory technician with experience in urinalysis (see Fig. 3-10).

If a positive result is discovered in the office, the patient should be referred to his primary health care provider, along with the results of the urinalysis and a report of any significant eye findings.

SPECIFIC LABORATORY TESTS FOR INFLAMMATION

Erythrocyte Sedimentation Rate (ESR)

For over 50 years, the ESR, or sed rate, has been used as a nonspecific but moderately sensitive measure of the presence of inflammation. It is elevated in infection, neoplasms, vasculitis, and most connective tissue disorders. It may be markedly elevated in giant-cell (temporal) arteritis and returns to normal upon disease treatment.

The ESR measures the rate at which red blood cells settle out of solution. The most common test ordered is the Westergren sed rate, which com-

bines a blood sample with a diluent. The sample is allowed to settle for 1 hour in a 200-mm long tube. The rate of erythrocyte settling is read as millimeters per hour. Inflammation causes the erythrocytes to clump together and settle out of solution faster. The normal sed rate is 0 to 20 mm/hr, but varies greatly depending on the patient's age and gender and the laboratory's reference range (Fig. 3-11).

The sed rate should be ordered on any patients suspected of having temporal arteritis or collagen-vascular disease. It can be ordered through your laboratory on a hematology form. A 5-ml sample of blood is drawn via venipuncture in the laboratory. The average cost of the sed rate is about $12.00.

Rheumatoid Factor (RF)

This is not actually a test specific for rheumatoid arthritis. It is in fact a test that indicates the presence of an antibody to gamma globulin (which is itself an antibody). Many patients have small amounts of rheumatoid factor. The test is positive in rheumatoid arthritis, chronic infections, cirrhosis, chronic pulmonary disease, and Sjögren's syndrome and has an increased incidence in the elderly. This test is particularly significant for the patient who presents with recurrent anterior uveitis of unknown cause because uveitic entities may be due to rheumatoid arthritis (see Chapter 18).

The RF is ordered on an immunology form supplied by the laboratory. A 7-ml blood sample is drawn via venipuncture following an 8-hour fast. RF is reported in 75% of clinically diagnosed rheumatoid arthritis cases. The cost of the RF test is about $17.00.

Antinuclear Antibodies (ANA)

Antibodies may exist that are reactive against tissue antigens. These are widely used in the diagnosis of autoimmune diseases. They are present at low levels in many healthy individuals and their family members and typically increase with age. The ANA is a helpful screening test for autoimmune diseases and systemic lupus erythematosus but is not specific for any one collagen-vascular

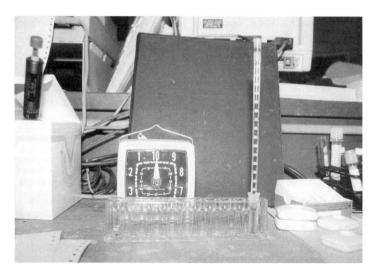

FIG. 3-11 The Westergren erythrocyte sedimentation rate (ESR): Note the capillary tube filled with a blood sample and the clock to measure the rate of sedimentation in one hour.

disease. The ANA should be ordered on patients presenting with recurrent anterior uveitis of unknown cause because collagen-vascular disorders may cause uveitis (see Chapter 7).

The ANA is ordered on an immunology order form available from the laboratory. Seven milliliters of blood is sampled by routine venipuncture, and the test requires the patient to fast. The average cost of an ANA test is $33.00.

HLA-B27

The HLA-B27 test helps in the diagnosis of seronegative collagen-vascular diseases such as ankylosing spondylitis and related disorders such as Reiter's syndrome and Crohn's disease. The HLA is a complex found on a chromosome, and it acts to control important immune functions. In theory it determines the patient's genetic tendency to develop these disorders.

Because it is not a mandatory test for ankylosing spondylitis, Reiter's syndrome, or Crohn's disease, the HLA-B27 test is not routinely performed. Furthermore, it is expensive and time-consuming, costing more than $60.00 and taking a considerable time to receive the results. Also, the HLA-

B27 antigen is found in 6% to 8% of the normal, white population, and its presence is of no diagnostic value in the absence of clinical disease.

The HLA-B27 test can be performed only by the immunology section of major reference laboratories. Most hospital and private laboratories refer the specimen to these facilities. A sample of 12 ml of whole blood is collected, as the test requires a large number of lymphocytes.

LABORATORY TESTING FOR COMMON INFECTIONS AND INFLAMMATION

Syphilis

Syphilis is a chronic, systemic infection caused by the spirochete *Treponema pallidum* (see Chapter 6). The battery of laboratory tests to help in the diagnosis are described as syphilis serology. These tests include the fluorescent treponemal antibody-absorption test (FTA-ABS), the venereal disease research laboratory (VDRL) test, the rapid plasma reagin (RPR) test, and the treponemal antibody hemagglutination (MHA-TP) test.

The FTA-ABS and MHA-TP tests depend on the presence of specific antitreponemal antibodies.

Because these antibodies may persist indefinitely, these two tests are often positive for life even after eradication of the disease. Nontreponemal serologic tests for syphilis include the VDRL and the RPR tests.

Fluorescent Treponemal Antibody-Absorbed Test (FTA-ABS). This test is used to detect early or late syphilis. It uses antigens derived from *T. pallidum* in order to detect antibodies from past or present infection. The FTA-ABS has largely been replaced by the MHA-TP test. Cost of the FTA-ABS is about $36.00.

Treponemal Antibody Hemagglutination (MHA-TP). This test is specific for treponema. It is not a screening test. The MHA-TP tests for the presence of *T. pallidum* antibodies, so once positive it is always positive, regardless of treatment. Seven milliliters of blood are sampled by routine venipuncture. The test is ordered on an immunology form available from your laboratory. Results take about 1 to 2 weeks. The MHA-TP replaces the FTA-ABS.

Venereal Disease Research Laboratory (VDRL) Test. This is a nontreponemal serologic test for syphilis. It has largely been replaced by the RPR test. The VDRL is still used to evaluate samples of cerebrospinal fluid.

Rapid Plasma Reagin (RPR) Test. This is a nontreponemal screening test for syphilis and is useful both for diagnosis of syphilis and in monitoring the patient following treatment. It also has a high false-positive rate, so all positive RPR results must be confirmed with a treponemal test like the MHA-TP.

This test detects antibodies to cardiolipin, not treponema. Because cardiolipin antibodies decrease with treatment, the patient may be monitored with the RPR test. Seven milliliters of blood are collected and the results are available in 24 hours. The RPR test is ordered on the immunology form. The cost of the RPR test is about $14.00.

Sarcoidosis

Sarcoidosis is a multisystem granulomatous disorder of unknown cause (see Chapter 11). Several laboratory tests may help in diagnosing sarcoid.

Alkaline Phosphatase. AP is a widely distributed enzyme tested by serum chemistry (SMA-12). It is frequently elevated in patients with infiltrative disorders of the liver such as sarcoidosis.

Serum Calcium. Serum calcium is also tested by chemistry (SMA-12). Twenty-five percent of patients with sarcoid show hypercalcemia. The elevated calcium levels fall with steroid therapy.

Angiotensin-Converting Enzyme (ACE). Angiotensin-converting enzyme is elevated in about 80% of patients with active sarcoid. Only about 5% of normal subjects have elevated ACE levels. The ACE level appears to reflect the activity of the disease. ACE decreases with steroid therapy. The ACE is a radiochemical assay test of serum samples. Two milliliters of serum are collected.

Gallium Scan. Abnormal gallium scans may occur in patients with granulomatous inflammatory disease such as sarcoidosis. The gallium scan is an imaging test. The patient is injected intravenously with gallium, which is a radiopharmaceutical. Gallium tends to bind to granulomatous lesions. Lung fields are imaged at varous times after injection and demonstrate granulomatous lesions if present in sarcoid. This test is ordered on a nuclear medicine form.

Histopathology. Lung biopsy confirms the presence of sarcoid in sampled tissues. This helps differentiate imaged sarcoid lesions from malignancies such as bronchogenic carcinoma. Conjunctival nodules may also contain sarcoid material and are easier to obtain for biopsy than lung tissue. The nodules are removed and fixed in formalin solution, and the biopsy results are interpreted by a pathologist.

Skin Hypersensitivity Test (Kveim). Skin testing for sarcoidosis is rarely done owing to the time it takes for results (several weeks) and the difficulty in appropriating sarcoid material for injection.

Tuberculosis (TB)

TB is a bacterial infection of the lungs which is commonly transmitted by airborne particles. Tests used commonly in the diagnosis of TB include the chest radiograph, acid-fast stain, a serum and sputum mycobacterial culture, purified protein derivative (PPD), and the Mantoux test.

Mycobacterial Culture. This body fluid culture detects the presence of mycobacteria from any number of samples, such as bone marrow, bronchial aspirate, cerebrospinal fluid, gastric aspirate, skin sputum, tissue, and urine.

Acid-Fast Stain. Acid-fast staining is a smear of one of the above samples studied under a microscope.

Sputum smears for acid-fast organisms are one of the most common techniques for diagnosis. This procedure uses yellow fluorescing dye and microscopy to detect acid-fast bacilli fluorescing against a contrasting background. Culturing is necessary to identify the species of mycobacterium. Acid-fast stain may require 48 hours for results. These tests are ordered on a microbiology order form.

Purified Protein Derivative (PPD). Delayed-type hypersensitivity skin testing uses antigens of purified protein derivative of tuberculin and evaluates the in vivo functional capacity of the T-cell immune system. The skin (usually of the forearm) is stuck with a syringe laden with inactive protein from the tuberculin mycobacterium. Patients with prior exposure to TB react within 24 to 48 hours with greater than 5 mm of skin errythema and induration. It is also referred to as the tine test.

Mantoux Test. This skin hypersensitivity test is similar to the PPD, except that the purified protein derivitive of the mycobacterium is injected subcutaneously.

Enzyme-Linked Immunosorbent Assay (ELISA)

In the past decade the ELISA has emerged from the research laboratory to become a significant diagnostic test in the detection of infectious agents. It is of particular use in establishing the diagnosis of rubella, herpes simplex, cytomegalovirus, adenovirus, human immunodeficiency virus (HIV), infection, gonorrhea, toxoplasmosis, and assorted parasitic infections. The ELISA is a serology test that detects small quantities of antibodies or antigens to infectious agents. The patient's serum is mixed with a known antigen, the anti–human immunoglobulin is mixed with an enzyme-linked alkaline phosphatase, and an enzyme substrate is added. The enzyme acts on the substrate to produce a color change in proportion to the amount of antibody fixed to antigen. The color change is read visually or with a spectrophotometer.

The ELISA is becoming an important method for the confirmation of HIV infection because of its high degree of specificity and sensitivity. It is also used to screen potential blood donors, units of blood for transfusion, and members of high-risk groups. To order an ELISA test, use the serology form available from the laboratory.

Bibliography

Ames Lab Guide: *Modern urine chemistry,* Ames Division, Miles Laboratories, 1979.

Bakken CL: *Interpretive data for diagnostic laboratory tests,* ed 2, Rochester, MN, 1981, Mayo Medical Laboratories.

The bio-science handbook—special diagnostic laboratory tests, ed 12, 1979.

Dougherty WM: *Introduction to hematology,* ed 2, St. Louis, 1976, Mosby–Year Book.

Free AH and Free HM: *Urinodynamics—concepts relating to routine urine chemistry,* ed 3, Ames Division, Miles Laboratories, 1978.

Hughes-Jones NC: *Lecture notes on haematology,* ed 3, Oxford, 1979, Blackwell Scientific Publications.

Lab User's Guide. Episcopal Hospital, Philadelphia, Department of Pathology and Radiology, Ohio, 1990, Lexi-Comp, Inc.

Reese RE and Douglas RG: *A practical approach to infectious disease,* Boston, 1983, Little, Brown and Co.

Stumacher RJ: *Clinical infectious disease,* Philadelphia, 1988, WB Saunders Co.

Tilkian SM, Conover MB, and Jilkian AG: *Clinical implications of laboratory tests,* ed 3, St. Louis, 1983, Mosby–Year Book.

Youmans GP, Paterson P, and Sommers HM: *The biological and clinical basis of infectious disease,* Philadelphia, 1985, WB Saunders Co.

4

Radiology

GEORGE E. WHITE
BARRY B. GOLDBERG
DANIEL A. MERTON

KEY TERMS

X-rays	Magnetic Resonance Imaging	Optic Canals View
Plain Films	Color Doppler Imaging	Basilar View
Tomography	Caldwell's View	Arteriography
Computed Tomography	Waters' View	Technetium Scan
Ultrasonography	Lateral View	

DEFINITIONS

X-Rays

X-rays are a form of radiant energy similar to visible light in several respects. They are produced by bombarding a tungsten target with an electron beam. They radiate from the source in all directions unless they are blocked by an absorbing or reflecting surface. Most x-rays are reflected, with a small portion absorbed. The fundamental difference between x-rays and light rays is in their range of wavelengths. Visible light rays have a longer wavelength than x-rays. Professor Wilhelm Conrad Roentgen of the University of Wurzburg developed the principles of radiology in 1895.

Plain Films

Direct imaging of the structures in question by radiation is referred to as plain films. This is quick and inexpensive and gives valuable information about the osseous structures of the body. However, it images other organs that are physically above or below it simultaneously. These are referred to as superimposition shadowgrams. They sometimes make interpretation difficult.

Tomography

Tomographic studies effectively slice the living patient so that one can study the shadows cast by certain structures free of superimposed shadows. The term *tomogram* is a general category. Different types of sectioning studies depend upon the results desired. The shadows intended for study and those purposely blurred are the essence of tomography. Only the structures in one plane are in focus in the tomogram, and all other structures are purposely blurred. Also, the thickness of the body slices may not match perfectly with the chosen plane of the study because the pivot point or selected focal point in the tomographic study is calculated arbitrarily for a certain distance in centimeters from the surface of the body, and body anatomy varies slightly with each patient.

Computed Tomography (CT)

Computed tomography (CT scan), or computerized axial tomography (CAT scan), was a major discovery. It was developed by adding a computerized program to tomography scans to better visualize cross-sectional anatomy of the body and most specifically the brain. The biggest advantage is the purposely blurred images of structures in slices on both sides of the plane chosen for study which add diagnostic confusion in plain films. The CT scan adds a computer program that gives focused radiologic information about one cross-sectional slice of the patient. Thus a CT scan gives a scheme of density values for a particular chosen slice of the patient which should be studied with regional cross-sectional anatomy in mind. CT scans are used clinically for all organ studies, but they are particularly useful in viewing the brain because other types of scans offer relatively limited diagnostic information.

Ultrasonography

Ultrasonography is included in most hospital radiology services as a diagnostic tool. It images a slice of organs of the body by directing a narrow beam of high-energy sound waves and recording the manner in which sound is reflected from the organs and structures. Ultrasound does not penetrate bone and therefore cannot be used for head scans. This is used ophthalmically when opaque media reduce conventional means of viewing the eye or when there is concern about retro-ocular soft-tissue abnormalities. Details about ophthalmic ultrasonography are included in this chapter.

Magnetic Resonance (MR) Imaging

MR scanning is one of the latest advances in imaging. It does not use ionizing radiation to image structure. The technique requires the patient to be placed within the bore of a powerful magnet. Radio waves are passed through the body in a particular sequence of very short pulses. Each pulse causes a characteristic responding pulse of radio waves to be emitted from the patient's tissues. The location from which the signals originate is recorded by a computer. This produces a two-dimensional picture representing a predetermined section or slice of the patient. This is used clinically in differentiating brain tumors.

Nuclear Medicine Imaging

This is another field included within the Department of Radiology in most hospitals. Nuclear medicine imaging is a branch of radiology which is based on the visualization of particular living organs and tissues after an injected radioactive isotope is taken up in that tissue. An image is obtained because the radioactive isotope emits gamma rays for a brief period of time. The emitted rays are recorded by a gamma camera and imaged on film. This is particularly useful in determining malignancies in certain organs.

HISTORY

Early experiments by Roentgen produced emission of x-rays as a by-product under laboratory conditions. He observed a chemically coated piece of cardboard which glowed with pale green light. This emission of visible light can be produced by a variety of methods by complex nuclear exchanges and is called fluorescence. This historic discovery of radiant energy passing through objects that are opaque to light was the first rudimentary x-rays. When a hand is placed between the source of the beam of energy and coated cardboard, the bones of the fingers within the hand are visible (Fig. 4-1).

INSTRUMENTATION

Photochemistry of X-rays

When light hits photographic film, an unusual photochemical process takes place in which metallic silver is precipitated in fine particles within the gelatin. This turns the film black when it is developed chemically. The places on the film which are not exposed to light remain white. When a "positive" paper print is made of this "negative" film, the values are reversed. The black or silver-bearing areas prevent light from reaching the photosensitive paper. Clear areas in the film permit the paper to be blackened.

The clinical x-ray film is equivalent to a photographic negative. X-rays, like light rays, precipitate silver in a photographic film, but they do so much less rapidly than light. This needs to be accomplished very quickly to eliminate long exposure time. Too much exposure to radiation is both dangerous and technically undesirable. A special film holder called a cassette was produced to speed up this technique.

The cassette contains a fluorescent screen that is activated by the x-rays. They in turn emit light rays that intensify the photochemical effects of the x-rays themselves upon the film. The silver-precipitating effect of the x-rays and the light rays they generate causes the blackening of the film. If an object placed between the x-ray beam source and the cassette has absorbed the rays, then no light activation of the fluorescent screen takes place. Neither the x-rays nor the light rays reach the film; thus, no silver is precipitated, and the film is white.

Fig. 4-2 shows a woman's right hand placed over the cassette and exposed to a beam of x-rays.

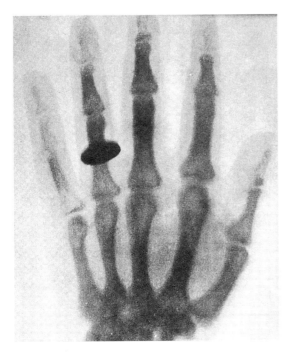

FIG. 4-1 Radiograph—actually a fluorograph—of a hand.

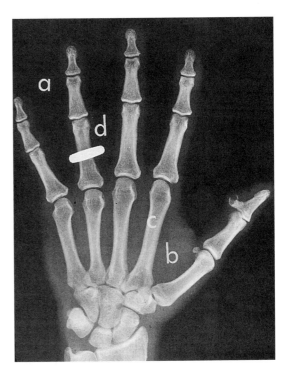

FIG. 4-2 Radiograph of a hand. Note that the gold ring on the third finger (**d**) totally blocks or absorbs all x-ray radiation and no exposure is seen. **b** shows the soft tissue of the hand.

Notice that the film not covered by any part of the hand has been intensely blackened. Therefore, very little of the beam was absorbed by the air, which was the only absorber interposed between the x-ray tube and the film. The soft tissue of the hand absorbed most of the beam so that the film appears gray. Very few rays reached that part of the film directly under the bones. The bones contain large amounts of calcium, are very dense, and absorb most of the x-rays. All metals absorb x-rays to an extent, depending on their atomic number and thickness. No x-rays at all pass through a gold ring on a finger, so the film underneath it is not altered photographically.

Electromagnetic Spectrum

The electromagnetic spectrum is a scaled arrangement of all types of radiant energy according to wavelength within the range used in diagnostic radiology (Fig. 4-3).

Technical Role

Plain Films. The x-ray technician is trained to select and use the particular wavelength suited to the penetrability and thickness of the scan that is ordered. This is accomplished by varying the kilovoltage. That is, the harder or more penetrating the beam required, the higher the kilovoltage required. The amount of beam radiation can be varied by altering both the milliamperage and the time of exposure. Thus, a thin object like the hand needs less radiation for a short time, and a dense object like the skull needs more radiation with slightly longer exposure.

Tomography. The scan is done by moving the x-ray tube and the film around the patient during the exposure. A thin, collimated beam of x-rays passes through the plane of the body chosen for study as the x-ray tube moves in a continuous arc around the patient. A pivot point is calculated to fall in the plane of the object to be studied. There-

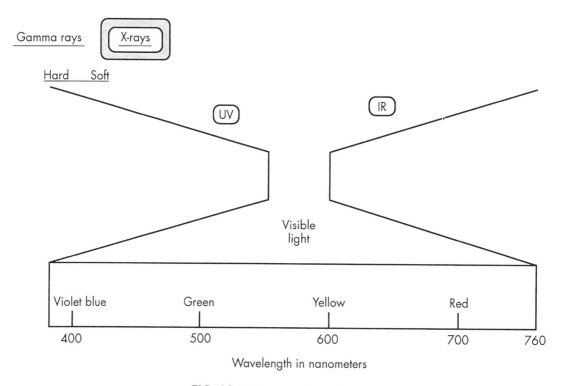

FIG. 4-3 Electromagnetic spectrum.

fore the shadows of all the structures not in the selected plane for study are intentionally blurred, because they are moving relative to the film. Thus, in Fig. 4-4 the object to be studied is in focus in the film while the shadows of the structures above and below are blurred.

CT Scan. Aligned directly opposite the x-ray tube are special electronic detectors that are a hundred times more sensitive than ordinary x-ray film. These detectors convert the exiting beam on the other edge of the body slice into amplified electrical pulses. The intensity depends upon the amount of the remaining beam of x-rays that has not been absorbed by the intervening tissues. Therefore, if the beam has passed mainly through dense areas of the body (such as bone), fewer x-rays emerge than when the beam traverses mainly low-density tissues (such as lung).

The photographic slice of the body can be conceived of as a flat mosaic of unit volumes. These volume units, called voxels, form a geometric grid. A single dense voxel (like the small black square in Fig. 4-5) absorbs none of the beam, in contrast to other, less dense neighboring voxels. Areas of the body that contain calcium produce such dense voxels.

This information is received by the detectors and is conveyed to a computer, which calculates the x-ray absorption for each voxel in the mosaic. The pictorial arrangement of absorption values makes up the final CT image. All tissues are given a specific absorption value. The absorption values are expressed in Hounsfield units (after one of the inventors of CT). Water was arbitrarily assigned the value of absorption of zero, and denser values range upward to bone or calcium, which can be +500 or more. Less dense structures range downward from fat to air, which can be −500.

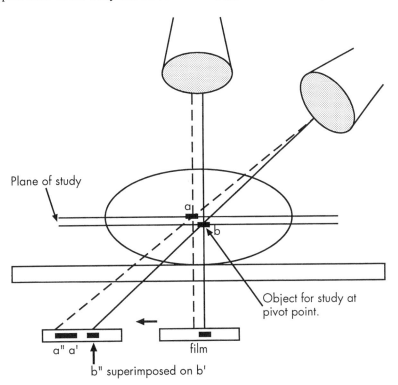

FIG. 4-4 Schematic of a tomogram, showing the movement of the film plane and the x-ray tube around the patient. The x-ray tube moves clockwise, and the film moves counterclockwise to purposely blur all areas except the object for study at the pivot point.

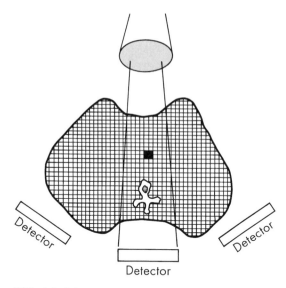

FIG. 4-5 Schematic of the CT scanner. Highlighted areas are the reference point and the detectors.

The attenuation number so obtained for each voxel in the mosaic matrix slice is converted into a dot on a television monitor screen. The brightness depends on the density of that unit volume and so reflects its anatomic structure. The picture produced is equivalent to a radiograph of that cross-sectional slice of the living patient.

Ultrasonography. Ultrasonography also gives an image of a slice of the body by directing a narrow beam of high-energy sound waves into the body and recording the manner in which sound is reflected from organs and structures. Ultrasound does not produce an image that is as sharp and clear as CT, but it has four singular advantages. First, it does not use ionizing radiation and produces no biologic injury. Second, it can be used in the transaxial or sagittal plane or at any chosen oblique axis required by the anatomic region being investigated. Third, it is far less expensive than CT or MR imaging. Fourth, it can even be performed at the bedside of very sick patients.

Ultrasound is sound above the range of human hearing (20 to 20,000 Hertz). Ultrasonography uses the principle of transmitting high-frequency sound waves into the body tissues and analyzing the returned echoes. Typical frequencies used for

diagnostic medical purposes are between 2 and 10 megahertz (million Hertz). Higher frequencies provide better detail resolution but less depth penetration. For ophthalmic scanning, only a few centimeters of penetration are required; therefore higher frequencies (7 to 10 MHz) can be used to provide optimal structural detail. Several types of diagnostic ultrasonography are in use today. The choice of which to use depends on the specific information desired.

Types of Diagnostic Ultrasonography. Various types of ultrasonography are used for ophthalmologic diagnoses. They are A-mode, B-mode (also known as two-dimensional gray scale), duplex Doppler, and *color Doppler imaging* (CDI). Doppler ultrasonography is used for the evaluation of blood flow.

A-mode or *amplitude mode* is a single point of sound that has only one dimension. Reflectors encountered along the path of the beam cause deflections of varying heights depending on the signal strength, and the deflections are displayed on an oscilloscope screen. Although use of this type of ultrasonography in other parts of the body has largely been replaced with two-dimensional gray-scale imaging, A-mode is still used in ophthalmology to obtain accurate measurements of orbital structures such as the thickness of the lens and retina.

B-mode or *brightness mode* is the most common form of diagnostic ultrasonography in use today. B-mode, or two-dimensional (2-D) ultrasonography is commonly used for evaluating anatomic structures such as the unborn fetus or the gallbladder (Fig. 4-6). Reflected echoes are displayed in shades of gray depending on their signal strength. Strong reflectors are displayed as white (on a black background), and progressively weaker echoes appear as gradually darker shades of gray (Fig. 4-7). Clear fluid such as that within the normal vitreous body contains no reflective particles and therefore is displayed as black. Updating the image very rapidly (faster than the eye can perceive) enables 2-D ultrasonography to show dynamic events, such as fetal heart motion, as they occur, resulting in *real-time* images. Two-dimensional ultrasonography is

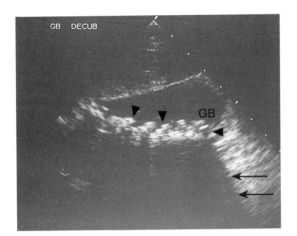

FIG. 4-6 Conventional long-axis B-mode ultrasound image of multiple gallstones *(arrowheads)* within the bile-filled gallbladder (GB). Note the acoustic shadow cast by the sound-attenuating stones *(arrows).*

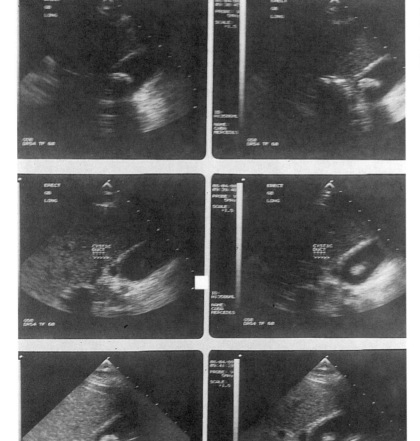

FIG. 4-7 Ultrasound, nonionizing source, viewing gallbladder, with no harmful biologic effects. Large dense white objects noted in each field represent gallstones.

best for obtaining information regarding normal and abnormal structures within the orbit and depicting their relationships.

Duplex Doppler imaging combines 2-D imaging with Doppler ultrasonography for the evaluation of blood flow. The Doppler effect allows us to "listen" to frequency changes that take place as the ultrasonic waves encounter moving structures. Using the 2-D image to identify the location of a vessel, a cursor called a *range gate* is positioned to provide blood flow information from a selected vessel segment. Doppler information can be in the form of an audible signal or can be visually displayed on the monitor via a spectral trace, allowing quantification of flow. Owing partly to the small size of the blood vessels supplying the eye, duplex Doppler ultrasonography has limited applications in ophthalmic scanning.

Color Doppler imaging (CDI) is a relatively recent advancement in diagnostic ultrasonography. CDI depicts nonmobile structures in gray scale, and moving structures, such as flowing blood, in color. Unlike duplex Doppler imaging, which provides flow information only from a single point on the image, CDI displays blood flow in color superimposed over the entire 2-D image. The operator can select colors, usually red and blue, to depict flow toward or away from the transducer, respectively. CDI allows rapid assessment of the presence and direction of flowing blood. By combining conventional ultrasonography with color Doppler, this valuable diagnostic tool provides both anatomic and physiologic information.

Although it is used throughout the body, the most common applications for CDI currently include echocardiography (ultrasonography of the heart), peripheral vascular (blood flow of the limbs), and cerebrovascular (blood flow to the brain). The eye and orbit region is a new area now being explored with CDI, with early research indicating that there are definite benefits of CDI over conventional ultrasonography for the evaluation of certain pathologic processes involving these structures. Because CDI can show blood in vessels that are beyond the resolution of conventional ultrasonography (approximately 1 mm), it can demon-

strate flow in even the tiny vessels supplying the eye such as the central retinal artery and vein located within the optic nerve (Fig. 4-8). The presence or absence of blood flow as depicted by CDI in an elevated portion of the retina can help differentiate retinal detachment from a tumor in this location (Fig. 4-9). This can be especially helpful in cases of intraocular bleeding. Suspected occlusions of the vessels supplying the eye can also be confirmed with this technique.

With its high sensitivity to blood flow, lack of harmful side effects, low cost, and relative ease of use, CDI promises to become an important diagnostic tool for the evaluation of orbital vasculature and pathology.

Magnetic Resonance Imaging. Different body tissues emit characteristic MR signals, which de-

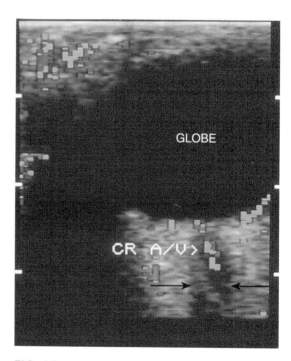

FIG. 4-8 Transverse color Doppler image demonstrating the normal central retinal (CR) artery and vein located within the hypoechoic optic nerve (*arrows*). Blood flow is also visualized at the back of the eye corresponding to flow in retinal and choroidal vessels. Red and blue indicate flow toward and away from the transducer, respectively.

termine whether they appear white, gray, or black on the final scans. Tissues that emit strong MR signals appear white in MR scans, whereas those emitting little or no signal appear black. The operator can vary the technique used by changing the sequence of pulses so that particular tissues can be viewed more clearly and easily. This may vary the appearance of the scan, but, in general, air and cortical bone as well as rapidly moving fluid, such as blood, appear black. Fat appears white. Slowly moving blood may or may not produce a detectable signal. Consequently, some venous structures and arteries imaged during diastole may return signals and appear in various shades of gray.

The thickness of the sections can be chosen as well as their orientation. In addition to the transverse sections of the body, MR imaging can be carried out in the sagittal and coronal planes and in various desirable oblique axes.

What the Patient Experiences during an MR Examination. The MR imaging scanner is composed of a large magnet housed in a dome-shaped machine that is hollow in the center. The patient is placed in a supine position on a sliding table that can be advanced into the hollow section of the magnet. Both eyes are imaged simultaneously with MR imaging, and the typical examination lasts about one hour. MR imaging is a painless procedure, but it may be necessary to position a small nonmagnetic coil on the skin surface around the orbit. This coil provides better detail of the eye and surrounding structures by improving the signal-to-noise ratio. While the examination is in progress it is important for the patient to lie as still as possible. Mirrors are positioned so that the patient can see his head and feet, and an intercom allows him to communicate with the doctor or technologist outside the magnet. After the images are obtained, they are interpreted by a specially trained radiologist. Fig. 4-10 is an example of an MR image in a patient with choroidal malignant melanoma of the left eye.

Nuclear Medicine Imaging. Radioactive isotopes are injected and taken up within the specific tissue being studied. This occurs because the selected chemical substance to which the isotope has been attached is involved in the physiologic metabolism of that organ. It should remain there long enough to be imaged. An image is obtained because the radioactive isotope emits gamma rays for a brief period of time. The emitted rays are recorded by a gamma camera during the period of gamma emission. A few hours or days later, the isotope stops emitting detectable rays as it returns to its stable state. The return to stability is measured in terms of its half-life, that is, the period until it is seen to be emitting half as much radiation as it did initially. Isotopes chosen for tagging are those that remain in the organ to be studied long enough to produce a usable image but with relatively short half-lives so as to minimize radiation to the patient's tissues.

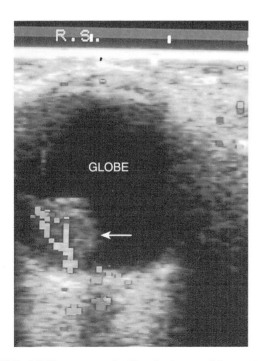

FIG. 4-9 Transverse color Doppler image of the eye in a patient with choroidal malignant melanoma *(arrow)*. Blood flow is detected from vessels in the tumor.

Industrial Uses

The industrial uses of x-rays are many and important. Flaws, cracks, and fissures in heavy steel can

FIG. 4-10 Axial magnetic resonance image of a patient with choroidal melanoma of the left eye *(arrows)*. MR imaging allows simultaneous evaluation of both orbits.

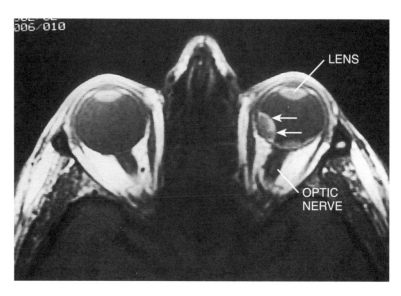

LENS

OPTIC NERVE

be shown by x-raying large building structures. Large-application industrial x-rays need equipment that is specialized to penetrate the density of buildings and similar structures. These are referred to as "hard x-rays." A clinical example of hard penetrating x-rays are those used in radiation therapy to kill malignant cells in cancer treatment. On the contrary, thin or delicate structures have special requirements to get an adequate scan also. For example, a radiograph of tissue sections of bone that measure 1 or 2 μ in thickness (microradiography) uses soft x-rays. These are very specific applications of x-rays. The typical x-rays used on a daily basis in a hospital setting fall somewhere between these two extremes.

CLINICAL PROCEDURES

How to Interpret

Certain variables and terms need to be understood by the clinician to be conversant within the various forms of radiologic imaging of the patient. These include form, composite shadowgram, and density. Consider how form contributes to the detail of a radiograph. A sheet of any uniform composition, if it lies flat and parallel to the film, has a uniform x-ray density and casts a homogeneous shadow. If it is curved, those parts that lie perpen-

dicular to the plane of the film radiograph as though they were more dense. X-rays pass through complex objects such as the human organs and render a "composite shadowgram." This does not render a picture at all but a composition. The densities must be interpreted from the shadows projected on the film plane. If we radiograph a flower, specifically a rose, consider how density can affect the picture. A rose petal that lies perpendicular to the plane or the ray is equivalent to many thicknesses of petals laid upon one another. Therefore it is logical that it appears much more dense than a single sheet lying flat. Next consider the stem of the rose, which is a tubular structure of uniform composition. The margins are relatively dense because they represent long curved planes radiographed tangentially and the center area between them appears darker and more radiolucent.

The next area of consideration is the density of objects or relative radiodensities of various substances and tissues. This is a reference similar to a gray scale, with the least dense being black or completely allowing all x-rays to pass through. The most dense substances, such as metals, absorb all rays and show completely white appearance on the x-rays. Consider a cube of various substances of various densities such as steel, bone, muscle, vein, liver, adipose or fat tissue, water, and air

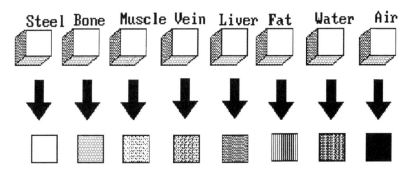

FIG. 4-11 Gray scale in order of densities of eight substances. At one end of the range are very dense substances such as steel and bone. These absorb most of the x-rays and the film is white. The less dense substances at the other extreme, such as air, absorb none of the x-rays and the exposure is black. Human organs fall in between.

(Fig. 4-11). Arranging these in order of radiodensity would be easy if they were all elements on the chemistry periodic chart. We could look them up by atomic number, and the list would be easy to generate. Intuitively we know that steel would have to be listed as the most dense. Air would be listed as the least dense.

Fig. 4-11 shows a density chart. Notice that it is difficult to categorize muscle, vein, and liver, because the gray scales for these three are almost the same. Human organs are not homogeneous and may be fluid-filled tissues with various densities. Because human tissue is not homogeneous with respect to thickness and form, viewing fluid-filled organs with or without pathology with regard to radiodensity is the basis for medical radiology.

X-ray films reveal a three-dimensional object or organ. This represents added densities of many layers of tissues. The most striking contrasts in radiodensity exist in the region of the chest. Air-filled lungs (radiolucent) on both sides, a radiopaque muscular chest, and a muscular fluid-filled heart occupy the inside of a bony rib cage. In studying Fig. 4-12, it is best to think three-dimensionally about such chest films by imagining the structures through which the x-ray beam passed from back to front—skin of the back, subcutaneous fat, a large amount of muscle encasing the flat blades of the scapulae, vertebral column, and posterior shell of the rib cage, then the vertebral column and the posterior shell of the rib cage, then the lungs and the heart and other mediastinal structures, the sternum and anterior shell of ribs,

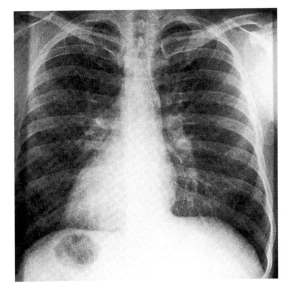

FIG. 4-12 PA view of the chest.

the pectoral muscles and subcutaneous fat, significant amounts of breast tissue in certain members of the species, and finally skin again.

Viewing Conventions

One of the conventions in handling and viewing films is how to put them up to the light box. This is the convention of viewing done by radiologists. Because films are transparent, one can look through them from either side. The film should be placed on the box as if one is looking face to face at the patient. Radiographs are usually marked right and left by the technician to indicate which is the patient's right side. In the chest films one can usually be somewhat independent of the marker because the left ventricle and the arch of the aorta cast more prominent shadows on the left side of the patient's spine.

Understanding Orientations of Scans: Posteroanterior, Anteroposterior, Lateral

Most chest films are made with the beam passing in a sagittal direction in a posteroanterior, or PA,

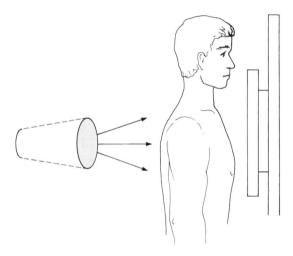

FIG. 4-13 Schematic of posteroanterior (PA) chest, showing the physical set-up with the x-ray tube behind the patient and the film plate in front of the patient.

view. This means that the x-ray tube is behind and the film is in front of the patient. This is the standard chest film taken today. It is customary to make a PA chest film of any patient who is able to stand and be positioned (Figs. 4-13 and 4-14).

Less satisfactory but often valuable AP films are made of the chest when the patient is too sick to leave his bed. The patient is propped up in bed and the film is placed behind him. The exposure is made with a portable x-ray machine at the foot of the bed. Thus the rays pass through the patient anteroposteriorly (Figs. 4-15 and 4-16).

After the standard PA film, the lateral view of the chest is the next most common. It is marked with an R or L according to whether the right or the left side of the patient was against the film. Most often a left lateral film is made because the heart is closer to the film and less magnified. Note in Fig. 4-17 how the ribs are parallel. Some pairs of ribs are superimposed by the beam, forming a single denser white shadow. Note how far the vertebral column projects into the chest. Large segments of lung extend farther back in the lateral view.

The chest film seen in Fig. 4-18 offers a test in three-dimensional thinking. It has an obvious artifact, or radiodensity. The shape of the metal suggests that it might be a bullet. The patient's his-

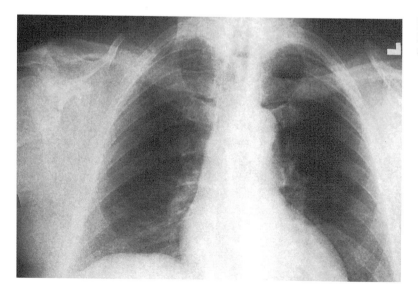

FIG. 4-14 PA chest radiograph. Note the clarity of the clavicles and the anterior ribs.

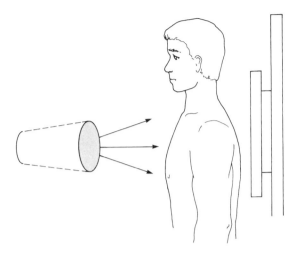

FIG. 4-15 Schematic of the anteroposterior (AP) chest radiograph showing the physical set-up with the x-ray tube in front of the patient and the film behind the patient.

tory indicated that he was a Vietnam war soldier who had been injured. After the surgeons viewed this film, they ordered a lateral film (Fig. 4-19) to determine the location of the bullet. If the bullet is located in the spinal cord or the trachea or in one of the major vascular structures at this level, surgical removal becomes more complicated. Actually the bullet was located harmlessly in the mediastinum and had caused no major injury to any vital structure. It was removed without incident.

One can never know precisely where a foreign body is located from a single radiograph. A film at right angles to the first study must be ordered. Foreign bodies of the extremities in the soft tissues are localized very accurately by a refinement of this procedure. Always ask for a right lateral chest film if the lesion is suspected to be on the right, so that the structure to be studied is as close as possible to the film.

Posteroanterior oblique views of the chest are sometimes used in studying the heart and hila of

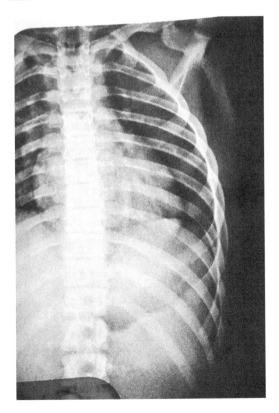

FIG. 4-16 AP chest radiograph. Note that the spinal column actually restricts the normal view of the chest. The AP view is usually used when the patient is not ambulatory and the portable x-ray machine is needed for the bedside.

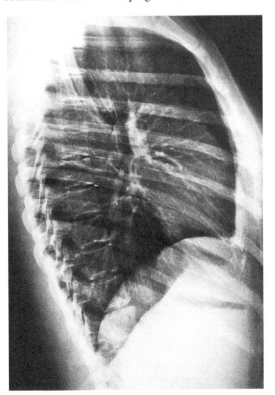

FIG. 4-17 Lateral view of the chest.

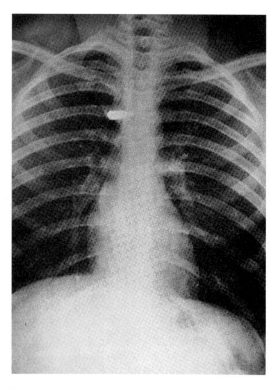

FIG. 4-18 PA view of a metallic foreign body in the chest.

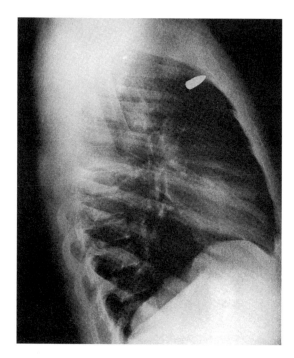

FIG. 4-19 Lateral view of the chest, cross-section showing the anterior level of the chest with the metallic foreign body.

the lungs. Another detailed study of the ribs is obtained by obliques made anteroposteriorly. Others designed for visualizing a particular structure in a particular way also offer anatomic information not otherwise available. Sometimes these views or procedures are carried out at the discretion of the radiologist. Many times the physician specifies the tentative diagnosis and wants the best study to rule out a particular disease.

Advantages of Plain Films versus Tomograms

The two films in Fig. 4-20 were made of the same patient. The left is a standard PA view of the chest. The right is a special-procedure film called a tomogram of the chest. A tomogram is helpful to get a clear view of a specific area under study. To understand how a tomogram works, imagine a cadaver cut in coronal slices, about 1 inch thick. A radiograph is made of each slice. Each film has

on it the shadows cast by the densities of the structures of that slice. There are no confusing superimpositions of the shadows of structures from other slices above or below to confuse the diagnosis.

Therefore, only the structures in the plane of the pivot point are recognizable. The shadows representing organs in front of or behind it are distorted so that shape and form are no longer recognizable. The blurred images of the unwanted structures are easy to ignore. Tomography is very helpful whenever detail is needed of a structure in the line of the x-ray beam.

Viewing Conventions

It is conventional to view the CT scan as though one were looking up at it from the patient's feet. It is important to hold the CT scan so that the patient's left side is presented as if the patient is facing the examiner (Fig. 4-21). Permanent images

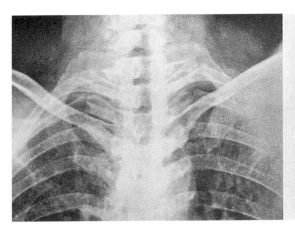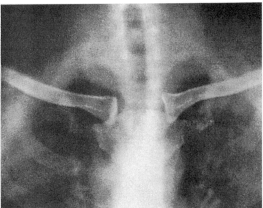

FIG. 4-20 PA upper chest on the right and the same area of the chest with a tomogram on the left. Note the clarity of the clavicles on the tomogram. All other areas are purposely blurred out.

are produced by photographing the monitor screen. The CT scan slices in sequence so that one slice can be linked to another. The slices above and below give additional information about a structure or an organ.

The usual CT series of scans consists of contiguous 10-mm-thick slices through the region requested, but slices as thin as 1.5 mm can be obtained when finer detail is needed for diagnosis. In ordering orbital scans, the slices are normally 2-mm-thick cuts through the tissue in question. The x-ray dose per slice varies from 1 to 4 rad (but only to the slice being imaged) and is comparable to the exposure for conventional radiographic studies of the area. (Rads are units of radiation.)

High-density materials such as barium or metal (hip prosthesis or metal surgical clips) may produce artifacts that look like bright stars with sharply defined geometric radiating white lines that degrade the image obtained and cause interference locally on the film. Motion also degrades the image. The movement of abdominal organs during respiration (about 1 to 2 cm) is enough to distort the images of smaller structures.

CT scanners require only 1 to 10 seconds to complete a slice, and a patient who cannot hold his breath may have motion artifacts on his scan. Most patients can hold their breath for 5 seconds repeatedly. However, unconscious, very ill, or

dyspneic patients and small children requiring CT studies may produce motion degrading of the image. Mild sedation and reassurance by the referring physician as well as by the radiologist may help.

The patient should be forewarned that the gantry or housing for the equipment is huge and may be frightening. Body CT scans can be produced with the patient supine or prone or lying on his side. Other planes or imaging, especially of the head and extremities, are possible.

Contrast Enhancements

Depending on the clinical condition under investigation, contrast media may be used during CT scanning to enhance the difference in density of various structures. The view that can be illuminated by giving the patient dilute contrast material helps distinguish stomach and bowel from other soft-tissue structures and masses. Intravenous administration of water-soluble contrast material produces a temporary increase in the density of vascular structures and highly vascularized organs. This is referred to as enhancement and is extremely useful. For example, a great vessel and the tumor mass encasing and constricting it appear as one homogeneously dense mass unless the vessel is enhanced with contrast material.

A significant number of patients are sensitive to

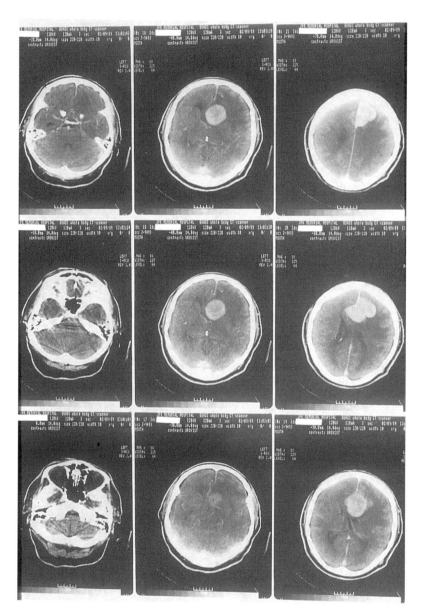

FIG. 4-21 CT scan of large tumor located in the cerebellum.

the contrast dye; therefore, its use needs extreme care by the radiologist.

Diagnostic Testing

Orbital Scanning. A scan can be ordered through the local hospital radiology department. A few steps are necessary. On a blank prescription pad or radiology form available from the local hospital radiology department, place the patient's name, age, and diagnosis clearly. A tentative diagnosis is adequate, and the type of scan desired should be indicated. If there are any questions, the radiologist will call you. Expect a call with any stat (or emergent) results so as to speed treatment. A routine interpretation and report follows in the mail in a few days.

The set-up for the CT scan of the orbits involves Reid's anatomic line. This runs from the rim of the orbit to the external auditory meatus. It is sometimes drawn on the face to help line the patient up in the ganty or opening of the CT scanner.

Orbital scans are done with level four or level five scans (Figs. 4-22 and 4-23). Level four cuts or slices are 10 mm apart and overlap, and level five cuts or slices are 8 mm apart and do not overlap. A level four or five scan with contrast takes about 20 minutes.

A radiologic work-up for a patient with orbital disease or ocular disease involves certain scans or plane films (Fig. 4-24). These include *Caldwell's view, Waters' view, lateral view, optic canals view,* and *basilar view*.

Caldwell's view is a coronal section. It allows one to view both orbits, the sphenoid wings and ridge, and part of the orbital floor (Figs. 4-25 and 4-26).

Waters' view is a transverse section (Fig. 4-27),

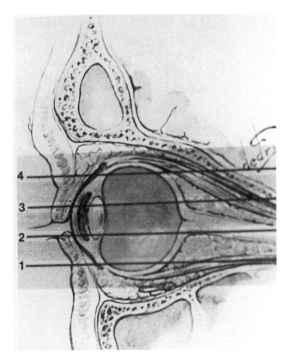

FIG. 4-22 Level four CT of orbits. This schematic shows approximately where the cuts are made. These do not overlap.

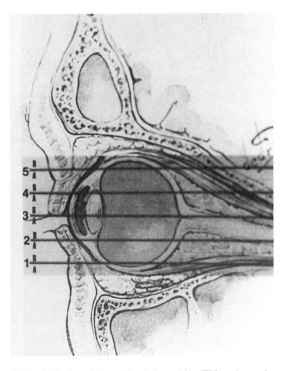

FIG. 4-23 Level five CT of the orbits. This schematic shows approximately where the cuts are made. These are overlapping.

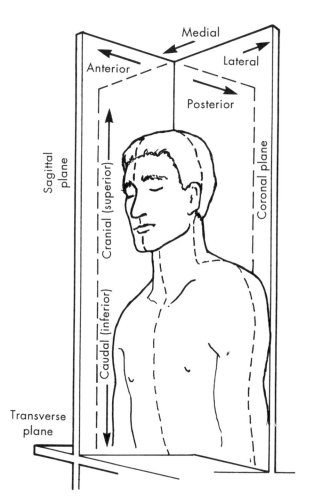

FIG. 4-24 Planes of the body.

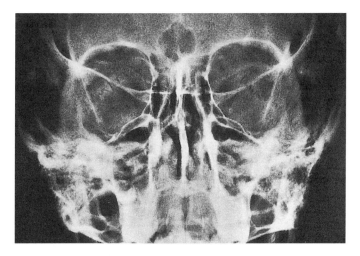

FIG. 4-25 Caldwell's view.

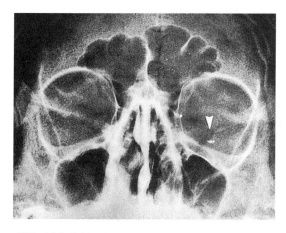

FIG. 4-26 Caldwell's view with a metallic foreign body in the orbit easily visualized.

which allows a view of the paranasal sinuses and floor and roof of the orbits and the maxillary antrum. This scan is used frequently by otolaryngologists and allergists. The ophthalmic application is limited to cases of suspected orbital floor fractures in trauma.

The lateral view is a cross-sectional view of the others from the side (Fig. 4-28). This should enhance subtle pathologic changes so as to indicate the depth of level of the lesion. The principle to remember in the use of this view is the same prin-

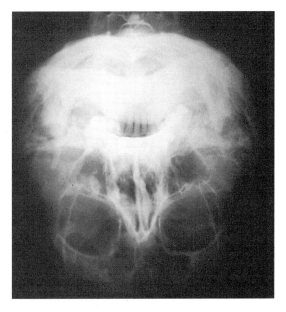

FIG. 4-27 Waters' view, a transverse scan. This allows for viewing of the paranasal sinuses and the roof and floor of the orbits.

ciple for measuring depth of a lesion in the cornea. For example, a corneal foreign body is located with direct illumination by slit-lamp examination. Then an optic section is used to determine how deep the foreign body has penetrated. Note that the arrow in Fig. 4-29 shows that the metallic

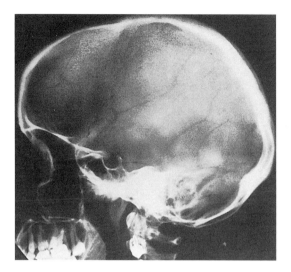

FIG. 4-28 Lateral view.

tip of the pencil embedded in the orbit is easy to identify. However, the wooden portion of the pencil does not show up very well on radiography.

Specialized scans are available to enlarge areas of particular interest. For example, the sella turcica is of particular interest in neurologic disease. Fig. 4-30 shows an enlargement used to view specific disease entities such as the empty sella syndrome and pituitary disease.

Scans of the optic canals are another view by which an enlargement of a very specific area within the orbit can be examined. Fig. 4-31 is an example of an optic canal scan.

The basilar view is a transverse scan. This allows the posterior wall of the orbit to be seen. The maxillary sinus and optic canals are also visualized in this scan (Fig. 4-32).

Arteriography

Arteriography is used to selectively show the vascular tree within an organ. The radiopaque dye is injected into the artery, and subsequent arteries are viewed based on the study in question. This is particularly helpful in malignancies because they are usually highly vascular in nature. It is also helpful in diagnosing aneurysms. It does, however, have a higher morbidity rate than CT. Therefore, it is done with caution and only when necessary, not

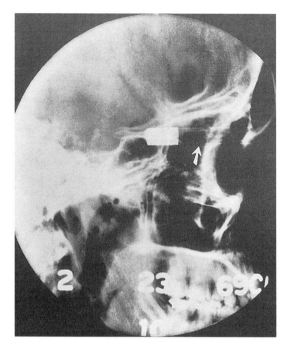

FIG. 4-29 Lateral view with pencil embedded in the orbit. Note the metallic cap of the pencil, which is easily identified as a foreign body on the radiograph. However, the wooden portion at the arrow is not easily seen.

as a routine test. Fig. 4-33 shows the vascular tree on lateral view. A large aneurysm of the internal carotid artery becomes visible with this scan.

Isotope Scans

Technetium has proved to be the most useful radioactive tracer, and it is linked to various physiologic substances that seek different organs. It is deposited temporarily in bone and is called a bone-seeker. The image obtained shows areas of more or less intensity of radiation related to the portion of the bone having increased turnover. Thus, "hot spots" showing markedly increased activity of bone are seen as dense black areas on a gamma camera or rectilinear scan of the whole skeleton (Figs. 4-34 and 4-35).

Unfortunately, this scan is very nonspecific and does not tell us the cause of the increased bone turnover. If they are located in symmetric joint areas, for example, they may be caused by acute in-

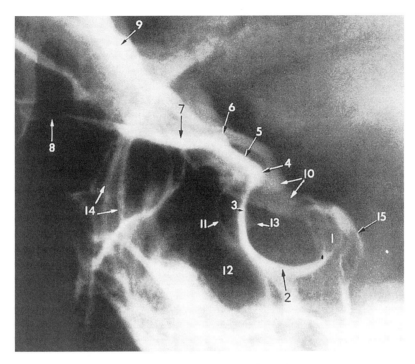

FIG. 4-30 Lateral view of the sella turcica, showing sella and anterior clinoids.

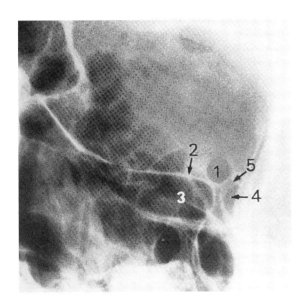

FIG. 4-31 Optic canals. A magnified specific scan can detail the foramen in the skull.

flammation secondary to arthritis. If they are located eccentrically, they may indicate the location of the bone metastases from the patient's known or suspected cancer. Therefore, this scan is not definitive but can be helpful with physical findings to aid in diagnosis.

Technetium may also be linked to a sulfur colloid that is normally picked up by the liver and remains there long enough to be imaged as a densely homogeneous, liver-shaped area of activity on the isotope scan of the abdomen. With any such radioactive pharmaceutical used, there may be areas on the scan where "cold spots" indicate physiologic uptake. These also are nonspecific in that they indicate only an area of less metabolic turnover. Thus, a large solitary cold spot in an otherwise homogeneously imaged liver might indicate the location of a large tumor metastasis or a benign cyst. An ordinary radiograph of a patient's abdomen might show his liver to be enlarged but would not differentiate the tumor-mass areas from

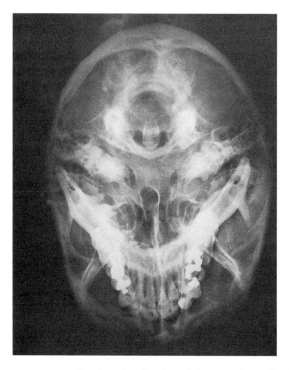

FIG. 4-32 Basilar view, a transverse scan allowing visualization of the posterior wall of the orbit, the maxillary sinus, and the optic canals.

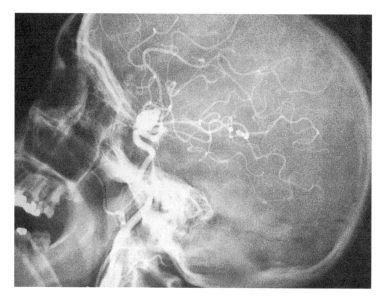

FIG. 4-33 Cerebral angiography. This shows the vascular tree on lateral view. A large internal carotid aneurysm is present.

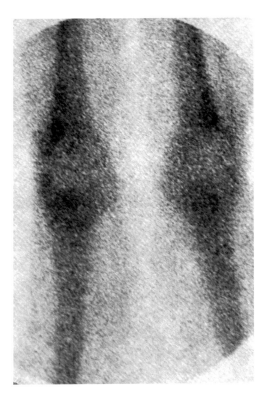

FIG. 4-34 Technetium bone scan. This is a radioactive tracer that can show "hot spots," which are usually indicators of metastases. Normal bone scan.

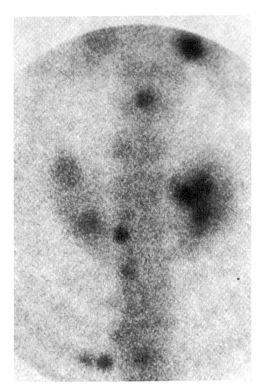

FIG. 4-35 Technetium bone scan. Dark spots on the scan show areas of uptake subsequently diagnosed as metastases.

normal metabolically active liver tissue around them. Isotope scans, like all other radiologic images, must always be interpreted in tandem with clinical information about the patient.

In the usual isotope scan, the image obtained is produced by gamma radiation from the entire thickness of the organ, not from the single slice as in CT, MR imaging, and sonography. Like fluoroscopy, plain radiography consists of continuous or intermittent observation of tissues penetrated by x-rays. This produces dynamic radiographic information. The motion of the fetal heart is routinely monitored by "real-time" sonography and is evidence that a quiet fetus is in fact alive. Dynamic studies using rapidly sequenced CT scans during the intravenous injection of contrast material produce time-lapse information about the vascularity of a liver mass. Similarly, sequential isotope scans

are used to document flow patterns such as blood flow through the heart chambers in a patient suspected of having a congenital heart anomaly.

DIAGNOSTIC IMPLICATIONS

It is important to learn how to enlist the help of a radiologist in planning which procedures ought to be included in the diagnostic work-up plan and the order in which they should be undertaken. CT and MR scans should usually be considered sophisticated and costly studies reserved for special problems. Less expensive procedures like plain films and ultrasonography should be used for routine evaluation. The important exceptions to this principle are traumatized patients and central nervous system emergencies. In head trauma the superior capacity of CT to recognize intracranial hemorrhage and organ rupture can speed diagnosis and often saves lives. CT much more efficiently informs managing clinicians about the order in which treatment procedures should be undertaken.

A suspected diagnosis is required to submit a patient for radiologic evaluation. The radiologist performs whatever testing is needed to rule out the suspected diagnosis. Written confirmation and test results are forwarded to your office.

ACKNOWLEDGMENTS

I would like to thank Dr. Max Cooper and Dr. J. Rajerum, radiologists at JFK Hospital in Philadelphia, PA, for their technical assistance in interpreting the scans; Tammi Anbari, radiologic technologist, for gathering the scans; Dr. Therese Deschenes for her technical drawings; and Dr. Christopher Rinehart for photographic support in copying the selected x-ray films.

BIBLIOGRAPHY

Abramson DH, Ellsworth R, and Kitchin S: Second non-ocular tumors in reinoblastoma survivor. *Ophthalmology* 91:1351, 1984.

Agarwal SK and others: Dose distribution from a Delta 25 head scanner. *Med Phys* 6:302, 1979.

Albert DM, Rubensstein RA, and Scheie HG: Tumor metastases to the eye: I. incidence in 213 adult patients with generalized malignancy. *Am J Ophthalmol* 63:723, 1967.

Alfidi FJ, Macintyre WJ, and Hoagan JR: The effects of biological motion on CT resolution. *AJR* 127:11, 1976.

Alper MG: *Endocrine orbital disease.* In Arger PH, editor: *Orbit roentgenology,* New York, 1977, Wiley.

Ambrose J: Computerized transverse axial scanning (tomography): Part 2. clinical application. *Br J Radiol* 46:1023, 1973.

Appleboom T and Durso F: Retinoblastoma presenting as a total hyphema. *Ann Ophthalmol* 17:508, 1985.

Arger PH: *Tumor and tumor-like conditions.* In Arger PH, editor: *Orbit roentgenology,* New York, 1977, Wiley.

Atlas SW and others: High field surface coil MR of orbital pseudotumor, *AJNR* 1986.

Bacon KT, Duchesnau PM, and Weinstein MA: Demonstration of the superior ophthalmic vein by high resolution computed tomography. *Radiology* 124:129, 1977.

Balchunas WR, Quencer RM, and Byrne SF: Lacrimal gland and fossa masses: evaluation by computed tomography of the orbits. *Neuroradiology* 14:89, 1977.

Bernardino ME and others: Computed tomography in ocular neoplastic disease. *AJR* 131:111, 1978.

Bilaniuk LT and Zimmerman RA: Computer-assisted tomography: sinus lesions with orbital involvement. *Head Neck Surg* 2:293, 1980.

Brant-Zawadski M and Enzmann DR: Orbital computed tomography: calcific densities of the posterior globe. *J Comp Assist Tomogr* 3:503, 1979.

Brismar J and others: Unilateral endocrine exophthalmos. Diagnostic problems in association with computed tomography. *Neuroradiology* 12:24, 1976.

Brooks RA and Dichiro G: Beam hardening in x-ray reconstructive tomography. *Phys Med Biol* 21:390, 1976.

Brooks RA and Dichiro G: Principles of computer assisted tomography (CAT) in radiographic and radioisotopic imaging. *Phys Med Biol* 21:689, 1976.

Brooks RA and Dichiro G: Theory of image reconstruction in computed tomography. *Radiology* 117:561, 1976.

Brown GC, Tasman WS, and Benson WE: BB-gun injuries to the eye. *Ophthal Surg* 16:505, 1985.

Bullock JD, Campbell RJ, and Walker RR: Calcification in retinoblastoma. *Invest Ophthalmol Vis Sci* 16:252, 1987.

Carlson RE and others: Exophthalmos, global luxation, rapid weight gain: differential diagnosis. *Ann Ophthalmol* 14:724, 1982.

Carson PL and others: Imaging soft tissue through bone with ultrasound transmission tomography by reconstruction. *Med Phys* 4:302, 1977.

Cohen BA and others: Steroid exophthalmos. *J Comput Assist Tomogr* 5:907, 1981.

Cohen G and Dibianca FA: The use of contrast-detail-dose evaluation of image quality in a computed tomographic scanner. *J Comput Assist Tomogr* 3:189, 1979.

Crooks LE, Ortendahl D, and Kaufman L: Clinical efficiency of nuclear magnetic resonance imaging. *Radiology* 146:123, 1983.

Davis KR and others: CT and ultrasound in the diagnosis of cavernous hemangioma and lymphangioma of the orbit, *CT: J Comput Tomogr* 4:98, 1980.

Dichiro G and others: The apical artifact: elevated attenuation values toward the apex of the skull. *J Comput Assist Tomogr* 2:65, 1978.

Duncan WJ: Color Doppler in clinical cardiology. Philadelphia, 1988, WB Saunders Co.

Edelstein WA and others: Spin ways NMR imaging and applications to human whole body imaging. *Phys Med Biol* 25:754, 1980.

Enzmann DR, Donaldson SS, and Kriss JP: Appearance of Graves' disease on orbital computed tomography. *J Comput Assist Tomogr* 3:815, 1979.

Erickson SJ and others: Color Doppler flow imaging of the normal and abnormal orbit. *Radiology* 173:511, 1989.

Erickson SJ et al: Stenosis of the internal carotid artery: assessment using color doppler imaging compared with angiography. *AJR* 152:1299, 1989.

Forbes G: Computed tomography of the orbit. *Rona* 20:37, 1982.

Forbes GS, Sheedy PF, and Waller RR: Orbital tumors evaluated by computed tomography. *Radiology* 136:101, 1980.

Groves AS Jr and others: Orbital fracture evaluation by coronal computed tomography. *Am J Ophthalmol* 85:679, 1978.

Guthoff R: *Ultrasound in ophthalmologic diagnosis.* New York, 1991, Thieme Medical Publishers.

Haik BG et al: Computed tomography of the nonrhegmatogenous retinal detachment in the pediatric patient. *Ophthalmology* 92:1133, 1985.

Hammerschlag SB and others: Blow-out fractures of the orbit: a comparison of computed tomography and conventional radiography with anatomical correlation. *Radiology* 143:487, 1982.

Haughton VM and others: Metrizamide optic nerve sheath opacification. *Invest Radiol* 15:343, 1980.

Hedges TR and others: Computed tomographic demonstration of ocular calcification: correlations with clinical and pathologic findings. *Neuroradiology* 23:15, 1982.

Hermon G: Demonstration of beam hardening

correction in computerized tomography of the head. *J Comput Assist Tomogr* 3:373, 1978.

Hesselink JR and others: Evaluation of mucoceles of the paranasal sinuses with CT. *Radiology* 133:143, 1979.

Hesselink JR and others: Radiological evaluation of orbital metastases with emphasis on computed tomography. *Radiology* 137:363, 1980.

Holland GN, Hawkes RC, and Moore WS: Nuclear magnetic resonance (NMR) tomography of the brain: coronal and sagittal sections. *J Comput Assist Tomogr* 4:429, 1980.

Hounsfield N: *Some practical problems in computerized tomography scanning.* In Ter-Pogossian MM and others, editors: *Reconstruction tomography in diagnostic radiology and nuclear medicine,* 1977, University Park Publishers.

Jacobs L, Weisberg LA, and Kinkel WR: *Computerized tomography of the orbit and sella turcica,* New York, 1991, Raven Press.

Johnson DL and others: Trilateral retinoblastoma: Ocular and pineal retinoblastomas. *J Neurosurg* 63:367, 1985.

Joseph PM: *Artefacts in computed tomography,* In *Radiology of the skull and brain: technical aspects of computed tomography,* vol 5, St. Louis, 1981, The CV Mosby Co.

Kak AC: Computerized tomography with x-ray emission and ultrasound sources. *Proc IEEE* 67:1245, 1979.

Krohel GB, Krauss HR, and Winnick J: Orbital abscess: presentation, diagnosis, therapy and sequelae. *Ophthalmology* 85:492, 1982.

Latchaw RE, Payne JT, and Gold LHA: Effective atomic number and electron density as measured with a computed tomography scanner: computation and correlation with brain tumor histology. *J Comput Assist Tomogr* 2:199, 1978.

Levi C and others: The unreliability of CT numbers as absolute values. *Am J Radiol* 139:443, 1982.

Lieb WE and others: Color Doppler imaging of the eye and orbit: technique and normal vascular anatomy. *Arch Ophthalmol* 109:527, 1991.

Lieb WE and others: Color Doppler imaging of the eye and orbit [abstract #4204]. Presented at the 6th World Congress in Ultrasound, Copenhagen, Denmark, September 1991.

Lieb WE and others: Color Doppler imaging in the demonstration of an orbital varix. *Br J Ophthalmol* 74:305, 1990.

Lieb WE and others: Color Doppler imaging in the management of intraocular tumors. *Ophthalmology* 97:1660, 1990.

Littleton JT and others: *Tomography: physical principles and clinical application.* In Robbins LL, editor: *Golden's diagnostic radiology*, sec 17. Baltimore, 1976, Williams & Wilkins.

Macree JA: Diagnosis and management of a wooden orbital foreign body: case report. *Br J Ophthalmol* 63:848, 1979.

Mafee MR, Peyman GA, and McKusick MA: Malignant uveal melanoma and similar lesions studied by computed tomography. *Radiology* 156Z;403, 1985.

Mancuso AA, Hanafee WN, and Ward P: Extensions of paranasal sinus tumors and inflammatory disease as evaluated by CT and pluridirectional tomography. *Neuroradiology* 16:449, 1978.

McCullough EC and others: On evaluation of the quantitative and radiation features of a scanning x-ray transverse axial tomograph: the EMI scanner. *Radiology* 111:709, 1974.

Meredith WJ and Massey JB: *The effect of x-ray absorption of the radiographic image.* In *Fundamental physics of radiology*, ed 2. Baltimore, 1972, Williams & Wilkins.

Merritt CR: Doppler color flow imaging. *J Clin Ultrasonography* 15:591, 1987.

Michael AS and others: Dynamic computed tomography of the head and neck: differential diagnostic value. *Radiology* 154:413, 1985.

Mitchell DG and others: Neonatal brain: color Doppler imaging part I—technique and vascular anatomy. *Radiology* 167:303, 1988.

Moore AT, Buncic JR, and Munro IR: Fibrous dysplasia of the orbit in childhood: clinical features and management. *Ophthalmology* 92:12, 1985.

Moore WS, Holland GN, and Kneel L: The NMR CAT scanner—a new look at the brain. *CT: J Comput Tomogr* 4:1, 1980.

Newton TH and Potts DG: *Radiology of the skull and brain, vol 5: Technical aspects of computed tomography*, St. Louis, 1981, The CV Mosby Co.

Nugent RA and others: Acute orbital pseudotumors: classification and CT features. *AJR* 137:957, 1981.

Osborn AG, Johnson L, and Roberts TS: Sphenoidal mucoceles with intracranial extension. *J Comput Assist Tomogr* 3:335, 1979.

Partain CL and others: Nuclear magnetic resonance and computed tomography. *Radiology* 136:767, 1980.

Peyster RG and others: Choroidal melanoma: comparison of CT fundoscopy and US. *Radiology* 156:675, 1985.

Peyster RG and others: Exophthalmos caused by excessive fat: CT volumetric analysis and differential diagnosis. *AJNR* 7:35, 1986.

Peyster RG and others: High-resolution CT of lesions of the optic nerve. *AJNR* 4:169, 1983.

Phelps ME, Hoffman EJ, and Ter-Pogossian MM: Attenuation coefficients of various body tissues, fluids and lesions at photon energies 18 to 136 Kev. *Radiology* 117:573, 1975.

Pickett IL: Instrumentation for nuclear magnetic resonance imaging. *Semin Nucl Med* 13:319, 1983.

Polak JF and others: Determination of the extent of lower extremity peripheral arterial disease with color-assisted duplex sonography: comparison with angiography. *AJR* 155:1085, 1990.

Powis RL: Color flow imaging: understanding its science and technology. *J Diagn Med Sonogr* 4:234, 1988.

Ramirez H, Blatt ES, and Hibri NS: Computed tomographic identification of calcified optic nerve drusen. *Radiology* 148:137, 1983.

Rothfus WE and others: Optic nerve/sheath enlargement. *Radiology* 150:409, 1984.

Rothfus WE and Curtin HD: Extraocular muscle enlargement: a CT review. *Radiology* 151:677, 1984.

Rutherford RA, Pullan BR, and Isherwood I: Measurement of effective atomic number and electron density using an EMI scanner. *Neuroradiology* 11:15, 1976.

Salvolini U and others: Computed tomography of the optic nerve. I. normal results. *J Comput Assist Tomogr* 2:141, 1978.

Sevel D and others: Value of computed tomography for the diagnosis of a ruptured eye. *J Comput Assist Tomogr* 7:870, 1983.

Sherman JL, McClean IW, and Braillier DR: Coat's disease: CT-pathologic correlation in two cases. *Radiology* 146:77, 1983.

Shields JA: Current approaches to the diagnosis and management of choroidal melanomas. *Surv Ophthalmol* 21:443, 1977.

Shrivastava PM, Lynn SL, and Ting JY: Exposures to patient and personnel in computed axial tomography. *Radiology* 125:411, 1977.

Simmons JD, LaMasters D, Char D: Computed tomography of ocular colobomas. *AJR* 141:1223, 1983.

Soloway HB: Radiation-induced neoplasms following curvative therapy for retinoblastoma. *Cancer* 12:1984, 1966.

Som PM: CT of the paranasal sinuses. *Neuroradiology* 27:189, 1985.

Som PM and others: Extracranial tumor vascularity: determination by dynamic CT scanning. *Radiology* 154:401, 1985.

Sorenson JA: Technique for evaluating radiation beam and image slice parameters of CT scanners. *Med Phys* 6:68, 1979.

Starr H and Zimmerman L: Extrascleral extension and orbital recurrence of malignant melanomas of the choroid and ciliary body. *Int Ophthalmol Clin* 2:369, 1962.

Switzer DF and Nanda NC. Doppler color flow mapping. *Ultrasound Med Biol* 11:403, 1985.

Towbin R and others: Post-septal cellulitis: CT in diagnosis and management. *Radiology* 158:735, 1986.

Trokel SL and Hilal SK: *CT scanning in orbital diagnosis.* In Thompson HS, editor: *Topics in neuro-ophthalmology.* Baltimore, 1979, Williams & Wilkins.

Turner RM and others: CT of drusen bodies and other calcific lesions of the optic nerve: case report and differential diagnosis. *AJNR* 4:175, 1983.

Unger J: Orbital apex fractures: The contribution of computed tomography. *Radiology* 150:713, 1984.

Unsold R, Degroot J, and Newton TH: Images of the optic nerve: anatomic CT correlation. *AJR* 135:767, 1980.

Unsold R, Newton TH, and Hoyt WF: Technical note—CT examination of the optic nerve. *J Comput Assist Tomogr* 4:560, 1980.

Wall BF and Green DAC: Radiation dose to patients from EMI brain and body scanners. *Br J Radiol* 52:189, 1979.

Weber AL and others: Malignant tumors of the sinuses. *Neuroradiology* 16:443, 1978.

Weisman RA and others: Computed tomography in penetrating wounds of the orbit with retained foreign bodies. *Arch Otolaryngol* 109:265, 1983.

Wells PNT: *Basic principles and Doppler physics.* In Taylor KJ, Burns PN, and Wells PNT: *Clinical applications of Doppler ultrasound.* New York, 1988, Raven Press.

Zimmerman RA and Bilaniuk LT: CT of orbital infection and its cerebral complications. *Am J Roetgenol Radium Ther Nucl Med* 134:45, 1980.

Zimmerman RA, Bilaniuk LT, and Littman PL: Computed tomography of pediatric craniofacial sarcoma. *CT: J Comput Tomogr* 2:113, 1978.

Zimmerman RA and Vignaud J: *Ophthalmic arteriography.* In Arger PH, editor. *Orbit roentgenology,* New York, 1977, Wiley.

PART II

Clinical Medicine in Optometric Practice

5

Ocular Allergy and Immunology

ALLAN LUSKIN

KEY TERMS

Allergy	*Immunoglobulins*	*Eosinophil*
Hypersensitivity	*B Lymphocyte*	*Prostaglandins*
Antigen	*Mast Cell*	*Cytotoxic Reactions*
Antibody	*Anaphylaxis*	*Immune Complex Reactions*
Plasma Cell	*Histamine*	*Cell-Mediated Reactions*

A llergic diseases of the eye affect a large segment of the population. Some of these dis-eases are common; others are rare. Like allergic diseases elsewhere, they are characterized by chronicity, inflammation, and recurrences. The most common are chronic, generally lasting more than six weeks and most much longer. There may be evidence of inflammation with redness, swelling, and discomfort. These diseases recur, waxing and waning over days, months, or years without therapy. Other common disorders mimic allergic eye diseases.

The normal and helpful protection offered by the host's defense mechanisms against infective agents is known as immunity. *Allergy* and *hypersensitivity* represent the possibly harmful results that occur when a host's immune reaction is exaggerated.

The immune system reacts to a foreign substance, or *antigen,* by producing antibodies or by activating T lymphocytes. The *antibody* is a protein produced by a special cell known as a *plasma cell.* Antibodies are *immunoglobulins,* five protein molecules designated IgA, IgD, IgE, IgG, and IgM. These immunoglobulins react with the antigen responsible for their formation in one of several ways. The antibody may neutralize a toxin or destroy a cell by lysis. T lymphocytes mediate a slower cell-mediated reaction which can also lyse cells and produce protective immune inflammation. However, harmful effects can occur by causing an allergic or hypersensitivity reaction.

The overall design of the immunoglobulin incorporates antigen-binding amino acid molecules that are specific to the offending agent. When an antigen, such as part of a virus, attaches to an immunoglobulin on the cell wall of a special lymphocyte (known as a *B lymphocyte*), the cell is stimulated to differentiate into a plasma cell. The plasma cell then produces antibodies that have a specific molecular structure, allowing them to react with the viral antigen to form an immune complex. This complex leads to the inflammatory response seen clinically.

One of the immunoglobulins, IgE, is intimately associated with atopic allergic disease. This allergy includes hay fever, asthma, and eczema. IgE has the capacity to attach to and sensitize cells that contain bioactive chemical mediators. The presence of a specific antigen binding to an IgE antibody on the cell wall causes the *mast cell* to degranulate and release mediators, which initiate the allergic response.

Four of the most common diseases involving the eye appear to require IgE as part of their pathophysiology. These are allergic (hay fever) conjunctivitis, vernal keratoconjunctivitis, giant papillary keratoconjunctivitis, and atopic keratoconjunctivitis. Allergic contact dermatitis, also commonly encountered, represents a classic cell-mediated immune response. A review of how immunologic hypersensitivity reactions can affect the eye and cause disease assists in a better understanding and treatment of ocular allergy.

THE PATHOPHYSIOLOGY OF THE IMMUNE RESPONSE

Type I Ocular Hypersensitivity Reactions

Immunologic hypersensitivity diseases can be mediated by four inflammatory mechanisms (Tables 5-1 and 5-2). Type I reactions occur in ocular

TABLE 5-1 *Ocular Hypersensitivity*

Type I

Ocular anaphylaxis (acute allergic conjunctivitis)

Allergic (hay fever) conjunctivitis

Type I and additional factors
(hyperinflammatory allergic diseases)

Vernal keratoconjunctivitis

Atopic keratoconjunctivitis

Giant papillary conjunctivitis

Type II

Pemphigus vulgaris

Cicatricial pemphigoid

Mooren's ulcer (peripheral corneal melting syndrome)

Type III

Erythema multiforme

Scleritis

Immune rings

Marginal ulceration

Type IV

Contact conjunctivitis

Phlyctenular keratoconjunctivitis

Corneal graft rejection

anaphylaxis and acute allergic conjunctivitis or in allergic (hay fever) conjunctivitis. Anaphylactic reactions are acute reactions that cause wheals and, in its most severe form, systemic shock.

Ocular anaphylaxis can occur as part of a systemic anaphylactic reaction or as isolated anaphylaxis of the eye, initiated by a systemically administered antigen or by topical application, accidentally or as a medicament, onto the eye. The acute IgE-mediated response results in a lid edema and marked dilation of the conjunctival vessels and, to some extent, the deeper episcleral vessels.

The most common immunologic ocular disease, allergic (hay fever) conjunctivitis, is also IgE mediated. In common allergic conjunctivitis, there are minimal mast cell infiltration, small amounts

TABLE 5-2 *Recognition*

Type	Name	System	Mediators	Diseases
I	Immediate	IgE-mast cell	Histamine Arachadonate products	Ocular anaphylaxis Allergic conjunctivitis
Ia	Immediate hyperin-flammatory	IgE-mast cell IgE-lymphocyte	Histamine Arachadonate products Multiple cytokines	Vernal keratoconjunctivitis Atopic keratoconjunctivitis
II	Cytotoxic	IgG/IgM	Complement	Pemphigoid syndromes Mooren's ulcer
III	Immune complex	IgG/IgM	Complement	Immune rings Erythema multiforme
IV	Delayed/cell-mediated	T cells	Lymphokines	Corneal graft rejection

of eosinophil collections, and mild lymphocytic infiltration. The disease resolves without scarring. Antigenic exposure, particularly when sustained, may lead to an IgE-mediated inflammatory reaction and chronic allergic conjunctivitis. In the hyperinflammatory allergic diseases—vernal keratoconjunctivitis, giant papillary conjunctivitis, and atopic keratoconjunctivitis—dramatic inflammatory events occur. The intense inflammation is responsible for the scarring potential of the conjunctival or corneal involvement.

Type I Hyperinflammatory Response

Three clinical illnesses involve Type I hypersensitivity in some major way, but additional factors are also involved. These are "hyperinflammatory allergic diseases." These diseases are vernal keratoconjunctivitis (VKC), giant papillary conjunctivitis (GPC), and atopic keratoconjunctivitis (AKC).

Type I hypersensitivity and atopy are usually part of the pathophysiology of these three diseases. However, marked inflammatory events occur with these syndromes that differentiate them from typical and more easily managed Type I hypersensitivity. For example, the corneal involvement that may accompany the conjunctival diseases differentiates these illnesses clinically from allergic (hay fever) conjunctivitis.

These three hyperinflammatory allergic reactions can be differentiated based on their present-

TABLE 5-3 *Cell Distribution: Normal Conjunctiva*

Cell Type	Epithelium (Cells/mm^3)	Substantia (Cells/mm^3)
Neutrophil	6,000	2,000
Lymphocyte	14,000	100,000
Plasma cell	0	45,000
Mast cell	0	5,000
Eosinophil	0	0
Basophil	0	0

ing signs. A patient with VKC develops giant papillae, thick ropy discharge, marked mucus production, and marked eosinophilic inflammation. GPC may appear clinically as a milder look-alike to vernal conjunctivitis. AKC presents as lid and ocular eczema.

The Mast Cell. The mast cell plays a central role in both typical Type I ocular allergy and the hyperinflammatory allergic diseases (VKC, GPC, and AKC). Mast cells are plentiful—50 million in each eye. More than 90% of them are localized to the lids and conjunctivae, about 5000 per cubic millimeter, mostly in the substantia propria of the upper and lower conjunctiva. There are very few in the normal conjunctival epithelium (Table 5-3).

In Type I reactions, the allergen dissolves in the tear film and brings preformed IgE onto the conjunctival mast cell, resulting in chemical mediator release. These mediators include *histamine, eosinophil,* and neutrophil chemotactic factors, and lipid mediators such as leukotrienes, *prostaglandins,* and platelet-activating factor (PAF). They are derived from activation of the mast cell membrane. These mediators are responsible for both the acute immediate symptoms of the early-phase hypersensitivity reaction as well as much of the inflammatory events that follow during the late-phase reaction. For example, histamine is the primary mediator responsible for the redness and itching of the early-phase allergic reaction.

IgE-Mediated Reactions—Early and Late Phase. The antigen-IgE complex on mast cells triggers histamine release and prostaglandin and leukotriene production, resulting in acute inflammation. There is recruitment of eosinophils, lymphocytes, basophils, and macrophages by mast cell-derived chemotactic factors (chemical mediators of inflammation). These cells then release cytokines and vasoactive mediators, including PAF, which reinforce the early-phase reaction as well as causing a late-phase inflammatory cell infiltrative reaction.

Ongoing chronic disease in the eye seems to consist of an early-phase reaction characterized by acute symptoms and a late-phase reaction characterized by inflammation (Fig. 5-1).

Early-Phase Pathophysiology. Antigen-challenged eyes in pollen-sensitive subjects reveal an inflammatory response characterized by predominantly neutrophilic infiltration at 20 minutes following challenge and a neutrophilic and eosinophilic infiltration at 6 hours. This may be followed by mast cell activation and proliferation, eosinophil proliferation, and increased local IgE production. Continued mediator release, including but not limited to histamine, over hours is a consequence of an IgE-mediated reaction.

Hyperinflammatory Pathophysiology. In the hyperinflammatory allergic IgE diseases a sustained recruitment of eosinophils and lymphocytes occurs. Patients with the most inflammation and those with hyperinflammatory diseases have the most dramatic eosinophilic response.

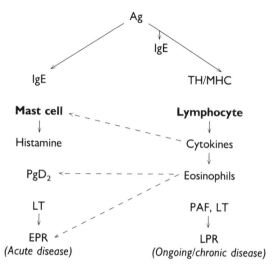

FIG. 5-1 Antigen-challenged eyes produce a biphasic reaction consisting of a mast cell–mediated acute response and a later onset inflammatory response. TH-MHC = T-helper/inducer cell–major histocompatibility complex; PgD_2 = prostaglandin D_2; LT = leukotrienes; PAF = platelet activating factor; EPR = early phase reaction; LPR = late phase reaction.

The factors that result in the sustained and increased inflammation are speculative, but a conjunctival epithelial defect may be involved. The normal eye has only a few mast cells in the conjunctival epithelium, and only a few more occur in patients with allergic conjunctivitis. This implies that antigen must diffuse to the substantia propria in order to cause significant amounts of mediator release. However, one of the characteristics of the hyperinflammatory allergic diseases is mast cell proliferation in the substantia propria and mast cell infiltration of the conjunctival epithelium (Table 5-4). A conjunctival defect would result in much greater mediator release from topically applied antigen. Studies indicate that this is the case. Tear histamine levels are normal or only modestly elevated in patients with hay fever conjunctivitis but markedly increased in those with VKC. The increased tear levels of major basic proteins in patients with VKC reflect the possibility that the eosi-

	Hay Fever	VKC	GPC	AKC
TABLE 5-4 *Hyperinflammatory Pathophysiology*				
Mast cells	+	+ + + +	+ + +	+ +
Eosinophils	+	+ + + +	+ +	+ +
Basophils	—	+ + +	+	+ +
Lymphocytes	+	+ +	—	+ +

VKC = vernal keratoconjunctivitis; GPC = giant papillary conjunctivitis; atopic keratoconjunctivitis
+ = minimal; + + = mild; + + + = moderate; + + + + = marked.

MEDIATORS IN EYE DISEASE

Normal:	Normal tear histamine
Hay fever:	Mildly elevated tear histamine
GPC:	Normal tear histamine
VKC:	Markedly elevated tear histamine
VKC:	Increased major basic protein

nophilic inflammation is most likely due to a conjunctival defect (see box above).

Giant papillary conjunctivitis may also be due to such a primary mucosal alteration. As many as one third of patients exposed to some suture material may develop GPC. The occurrence of GPC in previously asymptomatic persons with conjunctival irritation due to an exposed suture is suggestive of a requirement for some mucosal irritation or alteration. This conjunctival defect seems to initiate and perpetuate the cellular response leading to mast cell involvement.

Type II Hypersensitivity Reactions (the Cytotoxic Reactions)

In *cytotoxic reactions,* IgG and IgM immunoglobulins recognize antigens on the host's own cells or target cells. Antibodies are directed against this target cell and are very specific, but nearby cells may be damaged by the intense inflammation. Cytotoxic immunity is important in mitigating infections by microorganisms and in establishing tumor immunity. But because of its ability to attack antigens on the host's own cells, it plays a significant role in autoimmune disease.

Type II ocular hypersensitivity results in several diseases. These include sympathetic ophthalmia; the pemphigus diseases—pemphigus vulgaris and cicatricial pemphigoid; and Mooren's ulcer.

In patients with Mooren's ulcer, or peripheral corneal melting syndrome, an antibody directed against certain components of the cornea results in complement activation (augmenters of inflammation) and marked inflammatory cell infiltration. This may lead to blindness.

Cicatricial pemphigoid is a nonatopic immunologic inflammation characterized clinically by chronic conjunctivitis. Patients who have ocular cicatricial pemphigoid are generally elderly women. There is a genetic association, and the disease is more common in Jews. Patients often, but not always, have other mucous membrane disease and may have vaginal and oral symptoms as well as ocular disease.

Ocular involvement may, however, occur alone or prior to other mucosal manifestations. The ocular disease presents as a chronic relatively unremitting disease of the conjunctiva. The conjunctivitis is characterized by bulla formation. A skin, conjunctival, or mucous membrane biopsy reveals autoantibodies against the epithelial basement membrane that characterize pemphigus and ocular cicatricial pemphigoid.

Type III Hypersensitivity Reactions (Immune Complex Reactions)

Immune complex reactions occur after antibody-antigen complexes are deposited in the tissue. This immune complex causes subsequent inflammatory cell responses. Significant human diseases associated with immune complex disorders include serum sickness, vasculitis, and autoimmune diseases such as systemic lupus erythematosus and rheumatoid arthritis.

Type III hypersensitivity may result in disease in patients with adverse drug reactions of the erythema multiforme variety, particularly in its bullous form, and may result in scarring conjunctival disease. Sulfonamides and beta-lactam antibiotics are the most commonly implicated agents. As a rule, a patient with severe erythema multiforme should have an ocular evaluation at the time of diagnosis and then follow-up as needed. The ocular complications associated with the bullous form of erythema multiforme (Stevens-Johnson syndrome) can be severe.

Scleritis is seen with a variety of Type III diseases, particularly some collagen vascular diseases. Immune rings and marginal ulcerations are occasionally seen.

Type IV Hypersensitivity Reactions (Cell-mediated or Delayed Hypersensitivity)

Cell-mediated reactions depend on special sensitized lymphocytes (T lymphocytes) and not on antibody production. The term *delayed hypersensitivity* resulted from the observation that there is a delay of hours to days from the moment of antigenic challenge to observable reaction. In contrast, in antibody-mediated reactions the response by the host immune system is immediate and lasts only hours. Not all antigens produce a cell-mediated immune response.

Type IV hypersensitivity ocular diseases include

SYMPTOMS OF ALLERGIC CONJUNCTIVITIS

Early	Late
Itching	Foreign body sensation
	Lid swelling
Burning	Eye awareness
	Eye soreness
Redness	Cold feeling

---

contact conjunctivitis, corneal graft rejection, and phlyctenular keratoconjunctivitis. A phlyctenule is a whitish, heaped-up inflammatory infiltrate. In the past it was associated with a cell-mediated hypersensitivity to tuberculosis. Currently the most common antigen involved is of staphylococcal origin.

CLINICAL PRESENTATIONS OF ALLERGIC OCULAR DISEASES

Hypersensitivity and Hyperinflammatory Conditions (Type I)

The Type I immunologic diseases most commonly encountered are allergic (hay fever) conjunctivitis, atopic keratoconjunctivitis, marginal blepharitis, vernal keratoconjunctivitis, giant papillary conjunctivitis, and allergic contact dermatitis.

Allergic Conjunctivitis. Allergic conjunctivitis is ocular hay fever. The pathogenesis is that of a Type I hypersensitivity disease. Airborne allergens are the antigen. Degranulation of mast cells in the conjunctiva leads to release of pharmacologically active mediators, particularly histamine, causing itching, edema, and redness. Release of other mediators, just as in other atopic diseases, can lead to a late-phase inflammatory reaction and chronic allergic conjunctivitis.

In this disease, the symptoms are almost always greater than the signs (see box below, left). Patients may actually have very little in the way of ocular findings but may complain bitterly about their symptoms. The major symptoms are moderate itching, tearing, burning, and a watery discharge. These represent the early-phase, predominantly histamine-mediated, reaction.

Allergic conjunctivitis involves both an early and a late phase. The itching, burning, and redness tend to be symptoms of an early-phase reaction. A foreign body sensation, lid swelling, eye awareness, eye soreness (not pain), and a cold sensation in the eye represent late-phase inflammation. The history of patients with allergic conjunctivitis may allow the caregiver to divide the symptoms into predominant early-phase or late-phase reaction (see box on p. 89).

In a patient with rather acute early-phase reaction, minimal papillary reaction and mild conjunctival vascular reaction occur. A ciliary flush due to dilation of vessels may be present. Most of the redness is due to dilation of conjunctival vessels, but some dilation of episcleral vessels may occur. Chronic allergic conjunctivitis shows much more papillary reaction, redness, edema, and inflamma-

---

ALLERGIC (HAY FEVER) CONJUNCTIVITIS

Symptoms
    Itching
    Tearing
    Burning
    Watery discharge

Signs
    Occasionally none (symptoms greater than
      signs)
    Conjunctival edema
    Superficial conjunctival vessel dilation
    Minor lid swelling
    Mild papillary reaction

---

tion. The inflammation represents a chronic late-phase reaction. Mild conjunctival and subconjunctival edema (chemosis), often mild to moderate superficial conjunctival vessel dilatation, minor lid swelling, and a moderate papillary reaction all occur. Importantly, the cornea is free of disease. There is little or no photophobia or other symptoms or signs of corneal involvement (Fig. 5-2).

Diagnostically there are few or no eosinophils in conjunctival scrapings and no corneal involvement, and symptoms are often greater than signs. History is of great importance, with seasonal variation being very common with sensitivity to pollens. Indoor allergen sensitization, especially to dust mites or animal danders, may be associated with winter-time worsening in temperate regions. The offending antigen is usually apparent with a careful history. Occasionally allergy tests may be of assistance in guiding therapy in less obvious situations.

It is not common to have isolated hay fever conjunctivitis. Although many patients complain only of nasal or chest symptoms, it is unusual for a patient with hay fever conjunctivitis to have only ocular symptoms. In general, the eye symptoms associated with hay fever conjunctivitis, although

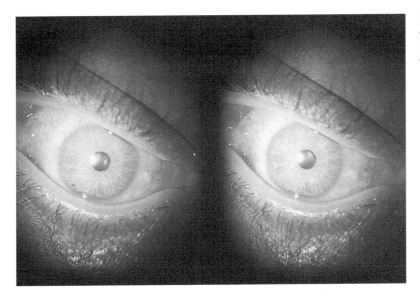

FIG. 5-2 Allergic conjunctivitis: Ocular hay fever—a type I hypersensitivity disease. *(Courtesy of Jane Stein.)*

very bothersome, usually occur in conjunction with nasal symptoms. A patient with only eye symptoms may have a nonatopic disease. Patients with predominant eye symptoms may have a hyperinflammatory allergic disease.

Therapeutically this disease is relatively easily handled with environmental control and simple pharmacologic therapy. Artificial tears are often helpful in eliminating mediators and allergen. Topical vasoconstrictors decrease edema (chemosis), and side effects including rebound are not clinically important when the drugs are used in low dose. Topical antihistamines are effective in reducing pruritus and may be combined with vasoconstrictors. Oral antihistamines are useful. Should these fail, cromolyn sodium may be helpful in preventing mediator release and attenuating both the acute and late-phase allergic response. Topical nonsteroidal antiinflammatory agents may provide significant symptom relief. Topical (ocular) steroids should be avoided, although topical nasal corticosteroids for associated allergic rhinitis often improve ocular symptoms without side effects. Immunotherapy may be of significant value for selective antigens if environmental control and pharmacotherapy fail to provide significant relief.

Atopic Keratoconjunctivitis (AKC). Atopic dermatitis affects 3% of the population. In the adult population, the most common presentation is ocular. The infantile form often "burns out" or leads to a childhood form with involvement of the flexor surfaces. This then often "burns itself out" but sometimes progresses into an adolescent and an adult form, which may present as hand and foot eczema. AKC is atopic dermatitis of the eye (Fig. 5-3).

The pathogenesis of this disease in some way involves a Type I hypersensitivity, but, as with atopic dermatitis elsewhere, a mild defect in cell-mediated hypersensitivity (Type IV) and neutrophil chemotaxis may be found. This disease generally affects postpubertal patients, often middle-aged. The reason for this, in a disease that is otherwise predominantly one of childhood, is unknown.

AKC is characteristically a chronic disease. Patients uncommonly complain of acute symptoms. Rather, they evidence "allergic eyes" with wrinkled, old-looking skin and eczema of the eyelids (Fig. 5-4). It is seen more commonly in men, usually in the third and fourth decades. There is a very strong genetic susceptibility; patients often have a bilateral family history of atopy. A history of previous or current involvement of other areas of the body with atopic dermatitis is almost always found. They usually have other atopic IgE-mediated disorders; no information is as yet available concerning a relationship with IgE-mediated

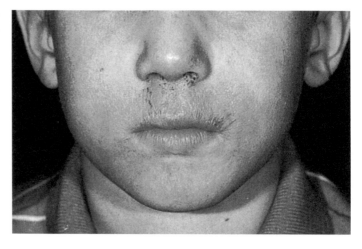

FIG. 5-3 Atopic dermatitis: Perioral involvement is common. The lips are dry and scaly. *(From Habif TB:* Clinical dermatology, *St. Louis, 1990, Mosby–Year Book.)*

reaction to foods or inhalants, as contrasted with the growing evidence of the exacerbating role of food allergy and mite sensitivity in the infantile form of eczema.

Mast-cell and T-cell–mediated inflammation recruits inflammatory cells; the cellular infiltrate is predominantly mast cell, basophil, eosinophil, and lymphocytic. This inflammation leads to chronic lid eczema. The eczema of the eyelids appears as chronic macerated, indurated, thickened lids. Patients have perennial, chronic symptoms. The oc-

ular symptoms include intense itching, burning, tearing—sometimes uncontrollable, and a mucoid discharge. The lid involvement is predominantly lower palpebral rather than upper palpebral (see box below).

Although patients complain about wrinkled, old-looking skin, AKC is not purely a lid disease. Conjunctivitis may be a prominent feature with dilation of both superficial and deep conjunctival vessels. Although ocular hay fever conjunctivitis does not scar the conjunctiva or lids, the inflam-

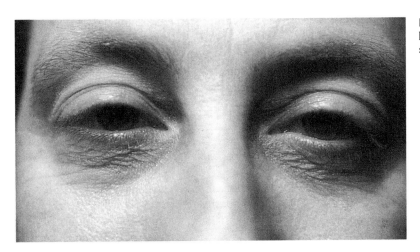

FIG. 5-4 Atopic dermatitis of lids: Note wrinkled, old looking skin in this 40-year-old male.

ATOPIC KERATOCONJUNCTIVITIS (AKC)

Symptoms	*Signs*
Perennial, chronic disorder	Lid eczema
History of other atopic respiratory symptoms	Induration, lichenification, maceration of lid margins
History of presence of atopic dermatitis elsewhere	Conjunctival inflammation/hyperemia may be scarring
Itching and burning	Corneal disease
Watery discharge, often uncontrollable	Atopic dermatitis
Mucoid discharge	Corneal disease
	Pannus
	Ulceration
	Punctate keratitis
	Neovascularization
	Scarring
	Atopic cataracts

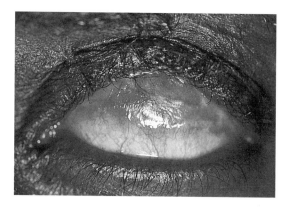

FIG. 5-5 Severe corneal involvement in atopic kerato-conjunctivitis with corneal neovascularization and pannus.

COMPLICATIONS OF ATOPIC KERATOCONJUNCTIVITIS (AKC)

Cataracts (10%-15%)
Retinal detachment
Conjunctival complications
    Keratoconus
    Pannus
    Ulceration
    Punctate keratitis
    Scarring

Infectious complications
    Herpes simplex keratitis
    Staphylococcus
        Infectious conjunctivitis
        Marginal immune ulcers
        Immune rings
        Phlyctenular keratoconjunctivitis

Marginal blepharitis

mation of AKC may cause scarring and subsequent distortion of the lower conjunctiva. The lid eczema, with induration, lichenification, and maceration of the lid margins, may scar while leading to fornical alteration.

Corneal involvement is frequent and should be suspected if photophobia is present. Corneal involvement ranges from mild to severe. Mild involvement is characterized by punctate keratitis without corneal vascularization. The moderate form is characterized by neovascularization growing in from the limbus a distance of 1 to 2 mm. Severe corneal involvement can be characterized by vascularization of the entire cornea and scarring with lipid material deposited in the cornea. Pannus formation and ulceration may occur. In addition, there is a 10% to 15% incidence of atopic cataracts. In this respect AKC is similar to significant atopic dermatitis elsewhere in the body; the development of atopic cataracts occurs by an unknown mechanism (Fig. 5-5).

Complications occur with AKC (see the box above, right). Atopic cataracts, anterior subcapsular cataracts with a "stretched bear rug" appearance, existed prior to the therapeutic use of corticosteroids and are not purely corticosteroid-induced phenomena. On the other hand, there certainly is suggestion that corticosteroids have increased the incidence and severity of this illness. It has an incidence of 10% to 15%. Fortunately,

in most patients, the cataracts do not interfere with vision.

Corneal complications, including keratoconus, pannus formation, ulceration, punctate keratitis, and mild corneal inflammation, scarring, and vision loss, may occur. AKC patients also seem more prone to herpes simplex keratitis. Symptoms that do not clear promptly should be viewed with caution. Corticosteroids may exacerbate herpes simplex keratitis. Other complications of AKC include conjunctival and lid scarring and retinal detachment.

Like atopic dermatitis elsewhere, patients with AKC have complications associated with the staphylococcal organism. Infectious conjunctivitis as well as several problems associated with hypersensitivity to staphylococci may occur. The immunologic complications include marginal immune ulcers, immune rings, and phlyctenular keratoconjunctivitis.

Marginal ulcers are shallow oval ulcerations typically seen at the 4 and 8 o'clock positions 1 mm from the limbus (Fig. 5-6). Dilation of adjacent vessels is seen. The ulcers are fortunately easy to treat, rarely leaving significant vision-impairing

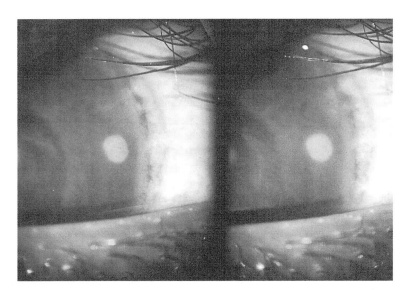

FIG. 5-6 Marginal ulcer due to atopic keratoconjunctivitis. *(Courtesy of Jane Stein.)*

scarring. Mild corticosteroids and attempts to eliminate the organism work well.

Phlyctenular keratitis appears as a whitish heaped-up area. A marked vascular reaction begins peripherally and moves centrally and may be vision-impairing if untreated. Potent steroids are required. The eye is usually acutely painful.

Phlyctenular keratoconjunctivitis is not a staphylococcal infection but rather a vascularized sterile inflammation associated with a cell-mediated hypersensitivity response to an antigen associated with staphylococcal blepharitis (Fig. 5-7). This disease may be seen occasionally in children. Therapy includes eradication of the antigen with antibiotics and suppression of the inflammation with topical corticosteroids.

Therapy of AKC is difficult and requires cooperative efforts to maximize therapy of the allergic inflammatory process and monitor for potential complications. Corneal involvement usually necessitates topical corticosteroids. These should be used in a "pulse" with rapid tapering over a week or so as healing occurs. Maintenance corticosteroids should be avoided if possible. Topical corticosteroid creams on the active lesions of the eyelids may be necessary.

Systemic antihistamines may decrease the itching and may be very helpful in decreasing the itch-

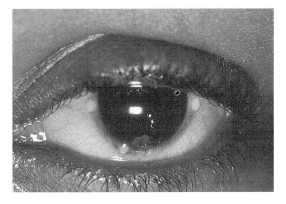

FIG. 5-7 Phlyctenular keratoconjunctivitis: Whitish, heaped up areas along the limbus represent a sterile inflammation associated with a cell-mediated hypersensitivity respond to an antigen.

scratch-rash cycle so prominent in these patients. Cromolyn sodium may decrease some or most of the conjunctivitis, but studies are inadequate to evaluate the long-term efficacy of this therapy. Dietary therapy, which may have a role in patients with severe generalized atopic dermatitis in childhood, probably has little role in the therapy of AKC, but this has not yet been explored.

Immunotherapy, particularly with dust mites, has been suggested for patients with atopic dermatitis. It has not yet been studied in patients with

AKC. Nevertheless, patients with AKC usually have concomitant allergic respiratory disease and allergic conjunctivitis, which often improve with immunotherapy. Environmental control for mite antigens has been reported to improve atopic dermatitis, and this mode of therapy certainly appears reasonable for sensitized patients with AKC.

Other diseases may cause blepharochalasis (lax, wrinkled eyelids) and mimic AKC (see box below). The presence of conjunctivitis, atopic disease, and atopic dermatitis elsewhere helps to diagnose AKC and to direct appropriate therapy.

Marginal Blepharitis. Marginal blepharitis is a common complication of atopic dermatitis, but it may exist alone. It often occurs in patients who have atopic skin. Like other patients with atopic disease, patients with AKC tend to be more susceptible to seborrhea, which leads to staphylococcal colonization. The chronic and inflammatory nature of AKC and the propensity of atopic patients for seborrhea may lead to the SSS syndrome (seborrhea, staphylococcal infection, and sicca). The sicca is not an autoimmune Sjögren's syndrome but a relative sicca. Patients with SSS may actually make normal amounts of tears but have so much debris that their eyes feel dry because the tears are insufficient to wash the scales away. Patients often note that their eyelids are caked together in the morning. The lid margins are scaly, and the lashes pull out easily. Ulcers may form at the lid margins.

Marginal blepharitis begins with seborrhea and scale formation, which then lead to granulated lids. Staphylococci then grow under the scales, ulcerating the lid margins. Large amounts of debris and perhaps a glandular abnormality then lead to blockage of the meibomian glands and chalazion. People who are prone to chalazion tend to have other atopic illnesses, atopic skin, and marginal blepharitis. The crusting and scales lead to complaints of dryness.

Therapy of marginal blepharitis must include lid care to treat the seborrhea. The initial therapy is mechanical. Patients may be instructed to wash their face in warm water, loosen the scales, and then use an ointment to assist the finger to scrape the scales. Initially done twice a day for the first few days, it can then be decreased to once or twice weekly. The initial eye redness and irritation subside rapidly. However, this is a chronic illness. Like "dandruff" or any other seborrheic condition, it is often a lifelong problem. "Artificial tears," because of the relative sicca, may be helpful. Antibiotic ointment and rarely mild steroids may be necessary.

Marginal blepharitis and SSS syndrome may be complicated by punctate keratitis, particularly of the lower third of the cornea. Both incomplete blinking (due to alterations of the blink reflex) and immunologic reaction to or direct toxic effect of staphylococcal exotoxins have been implicated in

---

DIFFERENTIAL DIAGNOSIS OF BLEPHAROCHALASIS

(Lax, wrinkled eyelid)

Recurrent lid edema
    Anaphylaxis
    Angioedema
Chronic lid edema
    Chronic conjunctivitis
Chronic dermatitis
    Atopic keratoconjunctivitis
    Allergic contact dermatitis
    Other
Obesity
Hypoglycemia
Nephrotic syndrome
Congestive heart failure
Acromegaly
Cutis laxa
Osteogenesis imperfecta
Congenital anomalies
    Spine
    Cardiac
    Renal
    Tracheobronchomegaly
T-cell lymphoma
Ascher's syndrome
    Double lip
    Endocrinopathies
Meretoja's syndrome
    Hereditary amyloidosis

punctate keratitis. Treatment of this complication includes artificial tears, occasional use of mild steroids, and encouragement of complete blinking. This is in addition to therapy directed at the seborrhea and staphylococcal colonization.

A less common complication is marginal immune corneal ulcers (Fig. 5-8). More painful than punctate keratitis, these are shallow oval ulcerations often at the 4 and 8 o'clock positions 1 mm in from the limbus. Dilation of adjacent vessels is seen. Pulse steroids are required for disease control. This complication is not usually vision-threatening, although some peripheral scarring may remain.

Vernal Keratoconjunctivitis. VKC is an extremely pruritic disease. It is characterized by intense itching, tearing, a hot tight sensitive feeling of the eyes, and photophobia. Its major signs are ptosis, conjunctival injection, giant papilla of the upper tarsal conjunctiva, and a thick ropy discharge (Fig. 5-9).

This disease is predominantly one of young males, with a male-to-female ratio of $3:1$. Eighty percent of patients have an onset of their disease before age 14, with almost all occurring after 3 years of age and before 25 years of age. As its name implies, it occurs in warm climates and has a seasonal variation.

Almost all patients complain of excessive mucus, and a thick ropy discharge is present. Although the conjunctival disease is not scarring, the corneal disease may be. Epithelial keratitis with punctate stippling may progress to a shieldlike vernal ulcer associated with neovascularization and vision loss.

Examination reveals moderately intense conjunctivitis, ropy discharge, and pronounced papillae on the upper tarsal conjunctiva. With time and rubbing on the cornea the papillae become flat, leading to a cobblestoned appearance. Conjunctival scrapings are virtually diagnostic, with two or more eosinophils per high power field seen in few other diseases. Trantas dots, collections of dead eosinophils and eosinophilic products, are often seen.

The pathogenesis appears to be of a Type I IgE-mediated reaction, most often directed against

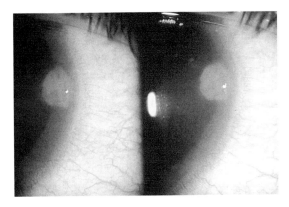

FIG. 5-8 Marginal immune corneal ulcers. *(Courtesy of Jane Stein.)*

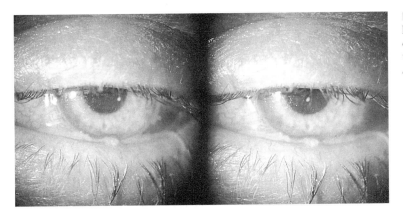

FIG. 5-9 Vernal keratoconjunctivitis: Note ptosis, conjunctival injection, and a ropy, thick discharge. *(Courtesy of Jane Stein.)*

grass pollens. An undefined mechanism sustains the recruitment of inflammatory cells and the intense inflammation.

The disease is markedly disruptive. However, it tends to last from 4 to 10 years and then disappears. Therapy must be vigorous and directed to minimizing the discomfort of the disease and controlling the corneal involvement. Cromolyn sodium is often extremely helpful and must be used frequently, particularly early in the disease. A "pulse" dose of steroids may be necessary to diminish the inflammation. Significant corneal involvement demands steroid therapy.

Giant Papillary Conjunctivitis (GPC). GPC in its later phases looks like vernal conjunctivitis with giant papillae and hypertrophy particularly of the upper tarsal conjunctiva. Mucus production is also increased. However, unlike vernal conjunctivitis, patients complain of only mild itching, and significant corneal involvement is generally absent. This disease is most often associated with soft contact lens wear. It is associated with coating of the contact lens and loss of lens tolerance (Fig. 5-10).

The pathogenesis appears to be coating of allergens of the contact lens associated with trauma of the upper conjunctiva by the foreign body and exposure of the upper lid to the allergens coated on the lens. An IgE-mediated reaction occurs that may be augmented and sustained by a Type IV reaction directed against the allergens or foreign proteins embedded on the lens surface. However, the disease may be seen in nonatopics and with sutures as the source of the irritation. The mast cell and eosinophilic inflammation is apparently a result of varying degrees of IgE response and irritation, which differ among affected individuals.

The therapy revolves around environmental control. Scrupulous lens care can virtually eliminate this disorder. Papain cleaning may be necessary, along with frequent replacement of lenses or use of disposable lenses. Use of cromolyn sodium often improves lens tolerance.

Allergic Contact Dermatitis. Ocular contact allergy is a contact dermatitis. It is a skin eruption characterized by redness and erythema, edema, fluid-filled vesicles, extreme pruritus, and, when occurring chronically, associated with scarring, hyperkeratosis, and lichenification. Although originally seen with plant extracts, it is now much more commonly seen with chemical sensitizers abundant in the environment.

It is indistinguishable from classic cell-mediated immune response in the skin, and all evidence points toward allergic contact dermatitis being a T-cell–mediated hypersensitivity reaction. The histopathology reveals invasion of the dermis by mononuclear cells, especially around blood vessels and sweat glands, and interepidermal vesicles filled with granulocytes and monocytes.

Sensitization occurs by initial exposure to or-

FIG. 5-10 Giant papillary conjunctivitis: Note large papules on upper palpebral conjunctiva. *(Courtesy of Jane Stein.)*

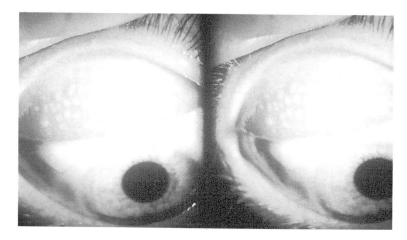

ganic or inorganic antigens. These may either be oleoresins from plants or chemicals in industry or the home. In general, these are small molecular weight molecules which are immunogenic alone. The immunogenicity appears to depend on the ability to penetrate skin (lipid-soluble) and form conjugates with tissue proteins in the malpighian layer of the epidermis.

Activated lymphocytes produce factors that, in concert with macrophages and monocytes, produce tissue inflammation and are recognized clinically as an eczematous inflammatory response. Contact allergy is usually manifested by occasional severe periorbital swelling. Although most diseases involving allergy are chronic, contact allergy is often characterized by symptoms that have been apparent for less than six weeks. There is usually no history of recent conjunctivitis. Often both eyes are equally affected; involvement of other facial areas is a major clue to the diagnosis.

Historical evidence of use of cosmetics, other eye medications, or fingernail polish may point to the cause for this Type IV hypersensitivity disorder. Chemicals contacted in the workplace may be transferred to the eyelid. These sensitive tissues may react clinically while the hands appear normal.

Patients generally are young to middle-aged. It is common throughout the population, occurring in both atopic and nonatopic individuals. There is no typical family history. Because this disease is caused by delayed hypersensitivity, onset of the rash from time of exposure is generally 4 to 72 hours, usually 12 to 48 hours. The incubation period for sensitization is widely variable; it may be as short as five days or may occur only after years of exposure. Interestingly, the site of initial sensitization may flare with reexposure at a distant site.

Patch testing often helps to confirm the causative agent. However, false-negative tests due to differential tissue sensitivity of the eyelid and the back make clinical suspicion, accurate history, and avoidance/challenge testing necessary.

Therapy. The therapy of the allergic eye is similar to therapy of allergic disease in other organ systems. Treatment of the underlying allergic dia-

thesis revolves around environmental control and immunotherapy.

Environmental control is the most effective therapy for allergic eye disease. In patients with allergic contact disorders, it is the only effective treatment; therefore, accurate diagnosis is necessary to properly educate patients as to which medications, preservatives, and cosmetics to avoid. Avoidance of inhaled allergens is more difficult but can be accomplished and often results in sufficient improvement to allow for discontinuation of regular medication in mild disease. Seasonal allergic conjunctivitis is almost always secondary to pollen, especially grass pollen, exposure. Keeping the windows closed in the home, car, school, or work and using air conditioning as much as possible are the most effective control measures.

Animal and dust control can also be simply accomplished. The reservoir for the allergens must be removed; therefore warm-blooded pets should be removed from the house or, in special circumstances, be allowed in but barred from the bedroom and bathed weekly. The dust mite is responsible for most dust allergy and lives in bedding, carpeting, and upholstered furniture. Therefore carpeting should be removed from the bedroom if possible and remaining carpet treated with a mitocide. Mattresses should be encased in airtight covers and linens washed in hot water weekly.

Immunotherapy, when needed, is very successful in controlling symptoms of both allergic con-

TABLE 5-5 *Allergic Conjunctivitis Therapy*

	Early-Phase Reaction	Late-Phase Reaction
Antihistamines	+ +	±
Cromolyn	+ + +	+ + +
Nedocromil	+ + +	+ + +
Topical corticosteroids	+ +	+ + + +
Nonsteroidal anti-inflammatory drugs	+	+ + +
Avoidance	+ +	+ + + +
Inhalation therapy	+	+ + +

junctivitis and concomitant rhinitis. It should be considered in patients whose symptoms are not optimally controlled on simple therapy, when symptoms are progressive, and when co-existing rhinitis is a major problem for the patient.

Pharmacotherapy is variously applicable to the early-phase reaction and late-phase reaction (Table 5-5). Antihistamines are entirely satisfactory for the early-phase reaction but have little effect on the late-phase reaction. Cromolyn or Nedocromil, both typically administered, attenuate the early-phase and late-phase reactions and the hyperreactivity with an outstanding safety record. They have been shown to reduce inflammatory cell infiltration in both classic and hyperinflammatory allergic disease.

Topical corticosteroids, when used acutely, have no effect on the early-phase reaction, but when used chronically may diminish the early-phase reaction as well as treat the late-phase reaction. However, topical corticosteroids cannot be used chronically in the eye, as they are in the nose or chest, because of the complications that can ensue.

Nonsteroidal anti-inflammatory drugs (NSAIDs) topically may decrease itching and may treat and prevent the late-phase reaction; more information is needed on their effect on hyperreactivity. These may be reasonable adjuvant-type drugs.

The pharmacotherapy of the ocular contact allergy patient is oriented toward symptomatic relief (see box below). Sometimes no therapy is needed if symptoms are mild. Over-the-counter (OTC) artificial tears may remove the antigen and media-

tors from the conjunctival sac. OTC or prescription vasoconstrictor/antihistamine topical therapy are reasonable drugs for mild symptoms.

Cromolyn or NSAID is the next line therapy. Although cromolyn often seems to work more promptly for allergic symptoms in the eye than for rhinitis or asthma, when patients have significant ongoing inflammation, onset of significant effect often takes days to weeks. Occasionally other therapy may be needed during this initial period. NSAIDs may be effective therapy.

Topical corticosteroids should rarely be prescribed for patients with hay fever conjunctivitis. Patients with active contact keratoconjunctivitis may benefit from a short course of potent steroid creams on the lid. Sometimes low-potency corticosteroid creams never adequately control the eczema even when used for long periods of time. Potent corticosteroids, applied carefully in a thin layer twice a day for three or four days, with repeated courses over several weeks, result in very reasonable control of the eczematous reaction. Corticosteroids are then discontinued entirely. Cromolyn sodium may be used regularly for concurrent conjunctivitis. Monitoring is required to evaluate the potential complications of those hyperinflammatory allergic illnesses, which are prone to vision-threatening complications. Immediate evaluation should be considered when patients have symptoms of photophobia (indicating corneal involvement), distortion of vision, double vision, loss of vision, pain (not itchiness, burning, awareness), halos around objects, or photophobia (see box below).

PHARMACOTHERAPY OF THE CONTACT ALLERGIC EYE

Nothing
Over-the-counter artificial tears
Vsoconstrictor/antihistamine
omolyn
Nonsteroidal anti-inflammatory drugs
Corticosteroids

SYMPTOMS SUGGESTIVE OF SERIOUS OCULAR PROBLEM

Blurred vision
Loss of vision
Pain (not itchiness)
Halos around objects
Photophobia
Double vision

Cytotoxic (Type II) Ocular Disease

Examples of cytotoxic ocular disease includes pemphigus vulgaris, cicatricial pemphigoid, and Mooren's ulcer.

Pemphigus Vulgaris. Pemphigus, of which vulgaris is the most common form, is a chronic, progressive disease characterized by the formation of bullae anywhere on the body. It is an autoimmune disease in which antibodies form against the intracellular cement substance, epidermal cohesiveness is reduced, and blisters or bullae form (Fig. 5-11). Its cause is unknown.

Clinically, blisters form on the skin and mucosa of a patient, usually between ages 50 and 70 years. Conjunctival inflammation is the most common ocular sign. Painful vesicles of the palpebral conjunctival surface may open but usually heal within one week. The skin eruptions show little tendency to heal (Fig. 5-12).

Treatment for pemphigus includes steroids and cytotoxic medications, which have greatly reduced the mortality rate from this disease. Topically, antibiotic corticosteroid therapy can be used to treat pemphigus conjunctivitis, with supportive mea-

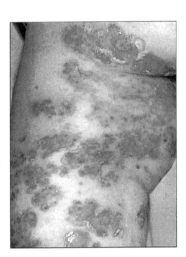

FIG. 5-11 Pemphigus vulgaris: Erosions and blisters rupture easily, with bleeding of exposed skin surfaces. *(From Lawrence CM and Cox NH:* Physical signs in dermatology: color atlas and text, *London, 1993, Wolfe.)*

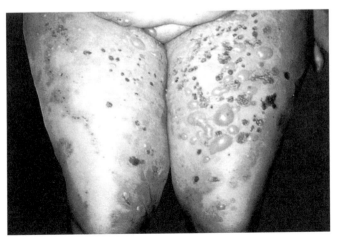

FIG. 5-12 Pemphigus vulgaris: Blisters on thigh of elderly patient show little tendency to heal. *(From Habif TB:* Clinical dermatology, *St. Louis, 1990, Mosby–Year Book.)*

sures including epilation of lashes if trichiasis occurs and artificial tears if tear abnormalities are noticed.

Cicatricial Pemphigoid. Known as ocular pemphigoid, this is a severe mucous membrane pemphigoid characterized by chronic bullous dermatosis. In its worst form, it can be debilitating and blinding (Fig. 5-13).

Systemic findings include blister formation mainly of the eyes and mouth. It occurs most often in women over the age of 60 years. The patient may experience a sore throat and difficulty swallowing due to pharyngeal inflammation.

Early eye symptoms include foreign body sensation and burning. Conjunctival findings include significant symblepharon formation with massive eradication of the fornices. Corneal involvement includes vascularization and ulceration (Fig. 5-14).

Systemic cicatricial pemphigoid is treated with corticosteroids, with some benefit noted. Topical corticosteroids have been used without much success. The dry eye associated with loss of goblet cells is managed with artificial tears, punctual occlusion, and bandage soft contact lenses.

Mooren's Ulcer. Also known as peripheral corneal melting syndrome, this ulcer is chronic and

progressive. It causes a marked marginal corneal degeneration. Autoimmune disease has been implicated in the immunopathology of Mooren's ulcer, but its cause remains unknown. Clinically, the

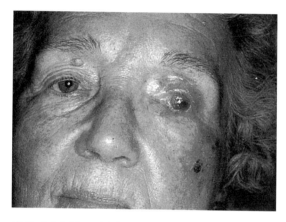

FIG. 5-14 Cicatricial pemphigoid: Symblepharon of the conjunctiva can be seen here in the lower cul-de-sac. *(From Habif TB:* Clinical dermatology, *St. Louis, 1990, Mosby–Year Book.)*

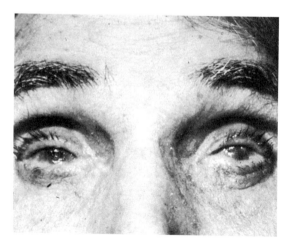

FIG. 5-13 Bullous dermatosis in cicatricial pemphigoid. *(From Bietta G:* Eye involvement in skin diseases. *In: Mausolf FA, editor:* The eye and systemic disease, *St. Louis, 1975, Mosby–Year Book.)*

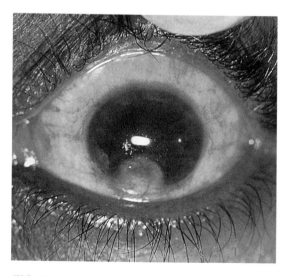

FIG. 5-15 Mooren's ulcer: Peripheral corneal melting syndrome.

ulcer begins as a gray peripheral infiltrate that progresses to a circular furrow (Fig. 5-15). Mooren's ulcer must be treated surgically, as medical management is usually not effective.

Immune Complex (Type III) Ocular Diseases

Immune complex hypersensitivity reactions are responsible for erythema multiforme, scleritis, immune rings, and marginal ulceration.

Erythema Multiforme. Erythema multiforme is characterized by acute skin and mucous membrane eruptions frequently caused by an infection (usually associated with herpes simplex) or a drug reaction (usually sulfonamides). There are two forms of the disease—a minor, mild form, and a major, severe form known as Stevens-Johnson syndrome. No cause for this disease has been established, although it is assumed to be a hypersensitivity reaction.

Clinically the patient experiences a period of fever and headache associated with joint pain. This prodrome persists for several days before the appearance of the skin lesions. These lesions are red and are usually found on the palms and soles of the feet. Typically the lesion appears as a "bull's-eye," with a bright red center surrounded by a pale, white ring. In the minor form the skin is usually involved, whereas in the major form the mucous membranes may show severe involvement (Figs. 5-16 and 5-17). The conjunctiva may show extensive blistering formation and conjunctivitis. Symblepharon may form with eventual entropion, ectropion, and trichiasis. There may be an associated dry eye, corneal desiccation, ulceration, and perforation.

Treatment of erythema multiforme usually involves systemic corticosteroids, with topical steroids used to manage active eye inflammation. Topical antibiotics should be used to prevent secondary infection when there is conjunctival blistering or corneal involvement.

Scleritis. Scleritis may be associated with rheumatoid arthritis in immune complex–type hypersensitivity reactions. The most common presenting symptom is eye pain, usually associated with conjunctival injection, tearing, and photophobia.

Clinically scleritis appears as an involvement of the deep episcleral vessels producing a reddish-blue conjunctival injection pattern (Fig. 5-18). With progression of scleral inflammation, uveal prolapse in possible along with corneal involvement.

Treatment of scleritis includes topical and usually systemic steroids or nonsteroidal anti-inflammatory medications. Thinning of the sclera may require scleral grafting, although this is not always necessary.

Immune Rings. These are known as Wessely rings and form in the corneal stroma. They are assumed to be antibody-antigen reactions that form an infiltrate concentric with the limbus.

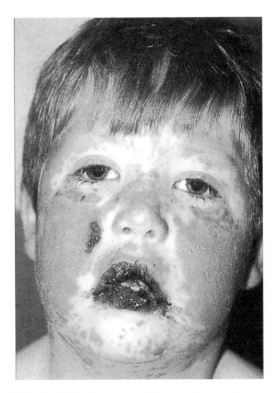

FIG. 5-16 Erythema multiforme: Stevens-Johnson syndrome with ulceration of mouth, eyes, nose, and genitals. *(From Lawrence CM and Cox NH: Physical signs in dermatology: color atlas and text, London, 1993, Wolfe Medical Publishers Ltd.)*

FIG. 5-17 Erythema multiforme: Note the red "bulls-eye" lesions with a surrounding pale white ring typically found on the palms and soles. *(From Habif TB: Clinical dermatology, St. Louis, 1990, Mosby–Year Book.)*

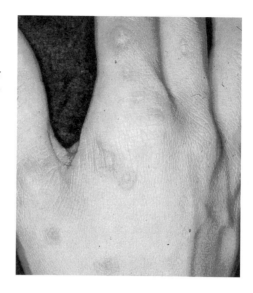

Cell-mediated (Type IV) Ocular Disease

Delayed immune responses include contact conjunctivitis (see Hypersensitivity and Hyperinflammatory Conditions Type I), phlyctenular conjunctivitis, and corneal graft rejection.

Phlyctenular Conjunctivitis. The phlyctenule is a white, nodular lesion usually present in the conjunctiva or cornea and may represent a delayed hypersensitivity reaction. This transient nodule is a response to any number of microbial agents, usually staphylococcal infection. They are usually found on the corneal limbus and persist for two weeks. They resolve with ulceration and leave a small scar with associated pannus.

Once associated with tuberculosis, phlyctenular keratoconjunctivitis was a leading cause of blindness due to corneal involvement. Topical steroids now reduce the risk of secondary scar formation and topical antibiotics may be used to address the staphylococcal infection.

Corneal Graft Rejection. There are several forms of corneal graft rejection.

Hyperacute rejection. Occurring within hours of the transplant, this form of rejection occurs as a result of the presence of pre-existing antibodies in the blood of the recipient. These antibodies react with donor antigen.

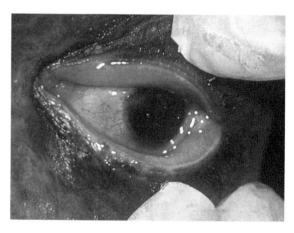

FIG. 5-18 Scleritis: Notice deep involvement of scleral vessels with reddish-blue conjunctival injection pattern.

Acute rejection. This occurs days to years after transplantation. In this case the recipient is nonsensitized and did not originally possess circulating antibodies to the donor tissue. The mechanism appears to be a cellular (Type IV) reaction.

Chronic rejection. This occurs years after transplant, and there is a gradual loss of function and tissue structure. It is most likely due to the presence of antibody. The therapy of graft rejection includes topical steroids, started just after corneal surgery.

SUMMARY

With a basic understanding of the nature of immunologic hypersensitivity diseases of the eye and the principles of therapy of allergic disease, adequate care for patients with allergic eye disorders can be delivered. Appropriate use of history and physical examination, environmental control, immunotherapy, and a stepwise approach to pharmacologic management lead to accurate diagnosis and therapy. Close monitoring when symptoms suggest a vision-threatening event and in diseases prone to significant corneal involvement minimizes complications and maximizes patient satisfaction.

Bibliography

Abbas AK, Lightman AH, and Pober PC: *Cellular and molecular biology,* Philadelphia, 1991, WB Saunders Co.

Allansmith MR and Ross RN: Ocular allergy and mast cell stabilizers. *Surv Ophthalmol* 30:229, 1986.

Barrett JT: *Medical immunology,* Philadelphia, 1991, FA Davis.

Bielory L: Immunology of the eye. *Allergy Proc* 12:364, 1991.

Bielory L and Frohman LP: Allergic and immunologic disorders of the eye. *J Allergy Clin Immunol* 89:1, 1992.

Friedlaender MH: Ocular allergy. *J Allergy Clin Immunol* 76:645, 1985.

Friedlaender MH: *Allergy and Immunology of the Eye,* ed 2. New York, 1993, Raven Press.

Hudson L and Hay FC: *Practical immunology,* Oxford, 1989, Blackwell Scientific Publications.

Muchnick BG, Dell W, and Ruggiero R: *Erythema multiforme: a review of clinical characteristics and ocular manifestations with case presentations. Clinical Eye Vision Care,* vol 2, no 1, Stoneham, Mass, 1990, Butterworths.

Niederkorn JY and others: The immunogenic privilege of corneal allografts. *Reg Immunol* 2:117, 1989.

Rahi AH and Garner A: *Immunopathology of the eye,* Oxford, 1976, Blackwell Scientific Publications.

Stites DD and Terr AJ, editors: *Basic and clinical immunology,* ed 7. East Norwalk, Conn, 1991, Appleton and Lange.

6

Infectious Diseases

JOHN A. McGREAL, Jr.
CONNIE L. CHRONISTER

KEY TERMS

Hepatitis	*Neuroparalytic keratitis*	*Immunofluorescent assay*
Hepatitis B	*Inclusion body*	*(IFA)*
Jaundice	*Spirochete*	*Enzyme-linked immunosorbent*
Herpesviridae	*Venereal Disease Research*	*(ELISA)*
Lymphadenopathy	*Laboratory (VDRL)*	*Protozoan*
Dendrite	*Rapid plasma reagin (RPR)*	*Parasite*
Varicella-zoster	*FTA-ABS*	*Cytomegalovirus retinitis*
Vesicle	*MHA-TP*	*Kaposi's sarcoma*
Postherpetic neuralgia	*Erythema migrans*	

HEPATITIS B

Hepatitis is a viral infection of the liver. There are five different types of hepatitis infection: hepatitis A, B, C, D, and E. Hepatitis A and E are transmitted via the fecal-oral route, and no Food and Drug Administration (FDA)–approved vaccine is available to prevent infection. Hepatitis B and C are caused by blood-borne pathogens. They can be transmitted by contact with infected blood or blood products and other body fluids such as genital secretions. Hepatitis D causes co-infection with hepatitis B. *Hepatitis B* is the only type of hepatitis that can be readily prevented by an FDA-approved vaccine. Therefore, the emphasis of this discussion is on hepatitis B.

The Centers for Disease Control and Prevention (CDC) have estimated that there are 750,000 to 1 million carriers of hepatitis B in the United States. These carriers are capable of transmitting hepatitis and about 25% go on to develop chronic active hepatitis. An estimated 300,000 persons per year contract hepatitis B infection in the United States. Approximately 25% become ill with *jaundice*, and more than 10,000 patients become ill enough to require hospitalization.

Hepatitis B is transmitted via inoculation of a

break in the skin or mucous membranes with infected body fluids. Body fluids potentially infected with hepatitis B include blood, blood products, breast milk, urine, semen, vaginal fluids, cerebrospinal fluid (CSF), saliva, and tears. Hepatitis is transmitted much more easily than human immunodeficiency virus (HIV). The modes of transmission and high-risk activities include sexual contact, needle sharing, needle stick, bite or scratch, sharing razors or toothbrushes, or any activity that causes exposure to infected body fluids. Based on the modes of transmission and the high-risk activities, the populations or persons at high risk for contracting hepatitis B become evident (see box below).

Hepatitis B infection can be obvious or elusive. The incubation period is 3 to 6 months. Acute hepatitis B infection occurs in 30% to 40% of those infected. The onset of acute infection is often insidious. Acute infection causes flulike symptoms of malaise, nausea, and fever. Most patients do not experience severe symptoms, but acute active infection can develop into a very severe liver infection. After the acute infection, the patient enters the jaundice phase, when symptoms improve and liver enlargement occurs. Some patients develop subacute active infection with minimal symptoms, but antibodies to HBV have been produced. Of those patients who develop acute infection, only 10% go on to become chronic carriers and carry the potential for reactivation of infection and for infecting others. Chronic carriers are at high risk of chronic liver disease with possible development of hepatocellular carcinoma. The CDC estimates that 5000 persons per year die of the complications of acute chronic hepatitis B virus infection.

Health care workers have a greater risk of contracting hepatitis B than the general population. Vaccination has greatly reduced the incidence of hepatitis infection among health care workers. Today three hepatitis B vaccines are utilized. Recombivax (Merck Sharp and Dohme) and Engerix-B (Smith Kline Beecham Pharmaceuticals) are both yeast-derived recombinant vaccines that are widely used for vaccination in the United States. These vaccines pose no risk of hepatitis infection because they are made through recombinant DNA techniques. Heptavax, a plasma-derived vaccine, is not as widely used as the recombinant, yeast-derived vaccines. In the United States, Heptavax is used for the vaccination of persons who have an allergy

---

HIGH-RISK GROUPS FOR CONTRACTING HEPATITIS B INFECTION

Homosexual/bisexual men
Intravenous drug users
Developmentally disabled or mentally challenged/
   institutionalized patients
Heterosexual partners of infected people
Persons with multiple sexual contacts/partners
Children of infected mothers
Health care workers
Public safety workers

GROUPS RECOMMENDED FOR PRE-EXPOSURE VACCINATION FOR HBV

Persons with occupational risk (health care and
   public safety workers)
Clients and staff of institutions for the developmentally disabled
Hemodialysis patients
Sexually active homosexual/bisexual men
Users of illicit injectable drugs
Recipients of certain blood products
Household and sexual contacts of hepatitis B virus
   carriers
Adoptees from countries of high hepatitis B virus
   endemicity
Other contracts of hepatitis B virus carriers
Populations with high endemicity of hepatitis B
   virus infection
Inmates of long-term correctional facilities
Sexually active heterosexual persons with multiple
   partners
International travelers who plan to reside for more
   than 6 months in areas with high levels of endemic hepatitis B virus

From Centers for Disease Control MMWR Recommendations and Reports, February 9, 1990 (RR-Z), p 5.

to yeast. The CDC recommends that persons who are at risk of contracting hepatitis receive a vaccine (see box on p. 105).

HERPES SIMPLEX

Herples simplex virus (HSV) is an enveloped DNA virus that is a member of the *Herpesviridae* family. There are two serotypes of herpes simplex: HSV type 1 and HSV type 2. HSV type 1 classically causes infection "above the waist" and more commonly causes ocular infection (Fig. 6-1). In contrast, HSV type 2 causes genital infection (Fig. 6-2) and less commonly affects the eye. Both types of HSV have been known to cause eye infection.

Ocular herpes is the leading cause of blindness due to corneal scarring and opacification. According to Pavin-Langston, more than 300,000 cases of ocular herpes are reported yearly in the United States.

Herpes virus infection is often used as a model for classic latent viral infection. Once a host is infected with herpes simplex virus, the virus always remains in a patient's system as either active or latent infection. The virus enters the host through mucous membranes or breaks in the skin. Transmission often occurs through sexual or intimate contact with an infected person. Primary infection occurs after a 2- to 12-day incubation period. Unfortunately, this infection is usually subclinical and the patient is unaware of infection. Primary systemic infection, if clinical, consists of aching, malaise, fever, and *lymphadenopathy*. Ocular infection includes vesicular, ulcerative lid lesions, acute follicular conjunctivitis, epithelial punctate keratitis, and subepithelial infiltrates. The virus often in-

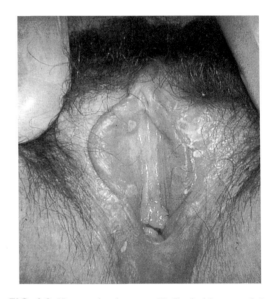

FIG. 6-2 Herpes simplex type II: Genital herpes of the vulva demonstrates a superficial red, sharply marginated ulceration that is painful and recurrent. *(From Habif TB: Clinical dermatology, St. Louis, 1990, Mosby–Year Book).*

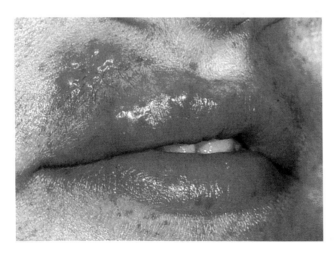

FIG. 6-1 Herpes simplex type I: Primary infection in children often includes gums with buccal ulceration and fever. Note skin lesions around lips. *(From Habif TB: Clinical dermatology, St. Louis, 1990, Mosby–Year Book).*

fects tissues of ectodermal origin such as skin, as well as autonomic and sensory nervous tissue (trigeminal nerve) (Figs. 6-3 and 6-4).

After resolution of primary infection, the virus migrates up the neuron to remain latent in the ganglia. Length of remission is variable. Stresses such as sunlight, fever, or immunosuppression trigger recurrences. Recurrent infection occurs when the virus is triggered to migrate down the axon to the nerve ending. Recurrent ocular infection usually follows the branches of the trigeminal nerve, and the cornea, skin of lid, and even skin around the lips are affected (Fig. 6-5). The cornea is the primary target of recurrent ocular herpes simplex infection.

Recurrent ocular herpes simplex can manifest in several ways. Epithelial infectious ulceration *(dendrite)* is the most common presentation (Fig. 6-6) of recurrent HSV infection. Within the ulcer-ation, HSV is actively infecting the epithelium of the cornea. The patient experiences varying degrees of pain, photophobia, and tearing. Recurrent attacks cause decreased corneal sensitivity. Because of this, corneal sensitivity. should be tested on patients suspected of having herpes simplex keratitis (Fig. 6-7).

Epithelial infectious ulceration begins as fine epithelial opacities that rupture and coalesce to form multiple branching dendrites. Swollen, virus-laden cells line the edges of the ulcer margin and cause the classic staining pattern with rose bengal.

Stromal disease results from an immune reaction to penetration of HSV into the corneal stroma, causing stromal inflammation. As a result, the stroma becomes edematous and develops infiltrates. Epithelium is usually intact, but dendrites may co-exist with stromal disease. The cornea develops areas of focal thinning in response to the inflammation. Uveitis or keratouveitis often occurs along with stromal disease. As with any intraocular inflammation, patients with herpes simplex

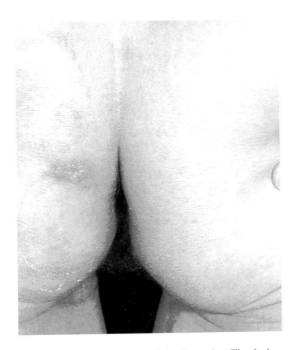

FIG. 6-3 Herpes simplex of the buttocks. The lesion consists of coalesced vesicles that have become pustular. *(From Habif TB:* Clinical dermatology, *St. Louis, 1990, Mosby–Year Book.)*

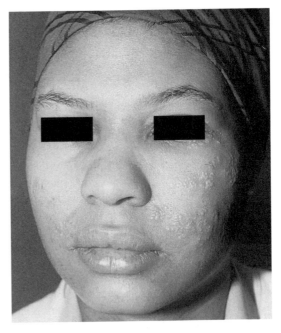

FIG. 6-4 Herpes simplex dermatitis. Note lesions on skin. *(Courtesy of Celeste Mruk, MD.)*

FIG. 6-5 Herpes simplex of the lips. There are clusters of small vesicles with surrounding pruritus and tenderness. These blisters rupture and leave serous crusts. *(From Habif TB:* Clinical dermatology, *St. Louis, 1990, Mosby–Year Book.)*

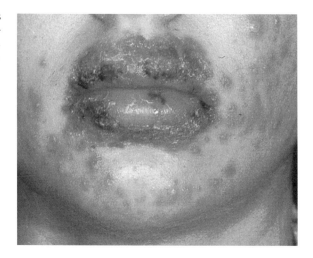

FIG. 6-6 Herpes simplex of the cornea.

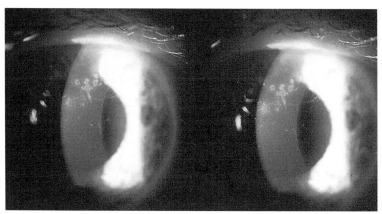

keratouveitis must be monitored for secondary glaucoma.

Diagnosis of ocular herpes simplex is often made on the basis of clinical presentation. The classic corneal dendrite is the hallmark of the disease. The clinician may opt to use laboratory tests to aid in diagnosis. Cytologic examination of conjunctival scrapings can be done with light microscopy and Wright-Giemsa stain. Viral culturing and isolation is the preferred test and can accurately differentiate between the different serotypes of herpes simplex (Types 1 and 2). It takes 1 to 4 days to get the results from viral culturing. Serologic tests for antibodies to HSV are faster but not as sensitive or specific as viral culturing.

Herpes simplex ocular infection is usually ini-

tially managed with topical antivirals. The common antiviral agents used are vidarabine (Vira A) ointment (four times per day) and trifluridine (Viroptic) solution (every 2 hours). Idoxuridine (IDU, Stoxil) ointment has been used in the past but often is not the current drug of choice. Acyclovir (Zovirax) ointment has been used experimentally by grant for deeper corneal infections and skin lesions. In severe infections and/or immunocompromised patients, oral acyclovir is used in conjunction with topical antivirals. Topical steroids should be avoided in all epithelial corneal HSV infections. However, occasionally, if there is stromal inflammation only, steroids can be carefully used to control the stromal inflammation caused by viral antigens.

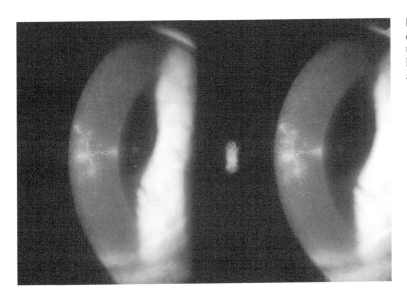

FIG. 6-7 Herpes simplex virus causing an epithelial infectious ulceration known as dendritic keratitis. Note "Christmas tree" appearance of stained lesion.

HERPES ZOSTER

Herpes zoster is a localized vesicular eruption that is limited to the dermatome of a single sensory spinal or cranial nerve. *Varicella-zoster* is a DNA virus belonging to the Herpesviridae family. Primary viral infection results in varicella (chickenpox), characterized by a mild disseminated vesicular eruption that is highly contagious. The virus remains dormant in the sensory ganglion once the infection has occurred. Zoster represents the reactivation of the latent virus. The mechanism of reactivation is unknown, but impairment of the host's cellular immunity plays an important role. Aging, malignancies, immunosuppression, acquired immunodeficiency syndrome (AIDS), local trauma, and irradiation predispose to zoster. The majority of cases occur in healthy adults.

Herpes zoster, or "shingles," is characterized by a unilateral vesicular eruption within a dermatome, commonly associated with severe pain. The dermatomes most frequently involved in order of frequency are thoracic (Fig. 6-8), cranial, cervical, lumbar, and sacral. Prodromal symptoms include pain, burning sensation, and hyperesthesia within a dermatome. These symptoms may precede the initial maculopapular rash by 48 to 72 hours. The

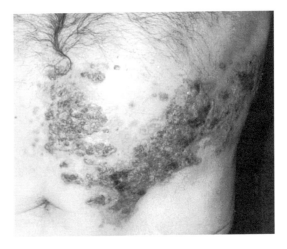

FIG. 6-8 Herpes zoster of the T7 and T8 nerve roots. Notice the clusters of small vesicles on a deeply erythematous background. There is usually surrounding edema. *(From Habif TB:* Clinical dermatology, *St. Louis, 1990, Mosby–Year Book.)*

rash becomes vesicular within 12 to 24 hours. The *vesicles* are filled with a turbid yellow fluid from which the virus may be cultured.

Herpes zoster affects the ophthalmic branch of the trigeminal nerve with a frequency second only to thoracic zoster (Fig. 6-9). Tender regional

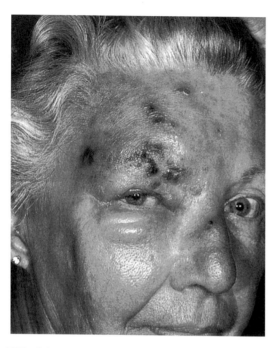

FIG. 6-9 Herpes zoster of the ophthalmic and maxillary fifth cranial nerve distribution. Eruption of blisters follows painful prodrome. *(From Habif TB:* Clinical dermatology, *St. Louis, 1990, Mosby–Year Book.)*

lymphadenopathy occurs early in ophthalmic branch involvement. Follicular conjunctivitis and punctate keratitis are self-limited. Mucous plaque keratopathy takes the form of dendritiform keratitis and is often associated with glaucoma, cataracts, and stromal infiltration (Fig. 6-10). Anterior uveitis is a common ocular manifestation, often seen accompanying corneal inflammation. Secondary glaucoma is not unusual. Retinal and optic nerve involvements complicate a small proportion of ophthalmic zoster. Acute retinal necrosis may be unilateral or bilateral and is more common in patients with AIDS. Ischemic optic neuropathy may be associated with meningoencephalitis. Corneal anesthesia may be pronounced, and normal sensation seldom returns. Neurotrophic keratitis then occurs and may be a persistent problem.

The ocular complications of varicella-zoster virus in patients infected with HIV are similar to those seen in immunocompetent patients but may be more refractory to treatment. As a result, prolonged treatment is often necessary.

After 2 to 3 weeks, the acute phase of the disease subsides. The more debilitating complication in both the normal and immunocomprised patient is the pain associated with acute neuritis and *post-*

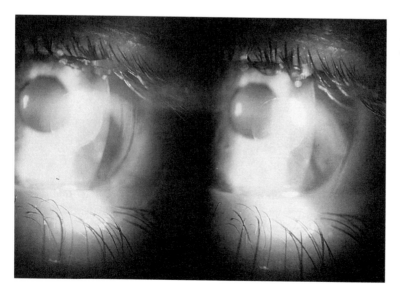

FIG. 6-10 Herpes zoster with corneal involvement. Note disk-shaped, discrete epithelial lesion of the cornea.

herpetic neuralgia. Up to 50% of patients over the age of 50 years with zoster develop this complication within 1 year of their diagnosis. Others are left with dysesthesia within a dermatome.

The diagnosis of varicella-zoster infection is based on clinical impression, and rarely is laboratory diagnostic evaluation necessary. Herpes simplex virus and coxsackievirus cause cutaneous eruptions that resemble zoster, but typically the history and physical examination allow proper differential diagnosis (Fig. 6-11).

Acyclovir is the antiviral agent active against the varicella-zoster virus. Oral acyclovir, 600 mg five times per day for 10 days, results in rapid resolution of clinical disease. It has no effect on the development of postherpetic neuralgia. Intravenous acyclovir is indicated for the treatment of acute retinal necrosis. The use of systemic corticosteroid treatments is controversial. Their use should be limited to severe inflammatory disease with accompanying pain. Prednisone, beginning with 40 mg/kg/day and tapering over 2 weeks, is customary. Topical corticosteroids are useful in the treatment of corneal disease, episcleritis, scleritis, and uveitis.

The management of acute neuritis and postherpetic neuralgia is often difficult (Fig. 6-12). Treatment may range from non-narcotic analgesics to narcotic derivatives. Codeine preparations are often effective in pain relief. Amitriptyline has demonstrated efficacy in recalcitrant cases. The use of topical capsaicin has recently come into favor for pain relief in postherpetic neuralgia.

Corneal complications often require surgical intervention. *Neuroparalytic keratitis,* exposure keratopathy, and resultant corneal scarring and ulceration can usually be effectively treated with lateral tarsorrhaphy.

CHLAMYDIA

Chlamydia trachomatis is the cause of the most common sexually transmitted infection in the adult world. It causes both adult and neonatal conjunc-

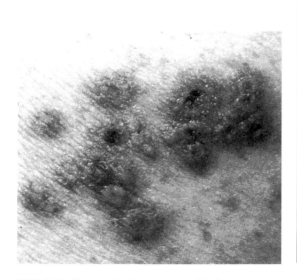

FIG. 6-11 Herpes simplex may resemble herpes zoster, as in this unilateral presentation of herpes simplex on the cheek. *(From Habif TB:* Clinical dermatology, *St. Louis, Mosby–Year Book, 1990.)*

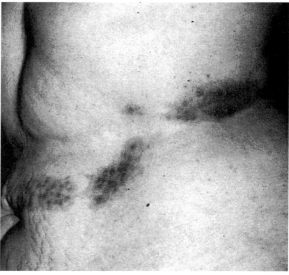

FIG. 6-12 Herpes zoster. Patchy distribution of lesion in the elderly may lead to postherpetic neuralgia for months or years. *(From Habif TB:* Clinical dermatology, Mosby–Year Book, *St. Louis, 1990.)*

tivitis. Genital chlamydial infection can lead to infertility in women, often without producing any symptoms before scarring has begun. If an adult patient has chronic follicular conjunctivitis, chlamydia should be considered as the cause—especially if the patient is sexually active and has multiple partners. Chlamydia should also be considered in neonates who have an acute conjunctivitis.

The CDC estimates that 3 to 4 million new cases of chlamydia occur in the United States each year. The occurrence of inclusion conjunctivitis in adults with genital infection is 1 in 300 cases for women and 1 in 100 cases for men. It is estimated that 30,000 new cases of adult inclusion conjunctivitis occur per year in the United States. Most patients who contract chlamydia are sexually active and are 15 to 40 years old, with a median age of 23 years.

In adults, chlamydia is transmitted through sexual contact. Transmission occurs via mucosal membrane contact with infected body fluids (genital secretions). Transmission usually occurs 2 to 4 months after sexual relations have been initiated. Chlamydia can also be transmitted via hand-to-eye or eye-to-eye contact. Neonates contract chlamydia by vaginal delivery through an infected cervix. The incubation period for chlamydia in neonates is 5 to 12 days after birth. It is estimated that 40% to 50% of exposed infants develop ocular disease.

Chlamydia trachomatis is an obligate intracellular parasite that has a 48-hour developmental cycle. It has the characteristics of both bacteria and viruses. Chlamydia attaches to and enters the host cell in order to utilize the host's contents to produce more DNA and RNA. An *inclusion body* or enlarged host cell is produced when the chlamydia is replicating within the host cell. These inclusion bodies can be seen in a scraping from a chlamydia-infected conjunctiva.

Chlamydia causes a classic chronic follicular conjunctivitis (Fig. 6-13). It can initially present as acute or subacute and appears 5 to 7 days after exposure. The follicular response is often more marked in the inferior fornix. Follicles can also be seen on the limbus, caruncle, and plica semilunaris. Occasionally there can be a mixed follicular

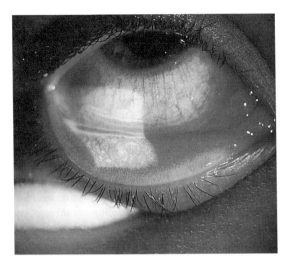

FIG. 6-13 Chlamydial conjunctivitis, a classic chronic follicular conjunctivitis.

and papillary response. Preauricular lymph node swelling is very common in this infection. Corneal involvement includes fine punctate epithelial keratitis that usually occurs 2 to 3 weeks after onset of the conjunctivitis. Subepithelial infiltrates can often be seen along the limbus or central cornea. Pannus with or without associated infiltrates can occur along the superior cornea of chronic untreated patients.

Patients with chlamydial keratoconjunctivitis experience foreign body sensation, tearing, redness, photophobia, lid swelling, and mucopurulent discharge. The infection can be unilateral or bilateral, with a mean duration of symptoms of 5 weeks. A patient can have ocular infection without experiencing any signs or symptoms of systemic genital infection.

Neonatal chlamydial keratoconjunctivitis is much more acute and severe than that seen in adult infection. Neonates present with a marked papillary conjunctivitis (little follicular). There is marked purulent discharge with pseudomembrane formation and lid edema.

Laboratory diagnosis of chlamydia includes examination of conjunctival scrapings with a light microscope. The presence of typical basophilic intracytoplasmic inclusion bodies (Giemsa stained)

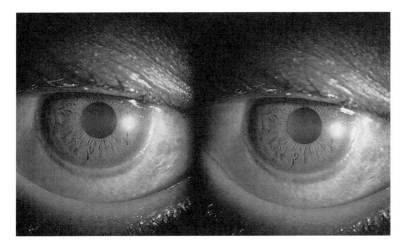

FIG. 6-14 Gonococcal conjunctivitis, a rapidly progressive, purulent conjunctivitis. *(Courtesy of Jane Stein.)*

is diagnostic of chlamydial infection. Another technique is to culture conjunctival swabs by inoculating infected material onto McCoy cells (mouse fibroblasts). Again, the presence of inclusion bodies within the McCoy cells is diagnostic. Fluorescent antibody techniques are more rapid and less expensive than culturing. The binding of fluorescent-tagged antibodies to the chlamydial inclusion body or surface antigen is diagnostic. A fluorescent microscope is used to view the bound fluorescent antibodies.

Chlamydial ocular infection can be treated with systemic tetracycline (adult dose, 250 mg four times per day) for 3 weeks. The treatment can be extended to 4 to 6 weeks if infection recurs. Milk or milk products and antacids prevent systemic absorption of tetracycline, and intake should be minimized during the treatment period. A 3-week treatment of doxycycline (adult dose, 100 mg four times a day) can also be used instead of tetracycline. Erythromycin has also been used to treat chlamydia in patients who are allergic to tetracycline. Topical medications are not necessary with systemic treatment, but topical erythromycin can be used. Usually, topical treatment alone is not effective. Topical steroids can occasionally be used to treat the infiltrates and/or a secondary uveitis.

GONORRHEA

Gonorrhea is an acute infectious disease of the urethra, endocervix, rectum, pharynx, and conjunc-

tiva caused by *Neisseria gonorrhoeae*. Complications include endometritis, salpingitis, peritonitis, bartholinitis, periurethritis, and epididymitis. Systemic manifestations include arthritis, endocarditis, hepatitis, and meningitis.

In recent years there has been a marked increase in the incidence of gonorrheal infections. Evidence suggests that the spread of gonorrhea, like that of syphilis and HIV, is associated with the exchange of sex for illegal drugs. Gonococcal conjunctivitis is the result of direct inoculation of the gonococcus onto the conjunctiva (involving sexual contact) or by passage through an infected cervix during delivery. The incubation period is 1 to 3 days. The disease manifests itself as a rapidly progressive, purulent conjunctivitis. Keratitis can develop quickly, progressing to ulceration and perforation. Untreated gonococcal ophthalmia is highly contagious and may rapidly lead to blindness (Fig. 6-14).

The diagnosis should be suspected in all cases of hyperacute purulent conjunctivitis. Gram's staining reveals typical gram-negative diplococci. Culturing is necessary to establish the diagnosis.

Widespread distribution of antimicrobial resistance to *N. gonorrhoeae* has led to recent changes in treatment recommendations. Penicillin and tetracyclines are no longer first-line therapies. The drug of choice is ceftriaxone, 250 mg in a single intramuscular injection for adults. This should be followed by a course of oral doxycycline, 100 mg orally twice per day for 1 week; tetracycline, 500

mg orally four times per day for 1 week; or erythromycin, 500 mg orally four times per day for 1
week. The sequential treatment is aimed at eradi-
cating chlamydial infections which often co-exist.
Infants should receive ceftriaxone, 25 to 50 mg/
kg/day in an intramuscular injection for 7 days.
Both parents should be treated for gonorrhea. Both
parents and infant should be tested for chlamydia.
For patients who cannot take ceftriaxone, specti-
nomycin, 2 g in a single intramuscular injection,
is an alternative drug. Ocular lavage is the only
topical ocular treatment required.

SYPHILIS

Acquired syphilis is a chronic systemic infection
caused by the *spirochete Treponema pallidum*. It
is usually sexually transmitted, but congenital infection can result if the spirochete passes across
the placenta of an infected mother. The incidence
of syphilis has dramatically increased in the late
1980s. This can be ascribed to the interaction of
substance abuse and sexual behavior. The
male:female ratio is decreasing. The incidence in
the black race has nearly doubled in the last 5-year
period.

The primary stage produces a chancre at the site
of inoculation. Regional lymphadenopathy is typical. If left untreated, the chancre spontaneously
resolves (Fig. 6-15).

Secondary syphilis has its onset weeks to
months after infection. The spirochete is widely
disseminated hematogenously in this stage. Generalized eruptions of the skin (Fig. 6-16) and mucous membranes (Fig. 6-17), fever, and diffuse
lymphadenopathy characterize this stage (Fig.
6-18). The rash is one of few known to affect the
palms of the hands and soles of the feet (Figs. 6-19
and 6-20). Uveitis is common in the secondary
stage. Optic neuritis, unexplained pupillary abnormalities, and retinitis may also be present in this
stage.

Latent syphilis is diagnosed with a positive
treponemal antibody test, normal CSF examination, and absence of clinical manifestations of
syphilis on physical examination. Approximately

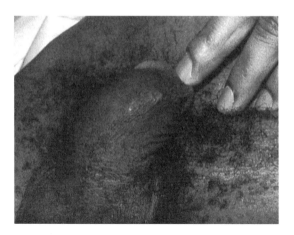

FIG. 6-15 Primary syphilis. Note change at site of inoculation. *(Courtesy of Celeste Mruk, MD.)*

70% of untreated patients with latent syphilis never
develop clinical evidence of late syphilis.

Late syphilis results if the secondary and latent
disease is left untreated. The disease may be
asymptomatic or may progressively involve the
central nervous system and aorta. This stage may
occur many years following the initial infection.
Symptomatic neurosyphilis includes the manifestations of general paresis and tabes dorsalis. Ocular manifestations of late (neurosyphilis) include
optic atrophy, pigmentary degeneration of the retina, and an Argyll Robertson pupil.

The diagnosis of syphilis can be supported with
serologic tests. Nontreponemal tests *(Venereal
Disease Research Laboratory [VDRL]* and *rapid
plasma reagin [RPR])* are quantitative measurements of reaginic antibody titer and assess the clinical activity of syphilis. They are also used to follow the titer in response to treatment. Treponemal
tests (fluorescent treponemal antibody absorption
[FTA-ABS], microhemagglutination for *Treponema pallidum [MHA-TP],* and *Treponema pallidum* immobilization [TPI]) are specific and are
used to confirm positive reaginic antibody tests.
They remain reactive even after therapy. Patients
suspected of late syphilis or those with infection
of more than 1 year's duration without treatment
should have a lumbar puncture for examination of

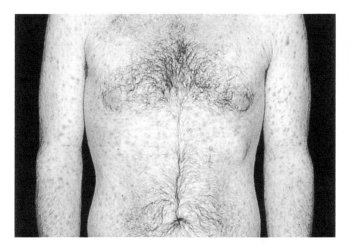

FIG. 6-16 Secondary syphilis of the chest and abdomen. Note red, scattered papules in this patient with malaise and lymphadenopathy. *(From Habif TB:* Clinical dermatology, *St. Louis, 1990, Mosby–Year Book).*

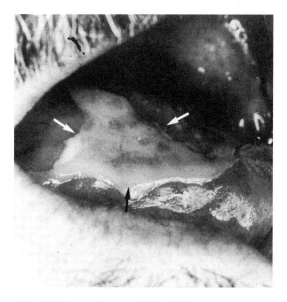

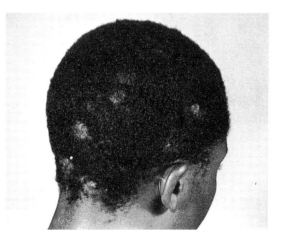

FIG. 6-18 Secondary syphilis with central clearing and a nodular margin with no skin irritation. Note alopecia of the scalp. *(From Habif TB:* Clinical dermatology, *St. Louis, 1990, Mosby–Year Book.)*

FIG. 6-17 Secondary syphilis of the mucous membranes of mouth. Note superficial erosions to the right of the tip of the tongue; scrapings of these lesions reveal treponemes. *(From Cawson RA and others:* Pathology: The mechanisms of disease, *St. Louis, 1989, Mosby–Year Book.)*

the CSF. Serologic tests should be repeated 4 to 6 weeks after the termination of treatment. Inadequate treatment or poor compliance are more likely to result in latent syphilis infection. Reinfection should always be considered. The occurrence of syphilis should alert the practitioner to the possi-

bility of other sexually transmitted diseases. Inquiries into sexual life style and substance abuse are relevant. Counseling and testing for HIV, gonorrhea, and chlamydia should be considered.

The treatment of primary, secondary, and early latent syphilis (less than 1 year's duration) is 2.4 million units of benzathine penicillin-G administered by a single intramuscular injection. For penicillin-allergic patients, tetracycline, 500 mg orally four times per day for 14 days, or doxycycline, 100 mg orally twice per day for 14 days,

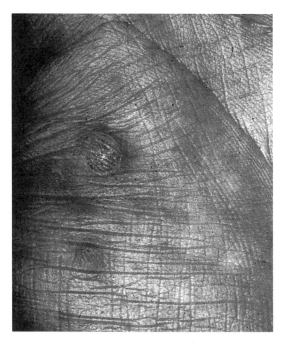

FIG. 6-19 Secondary syphilis. Note red papules on palm of hand. *(From Habif TB:* Clinical dermatology, *St. Louis, 1990, Mosby–Year Book.)*

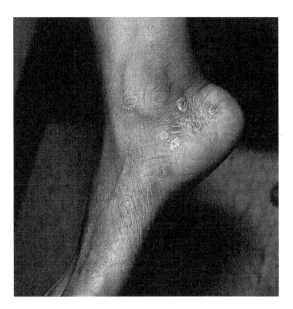

FIG. 6-20 Secondary syphilis. Note eruption of skin of ankle. *(Courtesy of Celeste Mruk, MD.)*

may be given. Ceftriaxone is also highly effective in a single dose and eradicates gonococcal infections, which often co-exist in patients infected with syphilis. Neurosyphilis requires a more intensive treatment consisting of 12 to 24 million units of aqueous penicillin-G administered intravenously for 10 to 14 days.

Recent studies point to the possibility of an altered behavior of syphilis in the HIV-infected patient. Conventional treatment of syphilis in HIV-infected patients seems to convert an acute infection into a chronic one. Some investigators recommend treating all patients with any manifestation of ocular syphilis and HIV infection with the regimen established for the treatment of neurosyphilis.

LYME DISEASE

Lyme disease is a tick-borne spirochetal illness caused by *Borrelia burgdorferi.* The major vector in the Northeastern United States from Massachu-

setts to Maryland and in the Midwest in Wisconsin and Minnesota is the *Ixodes dammini. Ixodes pacificus* is the vector in the western United States. The reservoir for the immature tick is the white-footed mouse, and the white-tailed deer for mature ticks.

Like other spirochetal diseases, Lyme disease occurs in stages, with different clinical manifestations associated with each stage. Stage I begins after an incubation period of 3 to 32 days following the tick bite. Many patients have no recollection of the bite. A characteristic expanding skin lesion, *erythema migrans,* begins at the site of the tick bite. Typically it begins as a red macule that expands to form a larger annular lesion (Fig. 6-21). The lesion is warm but not often painful. The rash is usually accompanied by flulike symptoms of headache, fever, chills, arthralgia, malaise, and fatigue. If untreated, these symptoms improve and resolve within weeks. Erythema migrans may be absent in 15% or more of clinical cases of Lyme disease.

Stage II develops after several weeks to months and often presents with frank neurologic abnormalities. These may include meningitis, cranial neu-

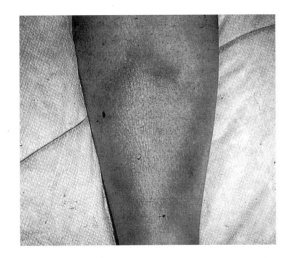

FIG. 6-21 Lyme disease rash. Note large annular lesion around a central light macule. *(From Habif TB:* Clinical dermatology, *St. Louis, 1990, Mosby–Year Book).*

ritis, and peripheral radiculoneuropathy. Cardiac involvement tends to be transient and can include atrioventricular block, left ventricular dysfunction, or cardiomegaly. Migratory musculoskeletal pain in the joints is common to this stage. Ocular findings include hemorrhagic conjunctivitis, keratitis, uveitis, retinal vasculitis, optic neuritis, and exudative retinal detachments.

Stage III occurs weeks to years after onset of infection and typically begins with joint pain. This may progress to arthritis and erosive synovitis. A common presentation is oligoarticular arthritis in large joints, with predilection for the knees. In some patients the arthritis becomes chronic. Chronic neurologic defects may also occur.

The diagnosis of Lyme disease is made clinically and supported with laboratory testing. Serologic tests, including *immunofluorescent assay (IFA)* and *enzyme-linked immunosorbent assay (ELISA),* detect class-specific immunoglobins directed against *B. burgdorferi.* Unfortunately, a significant number of false negatives still occur, and the serologic tests are neither sensitive or specific enough to provide conclusive results.

Treatment consists of tetracycline, 250 mg four times per day for 10 days in adults. Erythromycin, 250 mg four times per day for 10 days, is an alternative drug. Treatment should continue up to 30 days if symptoms persist. In children, amoxicillin, 50 mg/kg/day for 10 days, penicillin or, in penicillin allergy, erythromycin, 30 mg/kg/day for 15 days, can be used.

Later in the illness, parenteral antibiotics may be necessary. In meningitis or cranial neuropathies, penicillin-G, 20 million units intravenously for 14 days, or ceftriaxone, 2 g/day, is highly effective. In patients with established arthritis, doxycycline, 100 mg twice a day for 30 days, is effective. The response to antimicrobial therapy is frequently slow, and a repeat course of oral or intravenous treatment may be needed. The effectiveness of antibiotic treatment for the later manifestations of this condition has not been proven for systemic symptoms, let alone for ocular disease. Whether or not the organism is still present and is necessary for continued disease or the agent triggers an immune response against self components and is no longer necessary in the chronic stages of the disease is an important immunologic issue. In favor of an immunologic component is the association of HLA-DR2 and DR4 with severe chronic Lyme arthritis and history of previous antibiotic failure.

The response to treatment is best early in the illness. With later intervention, convalescence often requires months, and eventually the majority of patients have complete recovery. A substantial proportion of Lyme borreliosis cases are preventable. Mechanical techniques (long sleeves, long pants) and acaricidal chemicals are of established efficacy. The success of these measures depends on the assumption of responsibilities by individuals in endemic areas, public health authorities, educators, and health care workers.

TUBERCULOSIS

Tuberculosis is a communicable disease caused by *Mycobacterium tuberculosis.* Recently there has been an enormous increase in the occurrence of tuberculosis. At particular risk for tuberculosis are blacks, Hispanics, the elderly, and foreign-born persons from areas of the world with high prevalences of tuberculosis, such as Asia, Africa, and Mexico. Also at high risk are prison inmates, alcoholics, intravenous drug users, and household contacts of these at-risk groups. Recent outbreaks of tuberculosis in health care settings, including multiresistant strains of *M. tuberculosis,* have been reported. Patients with HIV infection have an inordinately high risk of tuberculosis. Transmission of tuberculosis is likely to occur from patients with unrecognized pulmonary or laryngeal infection who are not on effective antituberculosis therapy. The tubercle bacilli in respiratory secretions form nuclei for water droplets expelled during coughing, sneezing, and vocalizing.

Clinically, tuberculosis occurs primarily as a pulmonary infection. The bacillus may be hematogenously disseminated, in which case extrapulmonary manifestations may occur (Fig. 6-22). Ocular infection is rare but may affect any part of the eye. Primary ocular infection is commonly conjunctivitis, usually introduced into the eye by contaminated hands or by sputum particles con-

taining the tubercle bacilli. Secondary infection may be phlyctenular keratitis, granulomatous anterior uveitis, disseminated choroiditis, exudative retinitis, periphlebitis, or optic neuritis. Phlyctenular keratoconjunctivitis is the most common form of external ocular tuberculosis.

Diagnosis requires physical examination, tuberculin skin test, chest radiograph, and culture of sputum. Active tuberculosis is strongly suspected if the diagnostic evaluation reveals acid-fast bacteria in sputum, infiltration in the apical posterior segments of the upper lobes with cavitation on chest radiography, (Fig. 6-23), or symptoms highly suggestive of tuberculosis. These symptoms include productive cough, night sweats, anorexia, and weight loss. The diagnosis of tuberculosis in a patient with co-existing HIV infection is more difficult. Patients with HIV infection have cutaneous anergy and therefore have impaired responses to skin tests. They also have low sensitivity on sputum smears, and overgrowth of cultures with other mycobacterial strains such as *Mycobacterium avium* complex may occur. Additionally, radiographic presentations of pulmonary tuberculosis among patients with HIV infection may be atypical with diffuse infiltration.

Curative short-term systemic therapy for tuberculosis consists of isoniazid, 300 mg, and ri-

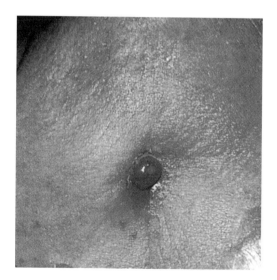

FIG. 6-22 Extrapulmonary manifestation of tuberculosis. *(From Lawrence CM and Cox NH:* Physical signs in dermatology: color atlas and text, *London, 1993, Wolfe Medical Publishers, Ltd.)*

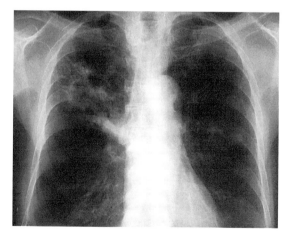

FIG. 6-23 Tuberculosis. Chest radiograph demonstrates cavitary destruction of upper lung fields. *(Courtesy of Celeste Mruk, MD.)*

fampin, 600 mg daily for 1 month. This should be followed by isoniazid, 900 mg, and rifampin, 600 mg twice weekly for 8 additional months. The daily regimen can be given for 9 months. Treatment regimens do not differ for pulmonary and extrapulmonary (ocular) manifestations.

Topical corticosteroids and cycloplegics may be necessary to control inflammation associated with keratitis and uveitis. In some cases, chronic inflammation requires maintenance therapy and long-term follow-up care. Rest, improved hygiene, and a well-balanced diet should be advised to patients on treatment. Close observation by an eye care practitioner is necessary to monitor both ocular therapeutic response and potential side effects, such as optic neuropathy, of the antituberculous medications.

When tuberculosis is diagnosed, public health authorities should be notified so the appropriate contact investigation can be performed. Chemoprophylaxis is necessary for household contacts. A 1-year course of isoniazid has been shown to be effective treatment in prevention.

Treatment failures are due to patient default with medications or the presence of drug-resistant strains. Periodic tuberculin skin tests should be performed on health care workers to identify those persons whose tests convert to positive. Health care workers involved in high-risk procedures (bronchoscopy, sputum induction) or those who are frequently exposed to patients with tuberculosis or AIDS should be retested at 6-month intervals.

TOXOPLASMOSIS

Toxoplasmosis is caused by the obligate intracellular *protozoan Toxoplasma gondii*. It has a predilection for the brain, eye, and muscle. Most infections are congenital in origin. Infants may present with convulsions, chorioretinitis, intracranial calcifications, strabismus, or nystagmus. Most infants survive the acute infection and have no sequelae. Many have healed scars in the fundus and are at risk for recurrent retinochoroiditis later in life.

Ocular toxoplasmosis may be acquired as an adult. Pregnant women should be advised to avoid cat litter, as this is a common mode of transmission of the toxoplasma *parasite*. Ingestion of partially cooked meats is also a mechanism of transmission. Acquired toxoplasmosis is a self-limited infection that usually goes unrecognized in immunocompetent adults and children. Cervical lymphadenopathy is the most common manifestation of *T. gondii* infection. Although the majority of patients with lymphadenopathy have no symptoms, some present with generalized malaise, fever, headache, fatigue, and myalgia.

Ocular disease is characterized by retinochoroiditis and usually reflects the late sequelae of congenital infection. Active retinal lesions are ill-defined yellow foci with a predilection for the posterior pole (Fig. 6-24). Panuveitis, vitritis, papillitis, and optic atrophy may also be present. Resolution of retinal inflammation results in the formation of discrete oval pigmented scars (Fig. 6-25).

Toxoplasmosis in immunosuppressed patients usually represents reactivation of a previously acquired infection. Although widely disseminated, it is the central nervous system involvement that is

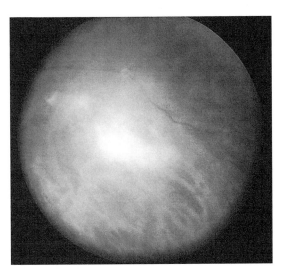

FIG. 6-24 Toxoplasmic retinochoroiditis. This active lesion obscures the fundus details.

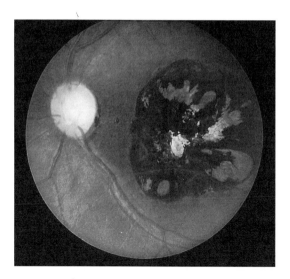

FIG. 6-25 Toxoplasmosis. Resolution of retinal inflammation results in the formation of discrete, macular, oval pigmented scars with severe loss of central vision.

associated with the highest morbidity and mortality. Intracerebral mass lesions, brain abscess, and meningoencephalitis are not infrequent in AIDS patients.

Serologic testing for anti-toxoplasma IgG antibody can be ordered using the Sabin-Feldman dye test, an IFA test, or a complement-fixation assay.

Immunologically intact children and adults seldom require treatment for acute *T. gondii* infection. The treatment of ocular disease depends on the location and severity of the retinal lesions. Large, macula-threatening lesions should always be treated. More peripherally located lesions may be observed without treatment. The best treatment for this infection remains a subject of controversy. Sulfadiazine is administered with a 2- to 4-g loading dose, followed by 1 g four times a day for 4 to 6 weeks. Pyrimethamine is given, 100 mg/day loading dose for 2 days, followed by 25 mg/day for 4 to 6 weeks. Clindamycin, 300 mg four times per day for 3 to 6 weeks, is gaining more favor as a drug of choice. Oral prednisone, 40 to 60 mg daily for 2 to 6 weeks, is indicated for active lesions threatening the macula or optic nerve. These four drugs may be used in multiple combinations, and often a synergistic effect is observed. For se-

vere cases, all four medications can be used concomitantly (quadruple therapy).

Topical corticosteroids are useful in treating anterior uveitis. Periocular corticosteroids are indicated in poor compliers and patients with intolerance or contraindications to oral corticosteroids. Adjunctive therapies include laser photocoagulation and cryotherapy.

Ocular toxoplasmosis in patients with AIDS usually responds favorably to antiparasitic therapy. The same medications are used for AIDS patients as for immunocompetent patients. Pyrimethamine is sometimes avoided because of pre-existing bone marrow suppression. Corticosteroid use is avoided to prevent further suppression of host immune mechanisms. There is also a high incidence of sulfonamide allergies among patients with AIDS. As is often the case in immunocompromised patients, toxoplasmosis tends to reactivate if antiparasitic therapy is discontinued. Maintenance therapy with full doses or lower, suppressive doses may prevent reactivations.

OCULAR MANIFESTATIONS OF HIV INFECTION

HIV infection and the opportunistic infections that result cause significant and varying ocular anomalies (Table 6-1). The most common ocular manifestations of HIV infection are retinal microvascular changes and cotton-wool spots. Many researchers (including Kestelym, Holland Freeman, Newsome, and Gabrieli) have reported that cotton-wool spots have been found in 45% to 100% of AIDS patients. Cotton-wool spots are areas of ischemia that occur from blockage of axoplasmic flow, swollen interrupted axons, and edema in the nerve fiber layer of retina. They can also be caused by diabetes, hypertension, anemia, and other diseases. These areas of focal ischemia (Fig. 6-26) resolve in 4 to 6 weeks. Pepose and Freeman have reported retinal hemorrhages in 8% to 40% of HIV-infected patients. In addition to hemorrhages and cotton-wool spots, microaneurysms and ischemic macular edema have been observed. The appearance of the aforementioned retinal microvascular changes is often likened to the microvascular changes seen in early diabetic retinopathy (Fig. 6-27).

The cause and pathogenesis of microvascular disease in HIV-infected patients remain uncertain, and many researchers have addressed this question. Ultrastructural retinal vascular changes that have been observed include loss and degeneration of pericytes, swollen endothelial cells, thickened basal lamina, and narrowed capillary lumina. HIV has been isolated in the endothelial cells that line retinal blood vessels. HIV may directly infect the retinal capillaries and cause microvascular disease. Circulating immune complexes that result from altered immunity seen in HIV infection may be deposited in the walls of capillaries and cause capillary occlusion. Other studies have looked at altered viscosity of blood and altered blood flow in HIV-infected patients. If the blood viscosity increases, retinal ischemia may result.

Regardless of the cause, it is known that the presence of cotton-wool spots in an HIV infected patient is a significant prognostic sign. Patients who exhibited cotton-wool spots were more immunocompromised and had lower CD4 counts than those with clear retinas. Cotton-wool spots are rarely found in HIV-infected patients who have had minimal to no signs of HIV infection. In contrast, in a study by Brezin, cotton-wool spots were found in 31% of AIDS-related complex (ARC) patients, and these patients were more likely to quickly develop full-blown AIDS than ARC patients without cotton-wool spots. The presence of cotton-wool spots indicates a compromised blood-retina barrier and compromised capillaries. As a result, opportunistic infections such as cytomegalovirus may more easily infect the retina by means of viremic seeding through the retinal arcades and capillaries. HIV-infected patients with cotton-wool spots should be monitored with routine fundus evaluation and/or retinal photography every 6 months.

Conjunctivae of HIV-infected patients also exhibit microvascular changes. Observations of alterations in blood flow of arterioles and venules of capillaries have included granular appearance of blood column, aggregation of red blood cells, decreased rate of blood flow, capillary dilation and microaneurysms, short vessel segments of irregular caliber, and isolated vessel fragments. Engstrom and others observed these changes to be most apparent on inferior, perilimbal, and bulbar conjunctivae. These changes have been reported in 75% of HIV-infected patients. Most likely, the cause of the conjunctival vessel changes is the same as the cause of the retinal cotton-wool spots.

HIV infects nervous tissue in all areas of the body, and the retina does not appear to escape. HIV has been isolated from retinal tissues, vitreous, and choroid. HIV has been found in all the retinal layers, but it infects primarily Mueller cells, the support cells of the retina.

Brodie and others and Quiceno and others have reported that some HIV-infected patients exhibit reduced acuity without any apparent cause. Although their retinas as well as ocular media appear clear, they exhibit reduced color vision and contrast sensitivity. These findings may be the result of HIV infection of Mueller cells, which are necessary for proper retinal function. As mentioned previously, HIV may be the cause of cotton-wool spots through infection of retinal vascular endothelial cells. More research is needed to confirm the effects of HIV's presence in the retina.

Cytomegalovirus (CMV) *retinitis* is the most common ocular opportunistic infection seen in AIDS patients. According to Holland and others and Henderly and others, CMV retinitis is the second most common ocular manifestation of HIV infection and is seen in 15% to 40% of AIDS patients. Once a patient contracts CMV, he or she is most likely very immunocompromised. CMV is seen very late in the course of HIV infection. It commonly affects vision when visually important structures such as the macula and optic nerve are infected with CMV.

CMV retinitis has a very characteristic appearance (Fig. 6-28). Many clinicians have referred to CMV retinitis as the "pizza fundus" or "cottage cheese and ketchup fundus." Active CMV infection causes granular white patches along the retinal vessels. The inflammation often follows the

TABLE 6-1 *Ocular Opportunistic Infections/Neoplasms*

Ocular Infection	Clinical Appearance	Treatment	Additional Comments
Viral infections			
Cytomegalovirus Retinitis	"Pizza fundus"—full thickness retinal necrosis and hemorrhage	Ganciclovir (IV) Foscarnet (IV)	Most common ocular opportunistic infection (20%-40%)
Herpes simplex Anterior segment Skin vesicles Follicular conjunctivitis Dendritic ulcer	Severe skin vesicles and corneal ulceration	Oral or IV acyclovir	Severe form in AIDS patients
Retinitis	Retinal necrosis Significant intraretinal hemorrhage	Vidarabine (Vira A) Trifluorothymidine (Viroptic) Foscarnet (IV)	
Herpes zoster Anterior Segment Conjunctivitis Keratitis Vesicular eruptions Uveitis	Severe skin vesicles and keratitis	Acyclovir (IV) (oral)	HZV in young patients indicates possible HIV infection. 4% of AIDS patients
Retinitis	Retinal necrosis		
Molluscum contagiosum (pox virus) "Warts" on eyelids	Benign epithelial tumor	Direct cautery, cryodestruction, surgical removal	Severe form in AIDS patients. Spread by direct or indirect contact
Protozoal			
Toxoplasmosis Chorioretinitis	Full-thickness necrosis Minimal hemorrhage, marked vitritis	Pyrimethamine Sulfadiazine Clindamycin	20%-30% AIDS patients (systemic infection) 1% chorioretinitis
Pneumocystis carinii Choroiditis	Choroidal inflammation Serous detachment	Pentamidine (IV) Methoprim (IV) Sufamethoxazole (IV)	Rarely causes eye infection

Bacterial				
Tuberculosis	Chorioretinitis	Mainly choroidal involvement Yellow-white choroidal nodule	Rifampin, pyridoxine, isoniazid, pyrazinamide, ethambutol	Rarely affects eye. Common cause of pneumonia
Syphilis	Uveitis, extraocular movement palsies, episcleritis, scleritis, neuroretinitis, optic neuritis	Great imitator (variable) Neuroretinitis Retinal necrosis	Penicillin (IV)	Variable presentation
Pseudomonas Staphylococcus *Neisseria gonorrhoeae* Capnocytophagia Chlamydia	Ulcer and conjunctivitis	Corneal infiltrate with excavation Red eye	Varies depending on causative agent	Always culture ulcers and conjunctivitis from HIV-infected patients
Fungal				
Cryptococcus neoformans *Candida albicans* *Sporothrix schenckii* *Histoplasmosis*	Chorioretinitis Endophthalmitis Keratitis	Endophthalmitis Small, white, fluffy infiltrates Spread to overlying vitreous Vitreal haze with white, fluffy lesions Vitreal abscess	Amphotericin B (IV) Flucytosine Ketoconazole	Fungal infections, although rare in general population, should not be overlooked in HIV-infected patients

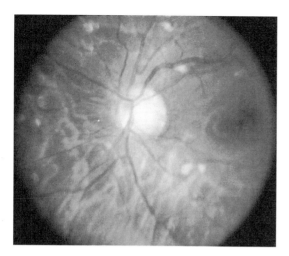

FIG. 6-26 Cotton-wool spots are the most common ocular manifestation of HIV infection.

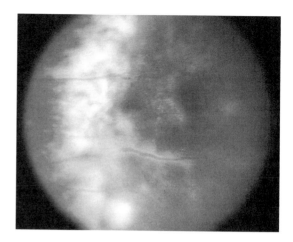

FIG. 6-28 Cytomegalovirus retinitis. Granular white patches along the retinal vessels and arcades.

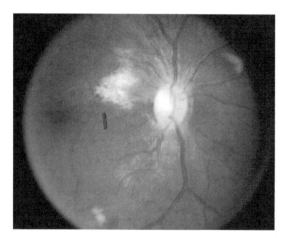

FIG. 6-27 Retinal hemorrhages, cotton-wool spots, microaneurysms, and ischemic macular edema in an HIV patient.

vascular arcades. The necrotic foci coalesce to form large patches of retinal necrosis with extensive edema, hemorrhage, and exudate. The infection spreads like a brush fire to invade the entire retina in 3 to 6 months. Untreated infection can lead to retinal detachment and blindness.

Two FDA-approved drugs are used to treat CMV—ganciclovir and foscarnet. These drugs treat ocular as well as other systemic infections

caused by CMV. Ganciclovir works by inhibiting the replication of CMV. It is an intravenous medication that requires hospitalization for the initial induction doses. An outpatient maintenance dose is needed to prevent reactivation of infection. Jabs reported improvement of the retinitis in 81% of treated patients, with complete remission in 61% of treated patients. Intravitreal injection of ganciclovir has been done experimentally Henry and others with varying results.

According to Weisenthal and others, the adverse effects of ganciclovir treatment include bone marrow suppression or neutropenia and long-term breakthrough progression of retinitis in 35% of treated patients. Because zidovudine (AZT) also causes neutropenia, great care must be taken in the administration of AZT with ganciclovir. Often a decision has to be made by both the patient and practitioner whether to administer ganciclovir to preserve vision or continue AZT therapy to control HIV infection. Because CMV patients are usually severely immunocompromised, the median survival of AIDS patients treated with ganciclovir is 8 months.

Fortunately, foscarnet, an alternative drug to ganciclovir, has been approved by the FDA. Foscarnet does not cause the same side effects as AZT, and therefore both drugs can be used simultaneously. Unfortunately, according to Fanning and others, foscarnet does not appear to be quite as effective against CMV as ganciclovir, and response to therapy was good in 47% of treated patients. Foscarnet is an intravenous drug that is administered in a similar manner to ganciclovir. It acts to inhibit the replication of CMV. Side effects of foscarnet include renal toxicity as well as anemia.

Many other drugs are being tried experimentally for the treatment of CMV retinitis. To enroll a patient in a clinical trial, call the AIDS clinical trial hotline: 1-800-TRIALS-A. As AIDS patients become more immunocompromised, they should be monitored every 3 months for the appearance and possible early treatment of CMV retinitis.

In the "non-AIDS" population, toxoplasmosis is the most common cause of infectious retinitis. Toxoplasmosis in the immunocompromised host is becoming a major cause of mortality, as it can cause life-threatening encephalitis, pneumonitis, or myocarditis. In AIDS patients, central nervous system infection is the most common manifestation of toxoplasmosis. Jabs reported that retinochoroiditis from toxoplasmosis occurs in 1% of AIDS patients and is the second most common form of retinal infection in that group. Its appearance is similar to that in non-AIDS patients except that new lesions often occur away from pre-existing toxoplasmic scars. This suggests acquired infection rather than activation of latent infection. Unlike CMV retinitis, toxoplasmosis rarely causes retinal hemorrhage. This difference usually assists the clinician in the differentiation of CMV from toxoplasmal retinal infection.

Active toxoplasmosis infection in AIDS patients can be difficult to treat. Treatment usually includes pyrimethamine, clindamycin, and sulfadiazine. Other ocular complications from toxoplasmosis include chronic iridocyclitis, cataract formation, secondary glaucoma, band keratopathy, cystoid macular edema, retinal detachment, and optic atrophy.

Herpes zoster can cause both anterior and posterior segment disease in HIV-infected patients. When herpes zoster infection is seen in patients younger than 40 years old, one should suspect HIV

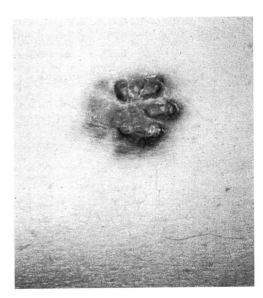

FIG. 6-29 Kaposi's sarcoma, a vascular malignancy common in AIDS patients. *(Courtesy of Celeste Mruk, MD.)*

infection. Many ocular opportunistic infections are seen in HIV-infected and AIDS patients. These infections are summarized in Table 6-1. Note that this list is not comprehensive, as new opportunistic infections are constantly being reported. Most of the ocular opportunistic infections seen in HIV-infected patients are similar in clinical presentation and appearance to those seen in other patients, but they are much more severe and more difficult to treat.

Dry eye syndrome has been reported in HIV-infected patients. In a study by Lucca and others, keratoconjunctivitis sicca was seen in 21% of HIV-infected men. It is hypothesized that HIV-infected patients develop a sicca complex similar to that seen in Sjögren's syndrome. Aggressive ocular lubrication is recommended for these patients.

Kaposi's sarcoma is a slowly progressive, vascular malignancy common in AIDS patients. Although it tends to be common in homosexual HIV-infected patients, it can be seen in any type of HIV-infected patient. According to Fujikawa, Kaposi's sarcoma occurs in 24% of AIDS patients. Ocular Kaposi's sarcoma causes a vascular malignancy commonly seen on the eyelids, caruncle, and conjunctiva (Fig. 6-29). Conjunctival lesions could easily initially be mistaken for a subconjunctival hemorrhage. Lack of regression of a red conjunctival lesion in an HIV patient should alert the practitioner to Kaposi's sarcoma. Treatment of Kaposi's sarcoma includes chemotherapy, immunotherapy, radiation therapy, cryotherapy, and excision.

HIV infection has numerous neuro-ophthalmic manifestations, many of which are due to the opportunistic ocular infections. If the retina becomes infected, HIV-infected patients may show extensive field loss. Optic nerve infection can result in vision loss as well as an afferent pupillary defect. HIV infection can also cause nerve damage that can present as a facial paresis or extraocular muscle paresis. Any neuro-ophthalmic abnormality should be carefully investigated in an HIV-infected patient.

Bibliography

Abrams J: The role of isoniazid therapeutic test in tuberculous uveitis, *Am J Ophthal* 94:511, 1982.

American Thoracic Society/Centers for Disease Control: Diagnostic standards and classification of tuberculosis, *Am Rev Respir Dis* 142:725, 1990.

Balfour HH and others: Acyclovir for herpes zoster: advantages and adverse effects, *JAMA* 255:387, 1986.

Banyas GT: Difficulties with Lyme serology, *J Am Optom Assoc*, 63:135, 1992.

Belec L and others: Peripheral facial paralysis indicating HIV infection, *Lancet* 2:1421, 1988.

Blumenkranz MS and others: Treatment of acute retinal necrosis with intravenous acyclovir, *Ophthalmology* 93:296, 1986.

Brezin A and others: Cotton wool spots and AIDS related complex, *Int Ophthalmol* 14:37, 1990.

Brodie SE and Friedman AH: Retinal dysfunction as an initial ophthalmic sign in AIDS, *Br J Ophthalmol* 74:49, 1990.

Cellini M and Baldi A: Vitreous fluorophotometric recordings in HIV infection, *Int Ophthalmol* 15:37, 1991.

Centers for Disease Control: Guidelines for preventing the transmission of tuberculosis in health care settings, with special focus on HIV related issues, *MMWR* 17:1, 1990.

Centers for Disease Control: Recommendations and reports, *MMWR* Vol 39:5, 1990.

Centers for Disease Control: Relationship of syphilis to drug use and prostitution. Connecticut & Philadelphia, Penna. *MMWR* 37:755, 1988.

Chess J: Zoster related bilateral acute retinal necrosis syndrome in a patient as a presenting sign in AIDS, *Ann Ophthalmol* 20:431, 1988.

Chronister CL: Dry eye in an HIV-infected female. *Clin Eye Vision Care* 4:61, 1992.

Corey L: *Herpes viruses*. In Sherris JC (ed): *Medical immunology*, New York, 1984, Elsevier.

Couderc LJ and others: Sicca complex and infection with human immunodeficiency virus, *Arch Intern Med* 147:898, 1987.

Craft JE: Antibody response in Lyme disease, evaluation of diagnostic tests, *J Infect Dis* 150:489, 1984.

de Smet MD and Nussenbatt RB: Ocular manifestations of AIDS, *JAMA* 266:3019, 1991.

Dobbie J: Cryotherapy in the management of toxoplasma retinochoroiditis, *Trans Am Acad Ophthalmol Otolaryngol* 72:364, 1968.

Eggleston M: Therapy of ocular herpes simplex infections, *Infect Control* 8:294, 1987.

Engstrom RE: Current practices in the management of ocular toxoplasmosis, *Am J Ophthalmol* 111:601, 1991.

Engstrom RE and others: Hemorrheologic abnormalities in patients with human immunodeficiency virus infection and ophthalmic microvasculopathy, *Am J Ophthalmol* 109:153, 1990.

Everetti A and Wong KL: Ophthalmic manifestations of AIDS, *Ophthalmol Clin North Am* 1:53, 1988.

Fanning MM and others: Foscarnet therapy of cytomegalovirus retinitis in AIDS, *J Acquir Immune Defic Syndr* 3:472, 1990.

Freeman WR and others: Prevalence and significance of acquired immunodeficiency syndrome–related retinal microvasculopathy, *Am J Ophthalmol* 107:229, 1989.

Freeman WR and others: A prospective study of the

ophthalmic findings in the acquired immune deficiency syndrome, *Am J Ophthalmol* 97:133, 1984.

Fugikawa L: Advances in immunology and uveitis, *Ophthalmology* 96:1118, 1989.

Gabrieli CB and others: Ocular manifestations in HIV-seropositive patients, *Ann Ophthalmol* 22:173, 1990.

Gagliuso DJ and others: Ocular toxoplasmosis in AIDS patients, *Trans Am Ophthalmol Soc* 88:63, 1990.

Ghantey K: Photocoagulation of active toxoplasmosis retinochoroiditis, *Am J Ophthalmol* 89:858, 1980.

Graham N: Prevalence of tuberculosis positivity and skin anergy in HIV seropositive and seronegative IV drug users, *JAMA* 267:369, 1992.

Grant ED: Acyclovir (Zovirax) ophthalmic ointment: a review of clinical tolerance, *Cur Eye Res* 6:231, 1987.

Gross JG: Longitudinal study of cytomegalovirus retinitis in acquired immune deficiency syndrome, *Ophthalmology* 97:681, 1990.

Haimovici R: Treatment of gonococcal conjunctivitis with single dose ceftriaxone, *Am J Ophthalmol* 107:511, 1989.

Hamed LM, Schatz NJ, and Galetta SL: Brainstem ocular motility defects and AIDS, *Am J Ophthalmol* 106:437, 1988.

Handsfield HH: Old enemies: combatting syphilis and gonorrhea in the 1990's, *JAMA* 284:1451, 1990.

Hanrohan JP: Incidence and frequency of endemic Lyme disease in a community, *J Infect Dis* 150:489, 1984.

Henderly DE and others: Cytomegalovirus retinitis as the initial manifestation of the acquired immune deficiency syndrome, *Am J Ophthalmol* 103:316, 1987.

Hennis HL, Scott AA, and Apply DJ: Cytomegalovirus retinitis, *Survey Ophthalmol* 34:193, 1989.

Henry K and others: Use of intravitreal ganciclovir (dihydroxy propoxymethyl guanine) for cytomegalovirus retinitis in a patient with AIDS, *Am J Ophthalmol* 103:17, 1987.

Holland GN: Ocular toxoplasmosis in patients with AIDS, *Am J Ophthalmol* 106:653, 1988.

Holland GN and others: Acquired immune deficiency syndrome: ocular manifestations, *Ophthalmology* 90:859, 1983.

Insler MS: AIDS and other sexually transmitted diseases and the eye, Orlando, FL, 1987, Grune and Stratton.

Jabs DA: Ocular toxoplasmosis, *Int Ophthalmol Clin* 30:264, 1990.

Jabs DA, Enger C, and Bartlett JG: Cytomegalovirus retinitis and acquired immunodeficiency syndrome, *Arch Ophthalmol* 107:75, 1989.

Jacobson MA and others: Foscarnet therapy for ganciclovir-resistant cytomegalovirus retinitis in patients with AIDS, *J Infect Dis* 163:1348, 1991.

Kaplowitz G and others: Prolonger continuous acyclovir treatment of normal adults with frequently recurring genital herpes simplex infection, *JAMA* 265:747, 1991.

Karabassi M and others: Herpes zoster ophthalmic survey, *Ophthalmology* 36:395, 1992.

Kaslow R: Current perspectives on Lyme borreliosis, *JAMA* 267:1383, 1992.

Kestelym P and others: A prospective study of the ophthalmic findings in acquired immune deficiency syndrome in Africa, *Am J Ophthalmol* 100:230, 1985.

Knox DL: *Syphilis and tuberculosis*. In Ryan SS (ed): *Retina*, St. Louis, Mosby–Year Book, 1989, p. 647.

Lakhanpal V: Clindamycin in the treatment of toxoplasma retinochoroiditis, *Am J Ophthalmol* 95:605, 1983.

Lee SF and others: Comparative laboratory diagnosis of experimental herpes simplex keratitis, *Am J Ophthalmol* 109:8, 1990.

Leport C and others: Treatment of central nervous system toxoplasmosis with pyrimethamine, sulfadiazine combination in 35 patients with AIDS, *Am J Med* 84:94, 1988.

Lipson BK and others: Optic neuropathy associated with cryptococcal arachnoiditis in AIDS patients, *Am J Ophthalmol* 107:523, 1989.

Lucca JA and others: Keratoconjunctivitis sicca in male patients infected with human immunodeficiency virus type 1, *Ophthalmology* 97:1008, 1990.

Luft B: Invasion of the central nervous system by *Borrelia burgdorferi* in acute disseminated infection, *JAMA* 267:1364, 1992.

Menage MJ and others: Antiviral drug sensitivity in ocular herpes simplex virus infection, *Br J Ophthalmol* 74:532, 1990.

McLeish W: The ocular manifestations of syphilis in the HIV infected host, *Ophthalmology* 97:36, 1990.

Newsome DA and others: Microvascular aspects of acquired immune deficiency syndrome retinopathy, *Am J Ophthalmol* 98:590, 1984.

Ostler HB: Ocular manifestations of herpes zoster, varicella, infectious mononucleosis and cytomegalovirus disease, *Survey Ophthalmol* 21:151, 1976.

Parker J: Update on treatment of gonococcal ophthalmia, *Arch Ophthalmol* 109:614, 1991.

Pavin-Langston D: Diagnosis and management of herpes simplex ocular infection, *Int Ophthalmol Clin* 12:15, 1975.

Pepin J and others: The interaction of HIV infection and other sexually transmitted diseases: *AIDS* 1989, 33-9.

Pepose JS: Herpes simplex keratitis: role of viral infection versus immune response, *Survey Ophthalmol* 35:345, 1991.

Pepose JS and others: Acquired immune deficiency syndrome. Pathogenic mechanisms of ocular disease, *Ophthalmology* 92:472, 1985.

Pomerantz RJ and others: Infection of the retina by human immunodeficiency virus type I, *N Engl J Med* 317:1643, 1987.

Quiceno JI and others: Visual dysfunction without retinitis in patients with acquired immunodeficiency syndrome. *Am J Ophthalmol* 113:8, 1992.

Regillo C: Ocular tuberculosis, *JAMA* 266:1490, 1991.

Raub W: Immunogenic basis of chronic Lyme arthritis identified, *JAMA* 264:117, 1990.

Rolfs R: Epidemiology of primary and secondary syphilis in the United States, 1981–1989, *JAMA* 264:1432, 1990.

Schwab IR: Oral acyclovir in the management of herpes simplex ocular infections, *Ophthalmology* 95:423, 1988.

Schwarcz SK and others: Crack cocaine as a risk factor for gonorrhea among black teenagers, presented at the 117th Annual Meeting of the American Public Health Association, Oct. 2-26, 1989, Chicago, IL.

Schwarcz SK and others: National surveillance of antimicrobial resistance in *Neiserria gonorrhoeae, JAMA* 264:1413, 1990.

Strauss SE and others: Varicella zoster virus infections, biology, natural history, treatment and prevention, *Ann Intern Med* 108:221, 1988.

Weisenthal RW and others: Long-term outpatient treatment of CMV retinitis with ganciclovir in AIDS patients? *Br J Ophthalmol* 73:996, 1989.

Wilson JD: *Principles of internal medicine,* vol 1, New York 1991, p 658, McGraw Hill.

Winward KE, Hamed LM, and Glaser JS: The spectrum of optic nerve disease in human immunodeficiency virus infection, *Am J Ophthalmol* 107:373, 1989.

Young TL and others: Herpes simplex keratitis in patients with acquired immune deficiency syndrome, *Ophthalmology* 96:1476, 1989.

7

Collagen-Vascular Disease

MARTIN JAN BERGMAN

KEY TERMS

Arthritides	*Diffuse Myalgia*	*Polyarticular Arthritis*
Arthropathies	*Sicca Syndrome*	*Pauciarticular Arthritis*
Podagra	*Sjögren's Syndrome*	*Onycholysis*
Monoarticular Arthritis	*Xerophthalmia*	*Raynaud's Phenomenon*
Borrelia burgdorferi	*Spondyloarthropathies*	*Amaurosis Fugax*

R heumatologic diseases can vary from the most benign forms of tendinitis and bursitis to the life-threatening forms of systemic lupus erythematosus and vasculitis. The common denominator is usually some degree of joint or muscle pain, often erroneously termed "arthritis." In fact, more than 100 forms of arthritis have been described, each with its own unique presentation, prognosis, and treatment. Although the term "arthritis" is usually associated with the most common disease, degenerative joint disease or osteoarthritis, other systemic forms exist and often involve the eye in their manifestations.

Arthritides can be broken roughly into two categories—inflammatory and noninflammatory. The noninflammatory diseases are usually localized and nonsystemic. When a joint fluid or effusion is present and analyzed, the fluid is of normal viscosity (that of thick motor oil), clear, and with less than 1000 white blood cells/mm^3 on microscopic examination. The inflammatory diseases are often systemic, involving not only the joints but also other organs, including the eye, and are characterized by a joint effusion (if present) that is of decreased viscosity (water-like), cloudy, and with more than 1000 cells/mm^3. Although the presence of a noninflammatory fluid does not preclude the diagnosis of an inflammatory or systemic illness, the presence of an inflammatory fluid cannot be attributed to a benign process such as trauma. The most common cause of noninflammatory arthritis is osteoarthritis.

OSTEOARTHRITIS

Osteoarthritis (OA, degenerative joint disease, DJD) is clearly the most common condition that results in pain, swelling, and loss of function of the joints. It is what most people think of when they hear the term "arthritis." Usually, it is a disease of aging and is thought to be a reflection of wear and tear of the joints, although recent evidence has suggested a role for heredity and metabolism in its pathogenesis. Although more common in the elderly, it is not exclusive to this group and can be seen at almost any age.

The hallmark of osteoarthritis is cartilage loss leading to the loss of the joint space. As a result, patients complain of pain, particularly with the use of the affected area, and of crepitus, or a grinding sensation on movement of the joint. In an attempt to distribute the forces at the joint, the body lays down new bone, resulting in the formation of an osteophyte, which is perceived by the patient as a lump or other disfiguring feature. Although theoretically possible in any joint, osteoarthritis occurs only in particular joints unless another cause, such as trauma or a metabolic disturbance like hemochromatosis, is also present. Joints classically involved are the proximal and distal interphalangeal joints of the hands and feet, the shoulders, the cervical and lumbar spine, the hips, and the knees. Conspicuously spared are the wrists, elbows, and ankles. When these latter joints are involved, one must either carefully look for an underlying cause such as a previous fracture or consider a different diagnosis.

Degenerative joint disease is not a systemic disease and as a result does not involve the eyes directly. Its significance to the optometrist is more in terms of decreased mobility in the patients, which could make routine examinations more difficult to perform, and in terms of toxicities to the medications used to treat the condition, than in direct ocular manifestations. The usual medications are the nonsteroidal anti-inflammatory drugs (NSAIDs); their blockade of prostaglandin synthesis may result in a tendency toward bleeding. Thus, conjunctival hemorrhage and even retinal hemorrhage may occur in these patients, and they may have a tendency toward prolonged bleeding following any invasive procedure.

The inflammatory *arthropathies* can be further divided into those caused by chemical agents (crystal arthropathies), those caused by infectious agents, and those of unknown cause (rheumatoid arthritis, for example). In addition, some forms of "arthritis" occur in which the joints are not involved but severe systemic manifestations may occur (temporal arteritis, for example).

GOUT

Gout is the classic crystal-induced arthropathy, caused by the accumulation of monosodium urate crystals in the joint and surrounding tissue. It has been described for centuries and was once thought to be a disease of the rich and their dietary indiscretions. It is now known to be a disease of all socioeconomic groups. Rare, hereditary forms exist which can cause gout in children, but for the most part, gout is a disease of the middle aged and older. Predisposing characteristics include heavy use of alcohol, particularly beer and Chianti wine, exposure to lead either through occupational activities or from moonshine distilled in lead-containing containers (saturnine gout), diuretic use, renal impairment, and neoplastic conditions resulting in rapid cell turnover such as leukemias and lymphomas. Many people, however, have no obvious predisposing cause whatsoever.

The classic gouty attack is of acute onset, usually at night, and involves the first metatarsal region of the great toe *(podagra)*. The joint becomes red, hot, swollen, and tender to even the slightest touch. The attack usually lasts for about 5 to 7 days and then resolves completely without residual pain. Any other joint can be involved, and multiple joints may be involved at the same time. In untreated cases, collections of monosodium urate known as tophi may appear at friction sites of the body, such as the elbow, and cause confusion with other diseases.

The diagnosis is best made by aspiration of the involved joint or tophus and by the demonstration of the monosodium urate crystals ingested by white cells when the fluid is viewed under compensated polarized light. Often the elevated serum uric acid level is used, but this is not consistently diagnostic, as low levels of uric acid may be seen during an acute gouty attack and high levels of uric acid may be seen in completely normal individuals.

Treatment of gout includes the use of NSAIDs, often indomethacin, and colchicine to relieve the acute attack and probenecid or hypouricemic agents such as allopurinol for the long-term treatment and the prevention of tophi or renal urate deposits. In patients in whom these medications may not be used, local injections of corticosteroids or even systemic steroids may be employed, and when all else fails, ice and narcotic analgesics are also helpful.

As with degenerative joint disease, gout rarely if ever directly involves the eyes. Indomethacin, when taken regularly for prolonged periods of time, however, can cause corneal deposits and retinal disturbances. For that reason, any patient on chronic indomethacin therapy for gout or any other reason should have regular screening examinations to check for those toxicities.

Calcium pyrophosphate dihydrate (CPPD) is another crystal that can deposit in joints and cause inflammatory symptoms, often referred to as "pseudogout." The symptoms and signs are often the same as in gout, and the definitive diagnosis can be made only by joint aspiration and the demonstration of the calcium pyrophosphate dihydrate crystals in the joint fluid. CPPD is also seen in a number of other diseases that warrant attention. The most common is degenerative joint disease, but CPPD can also be seen in patients with hypothyroidism, hyperparathyroidism, hemochromatosis, and hypophosphatasia. Anyone with the diagnosis of CPPD should be screened for these diseases by a complete physical examination and by appropriate laboratory testing.

Other crystals that can affect the joints include calcium hydroxyapatite, which can cause a bilateral swelling of the shoulders known as "Milwaukee shoulder," and calcium oxalate, which is seen in patients on chronic hemodialysis. From an op-

tometric standpoint, however, these crystals have little significance.

INFECTIOUS ARTHRITIDES

Any infection that can spread through the blood can eventually end up in a joint. Infectious arthritides can be rapidly destructive and must be treated aggressively with repeated joint aspirations and drainage and the institution of appropriate antibiotic therapies. Although staphylococcal and streptococcal species are the most common infectious agents involving the joints, special considerations must be kept in mind when dealing with certain age groups and patient populations. Infectious arthropathies are usually monoarticular or pauciarticular (involving less than four joints), and the joints are characteristically hot, tender, and swollen with signs of marked inflammation on synovial fluid analysis (white blood cell [WBC] counts as high as 150,000/mm^3). Unless another cause is known or demonstrated, any patient presenting with a monoarticular or pauciarticular inflammatory arthritis should be considered to have an infectious cause until proven otherwise.

Neisseria gonorrhoeae should be considered in any sexually active patient who presents with a *monoarticular* (single joint) inflammatory *arthritis*. Classically, the patient presents with a hot, tender, and swollen large joint (knee, wrist, ankle) and multiple petechial or pustular skin lesions. At this stage, cervical (or urethral in men) cultures are often negative, as are anal and throat swabs, and the diagnosis must be made on a clinical basis alone. Isolation of the microorganism from the blood or synovial fluid establishes the diagnosis, but it is not essential. As with all sexually transmitted diseases, both the patient and his or her partner(s) must be treated to prevent the recurrence of the disease after therapy has ended.

Patients who are intravenous drug users are also at high risk for the development of infectious arthritis. In these patients the clinician must be aware not only of the usual pathogens such as staphylococci and streptococci, but also of the gramnegative pathogens, such as pseudomonas. In these patients, or in any other patient who develops an inflammatory arthritis in the face of a recent bacterial infection, attention should be given to the presence of splinter hemorrhages in the conjunctival area and retinal infarcts, suggestive of a bacterial endocarditis. The ocular manifestations may be one of the earlier signs of this potentially fatal disease and may lead to early evaluation for the presence of cardiac valvular involvement and appropriate aggressive antibiotic therapy.

LYME DISEASE

Lyme disease is another disease in which joint involvement is one of the hallmarks. This disease is caused by the transmission of the *Borrelia burgdorferi* organism following a bite from the deer tick *Ixodes dammini* (see Chapter 6). The disease is divided into three stages: early localized disease, early disseminated disease, and late disseminated disease. In the early localized disease, which usually occurs about 1 week after the exposure to the organism, the patient complains of fevers and diffuse muscle aches *(diffuse myalgia)* and the presence of a slowly expanding red rash with a faded center, the erythema migrans rash. The rash is noticed by only 60% of patients, and even fewer may be aware of any tick bite at all. One of the other early signs of Lyme disease is conjunctivitis, and the presence of this ocular sign should prompt serologic testing for the disease.

In early disseminated disease, patients may develop cardiac involvement (heart block) or neurologic involvement. Meningitis may occur, but nerve palsies, particularly facial palsies but also palsies of the other oculomotor nerves, are more common. Optic neuritis has also been described at this stage. As with conjunctivitis, the presence of any oculomotor disturbance, Bell's palsy, or optic neuritis should prompt the clinician to obtain appropriate serologic studies to diagnose Lyme disease.

The most common disturbance of late disseminated disease is an inflammatory arthritis, usually monoarticular and usually involving the large, weight-bearing joints. Other manifestations at this stage include more severe neurologic deficits, including cognitive dysfunctions, optic neuritis, and chronic cutaneous changes.

Lyme disease is treatable and curable at all stages of disease, so correct diagnosis is essential. The most frequent laboratory test is a Lyme titer, done by an immunofluorescence or an enzyme-linked immunosorbent assay (ELISA) technique, and confirmation often involves the use of a specialized Western blot study. The presence of the classic erythema migrans rash alone is sufficient to make the diagnosis and requires no further testing. Because this rash may occur at the same time as the conjunctivitis, specific questioning for the presence of a rash in any patient presenting with acute conjunctivitis may lead to an early diagnosis and early institution of antibiotic therapy.

RHEUMATOID ARTHRITIS

The most common of the inflammatory arthropathies is rheumatoid arthritis, a disease that generally affects women of child-bearing age. This is a chronic disease that is characterized by symmetric swelling of multiple joints, usually of the hands, wrists, hips, knees, ankles, and feet. Classically spared are the distal interphalangeal joints of the hands and feet and the lumbar spinal region. Because it is long-standing and inflammatory, joint destruction, called erosions, can occur, resulting in loss of function and deformities.

Being a systemic disease, RA displays many signs and symptoms of nonarticular involvement. Patients may develop nodules, particularly at the elbows, which also signify a more severe disease. These nodules may affect the lungs, or the lungs may be involved separately, causing shortness of breath and a radiographic appearance that may be indistinguishable from lung cancer. Pleuritic involvement may also cause chest pain and discomfort. In more severe and usually long-standing disease, a vasculitis may develop. This inflammation of the blood vessels can cause infarction of the tissue perfused by that vessel and can result in localized tissue death and may even be fatal to the patient.

The eyes are often involved in rheumatoid arthritis, either as a direct result of the disease itself, due to conditions associated with the disease, or due to the medications used to treat the disease. Often this involvement is subtle and needs to be specifically looked for, before it becomes a more severe or permanent problem.

The most common problem is dry eyes, referred to as the *sicca syndrome.* In patients with rheumatoid arthritis, this is often caused by a related disease called Sjögren's syndrome. *Sjögren's syndrome* is an inflammatory disease of the exocrine or secreting gland system. It may exist in a primary form, not related to any other disease, or it may be seen in a secondary form, associated with another disease, such as rheumatoid arthritis. Nearly all of the inflammatory diseases seen by rheumatologists may be associated with Sjögren's syndrome, but it should be considered specifically in patients with rheumatoid arthritis, systemic lupus erythematosus, and primary biliary cirrhosis. The usual symptoms are related to failure of the exocrine glands to fulfill their primary function, that of lubrication. When it fails in the mouth, the result is dry mouth (xerostomia) leading to a burning sensation in the mouth, loss of taste, and dental caries. The infiltration of the glands by inflammatory cells may result in swelling of the parotid, the submandibular, and occasionally the lacrimal glands.

When this syndrome involves the eyes, it results in *xerophthalmia,* or dry eyes. Patients may not complain of this, so the examiner must specifically ask the patient about symptoms such as dry, itchy, scratchy eyes or the absence of tears. This absence of tears can be measured by a simple procedure known as Schirmer's test. A strip of filter paper is placed in the conjunctival sac and observed for 5 to 10 minutes. The extent of the wetting of the paper can be measured, with normal being 10 mm after 5 minutes and 20 mm after 10 minutes. Anything less than this is considered abnormal but is not diagnostic of Sjögren's syndrome. Other conditions that can cause dry eyes include medications, age, tobacco, and other diseases.

To be diagnostic, a patient must show changes of the cornea reflecting the damage done as a result of chronic dryness, defined as keratoconjunctivitis sicca. This requires a slit-lamp examination of the eye and the use of staining with either rose bengal or fluorescein. Properly treated with topical lubricants, keratoconjunctivitis sicca is little more than a nuisance for most patients, but untreated it can lead to a filamentous keratitis and corneal scarring.

Rarely, Sjögren's syndrome may affect the central nervous system, presenting a clinical scenario indistinguishable from multiple sclerosis. Thus, patients may have symptoms consistent with optic neuritis or extraocular muscle palsies. When this occurs, the disease is often treated aggressively with high-dose steroids and even cytotoxic agents.

Direct involvement of the eye in rheumatoid arthritis takes on three forms—episcleritis, scleritis, and scleromalacia—and usually occurs in patients with severe long-standing disease who test positive for "rheumatoid factors," IgM antibodies directed against IgG antibodies found in the blood of 85% of patients with rheumatoid arthritis. Episcleritis is a superficial inflammation of the sclera characterized by pain and redness, as well as a foreign body sensation. The involved area may be reddened or have a yellow, nodular quality and be easily movable using a Q-tip, reflecting its superficial nature. This condition often requires no therapy, but when it does, it generally responds to topical steroids alone.

As the lesion gets more severe and thus involves deeper structures, it becomes adherent to the sclera and is called scleritis. Biopsy of this lesion, as well as the lesion of episcleritis, is histologically similar to the nodules of the skin, so they both can be considered to be rheumatoid nodules of the eye. Scleritis is a potentially severe condition which, if untreated, can result thinning of the sclera (scleromalacia). When scleromalacia occurs, the uvea may bulge through the scleral defect (scleromalacia perforans), and the patient's vision may be threatened by the resulting uveitis. Scleritis is usually treated with a combination of topical and systemic steroids. If this fails to resolve the inflammation, aggressive treatments using immunosuppressive medications such as azathioprin or cyclophosphamide may be employed. (Figs. 7-1 and 7-2).

The two most common medications that may affect the eyes are systemic steroids (prednisone, methylprednisolone [Medrol], or "cortisone") and the antimalarial drugs (hydroxychloroquine [Plaquenil] and chloroquine). Cataract formation can occur in any patient taking steroids for a prolonged period of time and can result in decreased visual acuity, halos, or blurred vision. These cataracts are not generally reversible and may require surgical intervention. Glaucoma may also occur or may be worsened in chronic steroid therapy, so that monitoring intraocular pressures is essential.

The antimalarial agents affect the eye in two fashions: direct deposits in the cornea and a retinopathy, bull's eye maculopathy. Caught early, both of these complications of therapy are generally completely reversible with cessation of the medications, but ignored they can lead to decreased visual acuity and blindness. To monitor patients for this, eye examinations are recommended at 6-month intervals, and the examination should include formal visual field testing with a low-intensity (red dot) cursor.

JUVENILE RHEUMATOID ARTHRITIS

Juvenile rheumatoid arthritis is the most common connective tissue disease of childhood, and although it may have some similarities to its adult counterpart, it differs from the adult form in many ways. The disease is divided into three categories determined by the initial disease presentation: systemic, in which the initial signs and symptoms may not involve the joints at all; polyarticular, involving more than four joints; and pauciarticular, involving four or fewer joints. A fourth form of juvenile rheumatoid arthritis is sometimes described which is indistinguishable from the adult *spondyloarthropathies,* described below.

Systemic juvenile rheumatoid arthritis, also known as Still's disease, is, as its name implies, a systemic illness, with joint involvement sometimes being a less important feature than other systemic manifestations. These children may appear acutely ill, with high, spiking, hectic fevers, lymphadenopathy, splenomegaly, and strikingly high WBC counts, suggesting leukemia or lymphoma. In about half, a destructive arthritis develops which can lean to chronic deformities and disabilities. Fortunately, the eye is not a major organ affected, but it is not entirely spared. A chronic uveitis may develop (see Chapter 18) and may result in syn-

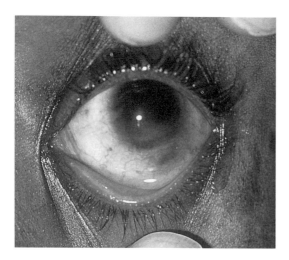

FIG. 7-1 Scleromalacia perforans secondary to rheumatoid arthritis. Note the dark gray uvea protruding through the sclera surrounded by the deep scleral injection, indicating scleritis.

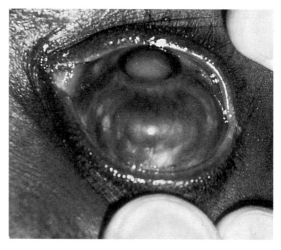

FIG. 7-2 Advanced scleromalacia perforans. Note dramatic protrusion of the uvea through a thinned-out sclera.

echia formation and loss of vision, much as in the pauciarticular form described below. Fortunately, in this form of juvenile rheumatoid arthritis, it is a rather rare occurrence.

The *polyarticular arthritis* in many ways mimics the disease of adults. Patients are frequently female, may have rheumatoid factors or antinuclear antibodies present in their serum, and may have a chronic, unremitting course with joint destruction, erosions, and early fusion of the growth plates. When the eye is involved, the presenting feature may be a chronic uveitis with an incidence that falls somewhere between that of the systemic disease and that of the pauciarticular form.

The *pauciarticular arthritis* has the gravest prognosis regarding the eyes yet overall has the best prognosis. In fact, the ocular manifestations of this disease cause the majority of the morbidity in these children. Chronic uveitis may develop in as many as 20% of patients, who are generally female and have a positive antinuclear antibody rather than a positive rheumatoid factor, as seen in adult rheumatoid arthritis. The uveitis is almost always anterior (iridocyclitis) and usually bilateral. Repeated bouts of uveitis can result in synechia formation, fibrous deposits in the anterior chamber, and band keratopathy. Cataract formation may also occur, both as a result of the chronic ocular inflammation and as a result of steroid therapy that may need to be employed. All can result in decreased vision and possible blindness but are easily treatable if the proper diagnosis is made and proper therapy begun. This usually takes the form of topical steroid preparations. Because of the frequency of uveitis in all children with juvenile rheumatoid arthritis, as well as the excellent resolution of the uveitis with proper treatment, constant and routine monitoring of these children with slit-lamp examination is an essential part of their treatment, regardless of which form of disease the child may have.

THE SPONDYLOARTHROPATHIES

The spondyloarthropathies constitute a group of diseases which have certain common features, including inflammatory arthritis, involvement of the sacroiliac joints to varying degrees, involvement of tendon insertion sites (enthesopathy), and genetic predisposition associated with the HLA-B27 gene. Likewise, they all have very similar extra-articular manifestations, including aortitis, cardiac conduction abnormalities, and uveitis.

Ankylosing Spondylitis

Ankylosing spondylitis is the prototype of this group of diseases. It is a disease of young men which usually begins insidiously as back pain and can result in fusion of the joints of the spine and the sacroiliac joints. Without proper monitoring of posture, these patients can become "hunched-over," unable to stand straight or look up. The HLA-B27 gene (see Chapter 3) is found in nearly 95% of these patients. Involvement of the axial skeleton is the hallmark of disease, and the peripheral skeleton is usually spared. Iridocyclitis is seen in about 25% of patients and may be the initial presenting feature of the disease. Because of the degree of pain that these patients may have, indomethacin is often employed in the treatment. Patients should be questioned concerning their drug use and screened appropriately.

Reiter's Disease

Reiter's disease is a peripheral arthropathy, often following a venereal disease but also following bouts of infectious diarrhea. A classic triad of arthritis, urethritis, and conjunctivitis is described, although an "incomplete" form is also commonly recognized. Besides frank arthritis, which is of the pauciarticular variety, tendinitis (often of the Achilles tendon) and a diffuse swelling of the entire digit (sausage digit) is common, usually involving the lower extremities to a greater degree than the upper extremities. Cutaneous involvement may be manifested by keratoderma blennorrhagicum (hyperkeratotic lesions of the foot which are indistinguishable histologically from psoriasis [Fig. 7-3]) and by circinate balanitis (ulcerations and hyperkeratotic lesions) of the penis. Oral and vaginal ulcerations may also occur. This disease, like ankylosing spondylitis, has a striking male predi-

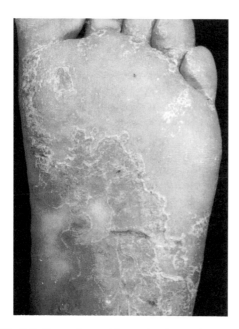

FIG. 7-3 Keratoderma blennorrhagicum. Hyperkeratotic lesions of the foot in Reiter's syndrome. *(From Habif TB:* Clinical dermatology, *St. Louis, 1990, Mosby–Year Book.)*

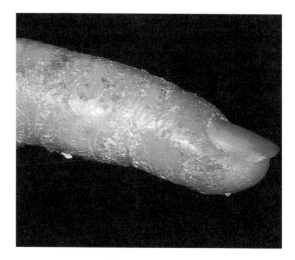

FIG. 7-4 Psoriatic arthritis. Psoriasis of the digits and fingernail pitting are hallmarks of this disease; this swollen joint is painful. *(From Habif TB:* Clinical dermatology, *St. Louis, 1990, Mosby–Year Book.)*

lection and a strong association with the HLA-B27 antigen. Besides the conjunctivitis, which is part of the diagnostic triad, these patients are also at risk for the development of uveitis and iritis. Recently, an association has been made between severe cases of Reiter's disease and HIV infection, so that patients presenting with uveitis and arthritis should at least be questioned for risk factors.

Psoriatic Arthritis

There are four forms of psoriatic arthritis: a symmetric polyarticular form that appears clinically to be essentially the same as rheumatoid arthritis, a predominantly distal form involving the distal interphangeal joints preferentially, an asymmetric oligoarticular (pauciarticular) form, and a very destructive form called arthritis mutilans, which can result in dissolution of the joint and surrounding bone, producing a shortened, "telescoped" digit. The common feature of all of these forms is the presence of psoriasis. The degree of psoriasis does not distinguish one form or another, and there is

no correlation between the severity of the skin disease and the severity of the joint involvement. The fingernails are frequently involved, showing pitting and even destruction *(onycholysis)*. As with the other spondyloarthropathies, psoriatic arthritis can be associated with both conjunctivitis and uveitis/iritis (Fig. 7-4).

Inflammatory Bowel Disease

Inflammatory bowel diseases such as Crohn's disease and ulcerative colitis (see Chapter 12) can also be associated with an oligoarthropathy, generally involving the larger joints of the lower extremities, as well as an enthesopathy, often involving the Achilles tendon. Patients may develop axial skeletal abnormalities indistinguishable from ankylosing spondylitis and have ocular involvement to much the same extent and degree.

SYSTEMIC LUPUS ERYTHEMATOSUS

Fortunately, some of the most severe systemic rheumatologic diseases have few or no ocular manifestations. Systemic lupus erythematosus (Fig. 7-5) is a disease usually of young women which can affect nearly all body systems. The most fre-

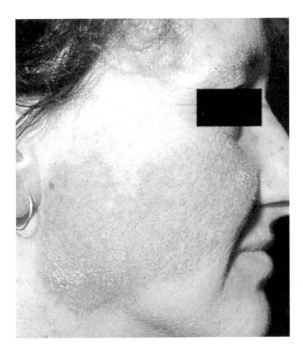

FIG. 7-5 Systemic lupus erythematosus of the face. Note the reddish "butterfly" rash across the cheek. *(From Lawrence CM and Cox NH:* Physical signs in dermatology: *St. Louis, 1990, Mosby–Year Book.)*

quently involved sites are the skin, where rashes, such as the butterfly facial rash and the scarring discoid rash, may occur; the joints, which may become swollen but not deformed; and the coverings of body cavities (serositis), resulting in pleuritic pain, pericarditis, and abdominal pain. Hematologic abnormalities are also common and may include anemia, low total WBC counts or specific defects in lymphocytes or granulocytes, and low platelet counts (thrombocytopenia). A coagulation defect may be noted on laboratory testing, but this so-called lupus anticoagulant, measured by the increase in the partial prothrombin time, may actually represent a tendency toward clotting and thrombosis rather than a bleeding tendency. The only common ocular manifestation is the cotton-wool spot, although conjunctivitis and uveitis may rarely occur.

The most feared complications involve the kidneys and the central nervous system. Kidney in-

volvement is often first noticed either on routine screening of the urine or by the new onset of hypertension. These patients may develop massive proteinuria, resulting in the nephrotic syndrome, may develop a rapidly progressive renal failure ending in the need for dialysis, or may have a more indolent course. Formal diagnosis often involves renal biopsy to determine the exact kidney lesion, and therapy is modified on the basis of these results.

The central nervous system manifestations are likewise diverse, ranging from mild cognitive defects to stroke. The more common problems encountered are seizures and frank psychosis, sometimes resulting in erroneous psychiatric hospitalizations. However, patients may develop infarction of the spinal cord, multiple brain infarcts, and inflammatory neuropathies, causing facial and oculomotor palsies and optic neuritis.

The diagnosis is made by the presence of the clinical signs and symptoms with the aid of specific antibody testing, most frequently the antinuclear antibody. Other antibodies often tested for are the anti–double-stranded DNA, the Smith and RNP antibodies, and antibodies to "Ro" and "La" (SS-A and SS-B). Some patients falsely test positive to the commonly used screening tests for syphilis (VDRL, RPR), so care must be used in diagnosing syphilis in patients who may have systemic lupus erythematosus.

The treatment depends upon the organ system involved and the severity of the involvement. When the disease is not life threatening, as with the arthritis, skin disease, or serositis, treatment is usually restricted to symptomatic relief using NSAIDs, with the addition of antimalarials, such as hydroxychloroquine. When the latter is used, routine ocular examinations are essential to monitor for the side effects of this medication.

As the disease manifestations become more severe, the therapies become more aggressive. Corticosteroids form the backbone of many of these therapies, but when life-threatening involvement of the kidneys or central nervous system is present, cytotoxic agents such as cyclophosphamide may be necessary.

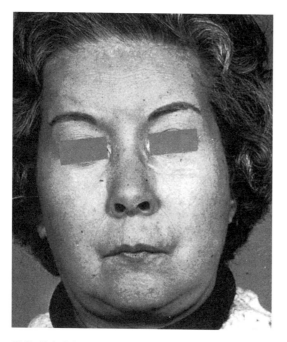

FIG. 7-6 Scleroderma. Note the classic signs of the tight skin over the forehead, nose, and cheeks, giving a "pinched" facial appearance and a reduced palpebral aperture size. *(From Cawson RA and others:* Pathology: The mechanisms of disease, *St. Louis, 1989, Mosby–Year Book.)*

DIFFUSE SYSTEMIC SCLEROSIS

Diffuse systemic sclerosis (scleroderma) is a chronic disease, predominantly of the skin, but also of the kidneys, the gastrointestinal tract, and the lungs, which also tends to affect younger women. *Raynaud's phenomenon,* or vascular spasm of the fingers and toes on cold exposure, may be the first symptom, but the patients may go on to develop a thickened skin that literally encases the body. A limited form (limited systemic sclerosis, CREST syndrome) also exists in which the skin thickening is restricted to the distal parts of the extremities and the face and tends to have less organ involvement. Fortunately, direct eye involvement is extremely rare, with the only common problem being the result of dryness due to the inability to fully close the tight and thickened eyelids (Fig. 7-6).

DERMATOMYOSITIS

Another rare disease that may have ocular manifestations is dermatomyositis, a disease of the skin and muscles, and its counterpart, polymyositis, which is identical expect for the lack of skin involvement. The common feature is proximal muscle weakness caused by inflammation of the skeletal muscles. As the disease progresses, more diffuse muscle involvement ensues and may result in difficulties with swallowing, aspiration, respiratory failure, and, rarely, involvement of the muscles of the eye and lid. Conjunctivitis, episcleritis, iritis, and uveitis have all been described, but the most common lesion, which distinguishes dermatomyositis from polymyositis, is the presence of a purple blush of the eyelid known as the "heliotrope" in the former (Fig. 7-7).

VASCULITIDES

A number of vasculitides (inflammatory disease of the blood vessels) may involve the eyes to varying degrees. Polyarteritis nodosa and Wegener's granulomatosis are two such diseases which can cause any number of inflammatory conditions of the eye ranging from conjunctivitis to uveitis and optic neuritis (Fig. 7-8).

GIANT CELL ARTERITIS

A more common form of vasculitis, one that the average practitioner is very likely to encounter, is temporal arteritis (TA, giant cell arteritis [GCA]). This is a disease of middle age and older which affects men and women equally. The presenting complaints include headache, usually in the temporal region, but not exclusively localized to this region, scalp tenderness, numbness of the tongue and jaw when talking or chewing (jaw and tongue claudication), and diffuse arthralgias and myalgias of the shoulder and hip girdle regions (polymyalgia rheumatica). *Amaurosis fugax* may occur, but all too frequently the presenting complaint is sudden onset of monocular blindness, which may be permanent, the result of infarction of the ciliary artery. Temporal arteritis is a medical emergency re-

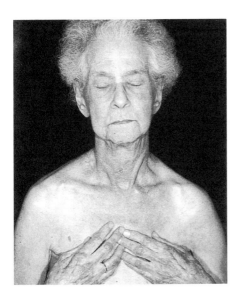

FIG. 7-7 Dermatomyositis. Erythema pattern in a symmetric distribution on the chest, face, and fingers. *(From Habif TB: Clinical dermatology, St. Louis, 1990, Mosby–Year Book.)*

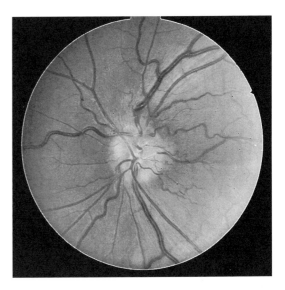

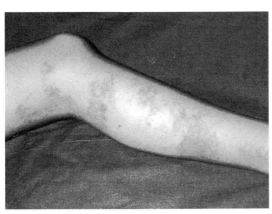

FIG. 7-8 Polyarteritis nodosa. Chronic painful ulceration of the leg, ankle, and foot in a patient with polyarteritis nodosa. *(From Lawrence CM and Cox NH: Physical signs in dermatology: color atlas and text, London, 1993, Wolfe Medical Publishers, Ltd.)*

FIG. 7-9 Swelling of the optic nerve head in a patient with temporal arteritis.

quiring immediate institution of corticosteroid therapy as soon as the diagnosis is considered. Failure to treat these patients promptly may result in irreversible blindness in the affected eye and blindness in the unaffected eye in 50% of patients, within 1 day to 3 weeks of onset of the first eye. The diagnosis is confirmed by an elevation of the erythrocyte sedimentation rate, but therapy should be begun even before test results are available (Fig. 7-9).

Bibliography

Cohen AS (ed): *Laboratory diagnostic procedures in the rheumatic diseases*, ed 3, Orlando, FL, 1985, Grune and Stratton.

Fassbender HG: *Normal and pathological synovial tissue with emphasis on rheumatic arthritis*. In Cohen AS and Bennett JC (eds): *Rheumatology and immunology,* ed 2, Orlando, FL, 1986, Grune and Stratton.

Leroy EC: *Scleroderma (systemic sclerosis).* In Kelly WR and others (eds): *Textbook of rheumatology,* ed 2, Philadelphia, 1985, WB Saunders Co.

McCarty DJ (ed): *Arthritis and allied disorders,* Philadelphia, 1985, Lea & Febiger.

Talan N: Sjögren's syndrome. In Rose N and Mackay I (eds): *The autoimmune diseases,* New York, 1985, Academic Press.

Wyngaarden JB and Smith LH Jr (eds): *Cecil textbook of medicine,* ed 19, Philadelphia, 1992, WB Saunders.

8

Dermatology

DAVID C. BRIGHT

KEY TERMS

Subcutaneous Tissue	Bulla	Atrophy
Dermis	Plaque	Excoriation
Epidermis	Wheal	Lichenification
Macule	Scale	Telangiectasia
Papule	Crust	Comedones
Nodule	Erosion	Urticaria
Tumor	Ulcer	Angioedema
Pustule	Fissure	Eczematous Dermatitis
Vesicle		

---

*T*he skin is the largest organ of the human body. Its tissue grows, differentiates, and renews itself constantly. The skin acts as an immune barrier between internal structures and the external environment, providing protection from mechanical and chemical trauma, microbial invasion, and thermal damage, and additionally allowing temperature regulation. The primary care optometrist is frequently faced with dermatologic conditions of the periorbital area and face. They occasionally occur as cutaneous manifestations of systemic disease but more often as benign or malignant skin lesions or growths. A working knowledge of dermatology is useful to the practitioner, both in recognition and in appropriate referral of various skin conditions.

The skin consists of three layers: subcutaneous tissue, dermis, and epidermis (from deepest to most superficial). The *subcutaneous tissue* is the site of the deep hair follicles, sweat glands, and lipid metabolism and storage. The *dermis* contains shorter hair follicles and sebaceous glands, as well as collagen, which contributes to the elasticity and support of the skin. Other structural elements include blood and lymphatic vessels, nerves, and eccrine sweat glands. Multiple cellular elements are present: lymphocytes, macrophages, mast cells, polymorphonuclear leukocytes, and eosinophils. The dermis ranges in thickness from 0.3 mm on the eyelids to 3.0 mm on the back. The *epidermis* is avascular, stratified squamous epithelium. Its basal layer lies deepest to the surface and is the site of basal cells, the germinal cells that give rise to all other cells of the epidermis as they progressively differentiate. Basal cells divide to form keratinocytes, produce insoluble protein, continuously flatten, and finally die as they reach the surface, forming the stratum corneum. The epidermis usually requires 3 to 4 weeks to replicate itself. Also present in the epidermis are melanocytes (located in the basal layer, producing melanin), Langerhans' cells (acting as immune sentinels), and Merkel cells (acting as mechanoreceptors). The epidermis ranges in thickness from 0.05 mm on the lids to 1.5 mm on the palms and soles.[16,96,222]

EXAMINATION

One component of dermatologic examination is the use of bright, white light. Daylight is best. If possible, position the patient in front of a window with natural light exposing the area to be evaluated.[240] In addition to gross examination, magnification using a transilluminator, direct ophthalmoscope, biomicroscope, and hand or head loupe is critical.[16]

Palpation is as valuable as observation. The examiner should carefully palpate the entity for texture, surface characteristics, firmness, depth, and attachment to any underlying structures. Additionally, regional lymph nodes should be palpated for any hard, discrete masses, suggesting metastasis from a malignant lesion.[246] The examiner should stretch out wrinkles, exposing lesions that may be concealed in shadow or within the concavity of a skin fold (particularly in the upper lids). Additional stretching is accomplished by folding down the ears, pulling aside the nose, and pushing back the hair.[240] A glass microscope slide or transparent plastic ruler is used to flatten the lesion being evaluated; blanching upon compression, followed by filling afterward, is characteristic of vascular lesions.[16] The evaluation of all ocular areas is important, including bulbar and palpebral conjunctivae, lid margins, and the fornices. Any crust or scale should be removed (when possible) with a moistened, sterile swab or forceps.[246] Examination of nonocular or facial skin sites, when possible, is valuable.

Dermatologic entities should be described by words, drawings, and photography. The following items should be noted[16,34,246]:

Type of lesion: primary, secondary, or special (see box on p. 143)
Color: hypo/hyperpigmentation, erythema, pallor
Size and shape
Elevation, firmness, consistency
Surface: color, questionable integrity, crust, scale, erosion, ulceration, telangiectasias
Location, distribution, any grouping
Surrounding skin: normal, traumatized, actinic damage, scarring
Associated ocular findings: hyperemia, madarosis, tearing

History of the dermatologic lesion and other information are most important.[16,19,246] They should include the following:

Awareness of the lesion
Duration (since birth or acquired)
Changes in size, shape, appearance, or sensation
Continuing infection, inflammation, or bleeding
Recurrence
Demographics: age, race, gender, general health, occupation, avocation, chemical/toxic exposure, sunlight exposure, geographic region during childhood/teen years
History of other malignancies or trauma

TYPES OF SKIN LESIONS

Primary lesions

Macule: circumscribed, flat discoloration, variety of colors

Papule: circumscribed, solid, elevated lesion; up to 5 mm diameter; variety of colors

Nodule: circumscribed, solid, elevated lesion; larger than 5 mm diameter

Tumor: large nodule

Pustule: circumscribed collection of leukocytes and free fluid

Vesicle: circumscribed collection of free fluid; up to 5 mm diameter

Bulla: circumscribed collection of free fluid; larger than 5 mm diameter

Plaque: circumscribed, elevated, superficial, solid lesion; larger than 5 millimeters diameter; often formed by confluence of multiple papules

Wheal: firm, edematous plaque; caused by infiltration of the dermis by fluid

Secondary lesions

Scale: excess dead epidermal cells, resulting from abnormal keratinization and shedding

Crust: dried serum, cellular debris (scab)

Erosion: focal loss of epidermis; no penetration beyond dermis

Ulcer: focal loss of epidermis and dermis

Fissure: linear loss of epidermis and dermis; sharply defined walls

Atrophy: depression in the skin, caused by thinning of epidermis or dermis

Scar: abnormal collection of connective tissue; damage to dermis

Special lesions

Excoriation: erosion resulting from scratching

Cyst: circumscribed lesion with a wall and lumen

Lichenification: thickened epidermis caused by scratching; furrowed surface (washboard)

Telangiectasia: dilated superficial capillaries or blood vessels

Comedones: sebaceous and keratinous material plugging the opening of a hair or sebaceous follicle

Adapted from Habif TP: *Clinical dermatology*, ed 2, St Louis, 1990, Mosby–Year Book.

Other family members with malignancies (dermatologic or other)

Evaluation of old photographs

ALLERGIC CONDITIONS

Urticaria and Angioneurotic Edema

Urticaria and angioneurotic edema (angioedema) are dermatologic manifestations of the Type I (immediate) hypersensitivity reaction. These conditions result from antigen-induced release of vasoactive substances from mast cells or basophils sensitized with immunoglobulin E (IgE) antibody and are typically of sudden onset, rarely lasting longer than 24 to 48 hours.

Urticaria consists of hives or wheals, superficial plaques that are either erythematous or white. Histamine and immune mediators cause capillary endothelial cell contraction; subsequent vasodilation and transudation of fluid into the surrounding tissue result in formation of hives (Fig. 8-1). Surface color of hives varies: uniform red or white, or a white plaque with a surrounding red or other colored border. Hives range in size from 2-mm papules to giant hives and itch in varying degrees.[96]

Angioedema refers to very thick plaques caused by edema extending into the dermal, subcutaneous, or submucosal tissue (Fig. 8-2). Angioedema causes burning and painful swelling but typically does not itch as severely as hives because fewer nerve endings are nearby.[96] Frequently the overlying epidermis is unaffected in cases of angioedema.[9]

There are many causes of urticaria (see box on p. 145). The majority of cases of urticaria are due to ingestion of either foods or medications. Penicillin is the most common offender among medications.[161,219] The causes of angioedema are somewhat similar to those of hives (see box on p. 145).

Urticaria and angioedema may occur as individual phenomena or simultaneously in any location. Angioedema commonly affects the face as well as other sites.[239] Periorbital tissue and eyelids are susceptible to angioedema owing to the spongy

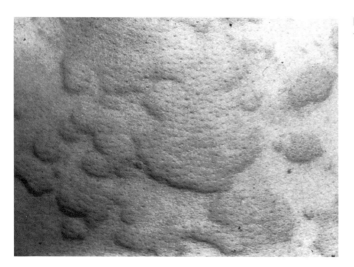

FIG. 8-1 Urticaria, with multiple hives of varying sizes.

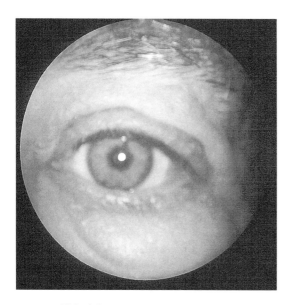

FIG. 8-2 Angioedema of the eyelid.

quality of the tissue and potential space for transudation of fluid.[80] Eyelids are the most frequent sites of ocular allergy due to the extreme thinness of the eyelid skin as well as their intimate relations with both palpebral and bulbar conjunctivae.[9,17]

Both hives and angioneurotic edema respond well to oral antihistamines, with resolution occurring within a period of hours to a few days. Sedating antihistamines may be desirable for the ad-

ditional relief they provide by inducing rest. Eyelid involvement may be also managed with cool compresses initially (inducing vasoconstriction and reducing transudation), then with warm compresses (enhancing drainage of fluid).

Allergic Contact Dermatitis

Contact with irritant or antigenic environmental substances may result in *eczematous dermatitis*. This reaction occurs most frequently with irritant substances such as strong soaps or industrial solvents, both of which extract lipid from the epidermis, but also with other chemicals that cause dehydration. A small group of patients are susceptible to allergic contact dermatitis, seemingly with a genetic predisposition. Irritant contact dermatitis is about three times more common than allergic contact dermatitis.[73]

The mechanism of the allergy process involves Type IV (cell-mediated or delayed) hypersensitivity, caused by one or more exposures to an antigenic substance (see box on p. 145). A low molecular weight hapten penetrates into the epidermis and combines with epidermal protein to form an antigen, which is then processed immunologically. Sensitized effector T lymphocytes are ultimately produced.[80] Depending on the sensitizing nature of the original antigen, the patient may require a single exposure to a small amount of a strongly sen-

CAUSES OF URTICARIA

Food—fish, shellfish, nuts, eggs, chocolate, strawberries, tomatoes, pork, cow's milk, cheese, wheat, yeast

Food Additives—salicylates, benzoates, aspartame (NutraSweet), dyes such as tartrazine

Drugs—includes penicillin, aspirin, sulfonamides

Infections of varying microbial causes
> chronic bacterial (sinus, dental, chest, urinary tract)
> fungal (dermatophytosis, candidiasis)
> viral (hepatitis B prodromal reaction, infectious mononucleosis)
> protozoal and helminthic (intestinal worms, malaria)

Inhalants—pollen, mold spores, animal danders, dust mites, aerosols, volatile chemicals, nasal sprays, insect sprays, feathers

Internal disease—includes serum sickness, systemic lupus erythematosus, hyperthyroidism, carcinomas, lymphomas, juvenile rheumatoid arthritis, polycythemia vera, rheumatic fever

Physical stimuli—dermatographism, pressure, exercise, water, solar exposure, temperatures (heat and cold)

Nonimmunologic contact—nettles, jellyfish, some medications (cinnamic aldehyde, compound 48/80, DMSO)

Skin diseases—urticaria pigmentosa, dermatitis herpetiformis, pemphigoid, amyloidosis

Hormones—pregnancy, premenstrual flare-ups (progesterone)

Insect bites and stings—mosquitoes, flies, spiders, caterpillars

Psychogenic stimuli—nervous stress, worry, fatigue

Adapted from Habif TP: *Clinical dermatology,* ed 2, St Louis, 1990, Mosby–Year Book, and from Sauer GC: *Manual of skin diseases,* ed 5, Philadelphia, 1985, JB Lippincott.

CAUSES OF ANGIOEDEMA

Severe allergy reactions (Type I)—food, drugs, stinging insect venom, pollen
Contrast dyes and aspirin—due to direct histamine release rather than immune mechanism
Serum sickness following exposure to:
> Heterologous serum
> Animal-derived vaccines
> Drugs (penicillin, sulfonamides, thiouracils, aminosalicylic acid, streptomycin, hydantoins, cholecystographic dyes)

Adapted from Habif TP: *Clinical dermatology,* ed 2, St Louis, 1990, Mosby–Year Book.

CAUSES OF ALLERGIC CONTACT DERMATITIS

Nickel—jewelry, scissors, door handles, watch bands, belt buckles
Chromium compounds—cement, leather gloves, leather shoes, metals, dyes, photographic processes
Balsam of Peru—perfumes, shampoos, hair products
Formaldehyde—cosmetics, wash and wear clothing, paper, glue
Topical anesthetics—sunburn and anti-itch preparations
Paraben mix—cosmetics, topical creams and ointments, topical corticosteroid preparations
Paraphenylenediamine—hair dyes, PABA sunscreens, sulfonamides
Rubber—shoes, elastic, adhesive bandages, condoms, surgical gloves
Acrylic fabrics
Other chemicals in personal care products—imidazolidinyl urea (preservative), wool alcohols, formaldehyde, quaternium-15

sitizing agent or multiple (or chronic) exposures to a weakly sensitizing one before sensitization occurs.[96] The induction phase of sensitization usually requires 14 to 21 days. Re-exposure elicits an inflammatory response in about 12 hours, peaking 48 to 72 hours later.[185] Upon re-exposure to the antigen (the original hapten or one similar to it), effector T lymphocytes release lymphokines, which recruit macrophages, which then secrete mediators of inflammation causing vasodilation and cellular changes of eczema.[73]

The clinical manifestations of contact dermatitis depend on the strength of the sensitizing agent. The most severe variety presents as acute eczema, with multiple, tiny, fluid-filled vesicles becoming confluent in a red plaque with a pebbled surface. This variety itches intensely. The most frequent causes of florid presentations are the oleoresins of plants of the *Rhus* genus (poison ivy, poison oak, poison sumac, as well as other members including mango, cashew, and Japanese lacquer trees).[96] Two ophthalmic medications, atropine and neomycin, promote similar, although slightly less florid, reactions, initially involving the conjunctiva and later involving lids and periorbital areas.[249] Other ophthalmic preparations may cause varying degrees of dermatitis; these drugs include antimicrobials[9] and glaucoma medications, particularly epinephrine and dipivefrin.

Most substances other than the *Rhus* plants and ophthalmic preparations typically produce subacute or chronic reactions, with eczema that is characteristically dry and scaly, with less erythema

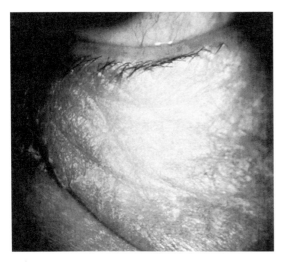

FIG. 8-3 Contact dermatitis of lower lid due to dipivefrin ophthalmic solution (Propine); chronic, with dry scaling.

and vesicular eruptions (Fig. 8-3). If the period of irritation is long-lasting, skin lines become enhanced, causing a *lichenoid* or "washboard" appearance. The skin may become fissured or excoriated, with risk of secondary infection.[34]

Cosmetic and personal care products deserve special mention as substances applied near the eyes, although they are usually weak sensitizers and are less common causes of allergic contact dermatitis. The delicate nature of eyelid skin often allows allergic contact dermatitis to present at that site alone, not provoking a reaction at the site of primary contact (fingers or hands).[184,249] Rubbing the eyes after handling cleansers, nail polish, or face creams may promote contact dermatitis. Eye cosmetics generally cause allergic reactions on the eyebrows and upper lids as a result of the method of application.[80]

Treatment of allergic contact dermatitis depends on the severity of the reactions. All manifestations require the identification of the antigen (where possible) and subsequent avoidance. Severe manifestations with vesicular eruptions, erythema, and itching warrant cool or astringent soaking, systemic steroids, and oral antihistamines.[185] The less severe, subacute or chronic manifestations require topical steroid ointments or creams, moisturizing lotions, and the "tincture of time." When allergic contact dermatitis occurs after use of ophthalmic medications, topical steroid solutions or suspensions are useful to reduce conjunctival inflammation; topical astringent soaking and oral antihistamines are also useful.

VIRAL SKIN DISEASES

Molluscum Contagiosum

Molluscum contagiosum results from viral infection of the epidermis, caused by an unclassified poxvirus that infects humans only.[46] The classic lesion is discrete, averaging 3 to 6 mm in diameter, smooth, dome-shaped, flesh-colored or pearly, and slightly umbilicated (Fig. 8-4) (see box on p. 147). As the virus infects epithelial cells, large intracytoplasmic inclusion bodies are produced and cell bonds are disrupted, resulting in a white, curdlike central core. Its center becomes soft and more depressed with time.[96]

Molluscum contagiosum occurs on the face, eyelids, trunk, axillae, extremities, and genital areas.[96] Lesions frequently appear in crops as a result of viral spread by autoinoculation. The lesion is active and infectious if its core material (containing infected cells) is being discharged.[34] Lesions can develop at any age, but many affected patients are children, often in settings of poor hygiene.[46,149] Up to 20% of symptomatic AIDS patients may have molluscum contagiosum, with solitary lesions often larger than usual (up to 10 mm) and frequently with large numbers of lesions (up to 100).[56,229]

When it involves the eyelids, molluscum contagiosum causes a variety of toxic conjunctival and corneal processes. The release of virus-laden debris into the tear film may result in chronic follicular conjunctivitis, epithelial keratitis, or a trachoma-like pannus.[46,188] Unilateral conjunctivitis should prompt the examiner to search for molluscum contagiosum as well as verruca.[19]

Molluscum contagiosum may mimic warts, varicella, and papillomas. Its central umbilication may mimic basal cell carcinoma and senile sebaceous hyperplasia, but these conditions typically appear in older individuals rather than in children. Molluscum lesions are known frequently to be self-limited, spontaneously clearing in 6 to 9 months in immunocompetent patients. If removal of a lesion is warranted, this can be achieved with either curettage or cryotherapy using liquid nitrogen.[149]

Verruca (Viral Wart)

Human papillomavirus (HPV) is a DNA virus that causes verrucae or warts, benign tumors commonly appearing on the skin or less frequently involving other epithelial tissue. At this time, 66 separate HPV serotypes have been isolated,[197] some of which have specific predilection for anatomic regions and clinicopathologic presentations (including cervical cancer and squamous cell carcinoma). Warts frequently appear in children and young adults but may occur at any age.[150]

Viral warts are limited to the epidermis and result from infection of basal cells or keratinocytes.[46] The infected cells expand and form cylindrical projections of varying lengths, either tightly or loosely fused together. On thick, tough skin the projections are fused tightly, giving the wart a lobular surface appearance.[96]

Common warts (verruca vulgaris) may appear on any skin surface but most frequently occur on the hands. They begin as smooth, flesh-colored papules that evolve into dome-shaped, slightly scaly, gray-brown hyperkeratotic growths (Fig. 8-5). Black dots may appear on the surface, which represent thrombosed capillaries. Common warts may occur in multiples and become confluent (mosaic warts).[150]

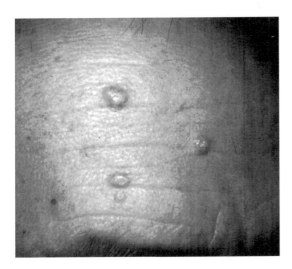

FIG. 8-4 Multiple molluscum contagiosum lesions, several with central umbilication.

CLINICAL CHARACTERISTICS OF MOLLUSCUM CONTAGIOSUM
Smooth surface
Dome-shaped
Flesh, pink, or pearly colored
Umbilicated
White, curdlike core
Single or in crops

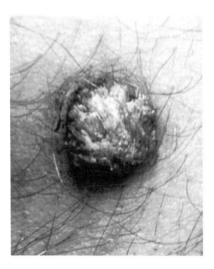

FIG. 8-5 Common wart (verruca vulgaris), with heavily keratinized, lobulated surface.

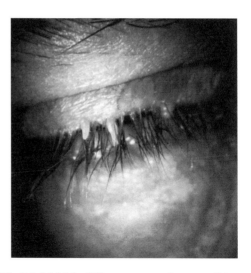

FIG. 8-6 Multiple filiform warts at the upper lid margin.

Filiform or digitate warts consist of finger-like projections emanating from a broad or narrow base (Fig. 8-6). They commonly appear around the mouth, eyes, and nose.[96] When they occur on the eyelids near the conjunctiva, they may cause sub-acute or chronic follicular conjunctivitis, possibly accompanied by superficial keratitis, due to release of viral toxins from the lesion.[188]

Flat warts (verruca plana) appear as flat-topped, smooth papules, typically flesh-colored or pink, with minimal or no surface scale (Fig. 8-7). They are usually 1 to 3 mm in size and are frequently numerous. Commonly affected areas are the fore-head, mouth, shaved areas (beard area), and backs of the hands[96] (Table 8-1).

Warts, particularly digitate and filiform warts, are often confused with skin tags and polyps. Warts typically lose fine skin lines as they grow[96] and often develop keratinized surfaces, to the ex-tent of cutaneous horns; this is not the case with skin tags. Warts can also be confused with sebor-rheic keratosis, squamous cell carcinoma, basal cell carcinoma, or keratoacanthoma.[46]

Reduction in cell-mediated immunity may ex-plain the increased severity and duration of verru-cae.[178] Warts are more common in patients with atopic dermatitis, lymphomas, and those taking

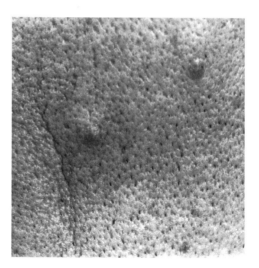

FIG. 8-7 Two flat warts (verruca plana) which are slightly elevated, papular, and flesh-colored.

immunosuppressive drugs.[96] Warts also occur more frequently, in greater numbers, and last longer in patients with AIDS.[89,138] Warts typically resolve in weeks to months. Because they leave little or no scarring after surgical removal, a con-servative therapy approach is best. Waiting for re-gression of the lesion is the least intrusive, but

TABLE 8-1 *Clinical Characteristics of Verrucae*

Warts	Characteristics
Common wart (verruca vulgaris)	Smooth papule (early) Closely lobulated surface (later) Scaly surface, hyperkeratosis Black dots Likeliest on hands
Filiform wart	Variably thick base Finger-like Multiple, loosely fused projections Located near mouth, eyes, nose
Flat wart (verruca plana)	Flat topped Smooth papule Flesh-colored or pink Minimal or no scale Located on forehead, beard area, hands

chemical cautery, cryosurgery, and carbon dioxide laser therapies are useful as well.

Herpes Simplex

Herpes simplex virus consists of two serotypes, causing both primary and recurrent mucocutaneous infections. The HSV-1 serotype is primarily associated with oral infections, and the HSV-2 serotype causes mainly genital infections.[104] Herpes simplex virus may remain dormant for life after the primary infection, living in a state of symbiosis with the human host, or may reactivate and travel down nerve fibers to re-establish skin infections. The recurrence of HSV infection appears to depend on both virulence of the specific virus[119] and host immunity.[48]

Primary or initial infection with herpes simplex virus occurs by direct exposure through mucocutaneous contact with an infected individual with primary or recurrent disease or with an asymptomatic carrier shedding the virus.[110] The most common form of primary infection is orolabial, with gingivostomatitis and pharyngitis, occurring in children aged 1 to 5 years. Symptoms occur 3 to

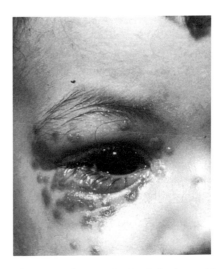

FIG. 8-8 Primary herpes simplex infection, with uniformly sized vesicles on an erythematous base.

7 days after contact, with fever, tenderness, pain, mild paresthesias, or burning. The classic presentation is vesicles of uniform size, grouped on an erythematous base (Fig. 8-8). Herpes labialis usually occurs on the mucocutaneous junction of the lips. The vesicles last 1 to 2 weeks and heal without scarring.[2] The virus then enters the nerve endings in the skin, ascending through the peripheral nerves to the ganglia.[119] Most primary infections are clinically insignificant; up to 90% of the infected adult population has experienced either a subclinical primary infection or one without clinical manifestations.[140]

Primary infection with HSV-2 presents with small grouped vesicles (similar to HSV-1 infection) that break and ulcerate within 2 to 4 days. Primary HSV-2 genital infections frequently present with painful enlarged inguinal lymph nodes and symptoms of pain, itching, dysuria, and vaginal and urethral discharge. The course of this primary genital infection is about 21 days.[2,49]

Recurrent herpes simplex infections are typically less symptomatic and of shorter duration than primary episodes.[52] Viral reactivation occurs in response to local skin trauma, to exposure to sunlight or cold wind, or to systemic conditions (the common cold, menses, fever, infection, fatigue, or "stress").[94,110,222] The usual number of recurrences is two or three per year.[96] Recurrent orolabial herpes simplex infection, known as "fever blisters" or "cold sores," is the most common recurrent manifestation, afflicting about one third of people in the United States.[52] This presentation of single or multiple eruptions on the vermilion border of the lip is due to virus traveling down the maxillary branch of the trigeminal (fifth cranial) nerve (see box below). If the virus travels instead down the ophthalmic branch from the trigeminal ganglion, recurrent ocular lesions such as vesicular[46] or erosive-ulcerative blepharitis,[63] corneal epithelial dendritic ulcers, and iridocyclitis result.[110,119]

Recurrent herpes infection most commonly presents in genital areas and is due to HSV-2 infection. Recurrent genital HSV-2 infections occur in more than 80% of patients within 12 months after the primary episode.[49] Genital recurrences are more frequent than orofacial recurrences.[244]

Acyclovir has proven to be remarkably effective in the treatment and management of many herpes simplex infections. Acyclovir ointment can be used topically for both orolabial and genital infections, either primary or recurrent, when they are mild to moderate in severity. Clinical experience with the topical form varies considerably; oral acyclovir, used in a 200-mg dose five times daily, is much preferred for mild or moderate infections.[196]

Acyclovir is most effective at decreasing the duration of viral excretion, new lesion formation, and vesicles, as well as promoting rapid healing in genital herpes infections.[28,49,169] Oral acyclovir, when used on a maintenance basis, may reduce the recurrences of some HSV-2 genital infections as well as the duration of the episodes, although its role in reducing recurrences is disputed.[52,206]

Herpes Zoster

Herpes zoster (shingles) results from the reactivation of latent varicella-zoster virus (VZV), acquired during a previous episode of varicella (chickenpox). After resolution of cutaneous varicella, the virus enters peripheral sensory nerve receptors and is then transmitted via retrograde spread[192] through sensory nerves to either the dorsal root ganglia of the spinal nerves or the extramedullary ganglia of the cranial nerves.[221] Cellular immunity blocks reactivation of the virus, but multiple factors may reduce that immunity[81,96,145,221] (see box below). With reduced cellular immunity, VZV replicates in the ganglion, enters sensory nerves, travels to the skin innervated by that particular dermatome, and enters dermis and epidermis, causing characteristic cutaneous lesions. The rash of zoster is likeliest in the dermatome(s) most densely affected during earlier

---

CLINICAL CHARACTERISTICS OF HERPES SIMPLEX

Grouped vesicles
Uniform size
Erythematous base
Mucocutaneous junction of lips
Periocular area
Genitalia
Progression of vesicles
   Turbid fluid
   Umbilicated center
   Rupture
   Eroded surface
   Crusted surface

FACTORS RELATED TO HERPES ZOSTER

Increasing age
Trauma
Fatigue
Emotional upset
Infection
Surgery
Bone marrow transplantation
Chronic illness
Malignancy
Radiation therapy
Chemotherapy
Immunosuppressive therapy
HIV infection

varicella infection, which presumably allowed larger amounts of virus to be transmitted to the corresponding sensory ganglia.[189] The dermatomes most frequently affected are the thoracic (50% to 55%), cranial (15% to 20%), cervical (10% to 15%), lumbar (10% to 15%), and sacral (2% to 5%).[145]

Herpes zoster is a common dermatologic condition, occurring in the lifetime of 10% to 20% of all individuals.[245] Although all ages may be affected, incidence of herpes zoster rises in the aging population.[200] This increase is likely due to decreases in cellular immunity, with less containment of the virus immunologically over time.[174,262] Hope-Simpson calculated that in a cohort of 1000 individuals who lived to be 85 years of age, 500 would have had one attack of zoster, but only 10 would have had a second attack.[108] Zoster is also more frequent in immunosuppressed patients, both those with hematopoietic or reticuloendothelial cancer and those undergoing cytotoxic or immunosuppressive therapy.[263]

Although one would expect to find an increased incidence or prevalence of cancer in those with zoster (owing to putative reduced immunity), these patients are at no greater risk for cancer than any other group.[201] Young individuals are less likely to contract herpes zoster. When zoster occurs in young, healthy patients without a known cause of immunosuppression, HIV infection should be suspected.[47,81,121,190] Herpes zoster ophthalmicus, often presenting with significant ocular complications, may be the first manifestation of HIV infection.[220,229]

The prodrome of zoster is characterized by headache, malaise, fever, and lymphadenopathy, followed by increasing pain in the involved dermatome. The pain or neuralgia, resulting from inflammation of neural tissue, varies from superficial itching, tingling, or burning to a severe, deep, boring, stabbing pain that may be constant or intermittent.[144] Prodromal pain, occurring without suggestive skin eruptions, can be mistakenly attributed to migraine headache, myocardial infarction, appendicitis, or other conditions.[245] The prodrome typically precedes the cutaneous rash by 2

or 3 days, which initially manifests as a maculopapular rash, evolving into a vesicular presentation within 24 hours. Vesicles, variable in size, are closely grouped on an erythematous base rather than being randomly distributed as in chickenpox (see box below). Clear vesicular fluid turns turbid and purulent within 3 to 4 days. Vesicles either umbilicate or rupture before crusting in 7 to 10 days; crusts fall off in 2 to 3 weeks (Fig. 8-9). The rash of zoster is typically worst in older patients, with more extensive inflammation and eruptions, and is of longer duration.[189]

Involvement of the first division (ophthalmic) of the trigeminal nerve is called herpes zoster ophthalmicus (HZO), regardless of ocular involvement.[94] The skin rash of HZO may extend from the vertex of the skull to the eye and nose but does not cross the midline. The ophthalmic division of the trigeminal nerve has three main branches: frontal, lacrimal, and nasociliary. The frontal branch, with two subdivisions (supratrochlear and supraorbital), is the most commonly affected nerve in HZO.[62] Involvement of the nasociliary branch is typically signaled by a rash on the nose or tip of the nose (Hutchinson's sign) and is significantly correlated with ocular complications. Ocular involvement occurs in about 50% of patients with

---

CLINICAL CHARACTERISTICS OF HERPES ZOSTER

Prodrome (headache, malaise, fever)
Neuralgia (pain, itching, burning)
Dermatome involvement
Maculopapular rash
Grouped vesicles
Variable sizes
Erythematous base
Midline honored
Progression of vesicles
    Turbid fluid
    Purulent fluid
    Umbilicated center
    Rupture
    Crusted surface

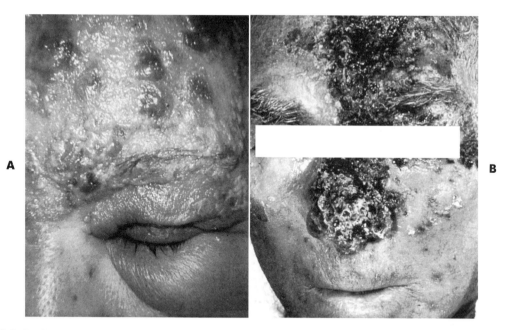

FIG. 8-9 A, Herpes zoster ophthalmicus, with vesicular and pustular eruptions. **B,** Herpes zoster ophthalmicus, with extensive crusting.

HZO[144] but can be as high as 71%.[268] Complications involve virtually all parts of the eye, including lids, conjunctiva, orbit, cornea, uvea, retina, and optic nerve.[143,144]

Treatment of herpes zoster involves a variety of medications and regimens. Treatment goals should be directed toward patient comfort, local skin care with prevention of secondary infection of the lesions, prevention of postherpetic neuralgia, and preservation of vision (with ophthalmic zoster). Non-narcotic analgesics and codeine-like analgesics are frequently used to control mild pain. Topical management of skin lesions includes wet compresses with Burow's solution or tap water as well as possible use of topical antibiotics for prophylaxis of infection.[266] Calamine lotion may be helpful to reduce itching.[148] Systemic corticosteroids, while controversial, have generally proved to be helpful in reducing pain duration.[145] Stellate ganglion blocks are quite effective in relieving the acute pain of HZO if used within 2 weeks of the appearance of the rash.[144] Cimetidine was initially

found to provide relief of itching and pain as well as enhanced resolution of cutaneous lesions,[162] but these benefits were not borne out in a larger, controlled study.[141] Cycloplegics and topical steroids are very useful in the management of ophthalmic zoster, for both uveitis and keratitis.

Acyclovir, in oral and intravenous forms, is the most promising antiviral agent at this time,[67] with the ability to reduce new lesion formation, reduce viral shedding, speed healing time, reduce rates of dissemination to the skin, and reduce acute pain.[10,165,179,195,269] The role of acyclovir in reducing complications of ophthalmic zoster is unequivocal,[43,44,45] although its value in nonophthalmic zoster is controversial because its cost may outweigh its benefits.[196]

Postherpetic neuralgia (PHN) is defined as pain persisting in a dermatome 4 to 6 weeks after the vesicular eruption has healed. It is characterized by constant burning and aching and is always present to some degree (although possibly fluctuating in intensity), occurring spontaneously or exacerbated by cutaneous stimulation.[148] PHN is more frequent in older patients, particularly those over 80 years of age.[98]

Management of PHN is very difficult because no modality is consistently effective. Although some reports have found no significant reduction in PHN with oral acyclovir,[10,44,45,269] other studies, emphasizing both prompt initiation and sufficiently high doses (800 mg five times a day), have noted significant reductions in the intensity of PHN in both generalized zoster infection[109,179] and HZO.[106] Oral steroid therapy may also reduce the severity and/or incidence of PHN, perhaps by its inhibition of perineural inflammation and fibrosis.[266] Low-dose regimens of tricyclic antidepressants, particularly amitriptyline, have been helpful in some patients.[163,258] Their benefit is possibly due to their effects on monoamine neurotransmitter metabolism.[257]

Capsaicin is the first of a group of neuropeptide active agents able to reduce chronic pain of PHN, diabetic neuropathy, and arthritis. Capsaicin appears to act on nociceptive (pain-related) type C sensory neurons by depleting substance P, a neuropeptide responsible for the mediation of pain impulses from the peripheral to central nervous system.[113,114,166] Substance P levels are elevated in sensory nerves supplying localized sites of chronic inflammation.[139] Capsaicin cream has provided significant relief of PHN pain in several studies.[13,14,29] Finally, encouragement and support can be as valuable to the patient as pharmaceutical modalities in dealing with the discomfort of PHN.

BENIGN SKIN TUMORS

Inclusion Cyst

Inclusion cysts comprise a variety of cystic lesions occurring on the eyelids or in the periorbital area: milia, epidermal cysts, sebaceous cysts (from glands of Zeis or sebaceous glands near hair follicles), and senile sebaceous hyperplasia (Table 8-2).

Milia are small, elevated lesions occurring on the eyelids. They are typically 1 mm in size, ei-

TABLE 8-2 *Clinical Characteristics of Inclusion Cysts*

Cysts	Characteristics
Milia	Small (1 mm)
	Elevated
	Flesh-colored, yellow, or white
Epidermal cyst	Central orifice or channel
	Firm, rubbery
	Yellow
	Keratin debris
Sebaceous cyst	Firm, rubbery
	Yellow
	Glands of Zeis, eyebrows
Senile sebaceous hyperplasia	Yellow or flesh-colored
	Elevated papules
	Umbilicated
	Doughnut-shaped

ther skin-colored, yellow, or white, and derive from occlusion of the pilosebaceous follicle.[19] Often they have no apparent cause, but milia may occur after trauma or acute contact dermatitis.[222]

Epidermal cysts result from an invagination of epithelium into the dermis, sometimes related to trauma. The trapped stratified squamous epithelium produces keratin, so that these contain keratin debris.[222] Epidermal cysts communicate with the surface via a narrow channel, often appearing as a round orifice resembling an open comedo (blackhead).[96] Epidermal cysts are firm and rubbery in texture, typically yellow, and clinically indistinguishable from sebaceous cysts (Fig. 8-10). In addition to the face, epidermal cysts also occur on the scalp, back, axillary and inguinal areas, and retroauricular regions.[26]

Sebaceous cysts typically derive from glands of Zeis or sebaceous glands near hair follicles, eyebrows, or other periorbital structures. They present as firm, rubbery masses, yellow when superficial and indistinguishable from overlying skin when lying deep.[34] Sebaceous cysts are most common on the scalp[222] and are much less common on the lids

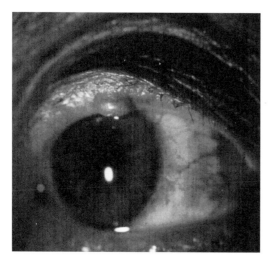

FIG. 8-10 Epidermal cyst on upper eyelid, with firm texture and small, central drainage channel.

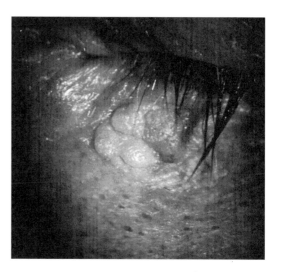

FIG. 8-11 Senile sebaceous hyperplasia, with multiple, lobulated papules.

than are epidermal cysts. They contain amorphous sebaceous material rather than desquamated keratin.[76]

Senile sebaceous hyperplasia typically occurs on the lower lids, forehead, cheeks, and nose in older patients. These lesions consist of enlarged sebaceous glands, forming yellow, slightly elevated papules (Fig. 8-11).[16] Their centers may depress, causing doughnut shapes, with telangiectatic vessels occurring in the valleys between the lobules. These benign, umbilicated growths may be confused with the malignant basal cell carcinoma, although the malignancy has telangiectasias distributed haphazardly over its surface.[96]

Sudoriferous Cyst

Sudoriferous cysts, when occurring on the lids, are likely due to ductal occlusion of the glands of Moll, associated with eyelash follicles.[102] These cysts are typically tense in texture upon palpation, retaining the surface quality of the overlying skin, and appearing somewhat translucent (Fig. 8-12).[26] They are also called hidrocystomas.

Another variety of sudoriferous tumor occurring in the periorbital area is *syringoma*. These tumors of sweat ducts are often filled with secretion and

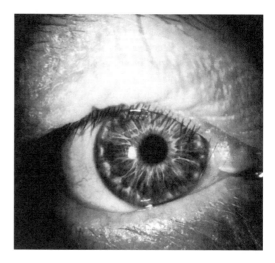

FIG. 8-12 Sudoriferous cyst at inner canthus; fluid-filled, translucent, with level of cellular debris.

typically occur in women during puberty and early adulthood. They appear as small, firm, skin-colored or yellowish papules on the lower lids, although they can also occur on the forehead and cheeks[156] (Table 8-3). Neither type of sudoriferous cyst has malignant potential.

TABLE 8-3 *Clinical Characteristics of Sudoriferous Cysts*

Cysts	Characteristics
Sudoriferous cyst	Tense
	Fluid-filled
	Translucent
	Glands of Moll
Syringoma	Flesh-colored
	Papules
	Lower lids
	Females (teens, 20s)

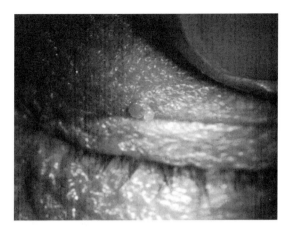

FIG. 8-13 Skin tag on upper lid; flesh-colored, sessile.

Papilloma (Skin Tag, Nonviral Papilloma, Achrocordon)

"Papilloma" is a nonspecific clinical term referring only to an epithelial lesion of no particular cause, consisting of papillae or finger-like projections, attached to the skin with a stalk of varying thickness. When the papilloma is noninfectious (contrasted with the wart or viral papilloma), it exists as a redundant flap or tag of skin with a cauliflower-like surface. Skin tags begin as tiny, brown or flesh-colored oval excrescences, attached by stalks of varying width and length, resulting in sessile (flat-based) or pedunculated lesions (Fig. 8-13). When the skin tag enlarges with a broad tip while retaining its narrow stalk, it is called a polyp[96] (Table 8-4). As the lesion enlarges, it may outgrow its blood supply and undergo necrosis.[34]

Both skin tags and polyps occur frequently on the eyelids as well as in the axillary region (most common site), neck, and inguinal region. Papillomas are cited in several studies as the most common benign dermatologic lesion of the eyelids.[102,261] Virtually any skin surface, except for the palms and soles of the feet, can be involved.[96] The differential diagnosis should include other papillomatous lesions such as verruca vulgaris (digitate projections, horny surface), dermal nevus, and seborrheic keratosis (keratinized, granular surface).[156] Skin tags or polyps irritated by patient manipulation can be easily removed by scissors excision or electrocautery.

TABLE 8-4 *Clinical Characteristics of Papillomas*

Papilloma	Characteristics
Skin tag	Flesh-colored or brown
	Variably thick stalk
	Sessile or pedunculated
	Lobulated surface (cauliflower-like)
Polyp	Flesh-colored or brown
	Narrow stalk
	Pedunculated
	Broad tip

Keratoacanthoma

Keratoacanthoma is a somewhat common, benign skin tumor without malignant potential, believed to derive from hair follicles. Its pathogenesis is not well understood. Numerous reports link the development of keratoacanthoma to both local trauma and skin conditions (including eczema, seborrheic dermatitis, psoriasis, and acne). It arises mainly in sun-exposed areas.[156] Eyelids, particularly lower lids,[20] are the fourth most common site for keratoacanthoma, after the cheeks, dorsa of the hands, and nose.[84]

Keratoacanthoma begins most often as a single, dome-shaped, red papule, growing to significant

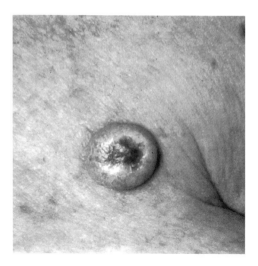

FIG. 8-14 Keratoacanthoma, typically presenting as a dome-shaped papule with a central keratin core.

CLINICAL CHARACTERISTICS OF KERATOACANTHOMA

Single lesion
Dome-shaped
Pink or red papule
Central crater or umbilication
Keratin cap
Less common: elevated, warty, ulcerated

size in a startlingly short period of time. Full growth is typically achieved in about 2 months. Typically keratoacanthoma develops a central crater or umbilication, usually covered with a keratin cap (Fig. 8-14) (see box above, right). Less often it may be elevated, with a warty or scaly ulcerated surface,[20] without a central keratin crater, or with increased pigmentation.[102] After reaching its full size (2.6 cm at the largest), the lesion remains quiet for several months to 1 year. It ultimately discharges its keratin, shrinks in size, and finally resolves, leaving a shallow, saucer-shaped scar.[84] Patients generally report an asymptomatic, rapidly growing lump, occasionally with redness, itching, or pain on pressure.[20]

Keratoacanthoma is interesting in that it grows quickly, resembling squamous cell carcinoma, but has no malignant potential. In fact, keratoacanthoma can so closely resemble squamous cell carcinoma that it has been used to illustrate this malignancy in textbooks and in classes on microscopic histopathology.[84] Keratoacanthoma may also be confused with basal cell carcinoma, verruca vulgaris, and papillomas.[20]

Because keratoacanthoma typically leaves a moderately disfiguring scar, there is no theoretical

advantage in waiting for the lesion to resolve spontaneously. Surgical procedures for the removal of keratoacanthoma are relatively simple, and the postsurgical result is acceptable, generally no worse than that of no surgical intervention at all.[96]

Seborrheic Keratosis

Seborrheic keratosis is an extremely common skin growth, likely the most common of all dermatologic lesions presenting on the face and eyelids.[7,76,248,251] Typically seen in middle-aged and older individuals, seborrheic keratosis has no known cause, and may occur more often in the patient with brown or black hair and an oily complexion.[222] The lesion originates and exists completely within the epidermis. Many, but not all, seborrheic keratoses occur in sun-exposed areas, although there is no relation to sun exposure in their development.[96]

Seborrheic keratosis varies in color from light tan or brown to a darker chocolate brown or black. The surface consists of multiple confluent papules laden with keratin (Fig. 8-15). Surface quality is granular and irregular, crumbling easily when scratched. "Horn pearls" are white or black pearls of keratin, often embedded in the surface of a dome-shaped seborrheic keratosis. This growth tends to be flat but is often elevated on the face, to the extent of being pedunculated on the eyelids and periorbital area.[26] The lesion may look like a wart, with prominent lobules. All lesions are characterized by a "stuck on," plaquelike appearance (see box on p. 157, left). Borders are always sharp but may be irregular, and colors may vary within

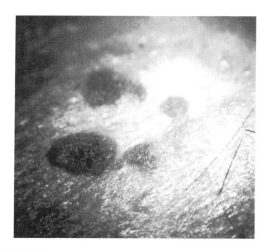

FIG. 8-15 Multiple seborrheic keratoses, with granular, crumbling keratinized surfaces.

CLINICAL CHARACTERISTICS OF SEBORRHEIC KERATOSIS

Variable tan to black color
Multiple confluent papules
Granular, keratinized, crumbling surface
Possibly multilobed or wartlike
Variable elevation (flat to pedunculated)
"Stuck on"
Sharp borders

the lesion, mimicking superficial spreading melanoma.[215] Seborrheic keratosis has no malignant potential, but other skin tumors have arisen infrequently within or adjacent to seborrheic keratosis, including basal cell carcinoma,[88] squamous cell carcinoma,[8] malignant melanoma,[270] and keratoacanthoma.[136] Histologic evaluation is mandatory for any seborrheic keratosis undergoing atypical changes (asymptomatic bleeding, ulceration, or rapid enlargement). Seborrheic keratosis may be removed for cosmesis or chafing from overlying clothing. Surgical removal is typically simple because of the superficial epithelial growth pattern.[156]

Actinic Keratosis

Actinic keratosis (solar keratosis or senile keratosis) is the most common premalignant skin lesion

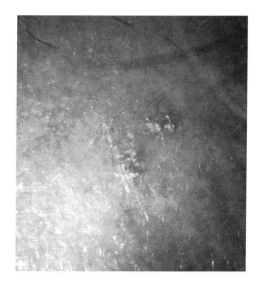

FIG. 8-16 Early actinic keratosis, slightly elevated, with roughened surface but without erythema.

CLINICAL CHARACTERISTICS OF ACTINIC KERATOSIS

Initially flat
Pink, increased vascularity
Increasing erythema over time
Increasing surface keratin over time

in white patients, affecting nearly 100% of the elderly white population.[250] It may also be seen in light-skinned people in their second and third decades who live in sunbelt regions.[223] The development of actinic keratosis depends on years of sun exposure and typically appears on the face and other sun-exposed regions.

Histologically actinic keratosis consists of hyperkeratotic epithelial cells with an abnormal basal layer.[215] Initially actinic keratosis presents as an area of increased vascularity with a slightly rough surface, similar to sandpaper (Fig. 8-16). Often the lesion is felt before it is seen by the patient. With time, the lesion develops increased erythema, heavier surface scale, and a variety of colors ranging from skin color to reddish brown or yellow-black. Some actinic keratoses develop cutaneous horns, a cylindrical projection of hyperkeratosis[223] (see box above).

Up to 25% of actinic keratoses have been said to develop into squamous cell carcinoma,[90] but this specific type of carcinoma is typically not aggressive, with a small risk of metastasis.[242] The actual risk of malignant transformation of a single actinic keratosis into squamous cell carcinoma within 1 year was calculated to be less than 1 in 1000.[158] Additional calculations based on these data provide a theoretical risk of malignant transformation of 6% to 10% for an average patient with multiple actinic keratoses followed over 10 years.[55] Malignant transformation is signaled by induration, increased erythema, erosion, bleeding, or growth spurt.[223]

Actinic keratosis is extremely common and is very likely to appear in older, fair-skinned patients. It can be confused with seborrheic dermatitis, which appears as scaly, dry, pinkish lesions,[215] and also with lentigo maligna, seborrheic keratosis, and pigmented melanocytic nevi. The presence of actinic keratosis in any patient should urge the examiner to search for other actinic-related skin conditions, such as basal cell carcinoma and squamous cell carcinoma.

Multiple treatment modalities exist for the management of actinic keratosis. Sun avoidance, use of sunscreens, and wearing protective clothing and hats may allow early lesions to spontaneously remit without further treatment. Up to 25% of actinic keratoses may remit spontaneously, particularly in persons who can reduce their sun exposure.[157] Topical tretinoin (Retin-A) may resolve mild lesions with only erythema and scaling.[191] Cryosurgery with liquid nitrogen, electrodesiccation and curettage, and the antimetabolite fluorouracil (2% and 5%) are also effective therapies.[96]

Cutaneous Horn

Cutaneous horn is a nonspecific, secondary tissue change that occurs with primary lesions. It consists of multiple concentric lamellae of keratin which form a conical, projecting nodule (see box). It may vary in size from a few millimeters to several centimeters. Cutaneous horn is most commonly seen with actinic keratosis. It may also occur with seborrheic keratosis, inverted follicular

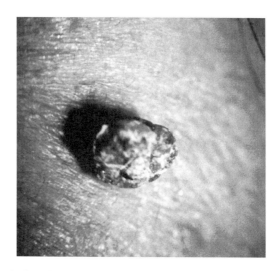

FIG. 8-17 Cutaneous horn developing on verruca vulgaris.

CLINICAL CHARACTERISTICS OF CUTANEOUS HORN

Keratin build-up
Possibly conical shape
Associated with a primary lesion

---

keratosis, filiform warts, squamous cell carcinoma, Bowen's disease,[18] and less commonly in basal cell carcinoma, sebaceous gland carcinoma, and Kaposi's sarcoma.[223] Because the lesion may develop in either benign or malignant conditions, the clinician must look for the primary lesion as the source of the cutaneous horn (Fig. 8-17).

Nevi (Melanocytic Nevi, Nevomelanocytic Nevi, Moles)

Melanocytes are cells capable of producing melanin pigment. Dendritic melanocytes manufacture pigment and transfer it to surrounding epidermal or epithelial cells, causing freckles, racial pigmentary differences, and suntans. Nevus cells, a contrasting subgroup of melanocytes, produce less pigment than dendritic melanocytes and do not transfer pigment to surrounding cells. Melanocytic nevi (nevi, moles) are formed of collections of ne-

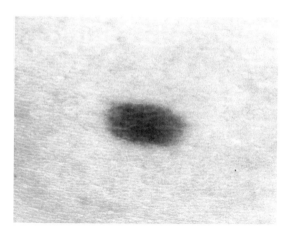

FIG. 8-18 Junction nevus, with smooth surface, regular borders, and little elevation.

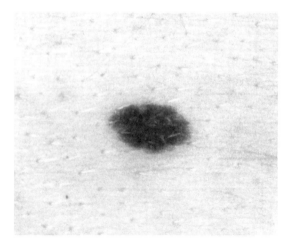

FIG. 8-19 Compound nevus, with elevated contour, slightly lobulated surface, and regular borders.

vus cells which lie at or near the dermoepidermal junction.[112]

The great majority of nevi are acquired after the first 12 months of life. Only about 1% of newborns have nevi present at the time of birth (congenital nevi).[33] Nevi increase in incidence throughout infancy and childhood. They may increase in number or darken at certain times of life, particularly during puberty and pregnancy.[208] It is possible for nevi to appear throughout life, although this is uncommon. The cause of nevi is uncertain. Ultraviolet light is postulated to be a proliferative stimulus to the melanocyte system, but the relationship is complex and is disputed in some studies.[6,91,202] Except for large congenital nevi and dysplastic nevi, most nevi possess a very low potential for malignancy.

Nevi have been classified into three clinical subtypes: junction, compound, and dermal. These three types correspond to the location of nevus cells as well as stages of development in the life cycle of a nevus.[96] Nevi generally begin as junction nevi, with nevus cells located at the dermoepidermal junction. As some cells migrate downward into the dermis, the nevus evolves into the compound type. Migration of all cells into the dermis results in the third type, the dermal nevus. As nevus cells move downward into the dermis, the mole becomes progressively more elevated and

nodular, losing its flat surface character.[194] Nevus cells decrease both in number and melanogenic activity with time.[205] Not all nevi progress from one stage into another, and progression along the developmental pathway may stop at any time.[92]

Junction nevi are typically flat or very slightly elevated. Pigmentation is usually uniform, ranging from light brown to black. Borders are regular, without notching, and shapes are symmetric, typically round or oval. Surface quality is usually smooth, without hairs (Fig. 8-18). Junction nevi typically present in early childhood and change into compound nevi after childhood.[92,208]

Compound nevi are more elevated than junction nevi, becoming even more elevated with time. They typically have a symmetric shape (round or oval) and maintain homogeneity of color, ranging from flesh tones to brown (Fig. 8-19). Surface quality is variable, ranging from smooth to wartlike, and sometimes includes hairs.[92,208]

Dermal nevi are the most elevated, possibly with warty or polypoid surfaces, and a variety of attaching stalks, ranging from thin and pedunculated to broad and sessile (Fig. 8-20). Colors are typically brown or black, but dermal nevi may become lighter or flesh-colored over time. Surface hairs are likely, possibly darker than the surrounding hair[92,208] (Table 8-5).

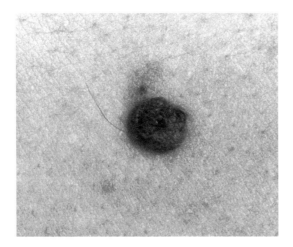

FIG. 8-20 Dermal nevus, with marked elevation, lobulated surface, and broad attachment.

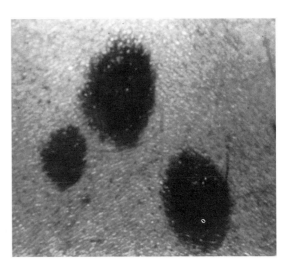

FIG. 8-21 Three dysplastic nevi, with symmetric shapes and regular borders; significant for their large size and dark color.

Nevi can be confused with freckles (ephelides), which are macular spots that darken with sun exposure and fade during the winter months. Freckles are caused by enlargement of melanocytes within the basal layer. They have no malignant potential but may serve as a marker for susceptibility to actinic damage.[194] Nevi can be mistaken for many other dermatologic lesions, including pigmented basal cell carcinoma, pigmented actinic keratosis, seborrheic keratosis, verruca, molluscum contagiosum, hemangioma, and Kaposi's sarcoma, among others.

Dysplastic Nevus (Atypical Mole)

Dysplastic nevus is a recently described variety of acquired melanocytic nevus, first reported in 1978,[42] and significant for its variable role as a precursor to malignant melanoma. Dysplastic nevus is a bizarre variety of melanocytic nevus, with irregular, ill-defined borders, variegations of colors, lacking the homogeneity and symmetry of other nevi (Fig. 8-21). More than one color is commonly present in dysplastic nevi, with haphazard distribution of multiple shades of brown and pink. Additionally, dysplastic nevi retain a macular component in addition to papular elevations, causing a pebbled or "fried egg" surface.[92,182,208] A recent study found that 60% of dysplastic nevi

TABLE 8-5 *Clinical Characteristics of Nevi*

Nevi	Characteristics
Junction nevus	Flat or slightly elevated
	Uniform pigmentation
	Smooth surface
	Regular borders
	Symmetric shape
Compound nevus	Slightly to moderately elevated
	Uniform pigmentation
	Variable surface: smooth, warty, hairy
	Regular borders
	Symmetric shape
Dermal nevus	Elevated
	Uniform pigmentation (lightest colored)
	Lobular or warty surface
	Variable stalk with pedunculation
	Regular borders
	Symmetric shape

evaluated had regular borders and two thirds were symmetric in shape. Elevation, multiple colors, "macular tan shoulders" (flat tan area extending beyond the central dark elevation), and complete lack of hypertrichosis were found in virtually all lesions[164] (see box). Normal nevi frequently appear on sun-exposed areas; dysplastic nevi occur in these areas as well as in atypical locations (scalp, buttocks, breasts). Dysplastic nevi typically begin to appear near puberty and new lesion development continues throughout life, in contrast to normal nevi, which typically appear only in childhood.[225]

Levels of risk for dysplastic nevi depend on personal and familial history of both dysplastic nevi and cutaneous melanoma. At greatest risk is the patient with dysplastic nevi with two or more first-degree relatives with both dysplastic nevi and melanoma (the familial dysplastic nevus syndrome); estimated lifetime risk of developing melanoma approaches 100%.[187] For the individual with dysplastic nevi *without* a personal or familial history of malignant melanoma (the sporadic dysplastic nevus syndrome), one estimate suggests a sevenfold increased relative risk and a 6% cumulative risk of malignant melanoma.[131,211] Some writers believe that most dysplastic nevi do not evolve into malignant melanoma but are more likely to regress with time.[225] Authorities universally acknowledge some increased risk of melanoma with dysplastic nevi but cannot agree on the magnitude of the risk.[57] In fact, the varying uses of the term "dysplastic nevus" have led to such controversy that the alternate term "atypical mole" has been proposed.[187]

NEOPLASTIC SKIN LESIONS

Basal Cell Carcinoma

Basal cell carcinoma (BCC) is the most common skin malignancy.[79,223] Up to 90% of all BCCs occur on the head and neck.[35] The nose is the single most common site (25% of cases), with an additional 29% presenting on the cheeks, temples, and forehead combined.[217] Up to 10% of BCCs occur on the eyelids.[183] Additionally, BCC comprises about 90% of *all* eyelid malignancies.[35,76,85,135] The patient prone to BCC is typically fair skinned and fair haired and has had multiple hours of exposure to ultraviolet radiation from work or avocation.[233] Other carcinogenic factors include large

---

CLINICAL CHARACTERISTICS OF DYSPLASTIC NEVI

Simultaneously flat and elevated
Pebbled or "fried egg" surface
Haphazard colors
Regular or irregular borders
Symmetric or asymmetric shape
"Macular tan shoulder"
No hypertrichosis

---

doses of x-rays (dermatologic therapy prior to 1950),[32,159] burn and vaccination scars,[116] intake of inorganic arsenic, and exposure to carcinogenic oils.[97]

BCC typically grows and expands by direct invasion of surrounding tissue, into dermis, periosteum, perichondrium, and other adjacent structures. Malignant basal cells depend on the support of surrounding stromal tissue; it is unlikely that they autonomously leave the primary site and metastasize by blood or lymphatic spread.[198] Metastatic BCC is thus extremely rare, with the highest reported incidence at 0.1%.[130] Metastatic BCC usually develops from progressively ulcerated, recurrent, large tumors and spreads to regional lymph nodes, lungs, bone, or liver.[74,175] It is usually encountered in older patients[199] but has been reported in a younger patient with AIDS with a preceding recurrent BCC.[231]

BCC typically grows slowly owing to few proliferating cells, prominent cell death, and host immune factors.[176] It initially appears as a smooth, nonspecific nodule in a variety of colors (flesh-colored, pink, red) that frequently develops in areas of normal skin (Fig. 8-22).[79] BCC often loses its fine skin lines and displays superficial telangiectatic vessels, although its surface is usually nonkeratinized.[85] It may remain nodular or may undergo central umbilication and erosion because its vulnerable, nonkeratinized cells afford little surface protection (Fig. 8-23).[32] Other features include pearly, rounded borders and a tendency to bleed and scab, leading the patient to believe that the lesion has "healed." BCC is rare in black patients, although it shares common features of head

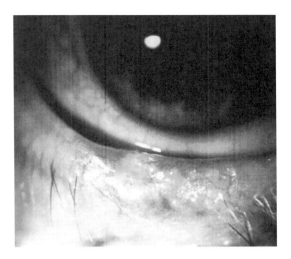

FIG. 8-22 Nodular basal cell carcinoma on lower lid, flesh-colored, with slight central umbilication but no erosion.

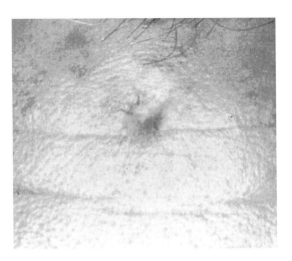

FIG. 8-24 Morpheaform (sclerosing) basal cell carcinoma, with appearance of scar tissue; lacking erosion or crusting.

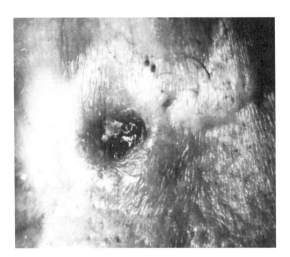

FIG. 8-23 Noduloulcerative basal cell carcinoma, with pronounced erosion and scabbing.

and neck locations, sun-exposed areas, surface telangiectasias, and a variety of shapes and clinical manifestations.[1,5]

The *nodular* and *noduloulcerative* types of BCC typically are the most frequently observed. One study found that 60% of eyelid BCCs were nodular and another 21% were noduloulcerative.[59] Two other types of eyelid BCCs described in this study

were *morpheaform* [fibrosing or sclerosing] (15%), typically appearing as a hard, pale, waxy patch of "scar tissue" with a significant connective tissue component (Fig. 8-24), and *multicentric* (4%), consisting of multiple nodules or lobes of tumor, separated by putatively "normal" tissue. The latter two types of BCC, although uncommon, deserve special mention because of their infiltrative nature, tumor spread beyond clinically apparent borders, frequency of misdiagnosis, difficulty of surgical removal, and likelihood of recurrence. The most atypical BCC is morpheaform because it lacks the characteristic rolled edges, ulceration, and crusting of the noduloulcerative type[59,85] (Table 8-6). Ocular basal cell carcinomas is found more often on the lower lids (66.9%) than the upper lids (12.3%) and at the nasal canthus (16.9%) more than the lateral canthus (3.8%).[11]

Three other types of BCCs have been described: *Superficial BCC* typically appears as an erythematous, scaly patch, lacking the smooth-surfaced nodular contour. These most often appear on the back, trunk, or extremities and are the least aggressive type of BCC.[96] *Pigmented BCC* is similar to the nodular type but brown or blue-black owing to deposition of melanin and hemosiderin.[53]

TABLE 8-6 *Clinical Characteristics of Basal Cell Carcinoma*

Basal Cell Carcinoma	Characteristics
Nodular	Smooth nodule Variable colors Superficial telangiectasias Possibly pearly surface
Noduloulcerative	Nodule Central umbilication, ulceration Pearly border Serosanguineous crust
Morpheaform/sclerosing	Scar tissue Hard, pale, waxy, "old ivory" Prominent telangiectasias No pearly borders
Multicentric	Nodules Variable color Possible telangiectasias "Normal skin"
Superficial	Erythematous Scaly, eczematoid
Pigmented	Nodular Superficial telangiectasias Pearly border Dark color (brown or blue-black)
Cystic	Translucent nodule Resembles epidermal cyst

Black individuals typically manifest pigmented BCC.[1,5] *Cystic BCC* is a translucent nodule with cystic degeneration of tumor cells in the center,[19] possibly resembling a benign epithelial inclusion cyst.[50]

Degrees of risk for BCC vary considerably with the type of lesion and its location. Sclerosing and multicentric BCCs are considered to be most difficult to manage because they extend beyond the clinically evident area, with significant dermal in-

volvement. They are also more likely to recur.[59] Dangerous locations are closest to periosteum and bone because the tumor grows by direct expansion rather than by metastasis and can ultimately extend into the orbit and central nervous system.[76,177] Orbital extension of any lid malignancy is suggested by diplopia on extreme gaze, upward or horizontal displacement of the globe, pain, tissue redness and chemosis, and an ulcerative lesion fixed to the underlying rim or surface of the orbit.[101] Some authors consider BCC of the lid the most difficult to manage, particularly at the medial canthus, owing to both the infiltrative nature of the tumor and its increased risk of recurrence.[35]

Multiple modalities exist for removal of BCC: cryosurgery, electrodesiccation and curettage, surgical excision, radiation, and Mohs' micrographic surgery. The Mohs' procedure is preferred for both sclerosing and multicentric BCC and for recurrent tumors, which tend to change architecturally from solid nests of tumor cells to infiltrating strands of cells in connective tissue.[97] The Mohs' procedure is also indicated for tumors near the nose, ears, and eyes because of the close juxtaposition of the skin to cartilage and bone. Tumor cells can easily invade periosteum or perichondrium; healing can occur over incompletely removed tumors, and deep invasion and lateral extension can go undetected.[96] In general, conventional surgery for periocular BCC is undependable, with up to 64% of tumors incompletely excised.[61,64,168] Mohs micrographic surgery is extremely effective in preventing recurrences.[177]

BCC can be easily confused with many other entities[50,59,76,116,177,222] (Table 8-7). Studies have found that correct diagnoses may be no more frequent than 60%.[59,193,261] BCCs may present with typical features, making their diagnosis straightforward, but many lesions are atypical. The usual patient with BCC is older, with greater cumulative amounts of ultraviolet light exposure, although up to 15% of BCCs occur in the 20-year-old to 40-year-old age group.[85] The clinician should not be lulled into a false sense of security when examining younger patients because typical BCCs have been overlooked in younger individuals simply because of their age.[180] Other BCCs in

TABLE 8-7 *Conditions Frequently Confused with Basal Cell Carcinoma*

Basal Cell Carcinoma	Conditions
Nodular	Epidermal cyst (inclusion cyst)
	Molluscum contagiosum
	Nevus (dermal)
	Papilloma
	Polyp (skin tag)
	Recurrent chalazion
	Seborrheic keratosis
	Senile sebaceous hyperplasia
Noduloulcerative	Keratoacanthoma
	Large comedones
	Molluscum contagiosum
	Senile sebaceous hyperplasia
	Squamous cell carcinoma
	Wart
Sclerosing (morpheaform)	Chronic blepharitis
	Dermatitis
	Ectropion
	Entropion
	Lid notching
	Lid retraction
	Madarosis
	Scarring
Cystic	Dermal nevus (nonpigmented)
	Epidermal cyst
	Molluscum
	Senile sebaceous hyperplasia
Pigmented	Dermal nevus (pigmented)
	Malignant melanoma (nodular)
Superficial	Dermatitis
	Eczema
	Psoriasis

young patients do not have the typical noduloulcerative appearance, but are erythematous, flat or slightly raised, often scaly, with surface telangiectasias and morpheaform structure.[183]

BCC demonstrates great variation from "textbook" presentations when observed on an individual basis.[34] The behavior of BCC cannot be predicted on clinical grounds, and both horizontal and vertical spread are unpredictable.[61] Finally, a lifetime cure is not achieved with successful excision of one BCC because the risk of both subsequent and recurrent BCCs is variably high.[36,71,264] Because more tissue is removed surgically than what is apparently involved, particularly in the riskiest locations, it behooves the clinician to be on the alert for BCC and to urge long-term (lifetime) follow-up.[233]

Squamous Cell Carcinoma

Squamous cell carcinoma (SCC) is believed to be the second most common skin malignancy in the United States,[16] although estimates of its incidence vary because neither BCC nor SCC is reported to tumor registries in the United States. The ratio of *nonocular* BCC to SCC ranges from 3:1 to 15:1[132,224]; a recent report proposes an average ratio of BCC to SCC of 7:1.[227] Sixty percent to 75% of SCC appears in the head and neck region.[233]

Like BCC, SCC most frequently develops on sun-exposed and sun-damaged skin,[242] although one study found that 40% of SCCs developed in skin that was clinically normal 1 year earlier.[158] SCC may appear on the scalp, pinnae of the ears, and backs of the hands, none of which are typical sites for BCC. Less frequent locations are areas of normal skin (appearing de novo) or "sick tissue" such as sites of radiation, chemical exposure (arsenic or tar), thermal burns, or chronically infected and draining sinuses and ulcers.[96,242] The most common precursor of the SCC is actinic keratosis; up to 25% of actinic keratoses may ultimately develop into SCC.[90]

It is accepted that SCC is less common than BCC on the eyelids. Some authors claim that overdiagnosis of eyelid SCC in the past has resulted in falsely high estimates of its incidence, and in 1963 they suggested a ratio of 38.6:1 for BCC to SCC.[135] A recent review of 33 studies of eyelid SCC, with incidences ranging from 2.4% to 30.2%, suggests that SCC averages 9.2% of all lid malignancies.[207] Reports have claimed SCC to be the second most common eyelid malignancy (after BCC),[3,7,135,193] third most common eyelid malignancy (after BCC and sebaceous gland carcinoma),[60] or fourth most common eyelid malignancy (after BCC, sebaceous gland carcinoma, and malignant melanoma).[248]

SCC is notorious for its wide variety of clinical forms[102] (see box). A typical, early appearance is a nonspecific, erythematous, rough, scaly patch (Fig. 8-25).[147] As SCC develops, superficial fissures and cracks appear with surface scaling. Beneath the scaling there is ulceration with bleeding and crusting, occurring sooner than in BCC.[207] Also typical is a hard, elevated border surrounding the ulceration.[76] In addition to its most typical presentation, SCC may also appear nodular or cystic[147] or as a wart or cutaneous horn.[102] SCC on the eyelids does not appear to have a predilection for either upper or lower lids.[207] About half the tumors in one study presented with central ulceration, and one fourth presented with intermittent purulent or bloody discharge.[60]

Surface scale of SCC depends on its development from a precursor lesion (actinic keratosis, cutaneous horn) and the type of skin from which it derives. SCC developing from actinic keratosis has thick, adherent surface scale. When developing in actinically damaged skin, SCC has little surface scale, appearing only as a firm, elevated mass.[96]

SCC is dangerous because of its ability to metastasize and spread to distant sites through nearby lymph channels. Likelihood of metastasis varies widely and depends on tumor size and location, degree of differentiation, depth of invasion, cause, and degree of anaplasia.[85] Rates of metastasis of SCC arising from actinically damaged skin are low, no higher than 3.6% in several studies.[37,118,152,242] One study cites a similarly low rate of metastasis (3.2%) from SCC of the eyelids,[60] but reports of lymph node involvement range from 1.3% to 21.4% with eyelid SCC.[85]

CLINICAL CHARACTERISTICS OF SQUAMOUS CELL CARCINOMA

Firm nodule
Flat patch
Erythematous

Variable surface scale
    Heavy, thick when deriving from actinic keratosis
    Mild when deriving from actinically damaged skin

Fissured surface
Ulceration
Bleeding, crusting
Purulent discharge, infection

Wartlike
Cystic
Cutaneous horn

No telangiectasias
No pearly borders

Rates from 0.5% to 16% exist for noninflamed or nondegenerated skin sites,[54] as high as 37% for the lower lip, and as high as 62% for genital and anal locations,[242] sites of mucous membrane or modified skin origin.[60]

No distinct clinical features easily establish the diagnosis of SCC. The superficial telangiectasias and pearly borders of BCC do not have clinical counterparts in SCC.[85] As a result, squamous cell carcinoma of the eyelids is frequently confused with other conditions[18,60,102,135] (see box on p. 166). The most common misdiagnoses include sebaceous gland carcinoma, morpheaform BCC, inverted follicular keratosis, keratoacanthoma, and pseudoepitheliomatous hyperplasia.[60] One study reported that only 12 of 115 presumed SCCs were confirmed as such.[135] It is thus possible that only 10% of a group of so-called SCCs are truly SCCs. Even though SCC is much less frequent than BCC on the eyelids and the risk for metastasis is low, the potential for misdiagnosis is considerable and prompt referral for biopsy is the most prudent

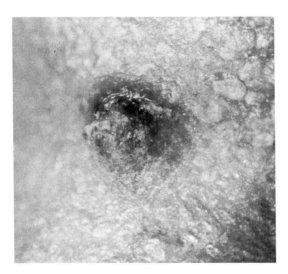

FIG. 8-25 Early squamous cell carcinoma, with erythema and elevated scale.

CONDITIONS CONFUSED WITH SQUAMOUS CELL CARCINOMA

Actinic keratosis
Adenoacanthoma
Adnexal carcinoma
Basal cell carcinoma (nodular)
Basal cell carcinoma (noduloulcerative)
Basal cell carcinoma (morpheaform)
Basal cell carcinoma with pseudoepitheliomatous
  hyperplasia
"Benign keratosis" (seborrheic keratosis)
Bowen's disease
Cutaneous horn
Inverted follicular keratosis
Keratoacanthoma
Papilloma
Pseudoepitheliomatous hyperplasia
Sebaceous gland carcinoma
Seborrheic keratosis with surface irritation
Wart (verruca)

course.[26] Additionally, there is a strong likelihood of other skin malignancies in the patient with SCC, particularly BCC.[18,37]

Merkel Cell Tumor

Merkel cell tumor, first described in 1972,[252] is now recognized as a particularly aggressive form of skin cancer. About 600 cases have been reported as of 1990,[124] and multiple reports describe its occurrence on the eyelids.[15,75,123,137,218,226] Although a rare condition, both on eyelid skin and elsewhere, it is extremely serious because of frequent misdiagnosis, quick growth, and likelihood of metastasis.

The Merkel cell is an oval cell found in the epidermis in several anatomic locations, notably the fingertips, toes, lips, and eyelids.[228] Although it is described as a slowly adapting mechanoreceptor that mediates the sense of touch and possibly the direction of hair movement, its precise function remains unclear.[232,267]

The most common site of Merkel cell carcinoma is the head and neck region.[226] One tenth of all cases appear in the eyelids or the periocular region,[124] with a special predilection for the upper lid.[218] Elsewhere in the body, the Merkel cell tumor tends to involve the extremities; only about

one tenth involve the trunk or mucous membranes.[230] Merkel cell carcinoma typically occurs in the elderly population, the average age of onset occurring in the seventh decade.[167] With ocular presentations, patients average 71 and 77 years of age for eyebrow and eyelid tumors, respectively.[124] There seems to be no particular gender predominance.[105] These tumors often arise in actinically damaged skin,[115] and a number of patients have histories of BCC, SCC, actinic keratosis, and other adnexal skin cancers.[87]

The tumor presents as a solitary dermal nodule, typically painless and nontender, protuberant, bulging, or dome-shaped. In the eyelid, it is often red, but hues range from skin color to blue, violet, and purple. Its surface is smooth and often shiny, frequently covered by dilated telangiectatic vessels.[15,137,226] The surface epithelium is rarely ulcerated[87] (see box on p. 167). The red color and dilated vessels may be related to the frequently observed inflammation and invasion of local lymphatic and vascular channels.[230] Merkel cell carcinoma is a fast-growing tumor,[115,255] with symptoms of less than 6 months' duration.[218]

Merkel cell tumor appearing on the eyelids may mimic lymphoma, amelanotic melanoma, cutane-

CLINICAL CHARACTERISTICS OF MERKEL CELL TUMOR
Solitary nodule Painless, nontender Protuberant, bulging, dome-shaped Variable colors (flesh, pink, red, violet) Smooth, shiny surface Surface telangiectasias Fast growth

DIFFERENTIAL DIAGNOSIS OF MERKEL CELL TUMOR
Lymphoma Amelanotic melanoma Cutaneous metastasis from primary malignancy Chalazion Basal cell carcinoma Squamous cell carcinoma Sebaceous gland carcinoma Kaposi's sarcoma

ous metastasis of carcinoma or lymphoma, or chalazion.[137,154] Less likely lid neoplasms in the differential diagnosis include BCC and SCC (both of which often ulcerate), and sebaceous gland carcinoma (which is often grossly yellow, involving the tarsus).[226] These latter three carcinomas also exist for more than 1 year before the patient's initial examination[218] (see box above, right). Electron microscopic studies provide definitive identification of the Merkel cell tumor; light microscopy alone has resulted in errors of diagnosis, including metastatic oat cell carcinoma, lymphoma, amelanotic melanoma, BCC, and metastatic neuroblastoma.[87,105,272]

Merkel cell tumors were initially thought to be tumors of low-grade malignancy. This is not the case: Local recurrences and satellite lesions occur in about one third of all patients, usually within 1 year of initial surgery. About two thirds of patients with Merkel cell carcinoma have had regional lymph node metastases, either at the time of diagnosis or within 18 months after initial therapy. Hematogenous distant metastases from these tumors have occurred in more than one third of cases.[230] Nearly one half of patients followed for 3 years or more have died of Merkel cell carcinoma, and the estimated 5-year survival rate is 38%. It appears that Merkel cell carcinoma, malignant melanoma, and sebaceous gland carcinoma are the three most malignant primary tumors of the eyelid.[124]

Merkel cell tumors demand prompt and aggressive therapy for a favorable outcome. Wide surgical excision of the primary tumor is desirable. Patients need regular follow-up for early detection of possible lymph node spread.[124] Because of the possibility of recurrence as late as 54 months after primary excision of the cutaneous tumor, lifetime follow-up at regular intervals is recommended.[218]

Sebaceous Gland Carcinoma

Sebaceous gland carcinoma (SGC) has been called "meibomian gland carcinoma" because meibomian glands are the most common ocular site of this neoplasm.[117,243] Other sebaceous glands of the ocular adnexa and periorbital area can be involved, including glands of Zeis and glands associated with the caruncle, eyebrows, and fine hairs on the lid surface.[21] Although it was previously considered a rare ocular tumor, incidences as high as 5.5%[199] and 6.4%[248] of all eyelid malignancies have been reported. SGC is more common in the eyelid area than in any other part of the body[155] and is perhaps more dangerous in ocular locations owing to its greater propensity for early metastasis from ocular sites than elsewhere on the skin.[117]

SGC is more common in individuals in their 50s and 60s, although carcinomas have been reported in younger individuals with a history of radiation exposure.[228] Caucasian patients present most frequently with SGC, although a strikingly high incidence has been reported in the Far East.[186] Upper lid involvement is two to three times more common than lower lid involvement.[21,186] Other sites include diffuse upper and lower lid involvement (18%) and the medial canthus and caruncle (5% each).[58] The cause of SGC is unknown.[117]

SGC frequently presents as a small, firm, slowly enlarging, painless mass. Although it frequently resembles a chalazion, SGC is rock-hard and nonmobile rather than rubbery and movable.[85] Superficial skin is typically normal and may display telangiectasias.[122] Ulceration usually occurs late in nodular presentations (unless at the lid margin), occasionally mimicking SCC or noduloulcerative BCC, both of which ulcerate earlier.[86] Tumors originating in the glands of Zeis are small, yellow nodules at the lid margin; those arising from the caruncle are subconjunctival, multilobulated yellow masses.[85] SGC may be yellow owing to its high lipid content and may cause atrophy of skin and extensive loss of nearby lashes, more severe than in chronic blepharitis[72,99] (see box below).

SGC can invade overlying palpebral conjunctiva, spreading diffusely throughout the conjunctival sac through the fornix ("pagetoid spread").[146] This phenomenon produces a clinical picture of chronic blepharoconjunctivitis and possibly thickened, hyperemic eyelids.[256] Spread of tumor cells within the conjunctival sac leads to considerable ocular irritation, and further spread within the corneal epithelium causes pannus.[146] SGC masquerading as chronic blepharoconjunctivitis is a common manifestation and may occur more often than its manifestation as a recurrent chalazion. Patients with either condition should have cytopathologic examination of eyelid scrapings or biopsy specimens to rule out SGC.[58]

SGC is infamous for the variety of clinical conditions it mimics[23,30,117,186,256] (see box below). Additionally, histopathologists are not exempt from diagnostic errors with SGC. The three most common errors in histologic diagnosis are SCC, BCC, and unspecified adenocarcinoma[204]; the most common clinical diagnosis at time of presentation is chalazion.[271] Boniuk and Zimmerman have proposed a series of clinical entities leading to a suspicion of SGC[21] (see box on p. 169, left). SGC should be included in the differential diagnosis of all lid lesions, and any clinically malignant lesion of the upper lid should be considered SGC until proven otherwise.[117,228]

Up to 36% of SGCs recur, either locally in the lid or orbit or at distant metastatic sites. Orbital invasion has occurred in up to 17% of cases, and involvement of regional lymph nodes has occurred in up to 28% of cases. The mortality rate for SGC has been calculated to be 15%.[117] Because this carcinoma frequently mimics benign inflammatory conditions, there is often considerable lag between onset of symptoms and diagnosis, contributing to the relatively high mortality.[78,99] Rao and coauthors have delineated multiple clinicopathologic features contributing to a poor prognosis in SGC[203] (see box on p. 169, right).

CLINICAL CHARACTERISTICS OF SEBACEOUS GLAND CARCINOMA

Upper lid involvement
Small, firm mass
Slowly enlarging
Painless
Rock-hard
Nonmobile
Normal surface
Superficial telangiectasias
Ulceration occurs late
Yellow color
Skin atrophy, madarosis
Chronic lid hyperemia, swelling
Conjunctival hyperemia, irritation
Corneal pannus

CONDITIONS FREQUENTLY CONFUSED WITH SEBACEOUS GLAND CARCINOMA

Chalazion
Basal cell carcinoma
Squamous cell carcinoma
Unilateral blepharitis
Unilateral blepharoconjunctivitis
Granulomatous lid lesions (from tuberculosis, sarcoid, syphilis)
Meibomitis
Superior limbic keratoconjunctivitis
Leukoplakia
Ocular pemphigoid
Carcinoma in situ
Cutaneous horn
Lacrimal gland tumor

Surgical management is advocated for all SGCs. If orbital spread has occurred, exenteration has traditionally been the treatment of choice.[117] Previous management of pagetoid spread of the conjunctiva has ranged from no additional treatment to exenteration for local control. Adjunctive cryotherapy has been used to control residual intraepithelial pagetoid spread while avoiding the use of exenteration.[146]

Malignant Melanoma

Malignant melanoma (MM) is well known as a very dangerous form of skin cancer. It comprises only 3% of dermatologic malignancies, yet causes two thirds of all deaths resulting from skin cancer[128] and is responsible for more deaths per year than any other dermatologic malignancy or disease.[127] In spite of earlier detection, better treatment, and improved survival rates, mortality from MM doubled between 1950 and 1980.[129] Incidence of MM has almost tripled in the last four decades[125] and is increasing at rates of 3% to 8% per year,[254] faster than any other malignancy.[237] MM, previously considered more common in older individuals, now shows both increasing incidence and mortality in young adults.[69] Estimates give a newborn in the United States a lifetime risk of MM of 1 in 135; if the incidence continues to rise as it has over the past 50 years, by the year 2000, 1 of every 90 Americans will have had MM in his or her lifetime.

Multiple causes exist for MM, including ultraviolet exposure, precursor lesions, a thinning ozone layer, skin type, genetic susceptibility, and immunologic defects.[27] Ultraviolet light, precursor lesions, and skin type have received the greatest emphasis, but factors of thinning ozone,[103,134] genetic susceptibility,[31,253] and immunologic defects[133,247] have only recently begun to be evaluated.

Numerous studies have evaluated the effects of ultraviolet light. Although it is a causative agent, it is not as clearly related to MM development as it is to the promotion of BCC and particularly SCC.[70] Sunburns at an early age and recreational ultraviolet exposure are implicated in the development of MM, although not conclusively or consistently.[65,107,126,142,153,234] Ultraviolet light is an important element in development of MM but must be considered with other causative factors.

Controversy exists on the role of precursor lesions. Junction nevi acting as precursors have been implicated in all cases of MM[4] as well as in no cases.[40] Often a history of a precursor nevus ac-

---

CLINICAL FEATURES LEADING TO A SUSPICION OF SEBACEOUS GLAND CARCINOMA

Any recurrent or atypical chalazion
Any yellow tumor of the lid margin with eyelash loss, particularly in the upper lid
Diffuse or nodular tumors involving the upper or lower eyelids
Any atypical unilateral blepharitis, meibomitis, or blepharoconjunctivitis, occurring with or without associated keratitis
Any orbital mass developing after removal of a tumor of the eyelid or caruncle
Any lid tumor following excessive radiation to the ocular tissues

Adapted from Boniuk M and Zimmerman LE: Sebaceous carcinoma of the eyelid, eyebrow, caruncle, and orbit, *Trans Am Acad Ophthalmol Otolaryngol* 72:619, 1968.

CLINICOPATHOLOGIC FEATURES ASSOCIATED WITH POOR PROGNOSIS IN SEBACEOUS GLAND CARCINOMA

Vascular invasion
Lymphatic invasion
Upper and lower lid involvement
Orbital invasion
Poor differentiation
Pagetoid invasion
Tumors larger than 10 mm
Highly infiltrative pattern
Multicentric origin (meibomian glands and glands of Zeis)
Duration of symptoms more than 6 months

Adapted from Rao NA and others: Sebaceous carcinomas of the ocular adnexa: a clinicopathologic study of 104 cases, with five-year follow-up data, *Hum Pathol* 13:113, 1982.

companies MM, yet histologic studies vary widely in the magnitude of nevus cells found in or adjacent to MM.[51,66,100,181] When MM develops in an acquired nevus, nevus cells do not undergo normal differentiation, which would ultimately result in the disappearance of the nevus. Instead, aberrant differentiation results initially in melanocytic dysplasia. If progressing to full malignancy, the precursor first grows radially, then vertically, with increasing metastatic potential.[39] In the setting of familial MM, most precursor lesions are dysplastic nevi.[92,93,182] Additional identifiable precursors are both small and large congenital nevi.[209,210]

Numerous studies suggest that fair skin, ease of burning, difficulty of tanning, likelihood of freckling, light eye color (blue or gray), and fair hair color (blonde or red) are associated with an increased incidence of MM.[65,68,82,151,234] Clustering of all these related phenotypic characteristics in an individual seems more important than any single feature in assessing melanoma risk.[126]

In evaluating the potential for MM, all risk factors must be evaluated. The most significant risk factor for development of MM is a persistently changed or changing nevus.[211] Simple clinical criteria allow the early detection of malignant change in more than 90% of cases.[235] These changes in nevi have been described by an "ABCD" mnemonic:[197]

A = Asymmetric shape of the lesion
B = Border irregularity (regressed or notched)
C = Color variegation involving half-tones or mixtures of red, white, and blue (plus black, brown, tan, red, and violet)
D = Diameter larger than 5 mm (size of a standard pencil eraser)

Of the "ABCD" changes in nevi, the most important features leading to suspicion of malignant transformation are changes in border irregularity and color.[236] Other suspicious features include changes in diameter and surface elevation, as well as itching, bleeding, and pain. Clinicians and patients are taught to notice pigmented lesions that have recently darkened, bled, ulcerated, become

tender, or enlarged; these changes typically apply to melanoma that has already deeply invaded the skin.[173,265] In addition to change in a nevus, other risk factors have been calculated for the development of MM (Table 8-8).

Three subtypes of cutaneous MM occur on the face: superficial spreading melanoma, nodular melanoma, and lentigo maligna melanoma. A fourth type, acral lentiginous melanoma, occurs almost exclusively on the extremities, specifically in nail beds, on palms and soles, and occasionally in mucous membranes. It is most common in blacks and Asians.[96,112,125] It is not discussed further because it never appears on the face.

Superficial spreading melanoma is the most commonly reported melanoma, about 70% of MM in the United States.[38] The hallmark of superficial spreading melanoma is a haphazard combination of colors. Shades of red, white, and blue in a brown or black lesion suggest malignancy; blue is the most ominous color.[173] Additionally, superficial spreading melanoma lacks symmetry in its shape and has irregular borders, with notching indicating interference with tumor spread by an immunocompetent area. Its surface is also irregular[40,171,172] (see box on p. 172, left). Superficial spreading melanoma typically grows horizontally or radially before progressing to a stage of vertical, penetrating growth, signaled by nodule development (Fig. 8-26).

Nodular melanoma is less common, between 12%[38] and 15%[128] of MM in the United States. Nodular melanoma is the most dangerous of melanomas owing to vertical growth without prior radial growth. Nodular melanoma typically presents as a raised, dome-shaped lesion. It may develop in a pre-existing nevus but more often arises in normal skin.[172] Abnormalities of melanin result in dark, elevated tumors, often with bizarre colors (Fig. 8-27). The surface of nodular melanoma may be irregular[40,171,172] (see box on p. 172, right). Nodular melanoma may be amelanotic (resembling a skin polyp) or pink or red (mimicking a blood blister or hemangioma). In fact, nodular melanoma is the most often misdiagnosed of the melanomas. Its hallmark is rapid growth, often over a period of

TABLE 8-8 *Relative Risks of Malignant Melanoma*

Factor	Relative Risk
Persistently changed or changing mole	Very high
Adulthood	88×
Dysplastic nevi	
With history of familial melanoma	148×
Without history of familial melanoma	27×
Lentigo maligna	10×
Large congenital nevi	17×
Caucasian race	
Compared with African Americans	12×
Compared with Hispanics	7×
Previous cutaneous malignant melanoma	5-9×
Cutaneous malignant melanoma in parents, children, or siblings of patient with malignant melanoma	2-8×
Immunosuppression (renal transplants, lymphoma, leukemia)	4×
Skin color	
Those who tan poorly, burn easily	3×
Those with multiple or severe sunburns	3×
Those with red or blonde hair	2-4×
Those who freckle with sun exposure	2×
Sun exposure	
Excessive sun exposure (childhood)	3×
Nonmelanoma skin cancer, actinic keratosis	5×

Adapted from Rhodes AR and others: Risk factors for cutaneous melanoma: a practical method of recognizing predisposed individuals, *JAMA* 258:3146, 1987.

weeks to months. The ABCD rule does not apply to nodular melanoma. Nodular melanoma should be included in the differential diagnosis of any pigmented lesion with a history of rapid growth.[125]

Lentigo maligna melanoma is the least common of the melanomas, between 5%[128] and 10%[38] of MM in the United States, but accounting for the majority of head and neck melanomas.[85] Lentigo maligna melanoma develops in elderly individuals in a premalignant precursor called lentigo maligna or Hutchinson's freckle. Lentigo maligna appears on the face in sun-exposed areas as a flat, discolored area with extremely irregular borders and varying brown tints, resembling a shoe polish stain.[40,41,171,172] Apparent migration of lentigo maligna is explained by expansion in one area accompanied by regression of another area.[235] Malignant transformation into lentigo maligna melanoma is signaled by surface irregularity, elevation, or a nodule within the lentigo maligna itself (Fig. 8-28)[41,171] (see box on p. 173). Because lentigo maligna usually grows radially for years to decades, only 5% or so ultimately develop into melanoma.[260] However, it has the potential for rapid progression (within months) and early excision must be considered as a management option.[120,170]

Although MM of the face makes up about 11% of all melanomas,[128] it is uncommon on eyelid skin, typically comprising about 1% of all eyelid tumors[102] and about 5% of eyelid malignancies.[248] MM can be considered a "rare" eyelid tumor compared with BCC, although its incidence is similar

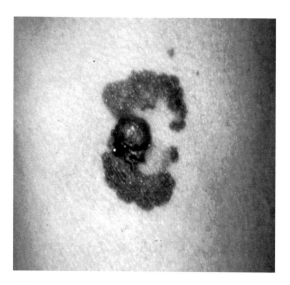

FIG. 8-26 Superficial spreading malignant melanoma, with regression and nodule development.

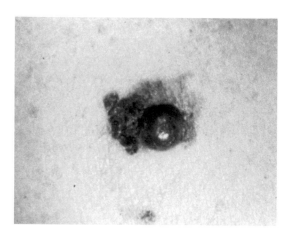

FIG. 8-27 Nodular melanoma, with surrounding flat component.

CHARACTERISTICS OF SUPERFICIAL SPREADING MELANOMA

Color variegation
  Tan, brown, dark brown
  Pink, rose, red (inflammation)
  Blue, blue-gray, purple
  White (regression)
  Haphazard arrangement of colors
  Disorganized combinations of brown

Borders
  Circular outline
  Usually irregular
  Increasing irregularity with enlargement
  Margins often elevated, palpable

Surface
  Irregularly elevated, palpable
  Possible nodules (pink-gray, dark gray)
  Possible yellow-brown, warty surface

CHARACTERISTICS OF NODULAR MELANOMA

Color
  Blue-gray
  Purple-blue
  "Thundercloud gray"
  Blue-black
  Reddish-blue
  Rose-gray
  Black
  Pale gray-blue (amelanotic)

Contour
  Spherical
  Polypoid
  Nodule (elevated)
  No flat component to the nodule
  Often symmetric shape
  Elevated, irregular, blue-black plaque (rare)

Surface
  Smooth
  Ulcerated
  Hyperkeratotic (uncommon)
  Irregular (uncommon)

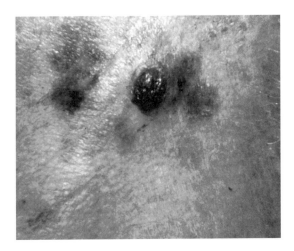

FIG. 8-28 Lentigo maligna melanoma, with irregular, flat areas of lentigo maligna (Hutchinson's freckle) and nodule with friable surface.

to that of SGC and SCC of the eyelids. Two studies agree on the most common melanoma subtype on the eyelids (nodular) but disagree on upper versus lower lid involvement.[83,95] Other recent information claims that superficial spreading melanoma and nodular melanoma are extremely rare on the eyelids, whereas lentigo maligna melanoma is the most frequent periorbital and eyelid melanoma.[85]

Differential diagnosis of MM includes melanocytic, nonmelanocytic, and vascular lesions[125,128,151] (see box, lower right). Melanocytic nevi may grow, darken, or increase in number at various times of life, particularly during puberty and pregnancy. Solar lentigines ("liver spots") are brown but more regular in color and smaller in size than lentigo maligna. Seborrheic keratosis, when darkly pigmented, has a "stuck on" appearance with a granular surface. Nodular melanoma, when darkly pigmented, can be confused with a pigmented BCC. Conversely, nodular melanoma, when presenting in shades of red or pink, resembles hemangioma (with or without surface trauma), Kaposi's sarcoma (typically violaceous in color), or Merkel cell tumor (typically red or violaceous).

The best predictor of survival in stage I melanoma (localized, without regional lymph node in-

CHARACTERISTICS OF LENTIGO MALIGNA MELANOMA

Color
　Usually variants of tan or brown
　White, gray-white (regression)
　Reticulated or flecked brown or black
　Variegation of colors

Borders
　Irregular everywhere on lesion
　Extremely convoluted

Surface characteristics
　Perfectly flat when lentigo maligna
　Largest surface area of melanomas

Signs of invasion
　Irregular surface
　Elevation
　Nodule (brown, black, blue-black)

DIFFERENTIAL DIAGNOSIS OF MALIGNANT MELANOMA

Acquired nevi
　Junction nevus
　Compound nevus
　Dermal nevus
Blue nevus
Halo nevus
Spitz nevus (benign juvenile melanoma)
Dysplastic nevus
Lentigo
　Lentigo simplex
　Solar lentigo
Dermatofibroma
Pigmented seborrheic keratosis
Pigmented actinic keratosis
Pigmented basal cell carcinoma
Merkel cell carcinoma
Hemangioma
Hemorrhage into cyst, nevus, or nailbed
Kaposi's sarcoma
Ulcerated pyogenic granuloma

volvement) remains the vertical thickness of the tumor.[214] Breslow used an ocular micrometer to quantitatively measure vertical thickness; this technique provides a better measure of prognosis than the level of invasion of the melanoma.[24,25] Favorable prognostic factors include radial rather than vertical growth phases; metastasis to skin or distant lymph nodes rather than to viscera; and lesions on arms, forearms, thighs, and legs rather than on the head and neck, trunk, hands, and feet.[212] Clinical types of melanoma may vary in their 5-year rates of survival. Nodular melanoma and acral lentiginous melanoma have poorer survival rates (about 65%) than do superficial spreading melanoma and lentigo maligna melanoma (85% to 90%), but the rates tend to equalize after controlling for differences in tumor thickness at the time of presentation.[125]

Once melanoma is suspected, excisional biopsy with a narrow margin of normal-appearing skin is performed. If MM is diagnosed, surgical excision is the treatment of choice. Thin melanomas (less than 1 mm thick) are excised along with a 1-cm margin of clinically normal skin and underlying subcutaneous tissue down to fascia, with the surgical margin histologically uninvolved by tumor.[187]

Treatment of patients with regional lymph node metastasis combines lymph node dissection with excision of the primary tumor. Adjuvant therapies are used to prolong survival in patients at risk for distant metastases, including chemotherapy, nonspecific immunotherapy, active specific immunotherapy, immunochemotherapy, and radiation therapy.[125,238]

Metastatic melanoma is generally incurable. Palliative treatment strategies have traditionally included chemotherapy, radiation therapy, and surgery. Experimental trials of innovative therapies are underway but are not conclusive. These newer therapies include high-dose chemotherapy followed by autologous bone marrow transplantation, colony-stimulating factors, interferon, monoclonal antibodies, and adoptive immunotherapy (using interleukin-2 to generated lymphokine-activated killer cells).[125]

CONCLUSION

It is impossible to estimate the true incidence of all benign and malignant eyelid lesions. The only available means is to study retrospectively all lesions submitted for pathologic evaluation. Studies of this nature are limited by patient motivation, economic factors, and over-referral by the surgeon. Nevertheless, studies find that benign lesions are three to five times more common than malignancies. Seborrheic keratoses, papillomas, chalazia, and inclusion cysts are the most common benign conditions; basal cell carcinoma is consistently the most common malignancy.[7,248] These same studies found that basal cell carcinoma comprised 18% to 19% of *all* lesions evaluated.

The high frequency of basal cell carcinoma on the eyelids is echoed by its high frequency elsewhere on the body. Nonmelanoma skin cancer (basal cell carcinoma and squamous cell carcinoma) is continually increasing. Estimates of more than 700,000 cases of nonmelanoma skin cancer were made for 1993;[22] together BCC and SCC account for more than half of all cancer diagnosed.[247] Malignant melanoma, although uncommon on the eyelids, is also increasing in incidence; about 32,000 new cases were estimated for 1993.[22] Because of its high risk, despite improvements in treatment, malignant melanoma is a public health problem. It is incumbent on the primary care optometrist to encourage increased patient awareness and prevention of skin cancer.

The value of early detection of skin cancer is indisputable.[160] Because so many of the lesions are mimicked by both benign *and* malignant entities and are subject to myriad clinical variations, the doctor must be alert to signs that suggest malignancy[34,50,240] (see box on p. 175). Suspicion of malignancy and appropriate referral are more important than the correct naming of a lesion; the danger is in doing nothing to a malignant lesion suspected to be benign.[248] Awareness of possible malignancy is important for any dermatologic lesion, but even more so for eyelid lesions, owing to increased risk of recurrence, difficulty of surgical removal, and complexity of restoring normal anatomic structure

FACTORS RAISING SUSPICION OF MALIGNANCY

Unpredictable behavior of lesion
Lesion not typical for patient's demographics
   Age
   Gender
   Race
History of dermatologic malignancy elsewhere
History of other malignancy or immunosuppression
Older patients
Excessive ultraviolet exposure
   Older patients
   Younger patients
   Geographic location
   Vocation or avocation
Family history of skin cancers
   Nonmelanoma skin cancer
   Malignant melanoma
   Dysplastic nevus syndrome
Fair-complectioned patients
Infection, inflammation
   Unresponsive to usual therapy
   Occurring in a previously stable lesion
Change in a previously stable lesion
   Color
   Border irregularity
   Size and shape
   Irregular or unpredictable growth
Other lesion characteristics
   Erosion, ulceration, bleeding
   Inflammation, infection
   Unusually large size
   Irregular tissue quality, poor surface integrity
   Telangiectasias
   Concurrent madarosis, conjunctival hyperemia, tearing

and function. One dermatologist claimed that he saw typical tumor only half the time; the remainder of diagnoses were based on a combination of patient risk factors and atypical behavior of the skin lesion.[240]

Both ultraviolet A (320 to 400 nm) and ultraviolet B (290 to 320 nm) are responsible for skin cancer,[12] but ultraviolet contributes more heavily to its development.[77] Ultraviolet light may reduce the immune response, both by suppression of Langerhans' cells and by induction of suppressor lymphocytes.[133] The loss of protective ozone, with resultant increase in amounts of ultraviolet B, may promote nonmelanoma skin cancer. One study proposed that a 1% depletion in the ozone layer per year will result in an increase of 2% in the incidence of skin cancer.[103] With a possible increase in ultraviolet B radiation in the coming years, protection becomes increasingly important. Regular use of sunscreens with SPF 15 during the first 18 years of life could reduce the lifetime incidence of nonmelanoma skin cancer by 78%.[241]

It behooves the eyecare professional to encourage prevention of actinic damage in all patients, particularly those at greatest risk. Several strategies have been proposed to specifically reduce the morbidity and mortality from squamous cell carcinoma, but their relevance extends to reducing risk for all skin cancer: (1) minimize ultraviolet radiation by preserving the stratospheric ozone layer; (2) reduce ultraviolet radiation exposure with sunscreens, sun avoidance during periods of most intense radiation, no sunbathing, and use of protective clothing and hats; (3) treat precursor lesions, such as actinic keratoses; and (4) encourage early detection and effective treatment of squamous cell carcinoma.[259]

ACKNOWLEDGMENTS

Special thanks goes to several individuals for their generous assistance with illustrations:
Joel I. Brown, O.D.
Marc D. Chalet, M.D.
Ronald L. Moy, M.D.
William V. R. Shellow, M.D.
The staff optometrists and residents of the Optometry Service, Department of Veterans Affairs, West Los Angeles Medical Center
Al Garcia, Southern California College of Optometry, for photographic reproduction

REFERENCES

1. Abreo F and Sansui ID: Basal cell carcinoma in North American blacks. Clinical and histopathologic study of 26 patients, *J Am Acad Dermatol* 25:1005, 1991.

2. Adam E: Herpes simplex virus infections. In Glaser R and Gotlieb-Stematsky T, editors: *Human herpesvirus infections,* New York, 1982, Marcel Dekker, Inc.

3. Aguilar GL, Egbert P: Eyelid tumors, *Curr Opin Ophthalmol* 3:333, 1992.

4. Allen AC and Spitz S: Histogenesis and clinicopathologic correlation of nevi and malignant melanomas: Current status, *Arch Dermatol Syphilol* 69:150, 1954.

5. Altman A and others: Basal cell epithelioma in black patients, *J Am Acad Dermatol* 17:741, 1987.

6. Armstrong BK, de Klerk NH, and Holman CDJ: Etiology of common acquired melanocytic nevi: constitutional variables, sun exposure, and diet, *J Natl Cancer Inst* 77:329, 1986.

7. Aurora AL and Blodi FC: Lesions of the eyelids: a clinicopathological study, *Surv Ophthalmol* 15:94, 1970.

8. Baer RL and others: Papillated squamous cell carcinoma in situ arising in a seborrheic keratosis, *J Am Acad Dermatol* 5:561, 1981.

9. Bartlett JD: *Diseases of the eyelids.* In Bartlett JD and Jaanus SD, editors: *Clinical ocular pharmacology,* ed 2, Boston, 1989, Butterworths.

10. Bean B, Braun C, and Balfour HH: Acyclovir therapy for acute herpes zoster, *Lancet* 2:118, 1982.

11. Bedford MA and Migdal CS: The management of eyelid neoplasms, *Trans Ophthalmol Soc UK* 102:116, 1982.

12. Berger RS: Sun protection and skin cancer, *NJ Med* 86:348, 1989.

13. Bernstein JE and others: Treatment of chronic postherpetic neuralgia with topical capsaicin, *J Am Acad Dermatol* 17:93, 1987.

14. Bernstein JE and others: Topical capsaicin treatment of chronic postherpetic neuralgia, *J Am Acad Dermatol* 21:265, 1989.

15. Beyer CK and others: Merkel cell tumor of the eyelid: a clinicopathologic case report, *Arch Ophthalmol* 101:1098, 1983.

16. Bezan D: An overview of dermatology for primary care providers, *J Am Optom Assoc* 61:138, 1990.

17. Bloomfield SE: *Clinical allergy and immunology of the external eye.* In Tasman W and Jaeger AE, editors: *Duane's clinical ophthalmology,* vol 4, Philadelphia, 1990, JB Lippincott.

18. Boniuk M: *Differentiation of squamous cell carcinoma from other epithelial tumors of the eyelid.* In Boniuk M, editor: *Ocular and adnexal tumors: new and controversial aspects,* St. Louis, 1964, Mosby–Year Book.

19. Boniuk M: Tumors of the eyelids, *Int Ophthalmol Clin* 2:239, 1962.

20. Boniuk M and Zimmerman LE: Eyelid tumors with reference to lesions confused with squamous cell carcinoma. III. Keratoacanthoma, *Arch Ophthalmol* 77:29, 1967.

21. Boniuk M and Zimmerman LE: Sebaceous carcinoma of the eyelid, eyebrow, caruncle, and orbit, *Trans Am Acad Ophthalmol Otolaryngol* 72:619, 1968.

22. Boring CC, Squires TS, and Tong T: Cancer statistics, 1993, *CA* 43:7, 1993.

23. Brauninger GG, Hood CI, and Worthen DM: Sebaceous carcinoma of lid margin masquerading as cutaneous horn, *Arch Ophthalmol* 90:380, 1973.

24. Breslow A: Thickness, cross-sectional areas and depth of invasion in the prognosis of cutaneous melanoma, *Ann Surg* 172:902, 1970.

25. Breslow A: Tumor thickness, level of invasion and node dissection in stage I cutaneous melanoma, *Ann Surg* 182:572, 1975.

26. Bright DC: Dermatologic conditions of the eyelids and face, *Optom Clin* 1(4):89, 1991.

27. Brown MD, Johnson TM, and Swanson NA: Changing trends in melanoma treatment and the expanding role of the dermatologist, *Dermatol Clin* 9:657, 1991.

28. Bryson YJ and others: Treatment of first episodes of genital herpes simplex virus infection

with oral acyclovir: a randomized double-blind controlled trial in normal subjects, *N Engl J Med* 308:916, 1983.

29. Bucci FA, Gabriels CF, and Krohel GB: Successful treatment of postherpetic neuralgia with capsaicin, *Am J Ophthalmol* 106:758, 1988.

30. Callahan MA and Callahan A: *Sebaceous carcinoma of the eyelids.* In Jakobiec FA, editor: *Ocular and adnexal tumors,* Birmingham, 1978, Aesculapius Publishing Company.

31. Cannon-Albright LA and others: Assignment of a locus for familial melanoma, MLM, to chromosome 9p13-p22, *Science* 258:1148, 1992.

32. Carter DM: *Basal cell carcinoma.* In Fitzpatrick TB and others, editors: *Dermatology in general medicine,* ed 3, New York, 1987, McGraw-Hill Information Services Company.

33. Castilla EE, Dutra MG, and Orioli-Parreiras IM: Epidemiology of congenital pigmented nevi: I. Incidence rates and relative frequencies, *Br J Dermatol* 104:307, 1981.

34. Catania LJ: *Primary care of the anterior segment,* Norwalk, Conn, 1988, Appleton & Lange.

35. Ceilley RI and Anderson RL: Microscopically controlled excision of malignant neoplasms on and around eyelids followed by immediate surgical reconstruction, *J Dermatol Surg Oncol* 4:55, 1978.

36. Chuang T-Y and others: Basal cell carcinoma. A population-based incidence study in Rochester, Minnesota, *J Am Acad Dermatol* 22:413, 1990.

37. Chuang T-Y and others: Squamous cell carcinoma. A population-based incidence study in Rochester, Minn, *Arch Dermatol* 126:185, 1990.

38. Clark WH and others: The developmental biology of primary human malignant melanomas, *Semin Oncol* 2:83, 1975.

39. Clark WH and others: A study of tumor progression: the precursor lesions of superficial spreading and nodular melanoma, *Hum Pathol* 15:1147, 1984.

40. Clark WH and others: The histogenesis and biologic behavior of primary human malignant melanomas of the skin, *Cancer Res* 29:705, 1969.

41. Clark WH and Mihm MC: Lentigo maligna and lentigo-maligna melanoma, *Am J Pathol* 55:39, 1969.

42. Clark WH and others: Origin of familial malignant melanomas from heritable melanocytic lesions: 'the B-K mole syndrome,' *Arch Dermatol* 114:732, 1978.

43. Cobo LM and others: Oral acyclovir in the therapy of acute herpes zoster ophthalmicus: an interim report, *Ophthalmology* 92:1574, 1985.

44. Cobo LM and others: Oral acyclovir in the treatment of acute herpes zoster ophthalmicus, *Ophthalmology* 93:763, 1986.

45. Cobo M: Reduction of the ocular complications of herpes zoster ophthalmicus by oral acyclovir, *Am J Med* 85(suppl 2A):90, 1988.

46. Cobo M, Ortiz JR, and Goins K: Viral diseases of the eyelids, *Ophthalmol Clin North Am* 5:177, 1992.

47. Cole EL and others: Herpes zoster ophthalmicus and acquired immune deficiency syndrome, *Arch Ophthalmol* 102:1027, 1984.

48. Corey L and Spear PG: Infections with herpes simplex viruses, (first of two parts), *N Engl J Med* 314:686, 1986.

49. Corey L and Spear PG: Infections with herpes simplex viruses, (second of two parts), *N Engl J Med* 314:749, 1986.

50. Crawford JB: *Neoplastic and inflammatory tumors of the eyelids.* In Tasman W and Jaeger AE, editors: *Duane's clinical ophthalmology,* vol 4, Philadelphia, 1990, JB Lippincott.

51. Crucioli V and Stilwell J: The histogenesis of malignant melanoma in relation to pre-existing pigmented lesions, *J Cut Pathol* 9:396, 1982.

52. Crumpacker CS: *Herpes simplex.* In Fitzpatrick TB and others, editors: *Dermatology in general medicine,* ed 3, New York, 1987, McGraw-Hill Information Services Company.

53. Davis NC and others: Pigmented skin tumors, *CA* 23:160, 1973.

54. Dinehart SM and Pollack SV: Metastases from squamous cell carcinoma of the skin and lip. An analysis of twenty-seven cases, *J Am Acad Dermatol* 21:241, 1989.

55. Dodson JM and others: Malignant potential of actinic keratoses and the controversy over treatment. A patient-oriented perspective, *Arch Dermatol* 127:1029, 1991.

56. Dover JS and Arndt KA: Dermatology [Contempo 1991], *JAMA* 265:3111, 1991.

57. Dover JS and Arndt KA: Dermatology [Contempo 1992], *JAMA* 268:342, 1992.

58. Doxanas MT and Green WR: Sebaceous gland carcinoma: review of 40 cases, *Arch Ophthalmol* 102:245, 1984.

59. Doxanas MT, Green WR, and Iliff CE: Factors in the successful surgical management of basal cell carcinoma of the eyelids, *Am J Ophthalmol* 91:726, 1981.

60. Doxanas MT and others: Squamous cell carcinoma of the eyelids, *Ophthalmology* 94:538, 1987.

61. Downes RN, Walker NPJ, and Collin JRO: Micrographic (Mohs') surgery in the management of periocular basal cell epitheliomas, *Eye* 4:160, 1990.

62. Edgerton AE: Herpes zoster ophthalmicus: report of cases and review of literature, *Arch Ophthalmol* 34:40, 1945.

63. Egerer I and Stary A: Erosive-ulcerative herpes simplex blepharitis, *Arch Ophthalmol* 98:1760, 1980.

64. Einaugler RB and Henkind P: Basal cell epithelioma of the eyelid: apparent incomplete removal, *Am J Ophthalmol* 67:413, 1969.

65. Elder DE: Human melanocytic neoplasms and their etiologic relationship with sunlight, *J Invest Dermatol* 92(suppl):297S, 1989.

66. Elder DE and others: *Acquired melanocytic nevi and melanoma: the dysplastic nevus syndrome*. In Ackerman AB, editor: *Pathology of malignant melanoma*, New York, 1981, Masson Publishing USA.

67. Elion GB: Mechanism of action and selectivity of acyclovir, *Am J Med* 73(suppl A):7, 1982.

68. Elwood JM and others: Pigmentation and skin reaction to sun as risk factors for cutaneous melanoma: Western Canada Melanoma Study, *Br Med J* 288:99, 1984.

69. Elwood JM and Lee JAH: Recent data on the epidemiology of malignant melanoma, *Semin Oncol* 2:149, 1975.

70. Elwood JM and others: Relationship of melanoma and other skin cancer mortality to latitude and ultraviolet radiation in the United States and Canada, *Int J Epidemiol* 3:325, 1974.

71. Epstein E: Value of follow-up after treatment of basal cell carcinoma, *Arch Dermatol* 108:798, 1973.

72. Epstein GA and Putterman AM: Sebaceous adenocarcinoma of the eyelid, *Ophthalmic Surg* 14:935, 1983.

73. Epstein WL: *Allergic contact dermatitis*. In Fitzpatrick TB and others, editors: *Dermatology in general medicine*, ed 3, New York, 1987, McGraw-Hill Information Services Company.

74. Farmer ER and Helwig EB: Metastatic basal cell carcinoma: a clinicopathologic study of seventeen cases, *Cancer* 46:748, 1980.

75. Fawcett IM and Lee WR: Merkel cell carcinoma of the eyelid, *Graefe's Arch Clin Exp Ophthalmol* 224:330, 1986.

76. Ferry AP: *The eyelids*. In Sorsby A, editor: *Modern ophthalmology*, ed 2, London, 1972, Butterworths.

77. Fitzpatrick TB and Sober AJ: Sunlight and skin cancer, *N Engl J Med* 313:818, 1985.

78. Foster CS and Allansmith MR: Chronic unilateral blepharoconjunctivitis caused by sebaceous carcinoma, *Am J Ophthalmol* 86:218, 1978.

79. Freeman RG: Histopathologic considerations in the management of skin cancer, *J Dermatol Surg* 2:215, 1976.

80. Friedlaender MH: Eczematoid reactions of the skin, *Ophthalmol Clin North Am* 5:195, 1992.

81. Friedman-Kien AE and others: Herpes zoster: a possible early clinical sign for development of acquired immunodeficiency syndrome in high-risk individuals, *J Am Acad Dermatol* 14:1023, 1986.

82. Gallagher RP and others: Risk factors for ocular melanoma: Western Canada melanoma study, *J Natl Cancer Inst* 74:775, 1985.

83. Garner A and others: Malignant melanoma of the eyelid skin: histopathology and behavior, *Br J Ophthalmol* 69:180, 1985.

84. Ghadially FN: *Keratoacanthoma*. In Fitzpatrick TB and others, editors: *Dermatology in general medicine*, ed 3, New York, 1987, McGraw-Hill Information Services Company.

85. Gilberg SM and Tse DT: Malignant eyelid tumors, *Ophthalmol Clin North Am* 5:261, 1992.

86. Ginsberg J: Present status of meibomian gland carcinoma, *Arch Ophthalmol* 73:271, 1965.

87. Goepfert H and others: Merkel cell carcinoma (endocrine carcinoma of the skin) of the head and neck, *Arch Otolaryngol* 110:707, 1984.

88. Goette DK: Basal cell carcinomas arising in seborrheic keratoses, *J Dermatol Surg Oncol* 11:1014, 1985.

89. Goodman DS and others: Prevalence of cutaneous disease in patients with acquired immunodeficiency syndrome (AIDS) or AIDS-related complex, *J Am Acad Dermatol* 17:210, 1987.

90. Graham JH and Helwig EB: Cutaneous premalignant lesions, *Adv Biol Skin* 7:277, 1967.

91. Green A and Swerdlow AJ: Epidemiology of melanocytic nevi, *Epidemiol Rev* 11:204, 1989.

92. Greene MH and others: Acquired precursors of cutaneous malignant melanoma: the familial dysplastic nevus syndrome, *N Engl J Med* 312:91, 1985.

93. Greene MH and others: High risk of malignant melanoma in melanoma-prone families with dysplastic nevi, *Ann Intern Med* 102:458, 1985.

94. Gross J, Gross FJ, and Friedman AH: *Systemic infections and inflammatory diseases.* In Tasman W and Jaeger AE, editors: *Duane's clinical ophthalmology,* vol 5, Philadelphia, 1990, JB Lippincott.

95. Grossniklaus HE and McLean IW: Cutaneous melanoma of the eyelid, *Ophthalmology* 98:1867, 1991.

96. Habif TP: *Clinical dermatology,* ed 2, St. Louis, 1990, Mosby–Year Book.

97. Hanke CW and Lee MW: Mohs' micrographic surgery for the treatment of eyelid malignancy, *Ophthal Plast Reconstr Surg* 4:137, 1991.

98. Harding SP, Lipton JR, and Wells JCD: Natural history of herpes zoster ophthalmicus: predictors of postherpetic neuralgia and ocular involvement, *Br J Ophthalmol* 71:353, 1987.

99. Harvey JT and Anderson RL: The management of meibomian gland carcinoma, *Ophthalmic Surg* 13:56, 1982.

100. Helwig EB: *Malignant melanoma of the skin in man,* NCI Monograph No. 10:287, 1962.

101. Henderson JW and Farrow GM: *Orbital tumors,* ed 2, New York, B.C. Decker, 1980.

102. Henkind P and Friedman A: *Cancer of the lids and ocular adnexa.* In Andrade R and others, editors: *Cancer of the skin,* Philadelphia, 1976, WB Saunders Co.

103. Henriksen T and others: Ultraviolet-radiation and skin cancer effect of an ozone layer depletion, *Photochem Photobiol* 51:579, 1990.

104. Hirsch MS: *Herpes simplex virus.* In Mandell GL, Douglas RG, and Bennett JE, editors: *Principles and practice of infectious diseases,* ed 2, New York, 1985, John Wiley & Sons.

105. Hitchcock CL and others: Neuroendocrine (Merkel cell) carcinoma of the skin. Its natural history, diagnosis, and treatment, *Ann Surg* 207:201, 1988.

106. Hoang-Xuan T and others: Oral acyclovir for herpes zoster ophthalmicus, *Ophthalmology* 99:1062, 1992.

107. Holman CD, Armstrong BK, and Heenan PJ: Relationship of cutaneous malignant melanoma to individual sunlight-exposure habits, *J Natl Cancer Inst* 76:403, 1986.

108. Hope-Simpson RE: The nature of herpes zoster: a long-term study and a new hypothesis, *Proc R Soc Med* 58:9, 1965.

109. Huff JC and others: Therapy of herpes zoster with oral acyclovir, *Am J Med* 85(suppl 2A):84, 1988.

110. Hyndiuk RA and Glasser DB: *Herpes simplex keratitis.* In Tabbara KF and Hyndiuk RA, editors: *Infections of the eye,* Boston, 1986, Little, Brown and Company.

111. Jakobiec FA: Conjunctival melanoma: unfinished business, *Arch Ophthalmol* 98:1378, 1980.

112. Jakobiec FA, Rootman J, and Jones IS: *Secondary and metastatic tumors of the orbit.* In Tasman W and Jaeger AE, editors: *Duane's clinical ophthalmology,* vol 2, Philadelphia, 1990, JB Lippincott.

113. Jessell TM: Neurotransmitters and CNS disease: pain, *Lancet* 2:1084, 1982.

114. Jessell TM, Iversen LL, and Cuello AC: Capsaicin-induced depletion of substance P from sensory neurons, *Brain Res* 152:183, 1978.

115. Jones EW: Some special skin tumors in the elderly, *Br J Dermatol* 122(suppl 35):71, 1990.

116. Jones WL: Basal cell carcinoma: a case of longstanding neglect and a case of early detection, *J Am Optom Assoc* 53:999, 1982.

117. Kass LG and Hornblass A: Sebaceous carcinoma of the ocular adnexa, *Surv Ophthalmol* 33:477, 1989.

118. Katz AD, Urbach F, and Lilienfeld AM: The frequency and risk of metastases in squamous-cell carcinoma of the skin, *Cancer* 10:1162, 1957.

119. Kaufman HE and Rayfield MA: *Viral conjunctivitis and keratitis.* In Kaufman HE and others, editors: *The cornea,* New York, 1988, Churchill-Livingstone.

120. Kelly JW: Following lentigo maligna may not prevent the development of life-threatening melanoma, *Arch Dermatol* 128:657, 1992.

121. Kestelyn P and others: Severe herpes zoster ophthalmicus in young African adults: a marker for HTLV-III seropositivity, *Br J Ophthalmol* 71:806, 1987.

122. Khalil MK and Lorenzetti DWC: Sebaceous gland carcinoma of the lid, *Can J Ophthalmol* 15:117, 1980.

123. Kirkham N and Cole MD: Merkel cell carcinoma: a malignant neuroendocrine tumor of the eyelid, *Br J Ophthalmol* 67:600, 1983.

124. Kivela T and Tarkkanen A: The Merkel cell and associated neoplasms in the eyelids and periocular region, *Surv Ophthalmol* 35:171, 1990.

125. Koh HK: Cutaneous melanoma, *N Engl J Med* 325:171, 1991.

126. Koh HK, Kligler BE, and Lew RA: Sunlight and cutaneous malignant melanoma: evidence for and against causation, *Photochem Photobiol* 51:765, 1990.

127. Kopf AW: Prevention and early detection of skin cancer/melanoma, *Cancer* 62:1791, 1988.

128. Kopf AW, Bart RS, and Rodriguez-Sains RS: Malignant melanoma: a review, *J Dermatol Surg Oncol* 3:41, 1977.

129. Kopf AW, Rigel DS, and Friedman RJ: The rising incidence and mortality rate of malignant melanoma, *J Dermatol Surg Oncol* 8:760, 1982.

130. Kord JP, Cottel WI, and Proper S: Metastatic basal-cell carcinoma, *J Dermatol Surg Oncol* 8:604, 1982.

131. Kraemer KH and others: Risk of cutaneous melanoma in dysplastic nevus syndrome types A and B [letter], *N Engl J Med* 315:1615, 1986.

132. Kricker A and others: Skin cancer in Geraldton, Western Australia: a survey of incidence and prevalence, *Med J Aust* 152:399, 1990.

133. Kripke ML: Immunology and photocarcinogenesis. New light on an old problem, *J Am Acad Dermatol* 14:149, 1986.

134. Kripke ML: Impact of ozone depletion on skin cancers, *J Dermatol Surg Oncol* 14:853, 1988.

135. Kwitko ML, Boniuk M, and Zimmerman LE: Eyelid tumors with reference to lesions confused with squamous cell carcinoma. I. Incidence and errors in diagnosis, *Arch Ophthalmol* 69:693, 1963.

136. Kwittken J: Keratoacanthoma arising in seborrheic keratosis, *Cutis* 144:546, 1974.

137. Lamping K and others: A Merkel cell tumor of the eyelid, *Ophthalmology* 90:1399, 1983.

138. LeBoit PE: Dermatopathologic findings in patients infected with HIV, *Dermatol Clin* 10:59, 1992.

139. Lembeck F, Donnerer J, and Colpaert FC: Increase of substance P in primary afferent nerves during chronic pain, *Neuropeptides* 1:175, 1981.

140. Leopold IH and Sery TW: Epidemiology of herpes simplex keratitis, *Invest Ophthalmol* 2:498, 1963.

141. Levy DW, Banerjee AK, and Glenny HP: Cimetidine in the treatment of herpes zoster, *J R Coll Phys London* 19:96, 1985.

142. Lew RA and others: Sun exposure in patients with cutaneous melanoma: a case control study, *J Dermatol Surg Oncol* 9:981, 1983.

143. Liesegang TJ: Corneal complications from herpes zoster ophthalmicus, *Ophthalmology* 92:316, 1985.

144. Liesegang TJ: Diagnosis and therapy of herpes zoster ophthalmicus, *Ophthalmology* 98:1216, 1991.

145. Liesegang TJ: The varicella-zoster virus: systemic and ocular features, *J Am Acad Dermatol* 11:165, 1984.

146. Lisman RD, Jakobiec FA, and Small P: Sebaceous carcinoma of the eyelids: the role of adjunctive cryotherapy in the management of

conjunctival pagetoid spread, *Ophthalmology* 96:1021, 1989.

147. Lober CW and Fenske NA: Basal cell, squamous cell, and sebaceous gland carcinomas of the periorbital region, *J Am Acad Dermatol* 25:685, 1991.

148. Loeser JD: Herpes zoster and postherpetic neuralgia, *Pain* 25:149, 1986.

149. Lowy DR: *Milker's nodules, molluscum contagiosum.* In Fitzpatrick TB and others, editors: *Dermatology in general medicine,* ed 3, New York, 1987, McGraw-Hill Information Services Company.

150. Lowy DR and Androphy EJ: *Warts.* In Fitzpatrick TB and others, editors: *Dermatology in general medicine,* ed 3, New York, 1987, McGraw-Hill Information Services Company.

151. Luce JK, McBride CM, and Frei E: *Melanoma.* In Holland JF and Frei E, editors: *Cancer medicine,* Philadelphia, 1973, Lea & Febiger.

152. Lund HZ: How often does squamous cell carcinoma of the skin metastasize? *Arch Dermatol* 92:635, 1965.

153. MacKie RM and Aitchison T: Severe sunburn and subsequent risk of primary cutaneous malignant melanoma in Scotland, *Br J Cancer* 46:955, 1982.

154. Mamalis N and others: Merkel cell tumor of the eyelid: a review and report of an unusual case, *Ophthalmic Surg* 20:410, 1989.

155. Mamalis N and others: Malignant lesions of the eyelid, *Am Fam Phys* 39:95, 1989.

156. Marines HM and Patrinely JR: Benign eyelid tumors, *Ophthalmol Clin North Am* 5:243, 1992.

157. Marks R and others: Spontaneous remission of solar keratoses: the case for conservative management, *Br J Dermatol* 115:649, 1986.

158. Marks R, Rennie G, and Selwood TS: Malignant transformation of solar keratoses to squamous cell carcinoma, *Lancet* 1:795, 1988.

159. Martin H, Strong E, and Spiro RH: Radiation-induced skin cancer of the head and neck, *Cancer* 25:61, 1970.

160. Masri GD, Clark WH, and Guerry D: Screening and surveillance of patients at high risk for malignant melanoma result in detection of earlier disease, *J Am Acad Dermatol* 22:1042, 1990.

161. Mathews KP: The urticarias. Current concepts in pathogenesis and treatment, *Drugs* 30:552, 1985.

162. Mavligit GM and Talpaz M: Cimetidine for herpes zoster [letter], *N Engl J Med* 310:318, 1984.

163. Max MB and others: Amitriptyline, but not lorazepam, relieves postherpetic neuralgia, *Neurology* 38:1427, 1988.

164. McBride A and others: Clinical features of dysplastic nevi, *Dermatol Clin* 9:717, 1991.

165. McKendrick MW and others: Oral acyclovir in acute herpes zoster, *Br Med J* 293:1529, 1986.

166. The Medical Letter of Drugs and Therapeutics, 34:62, 1992.

167. Meland NB, and Jackson IT: Merkel cell tumor: diagnosis, prognosis, and management, *Plast Reconstr Surg* 77:632, 1986.

168. Menn H and others: The recurrent basal cell carcinoma: a study of 100 cases of recurrent, re-treated basal cell epithelioma, *Arch Dermatol* 103:628, 1971.

169. Mertz GJ and others: Double-blind placebo-controlled trial of oral acyclovir in first-episode genital herpes simplex virus infection, *JAMA* 252:1147, 1984.

170. Michalik EE, Fitzpatrick TB, and Sober AJ: Rapid progression of lentigo maligna to deeply invasive lentigo maligna melanoma. Report of two cases, *Arch Dermatol* 119:831, 1983.

171. Mihm MC, Clark WH, and From L: The clinical diagnosis, classification and histogenetic concepts of the early stages of cutaneous malignant melanomas, *N Engl J Med* 284:1078, 1971.

172. Mihm MC, Clark WH, and Reed RJ: The clinical diagnosis of malignant melanoma, *Semin Oncol* 2:105, 1975.

173. Mihm MC and others: Early detection of primary cutaneous malignant melanoma, *N Engl J Med* 289:989, 1973.

174. Miller AE: Selective decline in cellular immune response to varicella-zoster in the elderly, *Neurology* 30:582, 1980.

175. Miller SJ: Biology of basal cell carcinoma (Part I), *J Am Acad Dermatol* 24:1, 1991.

176. Miller SJ: Biology of basal cell carcinoma (Part II), *J Am Acad Dermatol* 24:161, 1991.

177. Monheit GD, Callahan MA, and Callahan A: Mohs micrographic surgery for periorbital skin cancer, *Dermatol Clin* 7:677, 1989.

178. Morison WL: Viral warts, herpes simplex and herpes zoster in patients with secondary immune deficiencies and neoplasms, *Br J Dermatol* 92:625, 1975.

179. Morton P and Thomson AN: Oral acyclovir in the treatment of herpes zoster in general practice, *NZ Med J* 102:93, 1989.

180. Murray JE and Cannon B: Basal-cell cancer in children and young adults, *N Engl J Med* 262:440, 1960.

181. Nathanson L, Hall TC, and Vawter GF: Melanoma as a medical problem, *Arch Intern Med* 119:479, 1967.

182. National Institutes of Health Consensus Development Conference on Precursors to Malignant Melanoma: Precursors to malignant melanoma, *JAMA* 251:1864, 1984.

183. Nerad JA and Whitaker DC: Periocular basal cell carcinoma in adults 35 years of age and younger, *Am J Ophthalmol* 106:723, 1988.

184. Nethercott JR, Nield G, and Holness DL: A review of 79 cases of eyelid dermatitis, *J Am Acad Dermatol* 21:223, 1989.

185. Newcomer VD and Young EM: Recognition and treatment of contact dermatitis, *Drug Ther* 21:31, 1991.

186. Ni C and others: Sebaceous cell carcinomas of the ocular adnexa, *Int Ophthalmol Clin* 22:23, 1982.

187. NIH Consensus Development Panel on Early Melanoma: Diagnosis and treatment of early melanoma, *JAMA* 268:1314, 1992.

188. Ostler HB: *Blepharitis*. In Tasman W and Jaeger AE, editors: *Duane's clinical ophthalmology*, vol 4, Philadelphia, 1990, JB Lippincott.

189. Oxman MN: *Varicella and herpes zoster*. In Fitzpatrick TB and others, editors: *Dermatology in general medicine*, ed 3, New York, 1987, McGraw-Hill Information Services Company.

190. Palestine AG and Palestine RF: External ocular manifestations of the acquired immunodeficiency syndrome, *Ophthalmol Clin North Am* 5:319, 1992.

191. Papa CM: Tretinoin therapy for precancerous skin, *NJ Med* 86:361, 1989.

192. Pavan-Langston D and Dunkel EC: Ocular varicella-zoster virus infection in the guinea pig: a new in vivo model, *Arch Ophthalmol* 107:1068, 1989.

193. Payne JW and others: Basal cell carcinoma of the eyelids: a long-term follow-up study, *Arch Ophthalmol* 81:553, 1969.

194. Perniciaro C: Pigmented lesions of the eyelid and conjunctiva, *Ophthalmol Clin North Am* 5:287, 1992.

195. Peterslund NA and others: Acyclovir in herpes zoster, *Lancet* 2:827, 1981.

196. Petty BG: *Viral diseases of the skin*. In Rakel RE, editor: *Conn's current therapy 1990*, Philadelphia, 1990, WB Saunders Co.

197. Phillips TJ and Dover JS: Recent advances in dermatology, *N Engl J Med* 326:167, 1992.

198. Pollack SV and others: The biology of basal cell carcinoma: a review, *J Am Acad Dermatol* 7:569, 1982.

199. Purdy EP and Bullock JD: Eyelid tumors, *Curr Opin Ophthalmol* 2:271, 1991.

200. Ragozzino MW and others: Population-based study of herpes zoster and its sequelae, *Medicine* 61:310, 1982.

201. Ragozzino MW and others: Risk of cancer after herpes zoster, *N Engl J Med* 307:393, 1982.

202. Rampen FHJ and others: Prevalence of common "acquired" nevocytic nevi and dysplastic nevi is not related to ultraviolet exposure, *J Am Acad Dermatol* 18:679, 1988.

203. Rao NA and others: Sebaceous carcinomas of the ocular adnexa: a clinicopathologic study of 104 cases, with five-year follow-up data, *Hum Pathol* 13:113, 1982.

204. Rao NA, McLean IW, and Zimmerman LE: *Sebaceous carcinoma of eyelids and caruncle: correlation of clinicopathologic features with prognosis*. In Jakobiec FA, editor: *Ocular and adnexal tumors*, Birmingham, 1978, Aesculapius Publishing Company.

205. Reed RJ and others: Common and uncommon melanocytic nevi and borderline melanomas, *Semin Oncol* 2:119, 1975.

206. Reichman RC and others: Treatment of recurrent genital herpes simplex infections with oral acyclovir: a controlled trial, *JAMA* 251:2103, 1984.

207. Reifler DM and Hornblass A: Squamous cell carcinoma of the eyelid, *Surv Ophthalmol* 30:349, 1986.

208. Rhodes AR: *Neoplasms: benign neoplasias, hyperplasias, and dysplasias of melanocytes*. In Fitzpatrick TB and others, editors: *Dermatology in general medicine*, ed 3, New York, 1987, McGraw-Hill Information Services Company.

209. Rhodes AR: Pigmented birthmarks and precursor melanocytic lesions of cutaneous melanoma identifiable in childhood, *Pediatr Clin North Am* 30:435, 1983.

210. Rhodes AR and Melski JW: Small congenital nevocellular nevi and the risk of cutaneous melanoma, *J Pediatr* 100:219, 1982.

211. Rhodes AR and others: Risk factors for cutaneous melanoma: a practical method of recognizing predisposed individuals, *JAMA* 258:3146, 1987.

212. Rigel DS and others: Factors influencing survival in melanoma, *Dermatol Clin* 9:631, 1991.

213. Rigel DS and Kopf AW: The rate of malignant melanoma in the United States: are we making an impact? *J Am Acad Dermatol* 17:1050, 1987.

214. Rivers JK and Ho VC: Malignant melanoma: who shall live and who shall die? *Arch Dermatol* 128:537, 1992.

215. Rodriguez-Sains RS: The aging face: commonly encountered tumors and cutaneous changes, *Adv Ophthalmic Plast Reconstr Surg* 2:9, 1983.

216. Rodriguez-Sains RS, Jakobiec FA, and Iwamoto T: Lentigo maligna of the lateral canthal skin, *Ophthalmology* 88:1186, 1981.

217. Roenigk RK and others: Trends in the presentation and treatment of basal cell carcinomas, *J Dermatol Surg Oncol* 12:860, 1986.

218. Rubsamen PE and others: Merkel cell carcinoma of the eyelid and periocular tissues, *Am J Ophthalmol* 113:674, 1992.

219. Rudzki E: Contact sensitivity to systemically administered drugs, *Dermatol Clin* 8:177, 1990.

220. Sandor EV and others: Herpes zoster ophthalmicus in patients at risk for the acquired immune deficiency syndrome (AIDS), *Am J Ophthalmol* 101:153, 1986.

221. Satterthwaite JR and Tollison CD: Diagnosis and treatment of acute herpes zoster, *Drug Ther* 19:94, 1989.

222. Sauer GC: *Manual of skin diseases*, ed 5, Philadelphia, 1985, JB Lippincott.

223. Schwartz RA and Stoll HL: *Epithelial precancerous lesions*. In Fitzpatrick TB and others, editors: *Dermatology in general medicine*, ed 3, New York, 1987, McGraw-Hill Information Services Company.

224. Scotto J, Kopf AW, and Urbach F: Non-melanoma skin cancer among Caucasians in four areas of the United States, *Cancer* 34:1333, 1974.

225. Seab JA: Dysplastic nevi and the dysplastic nevus syndrome, *Dermatol Clin* 10:189, 1992.

226. Searl SS and others: Malignant Merkel cell neoplasm of the eyelid, *Arch Ophthalmol* 102:907, 1984.

227. Serrano H and others: Incidence of nonmelanoma skin cancer in New Hampshire and Vermont, *J Am Acad Dermatol* 24:574, 1991.

228. Shore JW and Bilyk JR: Clinical presentation, diagnosis, and treatment of eyelid tumors, *Curr Opin Ophthalmol* 2:579, 1991.

229. Shuler JD, Engstrom RE, and Holland GN: External ocular disease and anterior segment disorders associated with AIDS, *Int Ophthalmol Clin* 29:98, 1989.

230. Sibley RK, Dehner LP, and Rosai J: Primary neuroendocrine (Merkel cell?) carcinoma of the skin. I. A clinicopathologic and ultrastructural study of 43 cases, *Am J Surg Pathol* 9:95, 1985.

231. Sitz KV, Keppen M, and Johnson DF: Metastatic basal cell carcinoma in acquired immunodeficiency syndrome-related complex, *JAMA* 257:340, 1987.

232. Smith KR: The haarscheibe, *J Invest Dermatol* 69:68, 1977.

233. Sober AJ: Diagnosis and management of skin cancer, *Cancer* 51(June suppl):2448, 1983.

234. Sober AJ: Solar exposure in the etiology of cutaneous melanoma, *Photodermatology* 4:23, 1987.

235. Sober AJ, Fitzpatrick TB, and Mihm MC: Primary melanoma of the skin: recognition and management, *J Am Acad Dermatol* 2:179, 1980.

236. Sober AJ and others: Early recognition of cutaneous melanoma, *JAMA* 242:2795, 1979.

237. Sober AJ, Lew RA, and Koh HK: Epidemiology of cutaneous melanoma. An update, *Dermatol Clin* 9:617, 1991.

238. Sober AJ and others: *Neoplasms: malignant melanoma.* In Fitzpatrick TB and others, editors: *Dermatology in general medicine,* ed 3, New York, 1987, McGraw-Hill Information Services Company.

239. Soter NA and Wasserman SI: *IgE-dependent urticaria and angioedema.* In Fitzpatrick TB and others, editors: *Dermatology in general medicine,* ed 3, New York, 1987, McGraw-Hill Information Services Company.

240. Stegman SJ: Basal cell carcinoma and squamous cell carcinoma, *Med Clin North Am* 70:95, 1986.

241. Stern RS, Weinstein MC, and Baker SG: Risk reduction for nonmelanoma skin cancer with childhood sunscreen use, *Arch Dermatol* 122:537, 1986.

242. Stoll HL and Schwartz RA: *Squamous cell carcinoma.* In Fitzpatrick TB and others, editors: *Dermatology in general medicine,* ed 3, New York, 1987, McGraw-Hill Information Services Company.

243. Straatsma BR: Meibomian gland tumors, *Arch Ophthalmol* 56:71, 1956.

244. Straus SE: Clinical and biological differences between recurrent herpes simplex virus and varicella-zoster virus infections, *JAMA* 262:3455, 1989.

245. Straus SE and others: Varicella-zoster virus infections, *Ann Intern Med* 108:221, 1988.

246. Sturgis MD and Oshinskie LJ: Optometric management of eyelid malignancies, *J Am Optom Assoc* 58:307, 1987.

247. Taylor CR and others: Photoaging/photodamage and photoprotection, *J Am Acad Dermatol* 22:1, 1990.

248. Tesluk GC: Eyelid lesions: incidence and comparison of benign and malignant lesions, *Ann Ophthalmol* 17:704, 1985.

249. Theodore FH: Differentiation and treatment of eczemas of the eyelids, *Trans Am Acad Ophthalmol Otolaryngol* 58:708, 1954.

250. Tindall JP: Skin changes and lesions in our senior citizens: incidences, *Cutis* 18:359, 1976.

251. Tindall JP and Smith JG: Skin lesions of the aged and their association with internal changes, *JAMA* 186:1039, 1963.

252. Toker C: Trabecular carcinoma of the skin, *Arch Dermatol* 105:107, 1972.

253. Travis J: Closing in on melanoma susceptibility gene(s), *Science* 258:1080, 1992.

254. van der Esch EP and others: Temporal change in diagnostic criteria as a cause of the increase of malignant melanoma over time is unlikely, *Int J Cancer* 47:483, 1991.

255. von Domarus H, Johanisson R, and Schmauz R: Merkel cell carcinoma of the face: case report and review of the literature, *J Maxillofac Surg* 13:39, 1985.

256. Wagoner MD and others: Common presentations of sebaceous gland carcinoma of the eyelid, *Ann Ophthalmol* 14:159, 1982.

257. Walsh TD: Antidepressants in chronic pain, *Clin Neuropharmacol* 6:271, 1983.

258. Watson CP and others: Amitriptyline versus placebo in postherpetic neuralgia, *Neurology* (NY) 32:671, 1982.

259. Weinstock MA: The epidemic of squamous cell carcinoma, *JAMA* 262:2138, 1989.

260. Weinstock MA and Sober AJ: The risk of progression of lentigo maligna to lentigo maligna melanoma, *Br J Dermatol* 116:303, 1987.

261. Welch RB and Duke JR: Lesions of the lids: a statistical note, *Am J Ophthalmol* 45:415, 1958.

262. Weller TH: Varicella and herpes zoster: changing concepts of the natural history, control, and importance of a not-so-benign virus (first of two parts), *N Engl J Med* 309:1362, 1983.

263. Weller TH: Varicella and herpes zoster: changing concepts of the natural history, control, and importance of a not-so-benign virus (second of two parts), *N Engl J Med* 309:1434, 1983.

264. Wesley RE and Collins JW: Basal cell carcinoma of the eyelid as an indicator of multifocal malignancy, *Am J Ophthalmol* 94:591, 1982.

265. Wick MM and others: Clinical characteristics of early cutaneous melanoma, *Cancer* 45:2684, 1980.

266. Wilson FM: *Varicella and herpes zoster ophthalmicus*. In Tabbara KF and Hyndiuk RA, editors: *Infections of the eye,* Boston, 1986, Little, Brown & Co.

267. Winkelmann RK and Breathnach AS: The Merkel cell, *J Invest Dermatol* 60:2, 1973.

268. Womack LW and Liesegang TJ: Complications of herpes zoster ophthalmicus, *Arch Ophthalmol* 101:42, 1983.

269. Wood MJ and others: Efficacy of oral acyclovir treatment of acute herpes zoster, *Am J Med* 85(suppl 2A):79, 1988.

270. Yakar JB and others: Malignant melanoma appearing in seborrheic keratosis, *J Dermatol Surg Oncol* 10:382, 1984.

271. Yeatts RP and Waller RR: Sebaceous carcinoma of the eyelid: pitfalls in diagnosis, *Ophthalmic Plast Reconstr Surg* 1:35, 1985.

272. Zakzouk MS, Ramsay AD, and Buchanan G: Merkel cell tumor of the skin, *J Laryngol Otol* 100:561, 1986.

9

Cardiovascular Disease

DAVID S. KOUNTZ
JOHN H. NISHIMOTO

KEY TERMS

Systolic Hypertension
Hypercholesterolemia
ACE Inhibitors
Calcium Channel Blockers
Hypertensive Retinopathy
Arteriosclerosis

Angina
Nitrates
Beta-blockers
Myocardial Infarction
Streptokinase

Tissue Plasminogen Activator
Claudication
Transient Ischemic Attacks
Embolism
Endocarditis

---

*D*espite the proliferation of exciting techniques in the area of cardiology, patient history remains the most important tool in the evaluation of patients with suspected cardiovascular disease. In this chapter we review the major risk factors for the development of various cardiovascular disorders, including angina pectoris, acute myocardial infarction, peripheral vascular disease (intermittent claudication), and transient ischemic attacks. Each topic is preceded by a typical patient history and discussion that focus on important historical clues, physical examination findings, and key management issues for the optometrist.

HYPERTENSION

Case Study

A 75-year-old woman with a 25-year history of mild hypertension presents for follow-up of her bilateral cataracts. She relates a history of hypertension intermittently treated for the last 25 years. She is quite interested in her overall health care and is currently on no medication. She has seen four physicians in the last 12 months and at each office visit she has had a systolic blood pressure of more than 180 and a diastolic blood pressure in a range of 85 to 95.

The case above demonstrates a patient with isolated *systolic hypertension,* which is a systolic blood pressure of more than 160 mm Hg with a normal diastolic blood pressure. Isolated systolic hypertension is an important risk factor for cardiovascular and cerebrovascular complications.

No discussion of cardiovascular disorders should begin without mentioning the critical importance of hypertension. The size of the population of the United States affected with hypertension is staggering—roughly 20% of adults above the age of 18 have systolic blood pressures in excess of 140 mm Hg and/or diastolic blood pressure greater than 90 mm Hg. This figure is increased to 50% of the population over the age of 65 years.

Although many patients and some healthcare providers still believe the old philosophy that "a patient's normal systolic blood pressure is 100 + their age," this could not be further from the truth. It is now clearly recognized that all forms of hy-

pertension, including isolated systolic hypertension, should be treated, with the goal of reducing the systolic blood pressure to 160 mm Hg or less and the diastolic to 90 to 95 mm Hg or less. There is clear-cut evidence that all levels of elevated blood pressure should be treated for the purpose of reducing long-term cardiovascular events.

Risk Factors

One misconception common to practitioners and patients is the relationship between salt intake and the development of hypertension. In fact, an individual's prior or current salt intake is not a predictor of blood pressure level. It is true, however, that in some hypertensive patients excess salt does contribute to ongoing hypertension; therefore, salt restriction is a safe and usually effective means of nonpharmacologic management of hypertension, if patients can comply with the diet.

Because hypertension is essentially asymptomatic, the natural history is one of insidious damage that is often clinically silent for decades. The decision to treat a hypertensive patient should be made after great scrutiny of prominent risk factors such as *hypercholesterolemia,* cigarette smoking, and diabetes as well as a screening set of questions for secondary hypertension from an identifiable, treatable cause. For example, the optometrist may be involved with a patient with hypertension secondary to a pheochromocytoma, who may present with advanced retinopathy at a young age. Other disorders are listed in the box.

CAUSES OF SECONDARY HYPERTENSION

Renal vascular hypertension
Estrogen-induced hypertension
Primary aldosteronism
Pheochromocytoma
Drug-related (corticosteroids, sympathomimetics, recreational drugs)
Cushing's syndrome
Hyperthyroidism
Vasculitis

Diagnosis

Through the remainder of this decade, ambulatory blood pressure monitoring will become more common. This technique allows 24-hour reading of the blood pressure outside of the physician's office. Although not commonly employed at the present time, it may be important for several groups of patients, one of whom may be the labile hypertensive patients who have hypertensive readings in the office but who are not, in fact, hypertensive. These patients represent more than 10% of patients diagnosed as hypertensive at the first office visit.

Another group of patients who will benefit from ambulatory readings are those on once-a-day therapy to monitor the efficacy of therapy at the end of the dosing interval. Because most patients take their medication in the early morning, and there is a strong correlation between cardiac events (myocardial infarction) and the early morning rise in blood pressure, the importance of having 24-hour control is obvious.

Treatment

The treatment of hypertension should always begin with dietary modification and recommendations for modest weight reduction and aerobic exercise. Strict adherence to a low-salt diet has been shown to be very effective for reduction of blood pressure, but in reality this often does not occur because patients are unable to make such dietary changes.

Pharmacologic therapy for hypertension should not occur until 3 months of nonpharmacologic therapy have been tried. The agent to choose is often based on both concomitant diseases, such as asthma, and the efficacy of the drug. In most studies monotherapy in mild hypertensives is effective in approximately 60% of patients regardless of the drug that is used. Although there are some race and age differences, most drugs are effective for most patients. The goal is to achieve a systolic blood pressure of 140 mm Hg or less (in the elderly 160 mm Hg is acceptable) and a diastolic blood pressure of 90 mm Hg or less. To date, no evidence has supported aggressive antihypertensive therapy to levels below these; in fact, over-aggressive therapy may lead to an increase in cardiac events owing to reduced coronary perfusion. Antihypertensive therapy can also be quite expensive.

In the last 5 years we have seen an explosion in the use of two new classes of antihypertensive drugs—*angiotensin converting enzyme (ACE) inhibitors* and *calcium channel blockers*. Both of these classes of drugs represent significant advances in our treatment of hypertension. Primarily, these drugs offer an excellent quality of life profile, with patients feeling well while on therapy. The presence of side effects has always been the major limiting factor in compliance with antihypertensive drug therapy. Unfortunately, to date there have been no studies demonstrating long-term protective effects of these agents from cardiovascular complications.

Because of their beneficial effects on blood pressure and the absence of metabolic side effects, it follows that these drugs will protect the patient from cardiovascular events. Unfortunately, the scientific information to support this statement is lacking. Nonetheless, many primary care physicians consider these classes of drugs to be the first line of treatment for hypertensive patients.

The Ocular Manifestations of Hypertension and Arterioscleroses

In general, ocular changes are usually located in the retina, less commonly in the choroid and anterior segment. When the choroid and anterior segment are involved, there is a suggestion of renal disease or failure (see Chapter 10 on Renal Disease).

Signs and Symptoms of Hypertensive Retinopathy

Patients with *hypertensive retinopathy* may be asymptomatic and the early stages of retinal changes may not result in optic nerve or macular compromise. In more advanced stages patients may complain of decreased central vision (20/30 to 20/200, depending on the severity). Vision loss is painless and occurs over a 24- to 48-hour period.

Ocular manifestations of hypertension can vary depending on the degree (see box below). Initially, general vasoconstriction and glaucoma of the arterioles prevent vessel expansion and damage. This is especially true of pliable and nonsclerotic retinal vessels. With continued elevated pressure, damage to the blood-retinal barrier occurs, causing damage at the retinal pigment epithelium and endothelium of the retinal vasculature. At this point serous fluid and plasma leak into the retina, where hard exudates form and appear to have a "star-shaped" pattern surrounding the macular region. Also, there are flame hemorrhages from the blood collecting at the nerve fiber layer. In the malignant phase of hypertension, edema of the optic nerve head occurs. This may be a result of isch-emia or hypertensive encephalopathy with elevated intracranial pressure (Fig. 9-1).

Signs and Symptoms of Arteriosclerosis of the Eye

Arteriosclerosis is a general term referring to a hardening and thickening of the arteries. This is usually related to systemic hypertension. Characteristics are intimal hyalinization, medial hypertrophy, and endothelial hypertrophy.

Visually the patient may not have a reduction in vision by arteriosclerosis alone. However, vision can decrease, especially if there is edema, retinal hemorrhaging from a branch, or central retinal venous occlusion.

With long-standing hypertension, sclerosis of the vessel walls can result (see box below). Sclerosis characteristically shows hyalinization, endothelial hyperplasia, and medial hypertrophy and is initially seen ophthalmoscopically as a broadened light reflex along the central portion of the vessel which eventually obscures the true appearance of blood flow in the vessels. This can result in complications such as central retinal venous occlusion and branch retinal venous occlusion. The sclerosed arteriole is hard and inflexible, clamping down the pliable venule as it crosses over, impeding venous outflow. Other complications, such as cystoid macular edema and retinal neovascularization, can occur (Fig. 9-2).

Central Retinal Artery Occlusion (CRAO)

The central retinal artery usually becomes occluded from fibrinoplatelet or calcific plaque.

HYPERTENSION: DEGREE OF SEVERITY

General vasoconstriction and extenuation of arterioles (Grade +1 HR)
Hard exudates (Grade +2 HR)
Flame hemorrhages (Grade +3 HR)
Cotton wool spots/nerve fiber layer infarcts (Grade +4 HR)
Optic nerve head edema

HR = hypertension.

ATHEROSCLEROSIS

(From Long-Standing Hypertension): Degree of Severity

Broadened light reflex of arterioles (Grade 1 AS)
Vessel deflections at arteriovenous crossings (Grade 2 AS)
Copper wire appearance of arterioles (Grade 3 AS)
Silver wire appearance of arterioles (Grade 4 AS)
Note: Branch retinal venous obstruction is a consequence at any stage

AS = atherosclerosis.

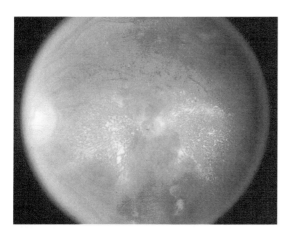

FIG. 9-1 Hypertensive retinopathy demonstrating hard exudates and flame-shaped hemorrhages. *(Courtesy of Jane Stein.)*

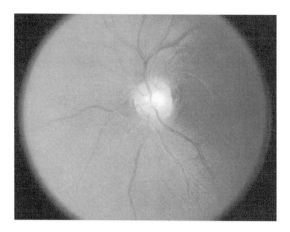

FIG. 9-2 Retinal arteriosclerosis secondary to long-standing hypertension. *(Courtesy of Jane Stein.)*

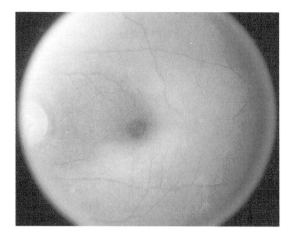

FIG. 9-3 Central retinal artery occlusion (CRAO) demonstrating the "cherry-red" macula. *(Courtesy of Jane Stein.)*

Other causes of CRAO include vasoconstriction of the artery from severe hypertension and vessel occlusion from inflammation in giant cell arteritis.

Signs and Symptoms. Diagnosis is actually quite easy. The usual symptom is sudden, painless loss of vision which may have been preceded by occasional amaurosis fugax. Visual acuities can range from 20/20 to no light perception. If the eye has a cilioretinal artery supplying the macular region, central vision may remain unaffected.

Depending on the time course from the occlusion, the appearance of the retina is varied. Within a few minutes of the occlusion the retina becomes edematous, especially in the posterior pole region. The foveal region appears red owing to the appearance of the unaffected, underlying choroid. With the surrounding whitish area the classic "cherry-red" spot to the fovea appears. After about 6 to 8 weeks the entire retina appears to be normal with the exception of optic atrophy and attenuated arterioles (due to better or no circulation through the vessels). Afferent pupillary defect can occur in the acute or later stages (see Fig. 9-3).

Branch Retinal Artery Occlusion (BRAO)

This condition (Fig. 9-4) appears similar to CRAO except that the occlusion has occurred in an area where only a portion of the retina became affected.

Signs and Symptoms. Amaurosis fugax can oc-

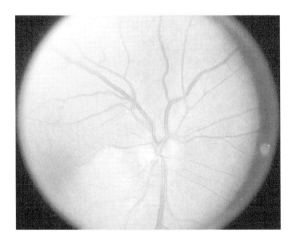

FIG. 9-4 Branch retinal artery occlusion (BRAO). *(Courtesy of Jane Stein.)*

cur prior to the occlusion. If the occlusion is in the inferior portion of the retina, the patient may be asymptomatic because it is not as common to look upward. Thus, the extent of ischemia and visual loss depends on the site of occlusion.

Management. CRAO is a medical emergency, especially if central acuity is lost. If retinal circulation is not restored within 90 to 100 minutes of the onset of obstruction, then retinal damage is irreversible and vision loss is permanent. Management attempts to try to dislodge the embolism to an area where central acuity is at least preserved or restored (a CRAO becomes a BRAO). The most effective method for dislodging the embolus appears to be to increase the arterial caliber size. By lowering the intraocular pressure, fewer forces from the outside compress the arterioles, thereby allowing the embolism to move. Attempts to quickly lower the intraocular pressure are usually performed by paracentesis of the anterior chamber, intravenous acetazolamide, or the use of topical beta-blockers.

Central Retinal Venous Occlusion (CRVO)

As a result of arteriosclerosis and hypertension, blood flow through the central retinal vein becomes more turbulent, especially at the site of the lamina cribosa, where there may be further compression of the central retinal artery over the central retinal vein (Fig. 9-5). This compression causes a back-up of venous blood into the retina.

Signs and Symptoms. There are typically two types of occlusion: nonischemic central retinal venous occlusion (NICRVO) and ischemic central retinal venous occlusion (ICRVO). NICRVO appears far less prominent than ICRVO. Patients are usually younger by approximately 5 years. Symptoms range from none to gradual (over a 24- to 48-hour period) with decreased vision and acuity varying from normal to 20/200.

Ophthalmologically, there is marked engorgement of the venules and there may be disc edema and retinal hemorrhages varying in appearance from peripheral only to prominent throughout the fundus. These findings are not marked, as the ICRVO neovascularization and capillary nonperfusion usually do not occur.

In ICRVO signs and symptoms are similar to those of NICRVO except much more extensive. There is gradual loss of vision over a 24- to 48-hour period except that visual acuity is usually better than 20/200. Ophthalmologically, significant hemorrhages and cotton wool spots dominate the findings. There is extensive nonperfusion and neovascularization of the iris (leading to neovascular glaucoma; occurs in 18% to 25% of all CRVOs).

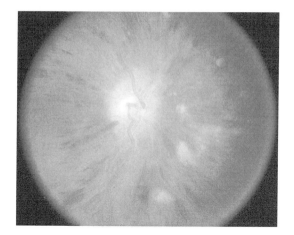

FIG. 9-5 Central retinal venous occlusion (CRVO). *(Courtesy of Jane Stein.)*

Usually, neovascular glaucoma occurs within 90 to 100 days of onset of CRVO.

Management. In NICRVO, the condition is self-limiting and findings usually resolve within 6 months. However, in some cases decreased vision may be permanent, poorer than 20/40. A follow-up examination on a monthly basis until resolution is reasonable to carefully monitor the condition and also to control the hypertension or systemic disease causing the condition. A laboratory test such as a complete blood count (CBC) may be useful in determining the underlying cause of hypertension.

In ICRVO anticoagulant therapy (e.g., heparin/ coumarin) may be used to improve circulation and prevent thrombosis. Studies have shown that anticoagulants can reduce the incidence of neovascular glaucoma. Panretinal laser photocoagulation has been shown to be useful in preventing neovascular glaucoma. Destroying retinal tissue decreases the demand for oxygen, thereby decreasing neovascularization. Follow-up visits every 3 to 4 weeks to closely monitor the condition are recommended.

Branch Retinal Venous Occlusion (BRVO)

BRVO is illustrated in Fig. 9-6.

Pathophysiology. The underlying cause of this condition is usually hypertension (77.7%). At the

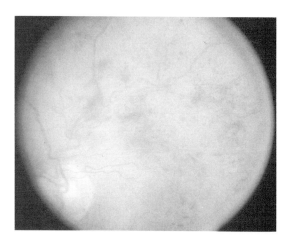

FIG. 9-6 Branch retinal venous occlusion (BRVO). *(Courtesy of Jane Stein.)*

site of an arteriovenous crossing, arteriosclerosis may distort and compress the venule, impeding venous outflow and causing an obstruction.

Symptoms vary from none to gradual loss of vision either superiorly or inferiorly, depending upon the location of the occlusion. Usually the condition is superior and temporal in the retina. Visual acuity may be decreased to 20/200, but many patients may not have decreased visual acuity if the macula is spread.

Ophthalmologically, retinal hemorrhages occur in a triangular configuration. The venules may be dilated and tortuous, and cotton-wool spots may be present. Retinal edema may spread into the macular region. Neovascular glaucoma is uncommon (1% of all BRVOs), but neovascularization in the retina (20%) occurs more often.

Management. Frequent follow-up visits (monthly until resolution) may be indicated for those conditions not affecting the macula. Argon laser photocoagulation may be indicated if macular edema exists. If the underlying systemic condition is under control, the fundus findings should disappear within 6 months.

Anterior Ischemic Optic Neuropathy

Occlusion of one of the posterior ciliary arteries can result in ischemia to some or all portions of the optic nerve.

Signs and Symptoms. The patient may complain of sudden loss of vision, which may occur especially upon awakening, because the likelihood of ischemia from decreased blood pressure is greatest during sleep. During the acute phase, the optic nerve head becomes swollen and edematous and visual fields can reveal an altitudinal field defect or complete loss of vision, or an afferent pupillary defect can occur. After about 2 months, optic atrophy occurs. The atrophy can be complete or segmented, depending on the extent of the ischemia.

Management. Because this condition is a sign of potential systemic compromise, an evaluation to rule out cardiovascular disease is indicated. A CBC and erythrocyte sedimentation rate (ESR) should also be performed to determine the cause as well as rule out giant cell arteritis.

Cranial Nerve (CN) Palsy

Atherosclerosis, including hypertension and diabetes, is the most common cause of CN III and VI palsies and the second most frequent cause of CN IV palsy (second only to trauma). The spontaneity of the palsy may be related to an interference with microvascular circulation to the nerve.

Signs and Symptoms. In acquired CN palsies involving extraocular muscles, the patient may complain of diplopia. In CN III palsy there may be an associated ptosis (approximately 2 mm), and the affected eye may be turned out and down because the superior oblique and lateral rectus muscles are not affected. In 80% of the patients the pupils are not affected. The diplopia may be intermittent. CN VI palsy reveals esotropia and restricted abduction on the affected side (from decreased function of the lateral rectus muscle).

In CN IV palsy, patients may complain not only of diplopia, but of head tilt to the side opposite the affected muscle (superior oblique). This is best diagnosed by the Bielschowsky head tilt test, in which the head is tilted to one shoulder and then to the other. The side that accentuates the hyperdeviation corresponds to the superior oblique muscle that is paralyzed.

Management. If the systemic condition is controlled, the palsy can resolve in 3 to 6 months. The

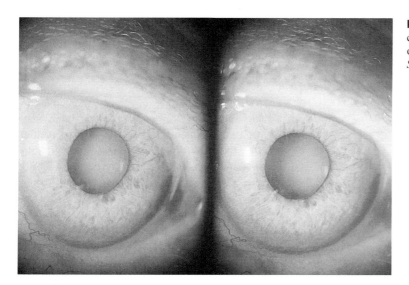

FIG. 9-7 Rubeosis iridis: Neovascular vessels can be seen coursing over the iris. *(Courtesy of Jane Stein.)*

use of a prism or occlusion can alleviate the diplopia.

Rubeosis Iridis

In severe peripheral vascular occlusive disease, especially in patients with carotid artery stenosis of greater than 70%, hypoxia and hypoperfusion occur, establishing the foundation for neovascularization at the iris to develop, leading to neovascular glaucoma. (Rubeosis iridis is illustrated in Fig. 9-7.)

Pathophysiology. Neovascular vessels usually develop at the pupillary margin between the 10 o'clock and 2 o'clock positions. In only rare instances do they occur initially at the angle. The neovascular vessels form a network across the iris and into the angle. The angiogenesis factor released to form the neovascularization creates a sticky surface to which the iris adheres, forming peripheral anterior synechiae.

Signs and Symptoms. Symptoms of rubeosis iridis itself usually occur only when neovascular glaucoma develops. When the intraocular pressure is elevated into the 40s and 50s, symptoms are similar to those of angle closure glaucoma (ocular pain, hazy/steamy vision, and red eye).

Signs include very small capillaries at the pupillary margin, sometimes mistakenly diagnosed as pigment, or the neovascular network is established. Then the shape of the pupil distorts and becomes oval (ectropion uveae). Gonioscopically, neovascular blood vessels appear to be approaching the angle. The iris closes the angle, creating closure and elevated intraocular pressure.

Management. Destroying hypoxic retinal tissue with panretinal laser photocoagulation has been shown to be successful in the prevention of neovascular glaucoma. If neovascular glaucoma does occur, management becomes difficult, and attempts to control intraocular pressure with beta-blockers (timolol maleate) or carbonic anhydrase inhibitors (acetazolamide) may be futile. Surgical control of intraocular pressure may be the only successful approach.

ANGINA PECTORIS

Case Study

A 55-year-old white man presents to an eye care practitioner for the fitting of contact lenses. His medical history is significant for hypertension, diabetes, and a strong family history of heart disease in his parents. On questioning, he mentions that he has been having squeezing, exertional chest pressure that he describes as a "heaviness" that does not travel and is relieved by rest. He assumes that this is indigestion. His blood pressure is found to be 180/110 mm Hg, and his eye fundus reveals Grade 2 and Grade 3 retinal changes.

Angina pectoris has been described since the eighteenth century. *Angina* is defined as the symptoms which, correlated with myocardial ischemia, occur when the oxygen demand of the heart exceeds the available vascular supply. Coronary stenosis or blockage is by far the most common cause of angina.

Angina is usually described by patients as a dull, ill-defined discomfort. Many atypical variances are described by patients, however, so one should have a high index of suspicion for other symptoms, including sharp, knife-like, or shooting pains. Other symptoms associated with angina include shortness of breath (due to left ventricular dysfunction and transient pulmonary edema), palpitations, fatigue, or difficulty in breathing.

Causes

Typically, angina is brought on by exertion and relieved by rest and is not related to meals or change in position. In addition to exertion triggering an anginal attack, coronary spasm may also play a role in contributing to angina.

In fact, most patients with stable and unstable angina have a combination of fixed atherosclerotic lesions and coronary vasospasm. Other disorders, including coronary artery embolism and vasculitis, can lead to angina by limiting cardiac output, thus restricting blood flow to the coronary circulation.

The natural history of patients with angina is well-defined. For patients with stable symptoms, the mortality is roughly 2% to 4% per year; for those with unstable symptoms, the mortality increases dramatically toward 10% per year. This distinction between stable and unstable is thus very crucial. Patients with stable angina have symptoms that are reproducible and predictable and do not increase in intensity. Those with unstable angina have symptoms that are new in onset, occur at rest or after a myocardial infarction, and are worse in character than those of stable angina. In these patients physicians should be particularly aggressive,

as they have a high annual risk of heart attack. The nature of the lesion has been recently recognized as predictive of development of a heart attack.

Diagnosis

Some investigators have developed techniques to actually look inside the coronary artery. It has been shown that the nature of the lesion may predict whether the patient will have a stable, uncomplicated course or a more aggressive course with his or her disease. Principles and management of patients with angina involve proper recognition of the syndrome, correction of any co-existing disorders such as hyperthyroidism or hypertension, and medical therapy that reduces coronary oxygen demand and increases coronary blood supply.

Treatment

The hallmark of therapy for angina is a class of medications called *nitrates*. Nitrates are smooth muscle relaxants that causes vascular dilatation, predominantly of the venous capacitance vessels. Nitrates are effective because they increase arterial supply by vasodilating coronary arteries. Nitrates can be given in multiple forms (oral, nitroglycerin spray, nitroglycerin patch, or sublingual forms).

Patients with angina should be instructed always to carry sublingual nitroglycerin, and it should be taken at the first signs of chest discomfort. Patients should be told that they should experience relief within 5 minutes; if no relief is obtained they should take a second tablet and then a third. If they have had no relief of their symptoms after 15 minutes, they should seek medical attention immediately.

Nitroglycerin ointment and topical patches are convenient ways to deliver this medication. One of the problems with nitroglycerin patches has been the occurrence of tachyphylaxis or nitrate tolerance after many hours. Most physicians are now recommending that their patients wear the patch for 12 hours during the day and remove the patch at night. In addition to nitrates, *beta-blocker* drugs such as metoprolol and propranolol are effective in angina. Unlike nitrates, which improve vascular supply, beta-blockers reduce myocardial oxygen demand by reducing contractility, blood pressure, and heart rate. The reduction in heart rate is conditionally beneficial because it allows more time for myocardial perfusion than occurs during filling or diastole.

Many studies have demonstrated the effectiveness of beta-blockers after a heart attack. They have also been clearly shown to improve mortality in patients with angina. Beta-blockers and nitrates nicely complement each other because beta-blockers can reduce the reflex tachycardia (increased heart rate) that may result from nitrate use, and nitrates help minimize any increase in left ventricular diastolic pressure that may ensue from beta-blockers' negative inotropic properties.

An important concern for the clinician considering the use of beta-blockers in patients with angina is their side effect profile. Because of the negative effects on pump function, patients with borderline cardiac function can develop heart failure on beta-blockers. In addition, because they reduce and affect the conduction system, various degrees of heart block can also develop on this therapy. Because beta receptors in the body are nonspecific, there is also an incidence of bronchospasm and asthma due to nonspecific beta-blockade in the lungs. Finally, in diabetics, beta-blockers have been shown to blunt the beta-adrenergic response to hypoglycemia and are to be used with great care in this population. Despite the relative contraindications in these patient subgroups, the beta-blockers should always be considered in patients with angina.

A newer class of agents, calcium channel blockers, have the benefit of providing many of the hemodynamic effects of beta-blockers without the complications. At present three main classes of calcium channel blockers are available which differ primarily in their effects on the conduction system of the heart. Calcium channel blockers inhibit calcium transport through the "slow" calcium channel of the cell membrane smooth muscle. Calcium channel blockers improve perfusion by causing coronary vasodilation in patients prone to spasm while arterial dilation and slowing of the

heart rate reduce myocardial work and oxygen demand.

In patients who are not candidates for surgical therapy for heart disease because of age or other conditions, calcium channel blockers have been used in conjunction with beta-blockers and nitrates to provide maximum medical therapy for the treatment of angina. Some of the relative properties of the first-generation calcium channel blockers are listed in Table 9-1.

An important adjunctive therapy in patients with angina is the use of antiplatelet agents such as aspirin. It has recently been recognized that the use of antithrombotic agents, including aspirin, warfarin, and heparin, improves survival in patients with unstable angina. The use of more aggressive thrombolytic therapy is discussed in the next section. Suffice to say, an aspirin every day or every other day seems prudent in patients with unstable angina in the absence of a contraindication.

Finally, surgical therapy for angina and unstable angina should be considered in patients who are refractory to medical therapy or at cardiac catheterization are found to have blockages in the left main coronary artery or significant lesions in all three of the main coronary vessels. A recent multicenter study has shown that in these two subgroups, patients do better over 7 years with surgical therapy than with medical therapy. The emerging view from these studies is that bypass surgery may prolong survival only in patients with the very worst prognosis. Work in this area is attempting to determine more precisely which patients do better with surgical intervention than with medical therapy.

Angioplasty is a technique that involves passing a balloon catheter into a stenosed vessel and inflating the balloon at the site of stenosis to widen the vessel lumen. Angioplasty has the advantages of a very short hospitalization and no opening of the chest as occurs with conventional bypass surgery. Patients with high-grade proximal stenosis (less than 70%) of a single vessel have been considered the best candidates for the procedure, although many studies are using the procedure in other settings, such as in multiple vessel disease.

TABLE 9-1 *Properties of First-Generation Calcium Channel Blockers*

	Diltiazem	Verapamil	Nifedipine
Mode of action	Reduces calcium entry into vascular muscle cells; decreases free intercellular calcium, reducing vascular tone, contractility, and peripheral vascular resistance		
Active within sinoatrial and atrioventricular nodes?	Y	Y*	N
Initial dosing ranges	90–180 mg/day	240–480 mg/day	30–60 mg/day
Major side effects	Nausea, ankle edema, headache, and rash	Constipation, postural dizziness, headache, nausea	Flushing, headache, postural dizziness, and ankle edema

*Verapamil, because of effects within the cardiac conduction system, is most likely to cause myocardial depression, excessive bradycardia, and atrioventricular nodal dysfunction. This drug should rarely, if ever, be used with beta-blockers.

The consensus is that angioplasty is an acceptable technique in experienced hands for many patients with occlusive coronary artery disease.

Summary

Angina pectoris is the symptom that correlates with occlusive coronary artery disease. The history should focus on pre-existing or concomitant conditions that may have exacerbated angina and a series of questions to determine whether the condition is stable or unstable. If unstable, recommendations for admission or referral to a cardiologist seem prudent. Stable angina is managed medically with nitrates, beta-blockers, antiplatelet agents, and calcium channel blockers. Close attention should be paid by all health professionals to risk factors in anginal patients, including recommending weight reduction, dietary modification if hyperlipidemia is present, stress reduction, and smoking cessation. Some patients are not candidates for ongoing medical management, and they should be considered for angioplasty or bypass surgery.

MYOCARDIAL INFARCTION

Case Study

A 68-year-old woman with a history of hypertension, diabetes, elevated cholesterol, and obesity presents to your office for annual evaluation of her cataracts. While rushing to keep her appointment, she develops crushing chest pressure in the parking lot. She is able to make it to your office, and she is found sitting in the waiting room. Her skin is cold and clammy and she is very short of breath, with severe, unrelenting chest pressure that travels into her left arm and up into her neck. She does describe episodes of chest pressure over the last several months and was given a prescription for nitroglycerin by her family physician. You immediately call for an ambulance while she takes nitroglycerin tablets sublingually. She experiences no relief of symptoms. You record a blood pressure of 100/60 mm Hg with many skipped beats when you feel her pulse. She continues to have severe chest pressure.

SIGNS AND SYMPTOMS OF ACUTE MYOCARDIAL INFARCTION (MI)

Symptoms

    Substernal squeezing or pressure sensation, often radiating into the neck or down the arms, lasting 15 minutes or longer.

    Discomfort may be localized just to the arm or neck without associated chest pain.

    Other symptoms include shortness of breath, weakness, diaphoresis, and nausea.

    Diagnostic difficulties may arise because one out of every five MIs is clinically silent or unrecognized. Only 23% of MIs (from the Framingham Heart Study) were preceded by a history of angina. Painless MI is more frequent in diabetic patients and in the elderly.

Signs

    Appearance: Normal to diaphoretic, pale, anxious.

    Vital signs: Mild to moderate increase in heart rate, blood pressure usually elevated; respirations may be increased. Low-grade fevers commonly seen.

    Lungs: Rales or overt pulmonary edema may be seen if left ventricular dysfunction is present.

    Heart: Gallop rhythms (S_4 and/or S_3) may be appreciated; new systolic murmurs may be heard, usually due to transient ischemia or infarction of the papillary muscles of the mitral valve apparatus.

Signs and Symptoms

The signs and symptoms of acute *myocardial infarction* are summarized in the box. Although most patients have some or all of the signs and symptoms listed, a sizable percentage of patients, particularly the elderly and diabetic, can have atypical symptoms or no symptoms at all. This condition is referred to as a silent myocardial infarction.

The diagnosis of acute infarction depends not only on signs and symptoms but on electrocardiographic changes and cardiac enzyme determinations. Creatine kinase (CK) level is the most sensitive blood marker of acute myonecrosis. This enzyme is released into the serum from injured skeletal or cardiac muscle. CK is present in several isoenzyme patterns—muscle specific (M) or brain specific (B). The "MB" form is specific for cardiac muscle. An MB fraction exceeding 7% to 8% of the total is indicative of acute myocardial infarction. Other techniques can also be used to support a diagnosis of suspected myocardial infarction such as echocardiography, which may reveal segmental wall motion abnormalities of the ventricle.

Management

The most important aspects of management of myocardial infarction include rapid transport to a coronary care unit and evaluation for thrombolytic therapy. The ultimate goal and a major determinant of survival in patients with acute myocardial infarction is thrombolytic therapy. If it can be done within 4 to 6 hours of the onset of symptoms, it limits the size of the infarcted area of the heart.

In the last 5 years two agents, *streptokinase* and *tissue plasminogen activator (TPA)*, have been shown to dramatically reduce the mortality and morbidity in patients with acute myocardial infarction. These agents, which should be given only by trained specialists in emergency medicine or cardiology, provide systemic fibrinolytic effects by degrading the fibrin clot and reversing thrombosis in a coronary artery. Initially, these drugs were given by an intracoronary route but now they are delivered through a normal intravenous catheter.

Both agents are effective in reducing complications from myocardial infarction, but they should be given with great care, as they have many relative contraindications as well as serious side effects, the most important being excessive bleeding. Along with the development of coronary care units in the 1960s, however, this is the most exciting advance in the treatment of acute myocardial infarction in the last 20 years.

Other important principles in the management of

patients with acute myocardial infarction include bed rest in a calm, quiet coronary care unit monitoring for arrhythmias and administering oxygen therapy, nitroglycerin, and beta-blockers.

Because of some of the measures mentioned, the in-hospital survival of patients with acute myocardial infarction has also improved (80% to 90%). In those patients with an uncomplicated course in the hospital, one of two options is available — either the performance of a cardiac catheterization to visualize the coronary anatomy or a more conservative approach with graduated exercise and the performance of a low level stress test before hospital discharge. If the stress test is abnormal, many physicians proceed with a cardiac catheterization before discharge.

Some patients need a more aggressive intervention in the hospital, and these include patients who develop congestive heart failure, serious arrhythmias, or recurrent angina. These patients should likely undergo cardiac catheterization, with the possible need for other interventions including angioplasty and bypass surgery.

Aspirin has now been shown to be very safe and effective for preventing second heart attacks. Additionally, beta-blocker therapy has also been shown to be effective, and this should be used in the absence of a contraindication. Even if patients undergo an aggressive form of therapy such as bypass surgery, the same risk factors can damage the new grafts, and patients need constant encouragement to stop smoking, achieve an ideal body weight, and lower their total cholesterol.

Many older patients may still consider acute myocardial infarction a preterminal disorder with excessive fears of incapacitation, altered self-image, and diminished self-respect. Every health care provider should help the patient deal with such fears and address the patient's concerns.

PERIPHERAL VASCULAR DISEASE

Case Study

A 44-year-old man presents to your office because of tearing in his left eye. During some informal questioning, he tells you of severe pain in his calves when he walks which is relieved with rest. His history is significant for heavy cigarette smoking of three packs per day and a family history of cardiovascular events. On examination of his legs you note a loss of normal hair pattern below his mid-calf and the absence of palpable pulses over the soles of his feet. The patient is afraid that he may need amputation and needs advice about this disorder.

Evidence of arteriosclerotic cardiovascular disease does not simply involve the heart. Other areas of the body, including the peripheral blood vessels in the legs and carotid arteries of the neck, can be affected by the same processes that involve the coronary circulation. Intermittent *claudication* is defined as the occurrence of exertional leg pain that is relieved with rest. It is akin to angina; it is a process of excessive oxygen demand with diminished vascular supply. Intermittent claudication is more common in diabetics and smokers.

In general, the development of claudication suggests a benign prognosis. In a recent study of 104 patients with claudication who underwent angiography to define the extent of their disease, almost 8% remained stable or improved during an average 2.5-year follow-up. The optometrist may see many of these patients, as they often have diabetes, and diabetics in general have more advanced vascular disease than nondiabetics.

Diagnosis of Intermittent Claudication

The physician can objectively measure the degree of claudication by comparing blood pressures in the arms and the legs. This ratio is often used in the office. The ratio should be 1:1, that is, similar systolic blood pressure in the arm and the leg, but as the claudication worsens, the blood pressure becomes higher in the arm than in the leg. As occlusion becomes more severe, the oxygen supply to the lower leg diminishes and the patients lose their normal hair pattern. Other findings of advanced disease include shiny skin and loss of peripheral pulses. Some patients describe a constant tingling sensation from chronic arterial insufficiency.

Treatment of Intermittent Claudication

The two most important methods of stimulating collateral circulation are the cessation of cigarette smoking and regular exercise. Smoking appears to hasten progression of atherosclerosis in men, in whom it impairs the development of collateral circulation. However, the mechanism is unproven.

Daily aerobic exercise also serves as a stimulus for the development of collateral circulation. Other methods such as careful attention to foot care and weight reduction to lessen workload by reducing metabolic demand on extremities are important. Treatment of hypertension and hyperlipidemia may also be of value in controlling the progression of atherosclerosis.

Drug therapy for this disorder is controversial. Certain classes of agents such as vasodilators would theoretically be beneficial but are unproven. A new agent, pentoxifylline, has been proven effective in some patients by increasing erythrocyte deformability to improve capillary blood flow. Because of the 100- to 120-day life span of red blood cells, therapy must continue for several weeks before any decision on efficacy can be made. Antiplatelet agents that are effective in coronary circulation have not been proven to have benefit in peripheral circulation.

In addition to smoking cessation, it is important to evaluate other medications that the patient is taking which may affect the peripheral circulation. These include beta-blocker drugs, which may worsen peripheral blood flow, as well as the use of ergot derivatives for migraines, which can induce ischemic symptoms.

Evaluation for surgery of patients with claudication is indicated when the patient has advanced ischemia resulting in ischemic ulcerations, gangrene, or pain at rest. These limbs are clearly at risk for amputation.

One new technique in the area of peripheral vascular disease has been angioplasty. As with coronary angioplasty, this technique employs a balloon catheter that can be inserted percutaneously at a remote site and manipulated fluoroscopically within the diseased segment of the artery. At the point of the occlusion the balloon is inflated to 4 to 6 atmospheres to expand the vessel lumen. As with coronary angioplasty, the technique is a viable alternative to bypass surgery in many situations.

Ocular Manifestations of Peripheral Vascular Disease

In general, hypoperfusion causing cerebrovascular incidents is usually due to embolic or distal circulatory flow failure. The classic sign is frequent amaurosis fugax in peripheral vascular disease from distal flow failure. Symptoms from carotid artery insufficiency including weakness, paralysis, numbness, tingling, and clumsiness, especially in fingers, hands, arms, and legs. Dysfunction can occur in speech behavior (higher cortical dysfunctions). Symptoms of amaurosis fugax depend on the origin of insufficiency. In carotid artery disease it is almost always monocular, most likely from ischemia to the corresponding retina and/or optic nerve. If the condition is of vertebrobasilar artery origin, symptoms of amaurosis fugax are usually bilateral because of ischemia to the occipital lobes.

Decreased circulation can affect the lower extremities, where findings such as intermittent claudication, peripheral nonhealing ulcers, and atherosclerotic renal artery disease result in severe hypertension.

Summary

Peripheral vascular disease is manifest by the symptom of intermittent claudication. Physician findings include depression or absence of peripheral pulses, loss of normal hair pattern, and a disparity in blood pressures between arm and leg. Frequent co-existing condition for claudication include cigarette smoking, diabetes, hypertension, and hyperlipidemia. Medical therapy has been most successful with pentoxifylline. Surgical management with angioplasty is a promising new modality. Surgical referrals should be considered when the patient has pain at rest.

TRANSIENT ISCHEMIC ATTACKS

Case Study

A 72-year-old right-handed man presents for evaluation of poor vision of his right eye. The patient describes "graying" of the vision in this eye accompanied by clumsiness of his right hand. These symptoms have occurred on and off for the last several days and are not associated with any pain or headache. The symptoms last for several minutes and then resolve spontaneously. His medical history is positive for hypertension. Physician examination is essentially normal at this time with the exception of poor blood flow in his right carotid artery circulation. His neurologic examination is normal at present.

Transient ischemic attacks (TIAs) follow the pattern similar to that of problems previously noted in this chapter. That is, they are a warning of more advanced vascular event. TIAs are defined as temporary focal cerebral dysfunction due to vascular disease. The onset is rapid, often less than 1 minute, and they last up to 24 hours. As with angina and claudication, the symptoms are completely reversible, but TIAs have been clearly shown to be a warning symptom for stroke. Coronary stenosis or blockage is by far the most common cause for this syndrome.

Background Information

The most common site for significant atherosclerotic changes is the extracranial circulation at the bifurcation of the carotid. Initially, an accumulation of lipids raises the endothelial cover, restricting blood flow. The initial lesion of atherosclerosis manifests itself as patchy accumulation of fatty materials in the arterial wall which becomes hard and calcified with age. Atherosclerosis commonly begins in childhood or adolescence, even before any degenerative processes begin.

Ocular Manifestations

One of the most common visual symptoms is amaurosis fugax (fleeting vision). This occurs with-

out warning in which the patient complains of a sudden "diminishing" or "graying" of the field of vision. The vision loss usually lasts 5 to 10 minutes. The source of this condition is usually an *embolism* formed from an atheromatous plaque in the cortical artery (see box below). The most common types of emboli are (1) cholesterol (Hollenhorst plaques), (2) a collection of fibrin and platelet (fibrinous-platelet plaques), and (3) calcific plaques (Fig. 9-8).

Hollenhorst, or cholesterol, emboli can be associated with carotid occlusive disease. When viewed ophthalmologically, they are shiny, refractile, and yellowish orange in appearance and because of this can appear larger than the actual blood vessel column. These emboli only rarely cause a retinal artery obstruction because of their flat shape and malleability, which allow blood to flow around the emboli. Because occlusion is rare, patients may not complain of amaurosis fugax.

ATHEROSCLEROTIC CHANGES

Hollenhorst plaque
Fibrinoplatelet plaque
Calcific plaque
Central retinal artery occlusion
Branch retinal artery occlusion

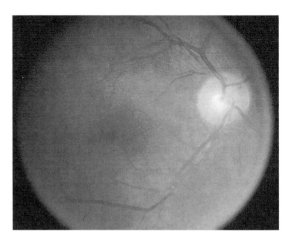

FIG. 9-8 Emboli in the retinal arterial vascular tree causing transient ischemic attacks. *(Courtesy of Jane Stein.)*

Fibrinoplatelet plaques consist of cholesterol and platelet aggregate from the atheromatous ulceration. These plaques appear to be the same size as vessels and are shaped like an elongated, segmented plug. The sticky nature of the fibrinoplatelet plaque allows adherence to the vessel, resulting in retinal arterial occlusion. However, these plaques can dissolve and can permit the return of normal blood flow. However, if occlusion lasts longer than 90 minutes, permanent damage with loss of vision can occur.

Calcific plaques, which begin predominantly from aortic or valvular heart disease, can also originate from atheromatous conditions. These emboli are individual and chalky or matte white in appearance. They travel to an arteriole and lodge near the optic disc, causing permanent retinal artery occlusion. In contrast to a Hollenhorst or fibrinoplatelet plaque, which can allow continuation or return of blood flow, a calcific plaque causes a permanent loss of blood flow past the occlusion.

Although atheromatous plaques can originate from areas other than the carotid artery, the importance of the finding of either cholesterol or fibrinoplatelet emboli as a sign of carotid artery disease has been well established. One study showed that 69% of patients with cholesterol emboli experience either a TIA or a stroke.

Diagnosis and Management of Occlusive Disease

Diagnosis and management should include a complete history and ocular examination. The status of the carotid artery should be determined. Each carotid artery can be palpated and the strength of the pulses compared. In the presence of complete or nearly complete occlusion (greater than 90%), the pulse may be reduced in strength.

Auscultation of the carotid arteries (see Chapter 1) to evaluate for bruit can indicate carotid stenosis of approximately 50% to 90%. However, the absence of a bruit may also indicate complete or nearly complete occlusion. In all cases in the presence of retinal emboli, urgent referral to a vascular surgeon or internist is advised, with a mild anticoagulant (one tablet of aspirin per day) pre-

scribed to improve circulation if there are no contraindications.

VALVE DISEASE

Endocarditis

Endocarditis occurs from infancy to old age, usually accompanied by a defect of tissue along the heart valves (see box below). Damage may be caused by abnormal hemodynamic conditions such as rheumatic valve disease, mitral valve prolapse, injection of foreign particles by intravenous drug abusers, or local immune complex deposition in disorders such as systemic lupus erythematosus. Retinal artery occlusion is the major ocular consequence of endocarditis.

There are two types of endocarditis: nonbacterial endocarditis and bacterial endocarditis. Nonbacterial endocarditis occurs when there is damage to the endothelial surface, causing a local deposition of fibrin and platelet. Bacterial, or infectious, endocarditis develops when circulating microorganisms adhere to the fibrin platelet vegetation of nonbacterial thrombotic endocarditis.

Pathogenesis, Signs, Symptoms, and Treatment. Infection of the lining of the heart is referred to as infectious endocarditis. Once a uniformly fatal disease, with the development of antibiotic therapy and cardiac surgery, 65% to 80% of patients survive. The most important aspect is to recognize those patients at risk for the development of endocarditis and to recommend appropriate prophylaxis.

Endocarditis develops in both normal and previously damaged heart valves. Prosthetic or artificial heart valves are very frequent targets for infection. The combination of a damaged endothelium and turbulent blood flow appears to provide the most fertile setting for the development of en-

---

VALVE DISEASE

Emboli-plaque formation in arterioles
Central retinal artery occlusion
Branch retinal artery occlusion

---

docarditis. In general, infectious endocarditis is more prevalent in the left-sided chambers of the heart because of higher pressures in the systemic circulation relative to those of the pulmonary circulation. Turbulent blood flow is also a reason why endocarditis is commonly seen in patients with certain congenital heart valve abnormalities such as ventricular septal defects. Over the last 10 to 20 years, a large increase in cases of endocarditis has been seen in patients who are intravenous drug abusers.

Endocarditis has been classified as subacute or acute. Subacute infectious endocarditis is a partially compensated disease lasting weeks or months in which the rate of healing never quite equals that of destruction. As the heart valve is eroded, new murmurs may appear and bits of infected tissue may embolize throughout the body, causing metastatic infections or infarctions. *Streptococcus viridans* is the leading cause of subacute infectious endocarditis. Acute infectious endocarditis is usually caused by *Staphylococcus aureus,* an invasive organism that can infect even normal heart valves. Acute infectious endocarditis is characterized by rapid valve destruction, the sudden appearance of new heart murmurs, extension of the infection to form myocardial abscesses, and hemodynamic compromise. Acute endocarditis is truly a medical emergency, often requiring emergency heart valve replacement.

The signs and symptoms of endocarditis can be nonspecific (malaise, fever, fatigue), cardiac (new or changing heart murmurs), or embolic (pulmonary or splenic emboli causing fleeting pulmonary infiltrates, splenomegaly, and left upper quadrant abdominal pain). The diagnosis of endocarditis is made by the finding of sustained bacteremia. Blood cultures provide a diagnosis in over 90% of cases. Approximately 10% of patients with endocarditis are considered culture negative because of prior antibiotic therapy, infection with fastidious organisms, or right-sided disease. Echocardiography plays a major role in determining the extent of valve damage, but it does not substitute for blood cultures in making a diagnosis.

The required duration of antibiotic therapy has not been studied prospectively; however, most authorities favor 4 to 6 weeks of intravenous therapy followed by another 2 weeks of oral antibiotics. Much of the therapy should take place in a hospital setting, as patients may deteriorate owing to arrhythmias, heart failure, or unexpected embolization. Clearing of blood cultures, normalization of ESR, and a falling titer of rheumatoid factor are all markers that can be followed for improvement in the patient's status.

Endocarditis is a very serious infection. Patients who may be at risk for endocarditis because of valvular heart disease should be referred to an internist or specialist who can make appropriate recommendations for prophylactic antibiotics. In many cases, endocarditis is a preventable disorder.

Mitral Valve Prolapse (MVP)

MVP is a retrograde displacement of one or more of the mitral valve leaflets. Several causes of MVP are known (connective tissue disorders, rheumatic and congenital heart disease, cardiomyopathy, and coronary artery disease), although in many cases no cause can be determined.

Pathogenesis, Signs, Symptoms, and Treatment. MVP (also known as Barlow's syndrome) is a common condition occurring in 5% to 7% of the adult population, mostly in women. There is evidence for autosomal dominant inheritance. Although most patients with this disorder are asymptomatic, occasionally patients present with atypical, nonexertional chest pain with evidence of excessive sympathetic nervous system activity, including sinus tachycardia and other arrhythmias. The cause of these symptoms is not known. MVP is often diagnosed as an incidental finding by the detection of a systolic click on cardiac auscultation. The diagnosis is confirmed by echocardiography.

The course of patients with MVP is usually benign, with patients asymptomatic throughout life. A small proportion of patients with MVP develop a more severe form of vascular heart disease known as mitral regurgitation, and on rare occasions this needs to be repaired surgically.

There is no specific treatment for patients with

MVP. The physician should reassure the patient that the condition is benign and has a very favorable prognosis. If MVP is suspected, an echocardiogram is recommended to determine the need for prophylaxis against infective endocarditis. Although controversial in patients with clicks only, patients with clicks and systolic murmurs should clearly receive antibiotics before dental work or other procedures.

Ocular Signs, Symptoms, and Treatment. The ocular associations of MVP may include ischemia because of intravascular thromboembolism because there is platelet stimulation from the abnormal hemodynamics around the valve surface. The ischemia results in central retinal, branch retinal, and choroidal arteriolar occlusion. There can also be an association with retinal venous occlusion because the increased platelet activity causes thickened blood flow through the venules. With these complications patients can complain of decreased vision and amaurosis fugax. Management of these patients can include a therapeutic trial of antiplatelet agents such as acetylsalicylic acid. Visual prognosis is favorable if management commences quickly.

Bibliography

Ameny A and others: Mortality and morbidity results from the European working party on high blood pressure in the elderly trial, *Lancet* 1:1349, 1985.

Hoshino PK and Gaasch WH: When to intervene in chronic aortic regurgitation, *Arch Intern Med* 146:349, 1986.

O'Neill W and others: A prospective, randomized clinical trial of intracoronary streptokinase versus coronary angioplasty for acute myocardial infarction, *N Engl J Med* 314:812, 1986.

Ross R: The pathogenesis of atherosclerosis—an update, *N Engl J Med* 314:488, 1986.

Willerson JT and others: Speculation regarding mechanisms responsible for acute ischemic heart disease syndromes, *J Am Coll Cardiol* 8:245, 1986.

10

Renal Disease

DAVID S. KOUNTZ
JOHN H. NISHIMOTO
BRUCE G. MUCHNICK

KEY TERMS

Hypervolemia	*Cystoscopy*	*Rhabdomyolysis*
Hypovolemia	*Azotemia*	*Uremia*
Plasma Creatinine	*Oliguria*	*Hemodialysis*
Blood Urea Nitrogen	*Polyuria*	*Elschnig spot*
Excretory Urography	*Hematuria*	

CHAPTER OUTLINE

*T*he kidneys serve a number of important roles in body homeostasis, including regulation of salt and water, excretion of toxic substances, regulation of acid balance, and production of hormones. The presence of renal disease is confirmed by the general internist by evaluating symptoms, urinalysis, and blood chemistry results.

Three goals of renal diagnosis are identification of the underlying disease, the determination of whether the disease is acute or chronic, and the determination of whether the disease process is reversible. Once the diagnosis has been established, appropriate supportive and specific treatment may be implemented for both the underlying disease and the renal insufficiency.

CLINICAL LABORATORY TESTING

A systemic approach to the determination of the presence of renal disease and its clinical evaluation includes a detailed history, urinalysis, imaging techniques, blood testing, and in some cases renal biopsy.

History

In evaluating the history, the clinician must be sensitive to the symptoms of both an underlying disease as well as renal pathology. First, a history of childhood renal involvement should be investigated. Next, previous examinations and urinalysis results should be reviewed. Any episodes of protein in the urine, exposure to toxins, or ingestion of poisons should be noted. The patient should provide a list of all medications that have been taken, even those considered over-the-counter, or "harmless."

Physical Examination

The physical examination of a patient with renal disease usually fails to pinpoint an underlying cause but often can assess such complications of kidney pathology as systemic hypertension, pericarditis, and *hypervolemia* or *hypovolemia*. A patient with volume depletion may develop renal failure and should have blood pressure readings taken in both the standing and sitting positions. If there is a large drop in blood pressure as the patient stands up, then volume depletion should be suspected. The physical examination should also include a pelvic and rectal examination to rule out masses that may cause voiding difficulties.

Urinalysis

To narrow the differential diagnosis of a patient symptomatic for renal disease urinalysis is invaluable to the clinician (see Chapter 3). Normal urine should be a light yellow color. Urine becomes reddish-brown if red blood cells are present or beets, red berries or candies, or phenothiazines were ingested. Pus in the urine may suggest infection, and a tea color results from the presence of bile in a jaundiced patient. Urine should be clear; turbidity may indicate a large number of red and/or white blood cells.

To analyze the wide assortment of chemicals in the urine, a test strip with reagents may be used. The important chemicals to evaluate in renal disease are albumin and hemoglobin, as well as a newer test to determine the presence of leukocytes. These tests to detect protein, hemoglobin, and leukocytes alert the clinician to the possibility of renal disease. The pH of the urine is also assessed on the test strip and if high (7.5 to 8.0) may indicate a urinary tract infection.

Following centrifugation, the urine is decanted, and the sediment at the bottom of the collection tube is examined under a microscope. Any red and white blood cells should be noted as well as casts and crystals. Red blood cells indicate involvement of the glomeruli, whereas casts indicate renal tubule involvement. White blood cells indicate urinary tract infection. Patients suspected of having a urinary tract infection should have their urine cultured for bacterial infection.

The presence of underlying systemic disease with renal involvement may cause increased protein concentrations in the urine. For this reason, the amount of protein in a 24-hour sampling of urine is determined. An elevated protein level in the urine is a useful test for renal abnormality.

Hematologic Testing

The significant blood tests to perform on suspected renal disease patients include *plasma creatinine* and *blood urea nitrogen* (BUN). Creatinine is the more useful of the two because plasma urea (a chief end product of protein metabolism) has a variable rate of production dependent on several factors. On the other hand, the production of creatinine is dependent on only one factor (muscle mass of the patient).

Renal Imaging Techniques

Imaging techniques in suspected renal disease includes diagnostic ultrasonography, *excretory urography* (intravenous pyelography [IVP]), plain film radiographs of the abdomen, computed tomography (CT), *cystoscopy,* and magnetic resonance imaging.

Ultrasonography has replaced many older studies because of the large number of patients suitable for the procedure, the lack of radiation and contrast medium, and its ability to study anatomic abnormalities in the kidneys and bladder in the supine and prone positions. Ultrasonography is useful for detecting the size, shape, and location of the kidneys as well as such abnormalities as cysts, renal stones, and infection. Ultrasonography may also help guide procedures such as percutaneous biopsy. Unfortunately, the use of ultrasonography depends on the skill of the operator and the radiologist and is difficult to perform on obese patients.

The plain radiograph of the kidney is limited in its usefulness by obesity and overlying gas shadows or fluid. It may aid in the determination of kidney size and location and detect renal stones or calcified masses.

The IVP requires an intravenous injection of water-soluble iodine-contrast medium to provide anatomic and physiologic information about the kidney. The IVP may be combined with a tomogram to provide information about the size and shape of renal masses. This test has the disadvantages of exposing the patient to radiation and the risk of an anaphylactic reaction to the contrast medium.

CT is helpful in evaluating renal masses or lesions, assessing renal trauma, and detecting calcified renal calculi. Although the patient is exposed to small doses of radiation, the major risk is concomitant use of contrast agents which can contribute to renal insufficiency if the patient is diabetic, elderly, or hypovolemic. While these are not contraindications to the use of contrast material, extreme caution must be exercised when using these agents.

To obtain direct visualization of the entire lower urinary tract, cystoscopy may be employed. In female patients the procedure is performed in the office with local anesthesia. In males cystoscopy is performed under general anesthesia, although some men can tolerate the procedure under local anesthesia.

Renal biopsy is the definitive procedure for diagnosing a renal lesion, but not all patients need to have it performed. The biopsy may be performed as an open surgical procedure or as a closed percutaneous technique with biopsy needle. In closed procedures ultrasonography may help guide the biopsy needle. It is useful in patients with suspected renal cysts or masses, acute renal failure, chronic renal failure, and systemic diseases affecting the kidneys.

RENAL DISEASE SYMPTOMATOLOGY

Symptoms are rare in most cases of renal disease. Commonly, kidney abnormalities are detected by blood and urine testing in patients who exhibit no renal symptoms. This makes the diagnosis of renal disease particularly challenging for the clinician.

The sudden elevation of blood urea nitrogen or creatinine level is termed *azotemia*. The clinician must determine if this is due to renal failure and, if so, whether it is acute or chronic. The cause of the renal failure, possible complications, and reversibility of the situation should likewise be determined.

In determining if the renal failure is acute or chronic, a detailed history is of utmost importance. Any historical evidence of previous kidney disease points toward the greater possibility of a chronic situation. The history may also reveal the cause of the renal failure by gathering information on drug use or toxic exposure or genetic disease in the family.

A chronic condition is also more likely if the patient appears to be well on a physical examination despite renal failure. An elevated blood pressure may lead to or be caused by renal failure, and its severity should also include kidney palpation to examine for tenderness or enlargement.

DIAGNOSIS OF RENAL DISEASE

If urine volume is too low to allow for appropriate excretion of nitrogenous waste products, then a concomitant state of renal failure may exist. This condition, known as *oliguria,* may be due to inadequate renal perfusion secondary to heart failure, obstructed urine outflow, or intrinsic kidney disease. Determination of the cause of oliguria is important when considering treatment options. Management of oliguria includes replacement of fluid deficiencies and in some cases stimulation of urine flow with diuretic therapy.

Polyuria is an increase in urine volume due to such conditions as diabetes, chronic renal disease, increased water intake, and other causes. The treatment of polyuria is based on the cause.

Blood in the urine is known as *hematuria* and should always be considered serious until otherwise proven. Blood may be seen grossly or detected in apparently normal samples by use of the test strip in urinalysis studies. It may be due to disease anywhere in the excretory system, including the kidney and urethra. Diagnostic testing when hematuria is present includes a careful history, urinalysis, a thorough physical examination, cytologic examination of the urine to rule out neoplastic cells, sickle cell testing in young black patients, an IVP, and, if necessary, ultrasonography and a CT scan. It is significant to recognize that 20% of patients presenting with gross hematuria are eventually found to have a tumor in the urinary tract.

Protein, such as albumin, should not appear in the urine, and when it does it is known as proteinuria. Almost all renal disease states produce proteinuria, and protein is detected on a dipstick test during urinalysis.

ACUTE RENAL FAILURE (ARF)

The sudden loss of renal function is termed acute renal failure. The most common cause is renal hypoperfusion, in which the kidneys fail as a result of ischemia or underperfusion. Other causes include toxic agents to the kidney such as heavy metals, aminoglycoside antibiotics, or other substances released when there is a breakdown of muscle tissue with concomitant release of muscle protein (myoglobin) into the urine *(rhabdomyolysis)*.

Another cause of ARF is postrenal obstruction. This is most commonly seen in older men with prostatic obstruction and older women with obstruction to urine flow because of ovarian enlargement. Systemic diseases such as lupus and endocarditis may produce direct inflammation of the kidney as a result of autoimmune disease.

The diagnosis of ARF is often made in a medical or surgical setting when a rapid decline in renal function occurs. This reduced kidney function is reflected in blood testing as a rise in serum creatinine and BUN.

It is important for the treating physician to examine the urine of the patient in suspected ARF. In the setting of acute hypoperfusion, urine sediment generally reveals epithelial cells and pigmented cellular casts. These and other laboratory indices can help the physician determine whether the cause of the ARF is hypoperfusion, obstruction, or intrarenal damage. This distinction is important, as therapy is different with each of these disorders.

Surgery

Surgery and trauma cause about one half of all cases of ARF, and pregnancy, medical conditions, and toxic reactions account for the remaining cases. These causes contribute to either prerenal cases of ARF, which lead to inadequate renal perfusion of blood; postrenal cases, in which there is urinary obstruction; or intrinsic renal disease. Treatment modalities are usually available for prerenal and postrenal disease, but only rarely if the cause is intrinsic to the kidney.

Treatment of ARF should be instituted in most cases by a nephrologist. Generally, intake of any substances excreted by the kidney should be limited. These include foods high in sodium and potassium and fluids of any kind. However, adequate caloric intake should be supplied either orally or parenterally. The treating physician should be careful to prevent any infection by avoiding catheterization and unnecessary intravenous lines. Finally, complex cases of renal failure may require peritoneal dialysis or hemodialysis.

CHRONIC RENAL FAILURE

Chronic renal insufficiency (see box on p. 208) is often the result of hypertension or diabetes and presents to the clinician a more common scenario than acute renal disease. These patients are more at risk for the full uremic syndrome, which includes metabolic and volume complications, than patients with ARF.

As a patient develops worsening renal function, no decrease in urine output may be detected. It is much more likely that the urine the patient is producing is less filtered than normal, so that the body retains toxic substances. As the patient's normal renal function worsens and the creatinine rises from a normal range of 0.5 to 1.0 mg/dl to 7 to 8 mg/dl, a number of complications develop, including worsening hypertension, abnormalities in calcium and phosphate metabolism, anemia, infec-

ASSOCIATED OCULAR CONDITIONS IN RENAL FAILURE

Hypertensive retinopathy
　　Flame hemorrhages
　　Cotton-wool spots (nerve fiber layer infarcts)
　　Optic disc edema

Diabetic retinopathy (especially advanced or proliferative)

Choroidal vascular changes
　　Elschnig's spots
　　Seigert's streaks
　　Serous detachment

Anterior segment
　　Band keratopathy
　　Calcium deposition in conjunctiva

Miscellaneous
　　Punctate lens opacities

tion, and fluid and electrolyte imbalances. The most dangerous of the electrolyte imbalances is hyperkalemia, which predisposes the patient to life-threatening ventricular arrhythmias.

Because of poorly functioning filtering abilities of the kidney, patients often lose immunoglobulins and other larger molecular weight substances such as albumin. It is in this setting that patients develop ankle edema and are prone to infections because of the lack of immunoglobulins for protection.

Stages of Renal Insufficiencies

There are three stages of chronic renal failure. The first and earliest stage demonstrates azotemia, which is an elevation of creatinine and BUN. There are no symptoms and the renal function remains well preserved.

As the azotemia increases the patient may experience nocturia, or increased urination at night. This second stage of chronic renal failure remains otherwise free of symptoms.

Uremia, the final stage of renal failure, is composed of a constellation of signs and symptoms,

including nausea, vomiting, hypertension, acidosis, hyperkalemia, and others affecting almost every part of the body. A significant complication of uremia is neurologic manifestations of chronic renal failure, including cerebrovascular accident, seizures, and encephalopathy.

Treatment

No single blood test tells the physician to consider alternate means of therapy for patients with renal failure; indeed, the course of chronic renal failure can be attenuated by the use of low-protein diets. Recently, certain drugs such as the ACE inhibitors have been found to slow the progression of renal disease in diabetic patients.

When a patient has renal dysfunction that is not compatible with life, one of three options for therapy are considered: organ transplantation, *hemodialysis,* or peritoneal dialysis. A renal transplant is the most successful replacement therapy with the longest survival; however, the patient must have a match (preferably a family member) and be willing to endure this type of surgery and subsequent immunosuppressive therapy.

Many older patients who develop renal failure as the result of long-standing diabetes or hypertension are not candidates for a transplant. In these patients hemodialysis is often used. In hemodialysis, patients are attached to a machine for 3 to 4 hours at a time through an arteriovenous fistula. Complications associated with hemodialysis include infection, graft closure, and anemia requiring frequent blood transfusion. This last complication has been addressed through the recent use of erythropoietin, a substance that stimulates the body to produce blood cells.

The third option, which is most useful for the young, motivated patient, is peritoneal dialysis. In this form of renal replacement therapy, the patient's own peritoneal membrane in the abdomen is used as the filter. Patients have a catheter placed through the abdominal wall and dialysate fluid is infused, often at bedtime. Over the course of the evening the toxic substances, through differences in charges and molecule size, are removed from the blood stream into their peritoneal fluid and the fluid is drained out by the next morning. This form of replacement therapy is more "physiologic" than hemodialysis and does not require the patient to be attached to a machine every other day. A problem associated with peritoneal dialysis is frequent bouts of peritonitis. Most patients are not candidates for peritoneal dialysis because they do not have the hand-eye coordination or the finances to afford this form of therapy.

OCULAR MANIFESTATIONS OF RENAL DISEASE

Renal Retinopathy

The most common ocular association with renal disease appears to be retinopathy similar to acute hypertensive retinopathy. These findings (discussed in greater detail in Chapter 9 on Cardiovascular Disease) include superficial retinal (usually flame-shaped) hemorrhages, nerve fiber layer infarcts (cotton-wool spots), arteriolar attenuation, arteriolar narrowing (focal and generalized), and arteriovenous crossing changes.

Clinical features of renal retinopathy distinguish it from true hypertensive changes. Studies have shown that the fundus in patients with renal failure is more severely affected than would be expected in patients with indirectly elevated diastolic pressures. Often, retinal and disc edema is present, as are numerous cotton-wool spots.

The fact that patients with advanced kidney disease have other problems in addition to true hypertension, such as metabolic imbalance, excess renin production, and hypervolemia with salt and water retention, may play an undetermined role in producing the significant findings. In addition, signs of choroidal circulatory deficiencies may appear as a consequence.

Posterior Segment

Nonrhegmatogenous Retinal Detachment. Localized, nonrhegmatogenous serous detachment of the retina appears as a complication of renal failure. The ophthalmoscopic appearance superficially may resemble central serous choroidopathy. The acute lesion may have an associated white area of retinal pigment epithelial necrosis. The resolution of the detachment may result in the formation of a small hyperpigmented or atrophic spot (called a chronic *Elschnig spot*). These detachments are usually bilateral and involve the inferior retina.

Elschnig Spots. When blood pressure control is not adequate, areas of serous detachment do not resolve as readily or quickly. In many of these eyes depigmentation or pigmentary clumping is seen at the level of the retinal pigment epithelium. These are called Elschnig's spots and are present in two forms. A chronic Elschnig's spot appears as a small circular area of hyperpigmentation surrounded by depigmentation. Acute Elschnig's spots may look like the serous detachment although much smaller and more whitish. There is a strong association with severe accelerated hypertension.

Seigert's Streaks. As a result of arteriosclerosis resulting from acute hypertension, the lumen of the choroid artery becomes obliterated and the entire walls become acellular and necrotic. Seigert's streaks are secondary to a patchy distribution of the sclerotic process of the choriocapillaris, consisting of hyperpigmentation that covers the affected vasculature. The streaks radiate into the periphery underneath the retinal vessels. Studies have indicated that these are associated with a poor prognosis for life.

Management of hypertensive choroidal vascular changes includes an urgent referral for control of the systemic condition. Once the systemic condition is controlled, and if controlled early, healing of the choroidal vascular endothelium and retinal pigment epithelium occurs with rapid disappearance of detachment. Minimal pigmentary change may be seen. However, if blood pressure is not controlled, detachment may still resolve because of decreased leakage from increased nonperfusion. Permanent loss of vision may occur as well as new detachments elsewhere.

Anterior Segment: Band Keratopathy

Anterior segment conditions associated with renal disease are relatively uncommon compared with posterior segment conditions previously mentioned. Hypercalcemia from renal failure can be manifested by band keratopathy, calcium deposits near Bowman's membrane. Band keratopathy presents as a hazy, "Swiss-cheese" appearance across the interpalpebral zone of the cornea. Symptoms include decreased vision and occasional foreign body sensation. Calcium can also deposit in the conjunctival epithelium and can be spread from the limbal interpalpebral region to the canthal region. Management for calcium deposition involves the cornea because treatment is removal of the deposition only if vision is affected.

OCULAR SIGNS IN RENAL TRANSPLANTATION

After renal transplantation, most ocular conditions are typically a result of medication. Posterior subcapsular cataracts are a common development. This condition appears to have a strong association with treatment with some type of immunosup-

---

ASSOCIATED OCULAR CONDITIONS IN RENAL TRANSPLANTATION (USUALLY IATROGENIC)

Bacterial, adenoviral infections
Herpes simplex keratitis
Posterior subcapsular cataracts

---

pressive medication, such as prednisone or azathioprine. Secondary infections include herpes simplex, keratoconjunctivitis, and bacterial and adenoviral infections (see box).

Patients with posterior subcapsular cataracts should be evaluated for extraction. It is more advisable to extract the cataract than discontinue the medication. Keep in mind that with transplantation the ocular manifestations that occurred with renal failure (such as advanced hypertensive retinopathy, Elschnig's spots, serous detachment) can be sharply curtailed.

Bibliography

Anderson S and Brenner BM: Effects of aging on the renal glomerulus (review), *Am J Med* 80:435, 1986.

Brezis M, Rosen S, and Epstein FH: *Acute renal failure.* In Brenner BM and Rector FC Jr, editors: *The kidney,* ed 3, Philadelphia, 1986, WB Saunders Co.

Eschbach JW: The anemia of chronic renal failure. Pathophysiology and the effects of recombinant erythropoietin. *Kidney Int* 35:135, 1989.

Ihle BU and others: The effect of protein restriction on the progression of renal insufficiency, *N Engl J Med* 321:1773, 1989.

Noble J: *Textbook of general medicine and primary care,* part XIX, chapters 136-141, pp 1827-1867, Boston, 1987, Little, Brown & Co.

Shemish O and others: Limitations of creatine as a filtration marker in glomerulopathic patients, *Kidney Int* 28:830, 1985.

Sirmon MD and Kirpatrick WG: Acute renal failure: what to do until the nephrologist comes, *Postgrad Med* 87:55, 1990.

Wyngaarden JB and Smith LH: Cecil *Textbook of medicine,* ed 18, part IX, chapters 74-93, Philadelphia, 1988, WB Saunders Co.

11

Pulmonary Diseases

MICHAEL R. SILVER

KEY TERMS

Forced Expiratory Volume	*Bronchiectasis*	*Adenosquamous Carcinoma*
Bronchodilators	*Dyspnea*	*Mesothelioma*
Tachypneic	*Squamous-cell Carcinoma*	*Hemoptysis*
Cyanosis	*Adenocarcinoma*	*Syncope*
Metered Dose Inhaler	*Large-cell Carcinoma*	*Isoniazid*
Methylxanthines	*Small-cell Carcinoma*	*Rifampin*
Cromolyn Sulfate		

CHRONIC OBSTRUCTIVE PULMONARY DISEASE

Chronic obstructive pulmonary disease (COPD) is the term applied to individuals with asthma, chronic bronchitis, or emphysema. All individuals with COPD have airflow limitation. When their disease is active, the amount of air an individual can exhale in one second (*forced expiratory volume*—FEV_1) is reduced in comparison with the total amount of air that an individual can forcefully exhale (forced vital capacity—FVC). The hallmark of COPD is a reduction of this ratio, FEV_1/FVC, which is normally greater than 70%. COPD affects more than 30 million Americans. Individuals with COPD often have components of more than one specific disease. The following is a description of the three major disease entities that comprise COPD.

Asthma

Definition. Asthma is a disease characterized by reversible airflow obstruction (reduced FEV_1/FVC). Improvement in airflow may occur spontaneously or as a result of therapy. A subset of patients with asthma may have a normal FEV_1/FVC but manifest hyperreactive airways. These individuals have a markedly increased sensitivity to certain inhalants (such as histamine or methacholine) with a resultant fall in their FEV_1/FVC.

Etiology and Epidemiology. Approximately 6% of the U.S. population carries a diagnosis of asthma. In the United States there are over 5500 deaths per year from asthma, many of them in individuals under 18 years of age. Asthma mortality has increased nationally and worldwide in the last decade. Suggested reasons for this increase include changes in the definition of asthma, inappropriate treatment, inadequate access to medical care, and changes in air quality. Given that asthma is a *reversible* disease, the fatalities associated with this disease become even more tragic.

Traditionally, asthma has been divided into extrinsic and intrinsic asthma. This was based on the observation that some asthmatics experienced acute exacerbations in response to extrinsic factors such as inhaled allergens (such as pollen, dust, animal dander, and perfume). Other individuals' disease would flare for unclear or intrinsic factors. Because the pathophysiology, clinical manifestations, and treatment of these two types of asthmatics are similar, the terms intrinsic and extrinsic are infrequently used. Although the terminology regarding asthmatic triggers has changed, the concept that certain factors may provoke an asthmatic attack remains quite important. Some of the precipitants of an asthmatic attack in susceptible individuals are listed in the box.

Pathophysiology. In the last several years there have been tremendous advances in the understanding of the pathophysiology of asthma. Previously, the airflow obstruction characteristic of the disease was thought to be caused by bronchial smooth muscle contraction. It now appears that contraction of the bronchial smooth muscle that circumferentially lines the respiratory airways is important, but not the sole explanation for the clinical manifestations of asthma. Inflammation of the bronchial wall leads to swelling of the bronchial mucosa. The circumferential narrowing caused by this swelling also leads to airflow limitation. The chronic airway inflammation that characterizes the

---

TRIGGERS OF AN ASTHMATIC ATTACK

Infection
   Viral
   Bacterial

Stress
   Exercise
   Emotion

Environmental
   Changes in weather
   Air pollution
   Cigarette smoke
   Formaldehyde

Inhaled allergens
   Animal dander
   House dust (mite *Dermatophagoides pteronyssinus*)
   Pollen
   Molds

Drugs
   Beta-blockers
   Aspirin
   Any drug precipitating an anaphylactic response

---

airways in some patients with asthma explains why therapy directed solely at bronchial smooth muscle relaxation is only intermittently effective. Influx of neutrophils, eosinophils, and mononuclear cells into the bronchial wall sustains the inflammatory response. Untreated, these leukocytes can amplify the initial allergic response, leading to clinical deterioration.

The dual mechanisms of airflow obstruction in asthma, early bronchial muscle constriction and late inflammatory response further narrowing the airways, have led to the terms *early-phase response* and *late-phase response*. The early-phase response is due primarily to bronchoconstriction and is amenable to treatment with acute *bronchodilators* such as beta$_2$-adrenergic agonists or theophylline. These agents do not have anti-inflammatory action and are ineffective in preventing the bronchoconstriction associated with the late-phase response. This late phase manifests hours after the initial exposure and requires anti-inflammatory treatment to prevent its development.

Clinical Manifestations. The appearance of an individual in the throes of an asthmatic attack is striking. Sitting upright, *tachypneic* and complaining of shortness of breath, asthmatic patients often have audible wheezing. In severe attacks they may be dusky, *cyanotic,* and unable to speak. A marked reduction in expiratory airflow (measured by a peak flow meter) is present, as may be a deterioration in both ventilation (an elevated Pco_2) and in oxygenation (decreased Po_2). In the early stages of an asthmatic attack, wheezing is first auscultated during the end-expiratory phase of respiration. As the airflow limitation increases, wheezing is heard earlier during expiration and eventually during inspiration. In severe attacks, no breath sounds may be heard at all owing to the lack of airflow during inspiration and expiration. The absence of breath sounds indicates impending respiratory failure.

Treatment. For individuals suffering from an acute asthmatic attack, acute bronchodilation is the goal of therapy. Sympathetic stimulation of the bronchial muscles effects bronchodilation. Bronchial muscle receptors are beta$_2$ selective, compared with cardiac beta-receptors, which are beta$_1$ selective. While children and young adults tolerate nonspecific beta-adrenergic stimulation with isoproterenol or epinephrine, older adults may have tachyarrhythmias or angina from cardiac stimulation associated with these drugs. In adults therefore, beta$_2$-agonists such as metaproterenol or albuterol are preferable to nonselective beta agonists such as isoproterenol or epinephrine. Most sympathomimetic agents are administered by inhalation using either *metered dose inhaler* (MDI) or by a medication nebulizer. MDIs are portable and inexpensive relative to a medication nebulizer, but they require either good patient technique to be effective or use of a spacer device for individuals unable to inhale and trigger the MDI simultaneously. Beta-agonists are also available as oral preparations and as subcutaneous injections. Both

of these forms are associated with more systemic side effects such as tremulousness, tachycardia, and tachyarrhythmias and should be used with caution in older adults.

Methylxanthines such as aminophylline and theophylline are also effective bronchodilators. Serum levels should be monitored because subtheraputic levels have little bronchodilator response, and elevated levels are associated with tremulousness, tachycardia, nausea, vomiting, tachyarrhythmias, seizures, and death. Recent use has diminished because of the availability of beta-adrenergic agents and because of the toxicity associated with elevated serum levels of theophylline.

For individuals with asthma regularly using beta-agonists, recent National Institutes of Health guidelines recommend the addition of an anti-inflammatory agent. Inhaled steroids are used to diminish the chronic airway inflammation characteristic of patients with moderate to severe asthma. When taken by inhalation, large local anti-inflammatory effects can be achieved with a marked reduction in systemic effects. For individuals with severe asthma, orally administered corticosteroids are the treatment of choice.

Inhaled *cromolyn sulfate* has been used to prevent asthmatic attacks, especially those precipitated by exercise. It is a useful adjuvant to patients receiving inhaled corticosteroids. Inhaled anticholinergic agents also may be useful adjuvant treatment for patients with asthma. They have no anti-inflammatory action but may directly cause bronchodilation. Administration of inhaled anticholinergic agents may be useful in treatment of acute bronchospasm secondary to beta-blockers or emotion, although they are more effective in patients with chronic bronchitis and emphysema.

Chronic Bronchitis

Definition. Individuals with a chronic productive cough for 3 months of a year for 2 consecutive years are considered to have chronic bronchitis.

Etiology and Epidemiology. Chronic bronchitis most often occurs in individuals exposed to cigarette smoke. Other respiratory inhalants, often found in manufacturing, may cause chronic bronchial irritation and result in development of chronic bronchitis. Most patients with chronic bronchitis also have some degree of air flow limitation as manifested by a reduced FEV_1/FVC. These patients are frequently less responsive to inhaled beta-adrenergic agents than are individuals with asthma. More than 10 million people in the United States carry the diagnosis of chronic bronchitis. Other causes of chronic bronchitis include local or systemic immune deficiencies, leading to colonization and recurrent infection of the bronchial tree. Abnormal mucus production in the lung (cystic fibrosis), decreased level of immune globulins (such as common variable immune deficiency), or local destruction (*bronchiectasis*) all predispose individuals to recurrent infections and recurrent symptoms of chronic bronchitis.

Pathophysiology. Bronchial colonization or infection may lead to increased airway obstruction. Local airway colonization leads to chronic airway inflammation and increased mucin production, contributing to airflow limitation. Recurrent infections cause chronic bronchial inflammation, increased mucin production, and mucus gland hypertrophy. Local destruction of the lung from previous infections allows bacterial colonization, making eradication of pathogenic bacteria more difficult.

Chronic bronchitis may also cause chronic hypoxemia. The increased mucin production leads to abnormalities of ventilation and perfusion of the lung. The resultant hypoxemia responds quite well to low-flow oxygen therapy. Interestingly, the exercise tolerance in patients with chronic bronchitis is not limited by their cardiopulmonary vascular reserve until late in their disease.

Treatment. Antibiotics remain the treatment of choice for individuals with chronic bronchitis and acute infection. Increase in sputum production, change in the quality of sputum, and increasing dyspnea are hallmarks of active infection. Antibiotic therapy with macrolides, semisynthetic penicillins, fluoroquinolones, or sulfamethoxazole-trimethoprim are all reasonable choices depending on the predominant microbiologic flora in the sputum. Sputum Gram's stain is the most useful test when attempting to determine empiric antibiotic choice. Other agents useful in the treatment of patients with chronic bronchitis include inhaled bronchodilators, oxygen if patients are chronically hypoxemic, and, in selected patients, corticosteroids.

Clinical Manifestations. Individuals with chronic bronchitis in the early stages of disease may appear entirely normal, with symptoms only of cough and increased sputum production. With time, these individuals may become plethoric from polycythemia, cyanotic from chronic hypoxemia, and have clubbing of their digits for unclear reasons. As the disease progresses, their cough and sputum production remain, but their *dyspnea* progresses from being present with exercise to eventually being present at rest. Smoking cessation can slow the disease progression but may not reverse existing damage.

Emphysema

Definition. Emphysema has been defined pathologically, not clinically. The most common definition, from the American Thoracic Society, states that emphysema is present when there is "an anatomical alteration of the lung characterized by an abnormal enlargement of the airspaces distal to the nonrespiratory bronchioles, accompanied by destructive changes of the alveolar walls."

Etiology and Epidemiology. The major cause of emphysema is exposure to cigarette smoke. Inhalation of cigarette smoke results in increased neutrophil influx into the lung. These neutrophils become activated and release proteolytic enzymes that cause destruction of lung tissue. Compounding this process is the reduction of circulating levels of antiproteases (most notably alpha$_1$-antitrypsin) in some smokers. Nonsmokers with a rare condition of hereditary alpha$_1$-antitrypsin deficiency develop emphysema, usually by age 60, whereas smokers with alpha$_1$-antitrypsin develop emphysema much earlier. It is not known why only a minority of smokers develop clinically apparent emphysema.

Pathophysiology. Ongoing destruction of lung parenchyma leads to reduced tissue elasticity. Reduced elasticity results in earlier airway closure during exhalation. This manifests clinically as wheezing. Destruction of alveolar walls also leads to coalescence of alveoli into bullae. These large, compliant airsacs are often ventilated but rarely perfused. The ventilation that they receive is therefore wasted, and inflation of these bullae may contribute to the hyperinflation of the lung in emphysema. Oxygenation is well preserved because pulmonary blood continues to flow to ventilated alveoli. The sense of breathlessness patients with emphysema experience may relate to hyperinflation and increased work of breathing.

Clinical Manifestations. Classically, individuals with emphysema are thin with wasting of peripheral muscle mass. They are "barrel-chested" from chronic hyperinflation, tachypneic, and may exhibit pursed lip breathing. Although breathless, they are not cyanotic. As the disease progresses, exercise tolerance is limited because they have very little pulmonary reserve. In severe cases, patients may become confined to bed and die of pulmonary insufficiency.

Treatment. The destruction of pulmonary parenchyma is irreversible. No therapy is available for smokers with emphysema. These people should be encouraged to quit smoking because smoking accelerates the loss of lung function. Individuals with alpha$_1$-antitrypsin deficiency can receive exogenously administered replacement therapy to halt disease progression. Replacement therapy must be given for an individual's lifetime and is quite expensive.

LUNG CANCER

Malignancies found in the pulmonary parenchyma may be either primary lung cancer or metastatic cancer. Primary lung cancer typically originates from uncontrolled proliferation of cells from bronchial wall, bronchial mucosal glands, or lung parenchyma. However, approximately 25% of all the malignant lesions found in the lung represent metastatic spread of malignancies from nonpulmonary tissues.

Primary Lung Neoplasms

Etiology and Epidemiology. Primary lung neoplasms are commonly classified by histologic characteristics of the tumor. The four major types of lung cancer are *squamous cell carcinoma, adenocarcinoma* (including bronchoalveolar carcinoma), *large cell carcinoma,* and *small cell carcinoma.* There is also a mixed form of primary lung neoplasm called *adenosquamous carcinoma.* Nearly 150,000 deaths from lung cancer are estimated to have occurred in 1992 in the United States. Lung cancer remains the most common cause of cancer death in men in the United States and has recently surpassed breast cancer as the leading cause of cancer deaths in American women. The biologic events responsible for malignant transformation of pulmonary cells is not known, but alterations in DNA expression may incite abnormal growth and proliferation. Epidemiologically, it is well recognized that the single most important cause of lung cancer is cigarette smoking. Other agents that are known to cause lung cancer include exposure to radon, ionizing radiation, vinyl chloride, and hydrocarbons. Exposure to certain forms of asbestos has also been strongly associated with development of lung cancer and cancer of the pleura *(mesothelioma).*

Clinical Manifestations. A minority of individuals with primary lung cancer are asymptomatic at presentation. Most of the symptoms patients with lung cancer experience are related to the local effects of tumor growth. The most common local effects from lung cancer are dyspnea, cough, intermittent hemoptysis, chest pain, and signs and symptoms of pneumonia. Radiographic abnormalities include mass lesions, pleural effusions, and persistent infiltrates. The infiltrates may be diagnosed and treated as pneumonia, but they fail to improve despite multiple courses of antibiotics.

Adenocarcinoma and squamous cell carcinoma tend to grow locally before metastasizing and are most often associated with local manifestations or direct extension into contiguous structures. Extension into the pleura may result in pleural effusions and dyspnea. Extension into the mediastinum may (1) involve the great vessels, causing superior vena cava syndrome; (2) cause hoarseness of the voice from involvement of the recurrent laryngeal nerve; and (3) result in esophageal obstruction. Horner's syndrome may also be seen with extension of these tumors superiorly.

Small cell carcinoma has a predilection toward early metastasis and is much more likely to present with distant organ symptomatology. Symptoms from brain metastases, including seizures and strokes, are common, as are hematologic manifestations such as anemia or polycythemia from bone marrow invasion by small cell carcinoma. In addition, small cell carcinoma has been associated with ectopic hormone production, giving rise to paraneoplastic syndromes such as Cushing syndrome (from excessive production of an ACTH-like substance), syndrome of inappropriate antidiuretic hormone secretions, and hypercalcemia.

Diagnosis. Diagnosis of lung cancer should be made based on microscopic examination of abnormal tissue. Heavy smokers with constitutional symptoms such as low-grade fever and weight loss who are found to have a mass lesion on chest radiograph have a high likelihood of having lung cancer, but treatment should not begin without a definitive tissue diagnosis. Examination of the sputum, biopsy of the lung mass, or inspection of the bronchial tree via bronchoscopy are all useful in diagnosing lung cancer.

Treatment. Treatment of lung cancer depends both on the cell type and the degree of spread of the disease. Modalities currently available for treatment include surgical removal, chemotherapy, and radiation therapy. For lesions that obstruct the bronchi, local treatment with either endobronchial radiation or laser removal of tumor may be possible. When there has been minimal or no spread to mediastinal lymph nodes, surgical removal of non–small cell carcinoma offers the best chance for cure. For non–small cell carcinoma not involving mediastinal structures, surgical resection of local disease has a greater than 50% 5-year survival.

As the tumor grows in size or metastasizes to regional and mediastinal lymph nodes, survival with surgery alone diminishes. The addition of either preoperative or postoperative chemotherapy and radiation has been reported in some studies to improve 5-year survival.

For patients with small cell carcinoma, optimal treatment is chemotherapy. Because small cell carcinoma has a tendency to metastasize early, surgical resection has less success than in similarly staged non–small cell lesions. Current chemotherapeutic regimens have more than doubled the median survival in this disease from 6 to 9 months to 15 to 22 months.

Metastatic Disease to the Lung

Patients who present with pulmonary complaints and abnormalities on chest radiograph suggestive of carcinoma of the lung may have neoplasms from other sources which have spread hematogenously to the lung. Malignancies with a high rate of pulmonary metastases include malignant melanoma and breast, colon, pancreas, hypernephroma, and thyroid carcinoma. Certain malignancies (breast, metastatic melanoma, Kaposi sarcoma) have a predilection toward metastasizing endobronchially as well as to the pulmonary parenchyma. An isolated mass lesion with malignant features could be either a primary lung neoplasm or a single metastatic lesion. Multiple pulmonary nodules of different sizes, especially in an afebrile individual, are strongly suggestive of metastatic cancer that has spread to the lung. Treatment is usually palliative and is dictated by the cell type of the primary cancer. Hormonal manipulation, chemotherapy, and radiation therapy may all have some role in treatment of metastatic cancer to the lung. Unless vital structures are involved or airway obstruction is present, surgical intervention is usually not indicated.

PULMONARY EMBOLISM

Etiology and Epidemiology. Pulmonary embolism is a disease caused by migration of venous thrombi from their site of origin to the pulmonary arterial circulation. For thrombi originating in the lower extremities, the clot travels up the inferior vena cava and through the right atrium and right ventricle and lodges in the pulmonary circulation.

It is estimated that in 1993 there were more than 500,000 deaths caused by pulmonary embolism in the United States. The source of the migratory venous thrombi typically is the deep veins of the lower extremities. Occasionally the clot can migrate from the pelvic veins or subclavian vein. Most lower extremity pulmonary emboli arise above the knee, although there is some debate as to the significance of venous thrombosis found in the calf. Several conditions are known to increase the likelihood of pulmonary embolism. These are described in the box.

Pathophysiology. Clot formation occurs when the vascular endothelium is disrupted, exposing underlying basement membrane. Platelet activation and activation of the clotting cascade occur, with resultant formation of a platelet-fibrin plug at the area of vascular disruption. Although this system is protective and generally beneficial, its inappropriate activation can lead to occlusion of vital structures such as coronary arteries (leading to myocardial infarction) or formation of clots in the vascular bed of the lower extremities. Many of the conditions listed in the box may alter the balance between clot formation and clot lysis, leading to inappropriate clot formation. The clinical symptoms and alterations in normal physiology with pulmonary embolism occur because of the hemodynamic effects of occlusion of the pulmonary vessels. Small recurrent pulmonary emboli over years may slowly obliterate the pulmonary vasculature with resultant pulmonary hypertension. Pulmonary hypertension occurs because the right ventricle slowly compensates for increased pulmonary vascular resistance. Larger clots in individuals without right ventricular compensation can lead to markedly elevated pulmonary pressures because of the marked increase in pulmonary vascular resistance. When this occurs, right ventricular output may fall markedly, resulting in decreased volume to the left ventricle. The right ventricle usually becomes acutely dilated. Decreased volume delivery

---

CONDITIONS ASSOCIATED WITH INCREASED RISK OF THROMBOEMBOLISM

Chronic congestive heart failure
Genetic predisposition toward clot formation
Immobilization
Neoplasms
Previous thromboembolic disease
Recent surgery
Use of birth control pills, especially in smokers

---

to the left ventricle can lead to reduced left ventricular output with resulting syncope or near-syncope. Acute right ventricular distention can lead to cardiac arrhythmias, including ventricular tachycardia or ventricular fibrillation with sudden death.

Clinical Manifestations. Clot formation in the lower extremities may be asymptomatic or may present with local effects such as lower limb swelling or pain. Pulmonary embolism typically has one of four clinical presentations—asymptomatic, dyspnea, syncope, and death. A subset of patients are entirely asymptomatic because of the small size of the clot. A second group of patients present with dyspnea as the classic symptom. The dyspnea is usually sudden in onset and may or may not be episodic. Other signs associated with dyspnea, although not with high frequency, include chest pain, wheezing, and cough. Most patients have an elevated respiratory rate, and many patients may have a low-grade fever (less than 100.5° F). Patients may have abnormal breath sounds or may be tachycardic.

A third group of patients with pulmonary embolism have a clot large enough to cause transient right ventricular distention and cardiac arrhythmias. This group manifests sudden loss of consciousness (syncope). If the cardiac system recovers, the person regains consciousness. The final group of patients suffer failure of the cardiac system to compensate for the sudden increase in pulmonary vascular resistance. These patients present with sudden death.

Diagnosis. Because pulmonary embolism has no classic signs or symptoms, diagnosis is made by demonstration of clot in the pulmonary vasculature or may be presumed when clot is found in the lower extremities in a patient with a history suggesting pulmonary embolism. A high index of suspicion is required because the disease is very common, but so are its nonspecific symptoms of shortness of breath. Demonstration of thrombosis in veins of the lower legs is sufficient grounds to begin anticoagulant therapy, the therapy of choice for pulmonary embolism. Demonstration of clot in the lung by either ventilation-perfusion scans (in the right clinical setting) or pulmonary angiography is sufficient evidence to begin anticoagulant therapy. Prolonged therapy without documentation of thrombus in the lower extremities or clot in the lung is ill-advised because of the morbidity and mortality of anticoagulant therapy.

Treatment. The mainstay of treatment of pulmonary embolism is the prevention of more pulmonary emboli. To achieve this, anticoagulation initially with heparin and then with warfarin therapy is the treatment of choice. Treatment modifications need to be made for pregnant women and individuals with congenital absence of clotting factors. The degree of anticoagulation has been reduced in recent years, thereby reducing the morbidity and mortality from excessive bleeding, although the possibility of significant bleeding still remains. Surgical removal of a pulmonary embolus is an aggressive intervention available in selected medical centers. This may be a useful approach in the treatment of some patients with severe pulmonary hypertension from recurrent thromboembolism. Direct visualization of the clot by an angioscope combined with laser therapy has the potential to be a corrective and definitive treatment for patients with pulmonary embolism.

SARCOIDOSIS

Definition. Sarcoidosis is a disease of unknown cause which is characterized by epithelioid cell granulomas in various tissues without any evidence of infection. No specific tests are diagnostic of sarcoidosis. It is a diagnosis made after excluding other disease entities with similar histologic and clinical characteristics.

Etiology and Epidemiology. Sarcoidosis has been diagnosed in virtually all age ranges, races, and ethnic cultures, and it affects both genders equally. In the United States it tends to affect blacks more frequently than whites, but in other countries whites are affected with the same incidence as blacks in the United States. The hallmark of sarcoid is epithelioid cell granulomas with or without caseation. The trigger for the formation of granulomas is unknown, but it is presumed to be a Type IV immunologic response to an unidentified antigen or antigens. Activation of T lymphocytes with subsequent production of interleukin-2 most likely initiates and maintains the inflammatory response leading to granuloma formation.

Pathophysiology. The triggers that are responsible for the development of sarcoidosis are unknown, as are the factors that frequently lead to spontaneous remission of afflicted patients.

Clinical Features. Sarcoidosis has been reported to affect virtually every organ and tissue in the body. The frequency of organ involvement and clinical symptoms at the time of initial presentation are shown in the box on p. 219.

Most patients at the initial time of diagnosis are either asymptomatic or complain of dyspnea and/or cough. Eye, skin, and lymph node involvement are common throughout the individual's history, but less frequent as the initial presenting complaint.

Clinically, sarcoidosis is classified according to the appearance of the chest radiograph. Stage 0 sarcoidosis is a normal chest radiograph in individuals diagnosed with sarcoidosis. Stage 1 sarcoidosis is bilateral hilar adenopathy on chest radiograph. Stage 2 sarcoidosis is bilateral hilar adenopathy and pulmonary infiltrate, and Stage 3 sarcoidosis is pulmonary infiltrates without hilar adenopathy.

Most patients never progress beyond Stage 2, but a subset of patients experience regression of their hilar and mediastinal adenopathy and develop pulmonary fibrosis related to the chronic inflammatory process in the lung parenchyma. These individuals may develop chronic respiratory failure

---

FREQUENCY OF ORGAN INVOLVEMENT AND CLINICAL SYMPTOMS AT THE TIME OF INITIAL DIAGNOSIS

Lung— 65%
Lymph node— 50%
Constitutional symptoms— 25%
   Anorexia— 12%
   Fever— 10%
   Weight loss— 8%
Eye— 12%
Liver— 7%
Skin— 4%
Endocrine— 2%
Central nervous system— 2%
Muscle— 2%
Heart— 1%
Genitourinary— 1%
Bone— 1%

---

with chronic hypoxemia and hypercapnea related to destruction of lung tissue. As with other interstitial lung diseases, these patients may ultimately die of respiratory failure.

The dermatologic manifestations of sarcoid typically are small, firm nodules located over the anterior surfaces of the lower extremity known as erythema nodosum. These lesions may regress spontaneously or may leave small scars. Diffuse symmetric lymphadenopathy also occurs with sarcoidosis. Hepatosplenomegaly, arthralgias, cardiomyopathy, and cardiac arrhythmias all have been reported to occur in patients with sarcoidosis. Sarcoidosis affects the central nervous system and can cause both hypopituitarism and diabetes insipidus from reduction in vasopressin release. Constitutional symptoms include fever and weight loss. Finally, endocrine abnormalities such as hypercalcemia also may occur and in severe cases may lead to increased calcium concentration in the urine and renal stone formation. In some unfortunate patients, transformation of sarcoidosis to lymphoma occurs.

Radiographic manifestations include bilateral hilar lymphadenopathy, mediastinal lymphadenopathy, pulmonary nodules, interstitial lung infiltrates, and cyst formation. With the exception of cyst formation, all of the changes represent potentially reversible disease.

Laboratory abnormalities include elevation of serum gamma globulins and occasional elevation of erythrocyte sedimentation rate. There can be marked hypercalcemia, although it occurs infrequently in patients with sarcoid. Serum angiotensin-converting enzyme is also produced by activated macrophages and granulomas in patients with sarcoidosis. Although it may be used as an indicator of disease activity, it is not useful for either prognosis or diagnosis.

Ocular Manifestations

Approximately 20% of patients with sarcoid have ocular involvement by sarcoid at some time during their clinical course. The activity of ocular sarcoid may not correlate with the activity of pulmonary sarcoid. Regardless of their symptoms, patients diagnosed with sarcoidosis need regular eye examinations to assess the presence or absence of ocular sarcoid. Ocular manifestations of sarcoid are listed in the box on p. 220. A discussion of many of these entities appears in Chapter 18.

Treatment. Treatment is not indicated for patients with asymptomatic hilar adenopathy, no evidence of organ involvement, and no constitutional symptoms. For individuals with significant pulmonary symptomatology, hypercalcemia, central nervous system involvement, and myocardial involvement, corticosteroids are generally used. No data strongly indicate that corticosteroid treatment of pulmonary sarcoidosis significantly alters the inevitable course of pulmonary disease. Steroids are definitely efficacious in ocular and central nervous system sarcoidosis. For individuals with dermatologic conditions, chloroquine has been used with some success.

PULMONARY INFECTIONS

Infections of the pulmonary system can be classified by site of infection or causative organism. The latter is used for the following discussion.

OCULAR MANIFESTATIONS OF SARCOID

Conjunctiva
    Conjunctival granulomas
    Conjunctivitis
    Calcification

Cornea
    Band keratopathy
    Keratitic precipitates
    Nonspecific keratitis
    Superficial punctate keratitis

Sclera
    Episcleritis
    Episcleral nodules

Uvea
    Anterior or posterior uveitis
    Acute or chronic iridocyclitis
    Anterior or posterior synechiae
    Koeppe's nodules (iris pupillary nodules)
    Busacca's nodules (iris stromal nodules)
    Secondary glaucoma

Retina
    Peripheral retinitis
    Periphlebitis
    Retinal edema

Vitreous
    Hemorrhage
    Nodular opacities

Lacrimal gland
    Dry eye (keratitis sicca)
    Lacrimal gland enlargement

External eye
    Pseudochalazia
    Cutaneous nodules
    Orbital tumors
    Extraocular muscle palsies

Optic nerve/visual disturbance
    Blurred vision
    Visual field defect
    Scotoma
    Optic neuritis
    Blindness

Bronchitis

Definition. Bronchitis is an infection with subsequent inflammation of the trachea, bronchi, and/or bronchioles. In normal individuals structures below the vocal cords (trachea and more distal tracheobronchial tree) are usually sterile.

Etiology and Epidemiology. In healthy individuals, most acute bronchitic episodes are related to a primary viral infection. Viruses such as coxsackie, rhinovirus, adenovirus, influenza, and parainfluenza may cause a primary inflammation of the bronchial epithelium.

In most parts of the United States these infections are typically more common in spring and fall. Because of the disruption of the protective epithelium, subsequent infection by bacterial adhesion and invasion may occur. Bacteria typically responsible for acute bacterial bronchitis include *Streptococcus pneumoniae, Haemophilus influenzae,* and *Moraxella catarrhalis.* Other gram-negative species and anaerobes may also play a role, especially if there has been prior treatment with antibiotics or abnormal host factors.

Pathophysiology. Colonization of the normally sterile tracheobronchial tree in chronic bronchitis may lead to airway inflammation. Infection of the airways usually leads to airway inflammation. Airway inflammation from microbial invasion is characterized by increased mucin production and bronchial wall edema, which often manifests as cough, shortness of breath, or increased sputum production.

Clinical Manifestations. Individuals with acute viral bronchitis typically present with a viral syndrome. They initially have a dry nonproductive cough, coryza, and sometimes associated myalgias. After several days of nonproductive cough, patients may develop a productive cough, signifying the beginning of a bacterial infection. This transformation from an acute viral bronchitis to an acute bacterial bronchitis is usually not associated with fever, leukocytosis, or radiographic changes.

Patients who carry a diagnosis of chronic bronchitis have airways colonized with organisms. Individuals who experience exacerbation of their chronic bronchitis typically experience an increase in sputum production or a change in the color or quality of their sputum. With changes in microbiologic flora, the normally white or gray sputum of bronchitis may become green or frankly purulent. With both acute and chronic bronchitis blood-streaked sputum *(hemoptysis)* may occur. Massive hemoptysis should prompt a search for other causes.

Treatment. Treatment of acute bronchitis both in the normal host and in the individual with a diagnosis of chronic bronchitis is similar. Antibiotic therapy when there is evidence of bacterial infection is efficacious. Antibiotic therapy for acute viral bronchitis does not alter the clinical course of the disease and may select resistant organisms that will subsequently colonize the tracheobronchial tree, making antibiotic treatment more difficult in the future.

Pneumonia

Definition. Pneumonia is defined as an inflammatory process secondary to infection that involves the respiratory bronchioles and alveoli of the lung.

Etiology and Epidemiology. Pneumonia can be caused by viruses, bacteria, mycobacteria, fungi, or protozoa. The determination of the cause of pneumonia is based both on clinical and radiographic grounds as well as culture of the causative agent. The most common cause of community-acquired pneumonia in a normal individual is *Streptococcus pneumoniae.* This is a gram-positive diplococcus known to colonize the upper airways of adults, especially in winter months. Other organisms also commonly responsible for pneumonia in normal hosts include *Haemophilus influenzae, Legionella pneumophila,* and *Mycoplasma pneumoniae. Haemophilus influenzae* is a gram-negative rod that commonly colonizes individuals with chronic lung disease. *Legionella* is so named because it was initially isolated as the cause of the 1976 epidemic outbreak at the American Legion Convention in Philadelphia. Identification of *Legionella* is difficult because the organism stains poorly with Gram's stain and does not grow in usual culture media. *Mycoplasma pneumoniae* is one of the smallest known free-living organisms and cannot be easily identified by sputum culture.

It may be responsible for as many as 15 million infections per year in the United States. The vast majority of these are a tracheobronchitis, with several million cases being asymptomatic and approximately 500,000 cases of pneumonia a year.

Individuals with a normal immune system but underlying lung disease may develop pneumonias from other organisms in the Enterobacteriaceae family such as *Klebsiella, Serratia,* and *Pseudomonas.* Patients with cystic fibrosis, bronchiectasis, or chronic antibiotic therapy are known to develop infection with *Pseudomonas.* Individuals with altered immune systems develop infections based on their specific immunologic defect. Individuals with immunoglobulin deficiencies have a tendency to develop *Streptococcus pneumoniae* infections. Splenectomized patients are more likely to develop infections with encapsulated organisms such as *S. pneumoniae* and *H. influenzae.* Patients with altered cellular immunity (chronic steroid therapy or HIV positive) may develop opportunistic infections. These are life-threatening infections that occur with organisms such as fungi or protozoa not typically pathogenic in immunologically normal human hosts.

Pathophysiology. In most patients with pneumonia, the infecting organisms trigger an inflammatory host response. An influx of activated neutrophils and monocytes leads to localized inflammation which may be radiographically evident. Activation of these white cells may lead to clinical symptoms such as fever and anorexia. As the inflammation continues, the area of involved lung becomes more edematous and more difficult to ventilate and oxygenate. When the infection is limited, the individual is able to use his pulmonary reserve to continue ventilating and oxygenating blood. For unknown reasons, some individuals develop a pattern of diffuse lung injury related to a localized inflammatory process. This diffuse injury can severely impair lung function, and patients may require artificial ventilation to survive.

Clinical Manifestations. Individuals with bacterial pneumonia typically have fever and a cough productive of purulent sputum. A rusty-colored sputum is classic for pneumonia from *S. pneumoniae.* If the infection involves the peripheral regions of the lung, patients may develop pleuritic chest pain related to inflammation of the visceral and parietal pleura. Other pleural manifestations include pleural effusions and chest pain related to musculoskeletal injury from coughing. Most patients have an elevated temperature and may experience rigors.

Bacterial pneumonias usually have a rapid onset, with only a 24- to 48-hour prodrome and an ill-appearing individual. The atypical pneumonias (*Legionella* and *Mycoplasma*) typically have a longer prodrome and clinical appearance of a less acutely ill patient with a nonproductive cough. Some individuals may have an elevated temperature, require life support, and even die as a result of these infections. Leukocytosis with expression of premature forms is much more common in a bacterial process than in cases of atypical pneumonia.

Opportunistic infection refers to pulmonary infections caused by fungi or *Pneumocystis carinii* (PCP) and can be more difficult to diagnosis than bacterial pneumonia. Patients with opportunistic infections often appear subacutely ill, and the diagnosis may be missed unless the clinician is suspicious of altered immune function. Fungal infections are indolent in nature and present after days or weeks of symptoms being present. Patients may have weight loss and fever but generally do not have a productive cough.

PCP infection often begins with dyspnea on exertion and gradually progresses to cough and dyspnea at rest. The time from initial symptoms to diagnosis is approximately 3 weeks. Although PCP may affect individuals on high-dose corticosteroids, it classically occurs in HIV-positive individuals. Even with PCP prophylaxis, virtually all patients who are HIV positive have at least one episode of PCP during their lifetime.

Diagnosis of pneumonia, like the diagnosis of acute bronchitis, is based on examination of the sputum. Presence of macrophages and absence of squamous cells ensure that the sputum sample is from the lower respiratory tract and not simply saliva. Gram's stain of the sputum guides empiric antibiotic therapy. Gram-positive cocci strongly suggest *S. pneumoniae* as the causative agent. Gram-negative rods suggest *H. influenzae, Klebsiella,* or, in the appropriate clinical setting, *Pseudomonas.* Presence of large number of inflammatory cells and absence of organisms strongly suggest either viral, *Mycoplasma, Legionella,* or fungal disease. Typically patients with PCP do not produce significant amounts of sputum.

Treatment. Because microbiologic culture results are not available for several days, treatment of pneumonia is often empiric. For immunocompetent patients with a community-acquired pneumonia who are not allergic to penicillin, semisynthetic penicillins, macrolides, or sulfamethoxazole-trimethoprim are acceptable agents. For individuals with gram-negative rods on sputum Gram's stain or those patients more likely to have gram-negative infections, cephalosporins, semisynthetic penicillins, or quinolones represent good oral antibiotic choices. Individuals exhibiting signs of systemic toxicity or debilitated individuals unlikely to tolerate respiratory compromise are best admitted to a hospital for intravenous antibiotics. Admission decisions cannot be based solely on the degree of temperature elevation or the nature of the sputum but must take into consideration the patient's pulmonary and clinical reserve as well as their clinical presentation. Outpatient oral antibiotics may not be possible for individuals with altered immune function or underlying lung disease. These patients should be referred for immediate evaluation to determine whether or not they need more aggressive diagnostic procedures or intravenous medication.

APPROACH TO SELECTED PULMONARY PROBLEMS

Tuberculosis

Although a number of species in the Mycobacteriaceae family can cause human disease, the comments below refer only to the organism *Mycobacterium tuberculosis.* Human infection with *M. tu-*

berculosis remains a problem worldwide, with more than 1 billion people infected with the organism. It is becoming an increasing problem in the United States. Increased frequency among patients infected with HIV and the frightening occurrence of multidrug-resistant tuberculosis are partially responsible. Tuberculosis is difficult to diagnose because its symptoms of weight loss, fatigue, cough, and low-grade fever are nonspecific. Skin testing for exposure to tuberculosis helps identify individuals infected with the organism, but is less useful in identifying patients who are contagious. The presence and number of tubercles in the sputum correlate with a person's infectivity. Prophylaxis with isoniazid for people with no evidence of active disease but positive skin test is routine up to 35 years of age. After this age the benefit of prophylaxis is outweighed by the risk of isoniazid hepatotoxicity in normal individuals. Patients with active tuberculosis need to be treated with multiple drugs. Current recommendations are isoniazid, rifampin, and pyrazinamide daily for 2 months and *isoniazid* and *rifampin* daily for 4 additional months. Individuals who are likely to have an organism resistant to one or more antituberculous agents should have at least one additional agent (streptomycin or ethambutol) added to their three-drug regimen. The resurgence of tuberculosis and the emergence of organisms resistant to all known antituberculous agents represent a significant threat to health care providers and the population as a whole.

Chronic Cough

Chronic cough can be defined as a persistent cough without clear cause for at least 4 weeks. Cough may be a manifestation of a co-existing disease. The causes of chronic cough are listed in the box. The most common of these diseases is postnasal congestion, in which mucus drains into the nasopharynx, oropharynx, and hypopharynx stimulating a cough response. Patients with asthma or gastroesophageal reflux may present with cough. Therapy should be directed at the specific disease entities present. Over-the-counter cough suppres-

---

CAUSES OF CHRONIC COUGH

Asthma
Chronic bronchitis
Gastroesophageal reflux
Hypothyroidism
Interstitial lung disease
Medication
    Angiotensin-converting enzyme inhibitors
Occupational factors
Postinfectious
Postnasal drip
Psychogenic
Unknown

---

sants are not particularly effective in suppressing cough. The most effective cough suppressants contain narcotics such as codeine and oxycodone. Patients with cough from a viral bronchitis should be advised that the cough associated with their illness can persist for 6 to 8 weeks.

Hemoptysis

Hemoptysis is defined as coughing up blood. The most common causes of this distressing symptom are acute and chronic bronchitis. In these cases the sputum is blood streaked or may contain small clots of blood. Some patients with hemoptysis have an underlying pulmonary malignancy or cavitary lung disease, but this is unusual. Patients with gross hemoptysis (500 ml of blood in 24 hours) frequently have a condition other than bronchitis. These individuals may have a malignant lesion that has bled, underlying interstitial lung disease with erosion into the pulmonary vasculature, or cavitary lung disease. This degree of hemorrhage can be life threatening—not from exsanguination but from asphyxiation. As little as 50 to 100 ml of blood may form a clot and clog a vital portion of the tracheobronchial tree, leading to a respiratory compromise and death. Treatment for patients with nonmassive hemoptysis is supportive. Cough suppressants may be beneficial because the recurrent coughing is responsible for the localized bleeding. The presence of massive hemoptysis demands urgent evaluation and treatment. These patients may undergo emergency bronchoscopy or other procedures to better localize the source of bleeding and to guide treatment. In some cases surgery or other interventions may be necessary.

Dyspnea

Dyspnea is a sensation defined as difficulty in breathing. Multiple disease processes lead to a complaint of dyspnea. There is no unifying explanation for the association of dyspnea with all these diseases. Some diseases such as asthma and emphysema may cause dyspnea by hyperinflation of the lung and mechanical disadvantaging of the diaphragm. Other individuals with pulmonary hemorrhage, congestive heart failure, or interstitial lung disease may experience dyspnea because of increased work of breathing. Even normal individuals may experience dyspnea at the end of a strenuous period of exercise when lactate production occurs and ventilatory requirements increase related to lactic acidosis. The duration of dyspnea may give some indication to possible disease processes that are responsible. Chronic dyspnea can be defined as shortness of breath for greater than 1 week and is more likely related to an underlying lung disease such as asthma, sarcoidosis, or interstitial lung disease. Acute dyspnea, especially with sudden onset of shortness of breath, requires more immediate attention. Congestive heart failure, myocardial infarction, asthma, and pulmonary embolism all may give rise to the fairly rapid (less than 24 hours) onset of intense dyspnea. As with other entities, the more rapid the onset of symptoms, the more urgent the need for diagnosis and treatment. Individuals with chronic complaints of dyspnea may also require significant medical evaluation, but this can usually proceed at a more measured pace.

Tobacco Use

Tobacco use has been characterized as the single greatest health hazard currently existing in the United States. An estimated 400,000 deaths in 1993 are directly related to the use of tobacco, primarily cigarettes. Most of these deaths occurred either from increased cardiovascular mortality or lung cancer. It is estimated that an individual who smokes one pack per day starting at the age of 15 loses approximately 7 minutes of life per cigarette inhaled. Individuals who smoke are at increased risk for heart disease and multiple different cancers, including cancer of the lung, tongue, larynx, esophagus, stomach, colon, cervix, and bladder. These individuals have a far greater risk than nonsmokers of developing chronic bronchitis and emphysema with resultant respiratory failure and death. Recently it has become recognized that inhalation of cigarette smoke from nearby smokers (passive smoking) also can be deleterious. Children whose parents smoke are at increased risk for development of asthma, morbidity related to asthma, bronchitis, otitis, and allergies. Adults who live with smokers also seem to be at increased risk for the development of cancer and possibly COPD.

Unfortunately, nicotine is addicting both physically and psychologically. Nicotine substitution with nicotine gum or with transdermal nicotine therapy has been somewhat successful in helping individuals quit smoking for the first several months. However, the recidivism rate for smokers remains quite high. One approach to counseling patients about smoking cessation is the five "As" as advanced by the National Cancer Institute: (1) Ask the patient if they have ever thought about quitting. (2) Assess their readiness for quitting. (3) Advise them about the benefits of quitting. (4) Assist them in quitting by providing pharmacologic support, developing treatment plans, and referring them to appropriate cessation programs. (5) Arrange for follow-up after they have quit. Helping patients find reasons for quitting and using these reasons to continually motivate them to quit smoking is very useful when counseling patients. Health care providers need to understand that the addiction to cigarettes is more than physical and as such requires ongoing support and attention to keep patients from smoking once they have successfully quit.

Bibliography

Becker DM, Philbrick JT, and Selby JB: Inferior vena cava filters. Indications, safety, effectiveness, *Arch Intern Med* 152:1985, 1992.

Burrows B: Airways obstructive diseases: pathogenetic mechanisms and natural histories of the disorders, *Med Clin North Am* 74:547, 1990.

Byrd JC: Environmental tobacco smoke. Medical and legal issues, *Med Clin North Am* 76:377, 1992.

Carney DN: Biology of small-cell lung cancer, *Lancet* 2:843, 1992.

Chapman KR: Therapeutic algorithm for chronic obstructive pulmonary disease, *Am J Med* 91:17S, 1991.

Corrigan CJ and Kay AB. The roles of inflammatory cells in the pathogenesis of asthma and of chronic obstructive pulmonary disease, *Am Rev Respir Dis* 143:1165, 1991.

Demers C and others: Thrombosis in antithrombin-III-deficient persons. Report of a large kindred and literature review, *Ann Intern Med* 116:754, 1992.

Dosman JA, Kania J, and Cockcroft DW: Occupational obstructive disorders: nonspecific airways obstruction and occupational asthma, *Med Clin North Am* 74:823, 1990.

Dresner MS, Brecher R, and Henkind P: Opthalmology consultation in the diagnosis and treatment of sarcoidosis, *Arch Intern Med* 146:301, 1986.

Goldhaber SZ and Morpurgo M: Diagnosis, treatment, and prevention of pulmonary embolism. Report of the WHO/International Society and Federation of Cardiology Task Force, *JAMA* 268:1727, 1992.

Hansen HH: Management of small-cell cancer of the lung, *Lancet* 2:846, 1992.

Hanson MA and Midthun DE: Outpatient care of COPD patients, *Postgrad Med* 91:89, 1992.

Haraf DJ and others: The evolving role of systemic therapy in carcinoma of the lung, *Semin Oncol* 19(Suppl 11):72, 1992.

Hirsh J: Antithrombotic therapy in deep vein thrombosis and pulmonary embolism, *Am Heart J* 123:1115, 1992.

Ihde DC: Chemotherapy of lung cancer, *N Engl J Med* 327:1434, 1992.

Johnson BE and Kelley MJ: Overview of genetic and molecular events in the pathogenesis of lung cancer, *Chest* 103(Suppl):1S, 1993.

Johnson DH: Treatment of the elderly patient with small-cell lung cancer, *Chest* 103(Suppl):72S, 1993.

Mammen EF: Pathogenesis of venous thrombosis, *Chest* 102(Suppl):640S, 1992.

Mulshine JL and others: Initiators and promoters of lung cancer, *Chest* 103(Suppl):4S, 1993.

Nesse RE: Pharmacologic treatment of COPD. Optimum therapy for ambulatory patients, *Postgrad Med* 91:71, 1992.

Niewoehner DE: What lies ahead? Future research and treatment for chronic obstructive pulmonary disease, *Am J Med* 91:41S, 1991.

Obernauf CD and others: Sarcoidosis and its ophthalmic manifestations, *Am J Opthalmol* 86:648, 1978.

Rosen RL and Bone RC: Treatment of acute exacerbations in chronic obstructive pulmonary disease, *Med Clin North Am* 74:691, 1990.

Roth JA: New approaches to treating early lung cancer, *Cancer Res* 52(Suppl):2652S, 1992.

Samet JM: The epidemiology of lung cancer, *Chest* 103(Suppl):20S, 1993.

Samtsov AV: Cutaneous sarcoidosis, *Int J Dermatol* 31:385, 1992.

Sharma OP: Sarcoidosis, *Dis Mon* 36:469, 1990.

Snider GL: Chronic obstructive pulmonary disease: a definition and implications of structural determinants of airflow obstruction for epidemiology, *Am Rev Respir Dis* 140:S3, 1989.

Souhami R: Lung cancer, *BMJ* 304:1298, 1992.

Turrisi AT III: Innovations in multimodality therapy for lung cancer. Combined modality. management of limited small-cell lung cancer, *Chest* 103(Suppl):56S, 1993.

Value of the ventilation/perfusion scan in acute pulmonary embolism. Results of the prospective investigation of pulmonary embolism diagnosis (PIOPED). The PIOPED Investigators, *JAMA* 263:2753, 1990.

Wanner A: The role of mucus in chronic obstructive pulmonary disease, *Chest* 97(Suppl):11S, 1990.

Zic JA and others: Treatment of cutaneous sarcoidosis with chloroquine. Review of the literature, *Arch Dermatol* 127:1034, 1991.

12

Gastrointestinal Disease

ANDREW S. GURWOOD
PHILIP GILMAN

KEY TERMS

Acetaldehyde	*Wernicke's Syndrome*	*Osteomalacia*
Gynecomastia	*Korsakoff's Psychosis*	*Crohn's Disease*
Jaundice	*Scurvy*	*Bilirubin*
Nutritional Optic Necropathy	*Rickets*	*Whipple's Disease*
Schilling Test		

ALCOHOLISM

Systemic Sequelae

Alcoholism is a worldwide health hazard. Excess alcohol intake has a number of effects on a variety of organs. The liver plays a very important role in alcohol (ethanol) metabolism. Ethanol initially undergoes oxidation by the cytosol enzyme alcohol dehydrogenase. *Acetaldehyde* is produced, and

NADH is generated from NAD (Fig. 12-1). Acetaldehyde is then converted to acetate by the mitochondrial enzyme aldehyde dehydrogenase. Another NADH is generated from NAD.

Acetaldehyde is toxic to the liver. It can bind to various hepatic proteins, causing inflammation and fibrosis. If fibrosis progresses, the liver can scar and develop cirrhosis. In addition, the increased ratio of NADH to NAD generated by ethanol metabolism can produce major changes in liver metabolism. One of the sequelae is fat accumulation (fatty liver).

The stomach also contains alcohol dehydrogenase, which can perform first-pass metabolism on ethanol consumed. Women have lower levels of gastric alcohol dehydrogenase than men. As a result, women have higher blood alcohol levels than men after consumption of equal amounts of ethanol. This may explain why women tend to be more susceptible to alcohol-induced liver injury than are men.

Ethanol can also undergo metabolism in the liver through the cytochrome P-450 system. This microsomal enzyme system is induced by ethanol. It is an important pathway when blood concentrations of ethanol are high and during chronic alcohol intake. When the P-450 system is induced by ethanol, it can increase the production of toxic intermediates of other drugs. For example, 90% of acetaminophen (Tylenol) normally undergoes a harmless conjugation with glucuronic acid or sulfate. When alcohol is ingested, more acetaminophen is metabolized through the cytochrome P-450 system to form toxic intermediates. Glutathione can then neutralize these toxic intermediates. When glutathione is overwhelmed, acetaminophen toxicity can lead to severe liver damage.

Systemic Examination

The clinician looks for stigmata of chronic liver disease such as palmar erythema (Fig. 12-2), *gynecomastia* (enlarged breasts), clubbing of the fingers, and spider angiomata, which are dilated vascular lesions on the skin that resemble spiders (Fig. 12-3). *Jaundice* and ascites are sought. Ascites is the accumulation of fluid in the peritoneal cavity. Other than chronic liver disease, ascites has a number of causes. A discussion of this condition is beyond the scope of this chapter.

Systemic Management

Treatment in alcoholic liver disease involves supportive measures. The clinician attempts to improve the patient's nutritional status and to treat

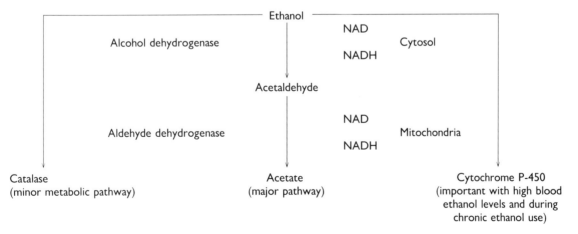

FIG. 12-1 Alcohol metabolism by the liver.

FIG. 12-2 Palmar erythema ("liver palms"). A clinical sign of chronic liver disease is this red discoloration of the palms. *(From Lawrence CM and Cox NH: Physical signs in dermatology: color atlas and text, London, 1993, Wolfe Medical Publishers, Ltd.)*

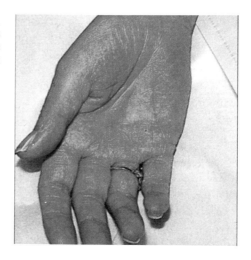

dehydration, electrolyte imbalances, or any complicating infections. A trial of prednisolone may reduce the mortality from severe alcoholic liver disease. Patients should undergo counseling regarding alcohol dependence or be referred to an alcohol treatment center.

Ocular Manifestations

Gastrointestinal and nutritional diseases have direct effects on the eye. Although both entities may act upon the tunics of the eye, adenexa, and nerves, nutritional deficiency is the most frequent cause for ocular consultation. In the United States and Europe the most frequent reason for optometric consultation, secondary to nutritional deficiency, is alcoholism.

Alcohol has the ability to affect the visual pathways and oculomotor system. Visual losses related to the effects of alcohol abuse are due to optic nerve dysfunction, atrophy, and death. In the past, these losses were classified as tobacco-alcohol amblyopias, but today the term *nutritional optic neuropathy* has gained a wider acceptance. Typically, affected patients experience an insidious loss of central vision over a period of 3 to 5 months, with equal losses in acuity and color perception in both eyes. Upon examination, the clinician should attempt to investigate several factors, as toxic/nutritional optic neuropathy is a diagnosis of exclusion.

In the earlier portions of this century, the ingestion of methanol (wood alcohol) was the principle precipitant for the onset of the nutritional optic neuropathies. The breakdown product, formaldehyde, causes severe poisoning marked by gastroenteritis, pulmonary edema, cerebral edema, and extensive retinal damage. Significant systemic absorption occurs principally through oral ingestion; however, toxic levels have been achieved through the inhalation of fumes and contact with skin (rare).

Systemic and related ocular symptoms range from acute weakness, nausea, vomiting, headache, acne rosacea, and Kussmaul respiration to long-term loss of central acuity, color perception, and visual field. Ocular signs and symptoms also include dense cecocentral scotomas, hyperemia of the optic disc, disc edema, papilledema, and, in severe chronic cases, optic atrophy. These may be outwardly seen during ocular examination as an afferent pupillary defect. The amount of pupillary unresponsiveness is proportional to the amount of nerve dysfunction. All findings are bilateral as a rule; however, asymmetry is common.

The mechanism of alcohol-related optic neuropathy is still unclear and poorly understood. Although the actual site of the lesions remains difficult to map, Smiddy and Green, in a 2-year postmortem study, found a particular preponderance for the destruction of maculopapillary bundles. Some authors (Heaton and others, 1958, Wokes,

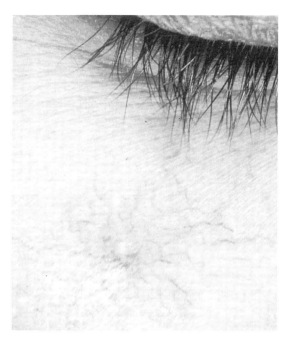

FIG. 12-3 Spider angioma (cheek nevus). Dilated vascular lesions of the cheek that resemble spiders due to chronic liver disease (hepatic cirrhosis). *(From Habif TB:* Clinical dermatology, *St. Louis, 1990, Mosby–Year Book.)*

1958) have hypothesized that excessive use of alcohol and tobacco renders a person vulnerable not only to the effects of the substance, but to vitamin-related deficiencies as well. Some evidence suggests that retinal ganglion cells, especially those responsible for central vision, are more susceptible; however, optic nerve axons sustain substantial damage as well.

Physicians have postulated that increased cyanide intake from heavy cigarette or pipe smoke is an additional contributing and often compounding factor because cyanide binds to the active form of vitamin B_{12}, hydroxycobalamine. Alcoholic optic neuropathy closely resembles vitamin B_{12} deficiency optic neuropathy. Alcohol itself is not toxic to the visual system, but the combinations of poor dietary intake and poor health maintenance contribute to vitamin B_{12} and folic acid deficiencies, which initiate neurologic tissue breakdown. Al-

though the mechanisms are poorly understood, the deficiencies in vitamin B_{12}, folate, and thiamine alter ATP formation, leading to stasis of neural axoplasmic flow, edema, and axonal death.

Ocular Examination

Examination begins with a full and complete history. If alcohol or substance abuse is suspected, the clinician should attempt to make careful observations regarding speech, patterns of communication (such as stuttering, redundancy, forgetfulness), physical appearance, and odor. Often these patients present for examination while inebriated. One of the hallmark signs of intoxication is endpoint nystagmus upon lateral gaze. This becomes apparent during extraocular muscle testing. The clinician must take care to complete a full dilated examination to rule out all other possibilities of neurologic disease.

Visual acuity is typically in the range of 20/50 to 20/400 when the patient seeks help. The stereotypical patient often reads the chart slowly, letter by letter, with an unsure tone of voice. These patients classically present in poor health with a chronic staphylococcal infection of the lower eyelids. As a rule, these patients give a long, convoluted history of being unsuccessfully treated by several ocular physicians for conjunctivitis. This stubborn, elusive disease description, along with the patient's history, should alert the clinician to the diagnosis of acne rosacea keratitis (Fig. 12-4).

In severe chronic cases, color vision is affected significantly, particularly in the red and green ranges. The red/green deficit indicates acquired dysfunction of optic nerve axons and associated maculopapillary damage. Visual field testing may reveal central and cecocentral scotomata. Ophthalmoscopically, the optic nerve may appear normal in cases that are detected early. Later the nerve may take on an edematous appearance with splinter hemorrhages. Long-standing cases show axonal atrophy from chronic congestion, appearing pale and atrophic.

The investigative work-up should include testing for inflammatory, infiltrative, ischemic, infectious, demyelinating, and compressive causes. Ap-

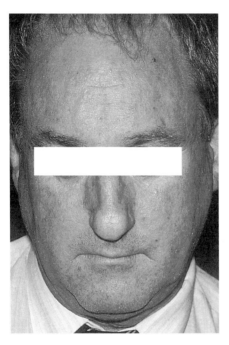

FIG. 12-4 Acne rosacea. The face shows red papules and pustules and lids reveal associated blepharitis. *(Courtesy of Jane Stein.)*

propriate blood testing may include complete blood count (CBC), fasting treponemal antibody absorption (FTA-ABS) test, erythrocyte sedimentation rate (ESR—Westergren), Lyme titer, and HLA-B27. Zinc, vitamin B_{12}, folate, and thiamine levels, along with liver function tests, should be ordered or suggested to the family physician. Radiographic studies may be used to rule out compression syndromes that would result in bilateral temporal optic nerve dysfunction. These include pituitary adenoma, chiasmal meningioma, and aneurysm. Computed tomography (CT) scans are considered adequate for lesions anterior to the chiasm, but magnetic resonance imaging (MRI) is an alternative modality. Arteriograms may be indicated in cases of suspected aneurysm and plane film chest radiography if infiltrative sarcoidosis is a diagnostic possibility. It is important to realize that alcohol-related nutritional optic neuropathy can extend into axons as deep as the chiasm.

Ocular Management

Fortunately, the prognosis for this condition is favorable. The current management for acne rosacea keratitis includes topical supportive therapy and topical antibiotic therapy when necessary. Acceptable medications include artificial tears and/or the antibiotic preparation of your choice four times per day in the affected eye. The patient diagnosed with acne rosacea requires an oral regimen of tetracycline, 250 mg four times a day by mouth. Doxycycline, a semisynthetic version of the medicine, may be substituted at 300 mg three times per day by mouth. In the event that these medications are contraindicated, because of age of the patient (do not dispense tetracycline to children because of the potential for adverse dental effects) or sensitivity, erythromycin can be substituted at a dosage of 250 mg four times per day by mouth. The removal of the toxic substance and return of deficient vitamins and minerals often bring about prompt and complete recovery.

Zinc sulfate, 100 to 250 mg three times per day by mouth, may promote the reversal of neuropathy. Because ethambutol results in the chelation of zinc and other metals necessary for normal optic nerve function, supplementation concurrent with removal of ethambutol may hasten recovery. This therapy is not yet approved by the Food and Drug Administration.

Once low serum levels of vitamin B_{12} have been documented, the patient should be given 300 mg of oral thiamine each week and 1000 µg of vitamin B_{12} intramuscularly for 10 weeks. Therapy alone does not reverse the neuropathy. The patient must be persuaded to eliminate the toxic substances and improve the quality of his diet. If the losses are permanent, low-vision aides may be suggested as an alternative to maximize functional acuity.

VITAMIN DEFICIENCY AND MALABSORPTION

Systemic Manifestations

Vitamins A, D, E, and K are fat soluble (see box on p. 231). A malabsorption state can result in a

VITAMINS

Fat soluble	A, D, E, K
Water soluble	B_1, B_2, B_3, B_5, B_6, B_7, B_9, B_{12}

CAUSES OF MALABSORPTION

Intestinal disease	Celiac disease Whipple's disease Tropical sprue Intestinal lymphangiectasia Radiation enteritis Crohn's disease Short-bowel syndrome
Pancreatic disease	Chronic pancreatitis Cystic fibrosis Pancreatic carcinoma
Cholestatic liver disease	Intrahepatic obstructive jaundice
Bacterial overgrowth	

deficiency of these vitamins. Malabsorption, in its strictest sense, should refer to an inability to properly absorb nutrients through the mucosa, as can be seen in intestinal mucosal disorders such as celiac disease, Whipple's disease, Crohn's disease, and radiation enteritis (see box above, right). It has also come to refer to an inability to properly digest nutrients, as may be seen with pancreatic disease. In pancreatic insufficiency secondary to chronic pancreatitis or cystic fibrosis, the pancreas cannot secrete an adequate amount of enzymes to break down the fats, carbohydrates, and proteins before intestinal absorption. Fat malabsorption can also occur with cholestatic liver diseases such as primary biliary cirrhosis, in which decreased amounts of bile salts enter the duodenum. Bile salts play an important role in fat digestion and in transportation of fats and fat-soluble vitamins to the small intestinal mucosal surface for absorption into the lymphatics and distribution in the body. A similar situation can be seen with mechanical obstruction of the common bile duct (as in pancreatic cancer). Steatorrhea, excessive amounts of fat in the stool, can result.

Vitamin A. Sequelae of vitamin A deficiency include epithelial changes throughout the body which render patients susceptible to respiratory tract infections, kidney stones, and urinary tract infections. A microcytic hypochromic anemia may also be seen.

Vitamin E. Vitamin E is an antioxidant. A deficiency state has been seen in cystic fibrosis and in children with chronic cholestatic disorders such as biliary atresia when bile flow is obstructed. Therefore, diminished bile flow into the small intestine can result in vitamin E malabsorption. In cystic fibrosis, pancreatic fibrosis with decreased function results from thick secretions obstructing the pancreatic ducts. Cholestatic liver disease is also a feature. The vitamin plays a crucial role in maintenance of neurologic function. Ophthalmoplegia, including limitation of upward gaze, is a feature. Other sequelae include diminished reflexes, decreased vibratory and proprioceptive sense, ataxia, and muscle weakness. Symptoms may improve after prolonged administration of high doses of oral vitamin E, although parenteral administration may be required. Abetalipoproteinemia is a disorder involving an inability to secrete β-lipoproteins, chylomicrons, and VLDL (all important in fat and fat-soluble vitamin transport). Vitamin E deficiency with progressive ataxia and pigmentary retinopathy develops.

Vitamin K. This fat-soluble vitamin plays an important role in blood coagulation. In the liver, it serves as a cofactor in the enzymatic carboxylation of glutamic acid residues located on the prothrombin complex proteins. A deficiency state, as seen with malabsorptive disorders and cholestatic liver disease, can result in bleeding problems. The serum prothrombin time is prolonged. Whether or not the prothrombin time corrects when a jaundiced patient receives vitamin K has some diagnostic value. If the prothrombin time does not correct in this situation, underlying advanced liver disease is likely. In this case the hepatocyte has lost some synthetic capacity. If the prothrombin time corrects, however, the patient most likely had vitamin K deficiency due to malabsorption from cholestatic liver disease.

Vitamin D. A deficiency of vitamin D can result from malabsorption, leading to decreased serum calcium levels. Serum calcium levels may also be reduced in malabsorptive states when calcium binds to unabsorbed intraluminal fatty acids.

Dietary intake of vitamin D plays a very small role as long as an individual receives adequate light exposure. Sunlight or artificial light convert D7-dehydrocholesterol to vitamin D_3. Vitamin D_3 is converted in the liver to 25-hydroxy-vitamin D_3. In the kidney, 25-hydroxy-vitamin D_3 is converted to 1, 25-dihydroxy-vitamin D_3. This is the active form of vitamin D. Parathyroid hormone facilitates this final conversion in the kidneys. The active form of vitamin D stimulates absorption of calcium and phosphate from the small intestine.

B Complex Vitamins. These vitamins are water soluble (see box, p. 231). Vitamins B_1 (thiamine), B_2 (riboflavin), B_3 (niacin), B_5 (pantothenic acid), B_6 (pyridoxine), and B_7 (biotin) are involved in intermediary metabolism of carbohydrates, fats, and proteins. Vitamin B_9 (folic acid) and B_{12} (cyanocobalamin) are involved in DNA production.

Vitamin B_1. Alcoholics are particularly likely to develop a form of vitamin B_1 deficiency called Wernicke's encephalopathy, which when fully developed consists of oculomotor abnormalities (especially nystagmus and bilateral abducens palsies), cerebellar ataxia, and mental confusion. It may be prevented by administering thiamine before the patient receives any glucose. Thiamine, because it is a cofactor in glucose metabolism, is further depleted from an already diminished body supply when glucose is administered first. Korsakoff's psychosis, an end stage of Wernicke's encephalopathy, includes confabulation, retrograde amnesia, and antegrade amnesia.

Vitamin B_2. Cheilosis (Fig. 12-5), glossitis (Fig. 12-6), and dermatitis have been associated with vitamin B_2 deficiency.

Vitamin B_6. A deficiency state can develop when a patient receives medication such as isoniazid (used to treat tuberculosis), which antagonizes pyridoxine. Manifestations includes cheilosis (angular stomatitis), glossitis, seborrheic dermatitis, blepharitis, lymphophenia, and a microcytic anemia.

Vitamin B_9. Folic acid is found in leafy green vegetables, liver, nuts, lentils, and fruits. It is also synthesized by the human intestinal flora. A deficiency state can develop from inadequate intake and from malabsorption. Drugs such as phenytoin (used to treat seizures) and sulfasalazine can inter-

FIG. 12-5 Angular cheilitis (angular stomatitis). Infected folds of skin at corners of mouth due to vitamin B_2 deficiency. *(From Habif TB:* Clinical dermatology, *St. Louis, 1990, Mosby–Year Book.)*

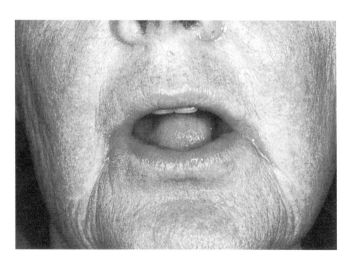

fere with folic acid absorption from the small bowel. A megaloblastic anemia results. This is related to difficulties in DNA production resulting from folic acid deficiency.

Vitamin B_{12}. Vitamin B_{12} is not found in vegetables or fruits but is found in liver, kidney, fish, and meats. Intestinal absorption of vitamin B_{12} depends upon several factors.

1. The ability of parietal cells located in the stomach to secrete intrinsic factor, which eventually binds to B_{12}.
2. The ability of the pancreas to secrete enzymes to partially degrade R proteins, which are secreted in gastric juice and bile. They bind to vitamin B_{12} much more avidly than does intrinsic factor. When R proteins are partially degraded, intrinsic factor can bind to vitamin B_{12}. The affinity of intrinsic factor for vitamin B_{12} increases in the more alkaline environment of the duodenum.
3. An intact terminal ileal mucosa is necessary for the vitamin B_{12}–intrinsic factor complex to attach to a receptor. Here vitamin B_{12} combines with transcobalamin II and is absorbed into the serum for transport.

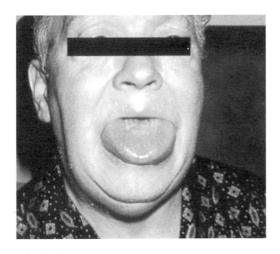

FIG. 12-6 Smooth tongue. This smooth, red, glossy appearance is due to loss of papillae in anemias, vitamin deficiency, and malabsorption syndromes. *(From Lawrence CM and Cox NH: Physical signs in dermatology: Color atlas and text, London, 1993, Wolfe Medical Publishers, Ltd.)*

A disturbance in any of these processes can result in vitamin B_{12} deficiency. For example, patients with pernicious anemia have gastric atrophy that results in an inability of the parietal cells to secrete hydrochloric acid (achlorhydria) and intrinsic factor. Vitamin B_{12} deficiency ensues with a macrocytic anemia and neurologic dysfunction (particularly posterior column signs). Vitamin B_{12} deficiency can also develop in patients with a diseased terminal ileum (as in Crohn's disease) or when the terminal ileum has been surgically removed. Patients with small intestinal bacterial overgrowth can develop vitamin B_{12} deficiency, as ingested vitamin B_{12} is consumed by intraluminal bacteria.

Systemic Examination

The Schilling Test. When vitamin B_{12} deficiency is suspected, a serum vitamin B_{12} level and *Schilling test* should be performed. The Schilling test helps delineate the mechanism of vitamin B_{12} malabsorption (presuming that it is not due to prolonged dietary deficiency).

Systemic Management

Stage I. Co-cyanocobalamin, 1 µg, is given by mouth. Simultaneously, 1000 µg of vitamin B_{12} is given by an intramuscular injection. This saturates the hepatic vitamin B_{12} biding sites and reduces the amount of radioactive vitamin B_{12} retained by the liver. Urine is then collected for 24 hours in order to determine the amount of radioactive vitamin B_{12} excreted. If it is less than 7% to 8% of the total radioactive vitamin B_{12} administered, vitamin B_{12} malabsorption exists.

Stage II. Intrinsic factor is administered along with radioactive vitamin B_{12} by mouth. If the amount of radioactive vitamin B_{12} excreted in the urine is corrected, pernicious anemia is the cause for vitamin B_{12} malabsorption. If excretion remains low, then stage III treatment is administered.

Stage III. Radioactive vitamin B_{12} is administered orally with pancreatic enzymes. This should correct the vitamin B_{12} malabsorption seen with pancreatic insufficiency or cystic fibrosis involving the pancreas. This should cause at least partial degradation of R proteins to allow vitamin B_{12} to combine with intrinsic factor. Although vitamin B_{12} malabsorption can be demonstrated in pancreatic insufficiency via the Schilling test, clinical vitamin B_{12} deficiency is exceedingly rare. If stage III does not correct vitamin B_{12} malabsorption, Stage IV treatment is administered.

Stage IV. The patient receives either metronidazole, 250 mg three times per day for 4 days, or tetracycline, 500 mg four times a day for 1 week, to treat a presumed small intestinal bacterial overgrowth state. If all four stages of the Schilling test remain uncorrected, vitamin B_{12} malabsorption is due to terminal ileal disease. The presence of renal disease can produce false-positive results.

Ocular Manifestations of Vitamin Deficiencies and Hypervitaminosis

Vitamins are defined in Dorland's Medical Dictionary as unrelated organic substances which are necessary in trace amounts for the normal metabolic functioning of the body. The principal vitamins are A, D, E, and K. Other important vitamins, with respect to ocular health, include vitamin B_1 (thiamine), vitamin B_6 (pyridoxine), vitamin B_{12} (hydroxycobalamin), and vitamin C.

Avitaminosis A. Vitamin A (all transretinoic acid) is one of the essential factors for epithelial growth and differentiation. Its ocular application is to stimulate goblet cell production within the palpebral conjunctiva. The goblet cells are responsible for the mucin component of tears, which are responsible for making the cornea more conducive to wetting. Vitamin A deficiency may result when cicatricial tissue replaces normally vascularized tissue. This results in a vitamin A–mucin deficient eye.

Ocular Examination. Ocular complications of avitaminosis A are principally related to dry eye (Fig. 12-7). Persistent dry spots on the cornea and conjunctiva can be observed as areas of nonwetting or recurrent tear-film break-up. In the conjunctiva, excessive dryness causes normal tissue to be replaced by scar tissue (cicatricial tissue).

In extreme cases the conjunctiva shrinks, scars, and develops abnormal adhesions to the eyelid. This is called cicatricial pemphigoid. The incidence is low (1:20,000), with women affected more often than men by a ratio of 7:3. The average age of presentation is 60 years. Continued worsening of the condition results in secondary complications such as symblepharon (Fig. 12-8), trichiasis, lagophthalmos, and exposure keratitis.

The significant anterior segment findings in cases of avitaminosis A are conjunctival xerosis

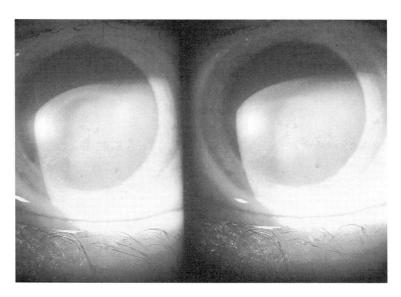

FIG. 12-7 Dry eye with superficial punctate staining. *(Courtesy of Jane Stein.)*

and keratomalacia (corneal softening). The clinical appearance may include corneal epithelial compromise (both positive and negative NaFl staining), corneal thinning, Bitot's spots (small, white, wedge-shaped elevations in the conjunctiva), and inflammation. Clinical changes may develop within the cornea as the disease progresses. Subepithelial infiltration, scarring, and loss of sensitivity are common sequelae. For completeness, the clinician should realize that secondary infectious diseases such as blepharitis and trachoma (dry eye with superior pannus secondary to *Chlamydia trachomatis* infection) may also become apparent.

Ocular management. Specific management includes referral to the internist for specific serologic testing. Topically, retinoic acid, 0.1% in peanut oil three times per day, has been shown to speed corneal healing. Although side effects are relatively minimal, larger doses have been associated with increased scarring. Vitamin A drops are available (Vit-A) along with many other supportive solution and ointment preparations. If ocular inflammation persists in the form of irritation or iridocyclitis, dilation and cycloplegia with cyclopentolate, scopolamine, or atropine once or twice per day, along with the administration of a topical anti-inflammatory preparations, may be indicated. This should be done cautiously in the wake of a compromised corneal epithelium. Mild preparations (FML) are available for early-stage disease, moderate preparations (0.12% Pred Mild) for developing cases, and full-strength (1% Pred Forte) for severe cases. Antimicrobial coverage may be accomplished through the use of topical antibiotic drops four times per day, lubricating antibiotic ointments at bedtime, or combination preparations such as Maxitrol or Pred-G four times per day.

The use of NaCl ointment at night or as needed to decrease corneal edema and promote epithelial adherence to the basement membrane is an additional modality that the clinician may employ after the disease has stabilized. Typically, one should attempt to avoid the use of ointments during the day, as they can blur vision. This author does not advocate the use of bandage contact lens application under these circumstances.

In cases of trachoma, topical preparations must be supported with oral antibiotics. The treatment of choice is systemic tetracycline or erythromycin, 1 g daily (250 mg q.i.d.) for 21 days or 2 g daily (500 mg q.i.d.) for 14 days. The usual contraindications for tetracycline apply. The maximum effect of therapy may not be realized for 10 weeks following commencement of treatment.

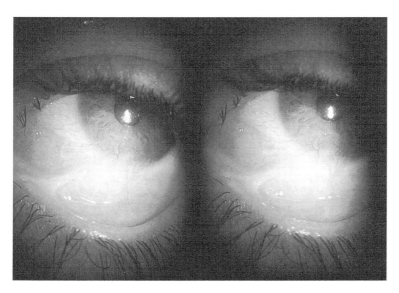

FIG. 12-8 Symblepharon: Adhesions of palpebral conjunctiva to bulbar conjunctiva. *(Courtesy of Jane Stein.)*

In the event of corneal ulceration, topical fortified antibiotics should be initiated aggressively (every hour) and alternated. A relatively new topical antibiotic called ciprofloxan (Cyloxin), a fluoroquinolone derivative, has proven to be extremely effective. Topical ciprofloxacin attacks microbes at the DNA level. The drug is applied every 1 to 2 hours. If the ulceration warrants special attention, referral to a corneal specialist is recommended.

Hypervitaminosis A

Ocular examination. A principal ocular complication that may result from hypervitaminosis A is pseudotumor cerebri. Individuals with this clinical entity often present with a history of using large doses of vitamins and supplements. The pathophysiology involves encephalopathy. The patients often present with intractable headache and in some cases diplopia secondary to compressive cranial nerve VI palsy. The funduscopic appearance of pseudotumor cerebri is bilateral swelling of the optic discs with a disappearance of the optic cup.

Ocular management. Pseudotumor cerebri is a diagnosis of exclusion. Patients must be worked up for intracranial mass by MRI or CT scan. The diagnosis hinges upon high opening pressure upon spinal tap and clear profile of recovered spinal fluid. Management of asymptomatic cases includes serial visual field measurements. Symptomatic cases should be referred to a neurospecialist for therapy with carbonic anhydrase inhibitors, systemic corticosteroids, and, in severe cases, optic nerve sheath decompression.

Vitamin B_1 (Thiamine) and B_2 (Nicotinic Acid and Riboflavin) Deficiency

Ocular sequelae. Vitamin B complex is subdivided into eight groups, but only the ocular manifestations of vitamin B_1 (thiamine) and B_2 (nicotinic acid and riboflavin) deficiency are discussed here. Vitamin B_{12} deficiency and its sequelae have already been discussed in the previous section on alcohol abuse. Although vitamin deficiency is a common complication of alcohol abuse, it is also a problem associated with malnutrition and worldwide hunger.

Vitamin B_1 is found in both animal and vegetable matter. Deficiency produces a systemic condition characterized by high-output cardiac failure, pleural and peritoneal effusions, and peripheral neuropathy. The condition is called beriberi. Seventy percent of these patients present with ocular abnormalities.

Vitamin B_2 is found in animals, vegetables, liver, yeast, and wheat germ. It is also associated with malnutrition and alcohol abuse. The clinical picture includes rosacea keratitis, limbal vascularization, seborrheic blepharitis, and optic atrophy with temporal disc pallor.

Ocular examination. The clinician should examine all patients with a history of malnutrition or alcohol abuse for signs and symptoms of vitamin B_1 or B_2 deficiency. Changes in the corneal epithelium and conjunctiva produce symptoms of dry eye and blurry vision. Visual loss with cecocentral scotomata is a secondary sequela of related optic atrophy. *Wernicke's syndrome* of delirium, stupor, ophthalmoplegia, ptosis, and nystagmus is a common result of vitamin B_1 deficiency. Patients may also report diplopia depending upon the severity of the ophthalmoplegia. The mental disturbance includes problems with memory, confusion, and disorientation. These signs and symptoms are collectively termed *Korsakoff's psychosis.* Wernicke's ophthalmoplegia may be horizontal or vertical and typically follows lateral rectus dysfunction. It must be differentiated from other forms of ophthalmoplegia such as internuclear ophthalmoplegia, downbeat nystagmus, and vertical gaze nystagmus.

Additional signs and symptoms may develop from therapy. Clinicians who frequently complete hospital rounds must maintain awareness that patients who are hospitalized for these conditions routinely receive intravenous glucose. These patients undergo metabolism that invariably exhausts stored thiamine. Thiamine must therefore be added to all parenteral feeds. Thiamine pyrophosphate is an important co-enzyme for the oxidation of glucose. When thiamine levels fall, the utilization of central nervous system glucose may be reduced by 50%. In these severe cases, funduscopic signs become apparent. Bilateral intraretinal hemorrhages, cotton-wool spots, Roth spots (white-centered hemorrhages), and papilledema are all reported sequelae.

Ocular management. Referral should be directed to the internist. Thiamine, given intravenously, often improves the ophthalmoplegia within hours. Full motility typically returns within 5 days, although the nystagmus may persist. Visual acuity usually exhibits rapid and marked recovery.

Vitamin C (Ascorbic Acid) Deficiency

Ocular sequelae and ocular examination. Vitamin C is found in fresh citrus fruits and green vegetables. Ocular manifestations result from the systemic lack of vitamin C, a condition known as *scurvy.*

Patients who present with scurvy are not always substance abusers. In fact, the disease is often the result of accidental malnutrition and poor dietary habits. Patients with scurvy have hemorrhagic lesions in a variety of sites such as the skin, mucous membranes, body cavities, and orbits. Hemorrhagic lesions may extend into the lids, subconjunctival space, anterior chamber, vitreous cavity, and retina (Fig. 12-9).

Ocular management. These patients should be referred to an internist or nutritionist. Treatment involves improvement of the diet, addition of vitamin C, and adequate amounts of citrus juice. The management of eye signs is generally supportive. Typically the hemorrhages resorb and any losses in acuity return. Resolution of the underlying problems produces success.

Vitamin D (Sterol Derivatives) Deficiency

Ocular Sequelae and Examination. The D vitamins are essential nutrients that work to maintain plasma calcium levels. The deficiency state exists mainly in children and causes the bone disease *rickets.* Deficiency in adults results in *osteomalacia.*

Patients with vitamin D deficiency also have decreased plasma calcium levels. This leads to a hypocalcemic tetany of the lens and results in cataracts. These opacities appear as white and colored crystals interdigitated with clear lens fibers within the layers of the anterior and posterior lens cortex.

Hypervitaminosis D

Ocular Sequelae and Examination. There is surprisingly little awareness of the adverse effects of excessive vitamin D intake. Hypervitaminosis D is well documented as being toxic to normal physiology. The incidence of this clinical entity has declined since the content of vitamin D in milk and

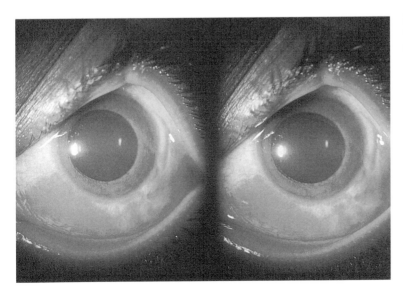

FIG. 12-9 Hemorrhagic conjunctivitis in vitamin C deficiency. *(Courtesy of Jane Stein.)*

other foodstuffs has been governmentally regulated.

In addition to systemic abnormalities, vitamin D has a substantial effect on the eye. Calcium deposits in the conjunctiva (concretions) and in the cornea (band keratopathy—Fig. 12-10) are most common. Strabismus, epicanthal folds, abnormalities within the bones of the orbit, nystagmus, sluggish pupillary reaction, iritis, and papilledema have all been documented.

Ocular Management. The patient should be referred to an internist or nutritionist to correct the underlying problem. Usually concretions require only patient education; however, they may need to be removed in symptomatic individuals. Removal is accomplished by curettage with a 27½-gauge needle or brisk massage with a cotton-tipped applicator under topical anesthesia. A small amount of bleeding is expected, so normal sterile and protective precautions should be observed. Organic waste and blood-contaminated materials should be disposed of appropriately. Copious use of prophylactic antibiotic ointment over the affected area prevents infection. Pressure patching is rarely necessary.

Treatment of band keratopathy consists of ablation of the corneal epithelium by curettage under topical anesthesia with a cotton-tipped applicator saturated with 0.01 M solution of EDTA, followed by irrigation with 0.37% EDTA for 20 minutes.

GENERAL MALNUTRITION

Ocular Sequelae and Examination

The medical complications of malnutrition are vividly demonstrated in countries with poor food supplies. Although the United States does not commonly see the effects of famine, it is a significant clinical problem for the impoverished masses of Asia and Africa.

There are five broad classes of nutrients recognized as necessary for human survival. These are proteins, carbohydrates, fats, minerals, and vitamins. Clinically, the absence of proteins and vitamins has the most profound effect.

The lack of protein intake results in Kwashiorkor syndrome. This is characterized by severe weight loss, dermatitis, alopecia, and impaired healing. The ocular manifestations include eyelid edema and chemosis with frequent conjunctival infection.

Patients should be questioned thoroughly during history taking. The clinician should record the frequency and onset of infectious conditions. Partic-

FIG. 12-10 Band keratopathy. Calcium deposits in the cornea in hypervitaminosis D. *(Courtesy of Jane Stein.)*

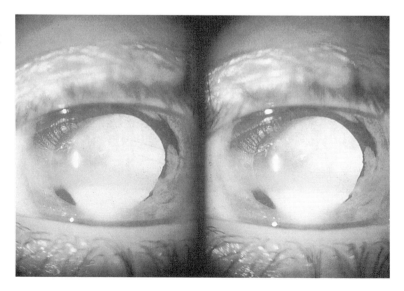

ular attention should be paid to the type of discharge (watery, stringy, or mucopurulent). Swollen preauricular nodes may provide information regarding a viral cause. Careful biomicroscopic examination should be completed noting eyelid debris, discharge, palpebral conjunctival papillae, follicles, and pseudomembranes.

Ocular Management

Treatment should include patient education on eyelid hygiene, lid scrubs, and topical antibiotic solutions and ointments where appropriate. If pseudomembranes (thin film of exotoxins anchored into the palpebral conjunctiva) exist, they should be removed by vigorous curettage with a cotton-tipped applicator under local topical anesthesia. These often bleed upon removal, so appropriate precautions should be observed. Prophylactic antibiotic ointment should be applied along with a cycloplegic following the procedure. Topical antibiotic/anti-inflammatory drops four times a day often hasten resolution. All organic waste should be disposed of in the usual appropriate manner. Follow-up should occur at 1 week for uncomplicated infections and 24 hours following any procedure. If corneal infiltrates are present, they may be treated with topical anti-inflammatory preparations depending upon their impact on visual acuity and patient symptomatology. If left untreated, corneal infiltrates typically resolve when the underlying cause is removed. If there is any evidence of internal ocular inflammation, dilation and cycloplegia may be necessary as well.

INFLAMMATORY BOWEL DISEASE

Inflammatory bowel disease has multiple causes. Underlying infections comprise most of the known causes. Prime examples include the colitis that results from a *Shigella* infection or the ileocecal inflammation that results when tuberculosis infects this part of the intestine. Inflammatory bowel disease of unknown cause includes ulcerative colitis and Crohn's disease. Ulcerative colitis, as its name implies, includes inflammation limited to the large intestine, most commonly the rectum and left co-

lon. *Crohn's disease,* on the other hand, may involve the gastrointestinal tract from mouth to anus. Combined ileocolonic involvement is the most common distribution in Crohn's disease. Involvement of the colon only or small bowel only can also be seen. Both disorders may have associated extraintestinal manifestations. Uveitis can be numbered among these.

Postulated Causes

The cause or causes of these two disorders remain unknown despite intensive research efforts by numerous investigators. Several theories and associations have been introduced:

1. An underlying infectious organism, such as an atypical mycobacterium in the case of Crohn's disease, may play a causative role. Atypical mycobacteria have been isolated from only a minority of the patients studied, however.

2. A genetic predisposition may exist. There is an increased prevalence of inflammatory bowel disease in first-degree relatives of patients with ulcerative colitis and Crohn's disease, with a tendency for a first-degree relative of an ulcerative colitis patient to have ulcerative colitis and for a first-degree relative of a Crohn's disease patient to have Crohn's disease. There may be an increased frequency of inflammatory bowel disease among Ashkenazi (Western) Jews.

3. Patients with ulcerative colitis may lack one subclass of colonic mucin (Type IV) that normally overlies the colonic mucosa. Its absence may decrease the integrity of the mucosa. Both ulcerative colitis and Crohn's disease may have increased intestinal permeability as a characteristic. This may be due to a primary genetic disorder. Increased intestinal permeability may eventually lead to bacterial invasion and inflammation.

4. Patients may have disturbances of immune regulation. For example, patients with Crohn's disease may have a disturbance in the balance between helper and suppressor T cells. A viral infection superimposed on inflammatory bowel disease results in interleukin-1 release, which

may affect the function of T cells, B cells, and natural killer cells.

5. There is an interesting association between cigarette smoking and inflammatory bowel disease. The risk for developing ulcerative colitis seems to be highest among former smokers and lowest in current smokers. In one small study, chewing nicotine gum brought on remissions in some patients with active ulcerative colitis. Patients with Crohn's disease, on the other hand, are more likely to be smokers than a matched control population. A causal relationship has been suggested here.

Mechanisms of Inflammation

Increased levels of mucosal prostaglandins derived from the cyclo-oxygenase pathway and increased levels of mucosal leukotrienes derived from the lipoxygenase pathway have been found in patients with inflammatory bowel disease. The cyclo-oxygenase derivative thromboxane B_2 may have detrimental effects, whereas the cyclo-oxygenase derivative PGE_2 may have protective effects on the mucosa. The lipoxygenase pathway metabolites such as leukotrienes and hydroeicosatetranoic hydroxy fatty acids (HETES) are known to cause neutrophil recruitment, aggregation, degranulation, and changes in macrophage function. Indeed, the observation that both Crohn's disease and nonsteroidal anti-inflammatory drug (NSAID)–induced bowel disease feature increased mucosal permeability suggests a common underlying mechanism. Because NSAIDs inhibit cyclo-oxygenase and divert arachidonic acid metabolism into the lipoxygenase pathway, increased intestinal levels of leukotrienes may be the common underlying mechanism. Mast cells may also help amplify the inflammatory process. The neutrophil and monocyte can generate toxic oxygen metabolites and hypochlorous acid, which can produce mucosal damage.

The end result is persistent inflammation and intestinal damage. There are, however, differences between ulcerative colitis and Crohn's disease with regard to the depth, distribution, and character of the bowel inflammation.

Comparative Pathology

The small and large intestines consist of four layers. From lumen (inside) to peritoneum (outside) the layers are mucosa, submucosa, muscularis, and serosa. Whereas the inflammation of ulcerative colitis involves only the mucosa and submucosa, the inflammation of Crohn's disease may involve all four layers (transmural inflammation). In ulcerative colitis, inflammation typically starts in the rectum and continues uninterrupted through the descending colon for a variable length of involvement. Crohn's disease is characterized by noncontinuous inflammation, in which bowel is interposed between areas of normal mucosa. In Crohn's disease, any part of the gastrointestinal tract from mouth to anus can be involved, whereas only the large intestine is involved in ulcerative colitis. The initial pathologic process in Crohn's disease appears to involve hyperplasia of lymphoid follicles. Granulomas can form and aphthoid (punched out) ulcers form over these aggregates of lymphoid tissue. Ulcerative colitis appears to begin with hemorrhagic and exudative inflammation of the mucosa. In Crohn's disease, adjacent organs may become involved because of the transmural nature of the intestinal disease. As a result, fistulas can form, for example, between the bowel and urinary bladder or bowel and skin.

Clinical Presentation and Systemic Sequelae

Ulcerative Colitis. The peak incidence of ulcerative colitis is in the 20 to 29 year age group. A second peak incidence occurs in the 50 to 89 year age group. It may also develop in children. The presenting signs and symptoms are variable and range from mild persistent bloody diarrhea when only the rectum is involved (ulcerative proctitis) to a fulminating course marked by severe bloody diarrhea, weight loss, fever, dehydration, malnutrition, anemia, and albumin concentration less than 3 mg/dl. This occurs when much greater lengths of large intestine are involved. This so-called fulminant colitis, which is seen in around 6% to 10% of ulcerative colitis patients, can result in toxic megacolon, in which abdominal distention is due to dilatation of the large intestine.

Bowel movement frequency may decrease and abdominal pain may develop with toxic megacolon. Colonic perforations, requiring emergent surgery, may result from fulminant colitis and/or toxic megacolon. After a brief period of 48 to 72 hours during which fluid and electrolyte restoration takes place, surgery has been advocated in toxic megacolon to avoid colon perforations and recurrences of toxic megacolon.

In most instances the patient with ulcerative colitis has a milder course characterized by recurrences of mild to moderate small-volume, blood-streaked diarrhea. There is great variability in frequency and severity of the flares.

Crohn's Disease. The peak incidence of Crohn's disease is in the 20 to 29 year age group, with a weaker secondary peak in the 69 to 79 year age group. The presentation of Crohn's disease can be highly variable because of its potentially extensive gastrointestinal tract involvement and its transmural nature. Right lower quadrant abdominal pain, diarrhea, and fever may be present when the distal small intestine is diseased. When the bowel wall becomes thickened, scarred, and narrowed, the patient may present with a bowel obstruction. Intra-abdominal fistulas and abscesses may be seen. Toxic megacolon can be seen with Crohn's colitis. Malnutrition may be seen with extensive small bowel disease, surgical removal of the terminal ileum, or severe terminal ileal disease. Disease in or removal of the terminal ileum may prevent the absorption of vitamin B_{12} or reabsorption of bile acids which, when secreted by the liver into the small intestine, play a role in fat digestion and absorption.

Children with Crohn's disease may have growth retardation as a major presenting feature. This is probably more common in Crohn's disease than in ulcerative colitis.

Extraintestinal Manifestations

Many of the extraintestinal manifestations associated with ulcerative colitis are thought to be seen in Crohn's disease when the colon is involved, but they may be seen with equal frequency when other areas of the bowel are involved. Peripheral arthritis, which tends to follow the bowel disease activity (although less so in Crohn's disease), usually involves large joints. Ankylosing spondylitis is also associated with inflammatory bowel disease. It affects the sacroiliac joints with eventual vertebral column fusion and skeletal deformation. It runs a progressive course unrelated to bowel disease activity. There is an association with the histocompatability antigen phenotype HLA-B27, as there is in ankylosing spondylitis unassociated with inflammatory bowel disease.

Eye findings are seen in 4% to 10% of patients and are frequently associated with joint findings.

Skin findings include erythema nodosum (Fig. 12-11) and pyoderma gangrenosum (Fig. 12-12). Both of these disorders can be associated with a host of other illnesses. Erythema nodosum lesions

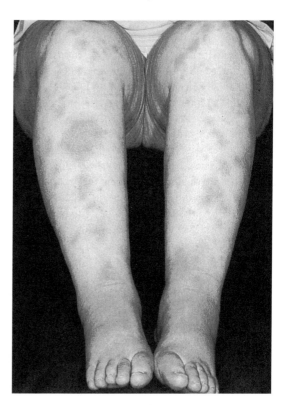

FIG. 12-11 Erythema nodosum. Bright red, raised, tender lesions, usually in the front of the shins. *(From Habif TB:* Clinical dermatology, *St. Louis, 1990, Mosby–Year Book.)*

FIG. 12-12 Pyoderma gangrenosum (thigh). An advancing crusted edge with irregular exudative ulceration and central healing with scarring. Associated with ulcerative colitis. *(From Habif TB:* Clinical dermatology, *St. Louis, 1990, Mosby–Year Book.)*

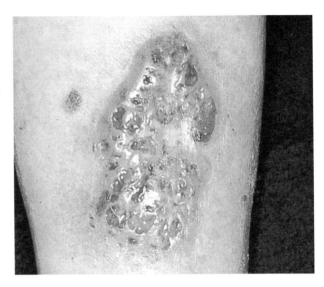

are raised, tender, erythematous nodules found on the extensor surfaces of the lower extremities. They tend to follow the bowel disease activity. Pyoderma gangrenosum is a chronic ulcer with necrotic bluish margins located at various skin sites, particularly on the pretibial surface. It may or may not follow the bowel disease activity.

Hepatobiliary disorders may be seen with inflammatory bowel disease. Among patients with Crohn's disease, there may not be a higher incidence of these disorders when the colon is involved. Sclerosing cholangitis (more common in ulcerative colitis; see section on jaundice in this chapter), bile duct carcinoma, and fatty infiltration of the liver may be seen. Gallstones develop commonly with ileal involvement in Crohn's disease. As previously discussed, bile salts are normally reabsorbed in the terminal ileum. When this area is diseased, fewer bile salts can be reabsorbed to return to the liver. As a result, the cholesterol concentration in the gallbladder bile increases. Eventually cholesterol precipitates out and cholesterol stones form.

Anemia, common to both disorders, can have multiple causes, such as iron deficiency secondary to chronic blood loss, vitamin B_{12} deficiency due to ileal disease, and folate deficiency due to drug-induced interference with folate absorption. Amy-

loidosis has been associated with Crohn's disease. Perianal complications such as fissures and fistulas are seen in Crohn's disease. These occur more frequently with Crohn's colitis or ileocolitis than with ileitis alone.

Systemic Diagnosis

The establishment of a diagnosis of either ulcerative colitis or Crohn's disease is based on the history (including any family history), physical examination in which one also looks for any extraintestinal findings, and compatible radiologic, endoscopic, and histologic findings (Fig. 12-13). The clinician must also rule out any infectious disorders that can mimic either form of inflammatory bowel disease.

Bacterial infections, such as *Campylobacter jejuni* infection or pseudomembranous colitis caused by *Clostridium difficile* (results from a variety of antibiotics), can mimic ulcerative colitis. Intestinal infections with *Yersinia enterocolitica* or tuberculosis can mimic Crohn's disease. Stools should be submitted for bacterial cultures, *Clostridium difficile* toxin, and ova and parasites. The HIV-positive patient could potentially be infected with a number of organisms that can mimic inflammatory bowel disease. A discussion of this problem is beyond the scope of this chapter.

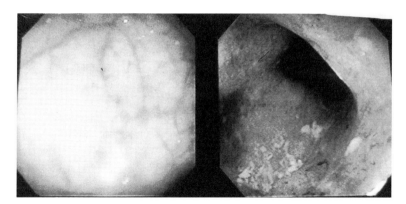

FIG. 12-13 Normally appearing colon with vascular integrity preserved *(left)* and the inflamed colon of a patient with inflammatory bowel disease revealing loss of normal vascular pattern along with small ulcerations and erythema *(right)*.

It is particularly important that an infectious cause for inflammatory bowel disease be ruled out, because corticosteroids, which are frequently used to treat inflammatory bowel disease, could potentially allow an infectious process to progress.

Systemic Treatment

In general, treatment is either surgical or medical in nature.

Medical Therapy

Supportive measures. These include intravenous hydration, restoration of electrolyte balance, administration of antibiotics to treat any complicating infections, blood transfusions when indicated, and nutritional support. In certain cases of Crohn's disease, nutritional therapy may be considered a specific therapeutic measure. The administration of elemental diets by way of nocturnal nasogastric feedings has brought on remissions and reversed growth retardation in children afflicted with Crohn's disease. Intravenous nutrition administered to inpatients with severe attacks of inflammatory bowel disease may prevent significant protein loses that have adverse effects on skeletal muscle functions.

Specific pharmacotherapy

Sulfasalazine. This has been used to treat inflammatory bowel disease for many years. It consists of 5-aminosalicylic acid (5-ASA) joined to sulfapyridine by an azo bond. Although the 5-ASA moiety is thought to be the active part of the drug, some investigators have suggested that sulfasalazine itself has additional activity against the inflammatory process. After oral ingestion, only 20% to 30% of intact sulfasalazine is absorbed in the upper gastrointestinal tract. 5-ASA is liberated in the distal gastrointestinal tract, where increasing numbers of bacteria (containing azo reductase) reside and break down the azo bond. So it appears that sulfasalazine is most effective in the colon. Sulfasalazine and 5-ASA may reduce inflammation by interfering with various stages of arachidonic acid metabolism to favor formation of protective prostaglandins such as PGE_2 and to inhibit the lipoxygenase pathway. Therefore, production of 5-HETE and leukotriene B_4 is inhibited. Sulfasalazine and 5-ASA may act as reactive oxygen scavengers. 5-ASA may also act as a hypochlorous acid scavenger. Both of these properties may help reduce intestinal inflammation.

Sulfasalazine is used in ulcerative colitis both to treat acute disease and to maintain a remission. Sulfasalazine may be beneficial in both Crohn's colitis and ileocolitis but is of no benefit or only modest benefit in ileitis alone. Sulfasalazine has not been shown to maintain remissions from active Crohn's disease.

Side effects are usually due to sulfapyridine, which gets absorbed into the bloodstream. Dose-related side effects include headache, vomiting, anorexia, and oligospermia. Idiosyncratic reactions include rash, hepatotoxicity, aplastic anemia, and a serum sickness–like illness. Folic acid deficiency can develop because sulfasalazine interferes with its absorption.

New oral 5-ASA drugs. Several 5-ASA preparations without an attached sulfa moiety are now available in order to avoid the potential side effects of sulfapyridine. These include two 5-ASA molecules joined to one another by a conjugated azo bond and either an ethylcellulose or an acrylic polymer coating the 5-ASA molecules. These forms allow maximum release of the active 5-ASA molecules in the distal small intestine and colon. Although side effects are few and mild, acute pancreatitis has been reported.

Topical preparations. Various topical corticosteroids and 5-ASA preparations in enema form are available to treat mild to moderate left-sided ulcerative colitis. These agents are thought to be less effective in treating Crohn's colitis. Newer agents, such as tixocortol pivalate, a nonglucocorticoid, nonmineralocorticoid derivative of cortisol, are currently under investigation. Tixocortol has the advantage of not having any of the systemic side effects seen with other topical corticosteroid agents.

Systemic corticosteroids. Systemic corticosteroids are used to treat both ulcerative colitis and Crohn's disease. They are usually administered in an oral form such as prednisone or prednisolone. Oral corticosteroids have proven beneficial in mild to moderate ulcerative colitis and Crohn's disease. In more severe illness, corticosteroids can be administered in intravenous forms such as hydrocortisone or methylprednisolone. They can be extremely beneficial in fulminant colitis. Intravenous ACTH may be of benefit to patients not recently exposed to corticosteroids but are not of any prophylactic benefit in quiescent Crohn's disease or ulcerative colitis. Corticosteroid side effects are well known and include hypertension, glucose intolerance, cataracts, muscle wasting, and osteoporosis.

Immunosuppressive therapy. The main agents used are 6-mercaptopurine (6-MP) and azathioprine. Azathioprine has an imidazolyl radical attached to a sulfur atom that is cleaved to form the presumed active agent 6-MP. These agents interfere with nucleic acid metabolism and reduce the natural killer cell population. The National Cooperative Crohn's Disease Study failed to demonstrate a good response to immunosuppressive therapy. One criticism of this study was that it was conducted over too brief a period of time for the immunosuppressive agents to be effective. On the average, it takes 3.1 months for these agents to show a favorable response. These agents are used predominantly in Crohn's disease but are beneficial in refractory ulcerative colitis. Some clinicians believe that it is unwarranted to subject patients with ulcerative colitis to the potential toxicities of these agents when surgery has the capability of producing a cure. Crohn's disease cannot really be cured with surgery because of its potential recurrent nature in any part of the gastrointestinal tract. While on immunosuppressive therapy, patients may be able to taper their doses of corticosteroids without any serious flares in disease activity. This reduces some of the long-term effects of corticosteroids.

The side effects of immunosuppressive agents include pancreatitis, bone marrow depression, and allergic reactions consisting of fever, joint pain, and a rash. Cholestatic liver disease has also been reported. Infectious complications and an increased number of malignancies may also occur. Although opinions vary on the subject, immunosuppressive agents may be safe during pregnancy, and there may not be an increased incidence of fetal abnormalities associated with their use.

Other drugs. Other drugs, such as plaquenil and methotrexate, are being tried in clinical studies of patients with inflammatory bowel disease. Metronidazole may be very helpful in treating perianal Crohn's disease, including sinus tracts and fistulas. A peripheral neuropathy can develop after long-term use of metronidazole.

Surgical Therapy

Ulcerative colitis. Surgery is indicated when fulminant disease is unresponsive to intensive medical measures, when bowel perforation secondary to fulminant colitis or toxic megacolon has occurred, when chronic disease of short duration is unresponsive to multiple medical regimens, when there is severe colonic hemorrhage, when dysplasia or cancer of the colon is found, and when early teenagers with disease fail to grow or develop secondary sex characteristics. In the latter case normal growth may resume when the colon and rectum are removed.

Removal of the entire colon and rectum cures the patient. Traditionally this required the construction of an ileostomy. The newest surgical procedure includes a colectomy, stripping of the rectal mucosa, and construction of an ileal pouch with an anastomosis to the anal sphincter. The ileal pouch behaves like a rectum. Continence should be preserved by attaching it to the anal sphincter. The patient may still have an average of six stools per day and one stool per night. Surgery is usually curative, but associated features such as pyoderma gangrenosum and primary sclerosing cholangitis may develop after colectomy.

Crohn's disease. Surgery may also be indicated for Crohn's disease in certain clinical situations, but, unlike in ulcerative colitis, it cannot be considered definitive therapy. Crohn's disease is marked by recurrences, especially at or just proximal to the prior surgical anastomoses. A conservative resection, in which only diseased bowel is removed, should be performed. The surgical indications include perforations, obstruction, bleeding, and intractability. Internal fistulas and intraabdominal abscesses may require surgical management.

Dysplasia and Cancer

Ulcerative Colitis. Patients with ulcerative colitis have an increased incidence of colon cancer compared with the general population. This risk of carcinoma developing in such a patient increases with greater duration of illness and greater length of colon involved. Older age at symptom onset may place the patient at greater risk for eventually developing cancer.

Surveillance colonoscopy has been recommended for patients with ulcerative colitis of extended duration. There is, however, some controversy regarding when and how often such surveillance should take place. There is also some controversy concerning just how high the risk of developing colon cancer in ulcerative colitis truly

is. One such recommendation is to have a patient with colitis involving greater than 60 cm of large bowel and of 10 or more years' duration undergo annual surveillance colonoscopy. A reduction in mortality due to colon cancer has yet to be demonstrated by screening colonoscopies.

During colonoscopy, multiple biopsies are systematically taken from one end of the colon to the other. The biopsies are viewed under a microscope in order to detect dysplasia—abnormal changes in the epithelial cells (in this case the colonic mucosa) that are thought to be premalignant in nature. Colonic strictures in patients with ulcerative colitis may pose a considerable risk of harboring dysplasia. Finding colon cancer, high-grade dysplasia, or low-grade dysplasia in a gross lesion on colonoscopic examination and biopsy is an indication for a total proctocolectomy. Finding low-grade dysplasia on repeated colonoscopic biopsies is also an indication for a proctocolectomy. Some experts are now recommending proctocolectomy after the initial finding of low-grade dysplasia.

Crohn's Disease. The risk of colon cancer in a patient with Crohn's colitis is increased but seems to be less than in ulcerative colitis. There are no current recommendations regarding colon cancer surveillance in Crohn's disease. There is, however, a very high risk of small bowel cancer in patients with Crohn's disease of the small bowel. This may be especially so for areas of diseased small bowel that have been bypassed rather than removed at the time of surgery.

Ocular Sequelae and Examination

The primary ocular complications of Crohn's disease include anterior stromal infiltrative keratopathy, episcleritis (Fig. 12-14), scleritis, uveitis, macular edema, central serous retinopathy, and proptosis from orbital pseudotumor. Secondary complications include cataract and scleromalacia caused by chronic oral prednisone use, glaucoma caused by topical anti-inflammatory use, exudative retinal detachment secondary to uveitis and scleritis, optic disc edema, vitamin A malabsorption and deficiency with its related problems, and endophthalmitis caused by parenteral infection.

Any patient who presents with idiopathic epis-

FIG. 12-14 Episcleritis associated with Crohn's disease. *(Courtesy of Jane Stein.)*

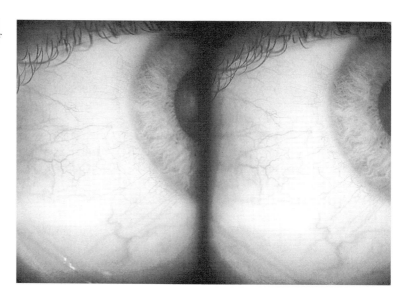

cleritis or uveitis should be questioned about gastrointestinal symptoms, such as cramping, diarrhea, and fever, as well as arthritis and psoriasis. Obtaining a history of extraintestinal complications of Crohn's disease such as arthritis, erythema nodosum (acute inflammation of skin), and hepatitis is noteworthy because it reveals an increased risk of ocular involvement. Patients being treated with systemic regimens of corticosteroids should be monitored for cataract formation and intraocular pressure elevation.

Visual symptoms are usually related to ocular irritation caused by episcleritis, keratitis, dry eye, and uveitis. In fact, episcleritis is the most common ocular finding in patients with Crohn's disease. These symptoms include itching, burning, tearing, pain upon change of gaze, photophobia from ocular inflammation, and vision loss from cataract formation or vitamin A deficiency. The clinician should carefully document any changes in the tear film, corneal epithelium, anterior chamber (cells and flare), lens (posterior subcapsular cataract formation), and posterior chamber. Serial monitoring of intraocular pressure is recommended for patients who are involved with corticosteroid (topical or oral) regimens.

Ocular Management

Prompt referral to the internist is necessary for the appropriate laboratory testing, diagnosis, and management of systemic condition. Modalities for managing ocular complications are simple. Periodic monitoring of the cornea, lens, and intraocular pressure, along with ocular lubricants four times per day, is a conservative modality. Therapy with the use of cycloplegics twice per day and topical anti-inflammatories four times per day may be required for controlling iridocyclitis and uveitis. Clinicians must formulate their uveitic therapies based on severity. In mild cases, 2% cyclopentolate twice per day with 1% prednisolone acetate four times per day may be adequate. More severe cases warrant 5% homatropine or 1% atropine twice per day, with topical steroids administered as often as every two hours. Cold compresses and over-the-counter analgesics may be suggested as supportive adjuncts.

LIVER DISEASE AND JAUNDICE
Systemic Sequelae

Jaundice can be a sign of liver disease. It has multiple causes. Because jaundice is due to an elevated serum bilirubin level, any disturbance in bilirubin metabolism and excretion from the liver can result in jaundice.

Bilirubin Metabolism. *Bilirubin* is produced from the breakdown of heme, an integral part of the hemoglobin molecule (from red blood cells). Heme is also found in myoglobin and many respiratory enzymes. Various disorders of excess breakdown of red blood cells, known as hemolysis, result in unconjugated hyperbilirubinemia and clinical jaundice.

Unconjugated bilirubin is normally taken up by the liver and undergoes conjugation with glucuronic acid. Glucuronyl transferase catalyzes this step. Gilbert's syndrome, a familial disorder, results from a mild disturbance in glucuronyl transferase. Mild unconjugated hyperbilirubinemia may be present. This usually develops during fasting or intercurrent illnesses. Severe glucuronyl transferase deficiency with marked unconjugated hyperbilirubinemia is characteristic of the Crigler-Najjar syndrome. Other than these isolated defects in glucuronyl transferase, liver function and histology are normal. Familial conjugated hyperbilirubinemia results when there is a problem with excretion of bilirubin from the hepatocyte into the biliary system after it has been conjugated. Dubin-Johnson syndrome and Rotor's syndrome are examples. Liver function is otherwise preserved in both of these disorders. Conjugated bilirubin is water soluble and can be detected in the urine when serum levels rise. Unconjugated bilirubin is bound to albumin and is not detected in the urine.

Jaundice secondary to hepatobiliary dysfunction consists predominantly of conjugated hyperbilirubinemia. This can result from various forms of hepatitis, including viral, drug-associated, and toxin-associated forms. Acute hepatitis, in which there is usually marked inflammation of the liver parenchyma, has markedly elevated aminotransferase levels. Jaundice with conjugated hyperbilirubinemia can also be seen with cholestatic liver disease, in which bile flow is decreased within the intrahepatic biliary system. This can be caused by various medications, sepsis, and underlying hepatic disorders such as primary biliary cirrhosis.

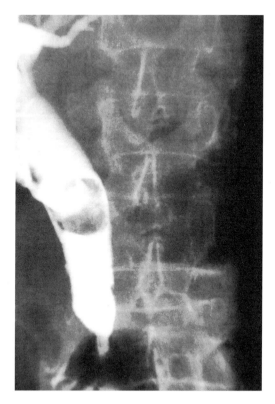

FIG. 12-15 Percutaneous transhepatic cholangiogram of a large common bile duct stone (central dark mass).

Extrahepatic cholestasis is caused by an obstruction in the bile duct. This can be caused by cancer of the pancreas or biliary tree, a stone impacted in the common bile duct (Fig. 12-15), or a bile duct stricture.

Systemic Diagnosis

The patient's history helps deduce the cause of jaundice. For example, viral hepatitis should be suspected when the patient presents with several weeks of anorexia, fever, and malaise prior to the onset of jaundice. The physical examination can also be helpful. A small liver is detected with cirrhosis of the liver (end-stage scarring) and in fulminant liver failure. A palpable gallbladder may be a clue to an extrahepatic obstruction from a malignancy.

Ultrasonography and CT of the liver are very

sensitive studies for diagnosing an extrahepatic obstruction. Dilated bile ducts are seen on these studies. Percutaneous transhepatic cholangiography and endoscopic retrograde cholangiopancreatography (ERCP) provide means to inject dye directly into the biliary system. These are the most accurate means of diagnosing an obstruction. They can identify the site and sometimes the cause of the obstruction. By applying special techniques, ERCP can provide a means for decompressing an obstructed bile duct.

Ocular Sequelae and Examination

The function and dysfunction of the liver represent significant segments of clinical gastroenterology. Ocular complications tend to occur as secondary sequelae to malabsorption of nutrients. Hepatocellular injury leads to functional insufficiency and ultimately hepatic failure. The systemic clinical picture includes weakness, anorexia, jaundice, and hepatomegaly. The jaundice occurs because bilirubin, derived from the normal breakdown of hemoglobin, cannot be excreted by the damaged liver as bile. This may first be detected by the eye care specialist because the excess bilirubin pigment is strikingly apparent against the white sclera. This accumulation of yellowish pigment in the thin bulbar conjunctiva is termed scleral icterus.

Any sign of scleral icterus should alert the eye-care specialist to urgently refer the patient to an internist for gastric and hepatic assessment. In addition to scleral icterus, the peripheral cornea has been cited as a location for the accumulation of pigment in cases of liver disease. In known cases of severe liver decompensation or Wilson's disease, copper metabolism and copper excretion into bile are blocked. This results in the accumulation of copper in peripheral tissues. The cornea prominently displays these circular deposits, which are known as Kayser-Fleischer rings.

The eye-care specialist must take great care to observe eyelid position in any patient who presents with a history of previous or active hepatocellular disease. A significant incidence of eyelid retraction (Dalrymple's sign) and eyelid lag (Graefe's sign) accompanies patients with acquired euthy-

roid Graves' disease secondary to hepatic cirrhosis. These patients also suffer from night blindness because of the intrinsic malabsorption of vitamin A that traditionally accompanies hepatic disease. These patients may have normal levels of stored vitamin A, but, they are unable to release it into the bloodstream, resulting in deprivation.

Ocular Management

Management of these conditions, outside of referral for correcting the underlying condition, is supportive. The management of avitaminosis A is covered in a previous section of this chapter. Management of euthyroid Graves' disease is accomplished by copious amounts of artificial tear solutions as needed and ointments at night. If signs and symptoms reach levels at which the cornea incurs substantial and chronic compromise, prophylactic antibiotic solutions may be required four times a day to guard against infection. These patients should be measured for congestive proptosis by Hertel exophthalmometry. A reading of 22 mm or more is considered positive by most authorities.

Patients suspected of having euthyroid Graves' disease should be assessed for appropriate blink rate and posture. Nightly eyelid taping, blindfolding, or the wearing of a Guibora moisture chamber along with lubricating ointments inhibits corneal desiccation. In the late stages of this disease, patients may complain of diplopia brought about by extraocular muscle restrictions or vision loss secondary to optic nerve compression. Therefore, visual field testing may prove to be an informative modality for monitoring progression. Patients presenting with sight loss warrant a referral to the neurosurgeon for optic nerve decompression or irradiation.

PANCREATIC DISEASE AND CYSTIC FIBROSIS

Systemic Sequelae

The pancreas is an organ composed of both exocrine and endocrine glands. The endocrine portion contains the islets of Langerhans, which secrete insulin. The absence or deficiency of insulin results in diabetes mellitus. The exocrine glands, which make up the majority of the organ's mass, secrete digestive enzymes. Pancreatic disease that compromises synthesis of enzymes results in maldigestion, malabsorption, and malnutrition.

Cystic fibrosis is traditionally categorized as a pancreatic disease although, by definition, it is actually a dysfunction of the exocrine glands. It is an autosomal recessive inheritance and occurs in approximately 1 in 2000 live births. The basic defect is in the body's mucus-producing glands, resulting in obstruction of gland lumina by viscous material. Clinically this produces malabsorption, secondary malnutrition, chronic bronchitis, and bronchopneumonia. Most cases are diagnosed early in childhood and carry a poor prognosis.

Ocular Sequelae and Examination

Pancreatic disease is associated with malnutrition and diabetes mellitus; therefore, ocular signs and symptoms are consistent with vitamin deficiencies and microvascular disease. The clinician must perform a dilated fundus examination on these patients and routinely scrutinize the retina for diabetic retinopathy and associated retinal vascular disease. Occasionally, acute pancreatitis can cause widespread dissemination of fat emboli caused by digestion of fat. This can cause retinal infarction (cotton-wool spots), superficial flame-shaped hemorrhages, and preretinal hemorrhages (Fig. 12-16). Some of these hemorrhages contain white fat emboli, appearing as white-centered hemorrhages called Roth spots. Patients presenting with Roth spots should have pancreatitis included in the differential diagnosis. The ocular signs and symptoms related to the secondary malnutrition caused by pancreatitis and cystic fibrosis are consistent with those described earlier in the chapter under vitaminoses and alcohol abuse. A detailed discussion of diabetes mellitus and diabetic retinopathy is covered in the chapter on endocrine dysfunction. Clinicians needing more information on the management of diabetic retinopathy should consult the Diabetic Retinopathy Study (Arch Ophthalmol 1979) and Early Treatment of Diabetic Retinopathy Study (Arch Ophthalmol 1985).

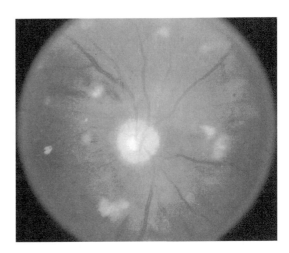

FIG. 12-16 Intraretinal flame-shaped hemorrhages and cotton wool spots in acute pancreatitis. *(Courtesy of Jane Stein.)*

WHIPPLE'S DISEASE

Whipple's disease is really more of a systemic illness than a gastrointestinal disorder. It can involve the gastrointestinal tract, lymph nodes, heart, joints, central nervous system, and other organ systems. It is characterized by periodic acid–Schiff (PAS) staining macrophages in a variety of body tissues. A rod-shaped bacillus is often found in these macrophages which can be identified by electron microscopy. Although this bacillus is still not believed to have been cultured from body tissues, it is the presumed infectious agent involved in the illness. The gene sequence of the bacillus has recently been identified.

Clinical Presentation

Patients can present in a variety of ways. Intestinal symptoms can be preceded for years by fever of unknown origin and migratory arthralgias. Cardiac involvement can take the form of endocarditis, myocarditis, and pericarditis. Chronic aortic regurgitation is the most common clinical manifestation of endocardial involvement. Congestive heart failure is not uncommon. Central nervous system involvement is characterized by personality changes, lethargy, headache, motor weakness, incoordination, optic nerve involvement (decreased visual acuity with papilledema), and cranial nerve III, IV, and VI palsies.

Gastrointestinal manifestations include chronic diarrhea, weight loss, and abdominal pain. Patients have malabsorption of fats, carbohydrates, and proteins. Gross and occult bleeding may also be seen on occasion. Anemia is common. It can have multiple causes, including gastrointestinal blood loss and malabsorption of iron, folate, or vitamin B_{12}.

Systemic Diagnosis

The diagnosis can be made by performing a small bowel biopsy. Intestinal villi tend to be broad and blunted. PAS-positive macrophages should be seen. PAS-positive macrophages have also been seen in small intestinal infection with *Mycobacterium avium-intracellulare (M. avium)* in AIDS patients. Acid-fast stain is positive in *M. avium* infections. In Whipple's disease the acid-fast stain of the small bowel should be negative. Electron microscopy should demonstrate the Whipple's bacillus both free in the extracellular space and within macrophages or epithelial cells.

Systemic Management

The current treatment recommendation is to administer antibiotics that penetrate the central nervous system very effectively. Although there is some lack of uniformity, specific recommendations are as follows:

1. Parenteral penicillin, 20 million units/day, and streptomycin for 2 weeks followed by trimethoprim (160 mg)-sulfamethoxazole (80 mg) twice a day for 1 year.
   or
2. Trimethoprim (160 mg)-sulfamethoxazole (80 mg) three times a day for 2 weeks, followed by the same dosage of trimethoprim-sulfamethoxazole twice a day for 1 year.

CNS relapses are very resistant to treatment.

Ocular Sequelae and Examination

Ocular signs and symptoms include the development of neuro-ocular complications and uveitis.

Supranuclear ophthalmoplegia characterized primarily by upgaze paresis has been reported on several occasions. Uveitis in Whipple's disease tends to present bilaterally with posterior uveal accumulations of cellular material in the vitreous and around the blood vessels. Some have compared the presentation to that of sarcoid uveitis.

The management of the systemic condition is best left to the internist or gastroenterologist. This is typically accomplished with systemic antibiotics. The uveitis resolves as the underlying condition is treated. Management includes meticulous recording of inflammatory signs (cell and flare) (Figs. 12-17 and 12-18) in both the anterior and posterior chambers. The grading scale is often subjective, with trace cells being the least, and Grade 4+ cells and flare or "plasmoid aqueous" being the most severe.

Ocular Management

The objectives in the treatment of uveitis are the following: (1) make the patient comfortable, (2) prevent posterior synechiae, and (3) determine the underlying cause. Treatment begins with dilation and cycloplegia. This places the ciliary body and iris at rest and reduces the subjective symptoms. The choice of cycloplegic depends upon the severity of the case. Clinicians may select a mild agent like tropicamide 1%, which provides cycloplegia for up to 6 hours; a moderate agent like cyclopentolate 1%; or stronger agent like homatropine 5%. Atropine 1% is the strongest cycloplegic, but it can cause the pupil to remain stagnantly dilated and vulnerable to posterior synechiae. Synechiae may form as easily at 8 mm as they do at 3 mm. Cycloplegics, under extreme circumstance, are most effective when used two or three times per day.

Anti-inflammatory therapy is most commonly administered in the form of topical suspension preparations. The most effective topical steroid is prednisolone acetate 1% because it easily penetrates the corneal epithelium to become bioavailable to the anterior chamber. Suspension preparations need vigorous shaking before use to resuspend the steroid in the vehicle. Again, dosage depends upon severity. In severe cases, treatment

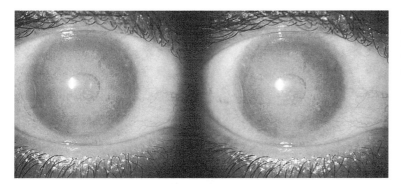

FIG. 12-17 Granulomatous uveitis displaying circumcorneal flush, and mutton-fat keratic precipitates on corneal endothelium. *(Courtesy of Jane Stein.)*

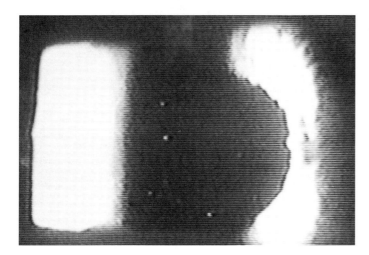

FIG. 12-18 Cells in the anterior chamber in Whipple's disease. Most often the type of uveitis is an iridocyclitis with vitritis and vasculitis.

every 2 hours while awake provides immediate results. Other recommended dosages include four, three, and two times per day. As mentioned, all patients placed on topical anti-inflammatories must be monitored for spikes in intraocular pressure.

Patients who present with posterior uveitis gain little benefit from topical preparations. These patients require oral, injectable, or nonsteroidal anti-inflammatory agents (NSAIDs). In addition to our previous three objectives, we must add (4) protecting the vitreous, (5) protecting retinal and macular function, (6) protecting the ciliary body, and (7) preventing cataract formation.

All steroidal regimens should be tapered to prevent the rebound phenomenon. All patients with suspicious, idiopathic, or recurring uveitides require blood work to rule out systemic causes. The commonly ordered tests include erythrocyte sedimentation rate (ankylosing spondylitis), chest radiography (tuberculosis, sarcoid), FTA-ABS (syphilis), HLA-B27 (arthritis, histoplasmosis, Reiter's syndrome), antinuclear antibody (juvenile rheumatoid arthritis), rheumatoid factor (arthritis), angiotensin-converting enzyme (sarcoid), and complete blood count (anemias).

BEHÇET'S DISEASE

Ocular Sequelae

The initial description of Behçet's disease was that of a triad of oral ulcers (Fig. 12-19), genital ulcers (Fig. 12-20), and ocular inflammation. Other organs can be involved. Included are esophageal ulcerations, intestinal ulcerations, pulmonary an-

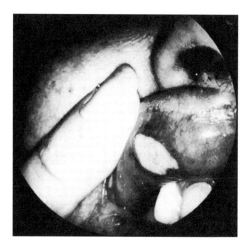

FIG. 12-19 Oral ulcerations associated with Behçet's syndrome. The condition presents with painful ulcers in the mouth and pharynx. *(From Blodi FC:* Ocular involvement in dermatologic disease. *In: Mausolf FA, editor:* The eye and systemic disease, *St. Louis, 1975, Mosby–Year Book.)*

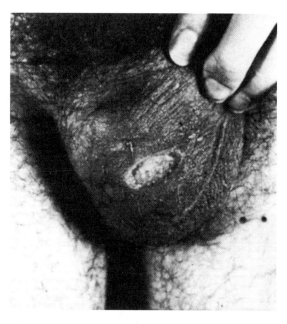

FIG. 12-20 Genital ulcerations associated with Behçet's syndrome. Recurrent orogenital ulceration. *(From Blodi FC:* Ocular involvement in dermatologic disease. *In: Mausolf FA, editor:* The eye and systemic disease, *St. Louis, 1975, Mosby–Year Book.)*

eurysms, thrombophlebitis, arthritis, and neurologic lesions.

Esophageal ulcers may be deep or shallow and present with odynophagia (pain on swallowing). Intestinal involvement frequently occurs in the ileocecal region. Bowel ulcerations, which tend to be deep, may perforate or fistulize and necessitate surgical intervention. The ulcers tend to be deeper than those seen in Crohn's disease and, unlike Crohn's disease, the ulcers are surrounded by normal tissue. Bowel ulcers may be localized or diffuse. Granulomas are absent, unlike Crohn's disease.

Corticosteroids may reduce some of the inflammation underlying Behçet's disease. Recently, azathioprine was found to prevent progression of ocular disease and to reduce the frequency of oral, genital, and joint disorders.

Behçet's disease is a rare multisystem disorder often causing gastrointestinal symptoms, colitis, painful genital ulcers, nonulcerative skin lesions, ulcers of the tongue and mouth, and ocular symptoms. The disease has a high incidence in Far and Middle Eastern populations and is characterized by four major criteria: oral ulceration, skin lesions, such as erythema nodosum, genital ulceration, and inflammatory ocular disease. The cause is still unknown, but evidence suggests a viral, immunologic, or hereditary condition.

Ocular Examination

The ocular findings associated with Behçet's syndrome are found in 75% of the cases and include nongranulomatous hypopyon (Fig. 12-21), uveitis, retinal vasculitis, cataract formation, and glaucoma. The retinal vascular components are severe, permanent, and swift if left untreated, with 50% resulting in blindness.

Ocular Management

The management of uveitis has been thoroughly described in the previous section (pancreatic disease). Treatment of recurrent conjunctivitis can be tackled with broad-spectrum topical agents such as

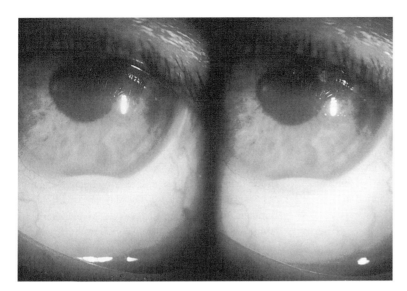

FIG. 12-21 Hypopyon in a case of Behçet's syndrome. *(Courtesy of Jane Stein.)*

polytrim, gentamicin, tobramicin, and neosporin. Not previously discussed, hypopyon is a collection of inflammatory cells, predominantly polymorphonuclear leukocytes with some mononuclear cells and macrophages. It is characteristic of secondary bacterial and fungal activity. The treatment is supportive with respect to the eye. The hypopyon resolves when the underlying condition is removed.

Cataract formation is often the result of chronic systemic oral corticosteroids. Patients must be followed closely with routine dilated examinations of the lens.

The most dangerous of the retinal vasculitides are central retinal vein occlusion (CRVO) and central retinal artery occlusion. Both are ocular emergencies. CRVO (Fig. 12-22) leaves the retinal tissue hemorrhagic and hypoxic. The underlying retinal profusion cannot be assessed because intraretinal blood blocks the view of sodium fluorescein dye. All the while, in ischemic CRVO, the retinal tissue craves oxygen. This, along with vasoproliferative substance released from venous blood, causes prompt and extensive neovascularization of the angle of the eye, or rubeosis iridis. The result is raised intraocular pressure from decreased outflow. To avoid this occurrence, patients must be

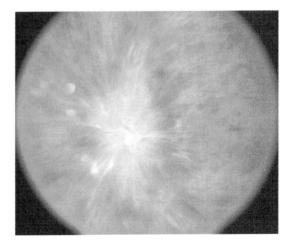

FIG. 12-22 Central retinal vein occlusion in a case of Behçet's syndrome. *(Courtesy of Jane Stein.)*

referred to a retinal specialist for immediate evaluation for panretinal photocoagulation. In ischemic cases, the oxygen-starved peripheral retina is photoablated in the hope of stopping the neovascular response. Although this may seem extreme, it is often successful in avoiding the tragic outcome associated with rubeosis — secondary neovascular glaucoma and blindness.

Bibliography

Adler DJ and Korelitz BI: The therapeutic efficacy of 6-mercaptopurine in refractory ulcerative colitis, *Am J Gastroenterol* 85:717, 1990.

Albert MB and Nochomovitz LE: Dysplasia and cancer surveillance in inflammatory bowel disease, *Gastroenterol Clin North Am* 18:83, 1989.

Allen R: Crohn's disease, *Med Int* 2:1049, 1986.

Arias IM and others: Chronic nonhemolytic unconjugated hyperbilirubinemia with glucuronyl transferase deficiency, *Am J Med* 47:395, 1969.

Astead EM and others: Safety of azathioprine in pregnancy in inflammatory bowel disease, *Gastroenterology* 99:443, 1990.

Baba S and others: Intestinal Behçet's disease: A report of five cases, *Dis Col Rect* 19:428, 1976.

Barresi BJ: *Ocular assessment: The manual of diagnosis for office practice,* Boston, 1984, Butterworths.

Bartlett J and Jaanus SD: *Diseases of the optic nerve.* In *Clinical ocular pharmacology,* ed 2, Boston, 1989, Butterworths.

Bennett RA and others: Frequency of inflammatory bowel disease in offspring of couples both presenting with inflammatory bowel disease, *Gastroenterology* 100:1638, 1991.

Bernstein LH and others: Healing of perineal Crohn's disease with metronidazole, *Gastroenterology* 79:357, 1980.

Binder SC and others: Toxic megacolon in ulcerative colitis, *Gastroenterology* 66:909, 1974.

Bjarnason I and Peters TJ: Helping the mucosa make sense of macromolecules, *Gut* 28:1057, 1987.

Bjarnason I and Peters TJ: Intestinal permeability, non-steroidal anti-inflammatory drug enteropathy and inflammatory bowel disease: an overview, *Gut Festschrift* 1:22-28, 1989.

Black M and Billing BH: Hepatic bilirubin UDP-glucurmyl transferase activity in liver disease and Gilbert's syndrome, *N Engl J Med* 280:1266, 1969.

Blumberg RS: Relapse of chronic inflammatory bowel disease: a riddle wrapped in a mystery inside an enigma, *Gastroenterology* 98:792, 1990.

Booth IW and Harries JT: Inflammatory bowel disease in childhood, *Gut* 25:188, 1984.

Bouchier IAD: Diagnosis of jaundice, *B Med J* 283:1282, 1981.

Boyko EJ and others: Risk of ulcerative colitis among former and current cigarette smokers, *N Engl J Med* 316:707, 1987.

Brandt LJ and others: Metronidazole therapy for perineal Crohn's disease: a follow-up study, *Gastroenterology,* 83:383, 1982.

Brourman ND, Spoor TC, and Ramocki JM: Optic nerve sheath decompression for pseudotumor cerebri, *Arch Ophthalmol* 106:1378, 1988.

Bruckstein AH: Whipple's disease—effective therapy, elusive etiology, *Hosp Pract* May:61-70, 1989.

Burnham WR and Lennard-Jones JE: Mycobacteria as a possible cause of inflammatory bowel disease, *Lancet* 2:693, 1978.

Calking BM: A meta-analysis of the role of smoking in inflammatory bowel disease, *Dig Dis Sci* 34:1841, 1989.

Carlier C and others: Prevalence of malnutrition and vitamin A deficiency in the Diourbel, Fatick and Kaolack regions of Senegal: epidemiological study, *Am J Clin Nutr* 53:70, 1991.

Catania LJ: *Primary care of the anterior segment,* Norwalk, CT, 1988, Appleton and Lange.

Chajek T and Faihar M: Behçet's disease: a report of 41 cases and a review of the literature, *Medicine* 54:179, 1975.

Chiodini RJ and others: Possible rate of mycobacteria in inflammatory bowel disease: an unclassified mycobacterium species isolated from patients with Crohn's disease, *Dig Dis Sci* 29:1073, 1984.

Chong SKF and others: Infantile colitis: a manifestation of intestinal Behçet's syndrome, *J Pediatr Gastroenterol Nutr* 7:622, 1988.

Chopra S and Griffin PH: Laboratory tests and diagnostic procedures in evaluation of liver disease, *Am J Med* 70:221, 1985.

Christie PM and Hill GL: Effect of intravenous nutrition on nutrition and function in acute attacks of inflammatory bowel disease, *Gastroenterology* 99:730, 1990.

Clementz GL and Schade SG: The spectrum of vitamin B_{12} deficiency, *Am Fam Physician* 41:150, 1990.

Collins RH, Feldman M, and Fordtran JS: Colon cancer, dysplasia, and surveillance in patients with ulcerative colitis, *N Engl J Med* 316:1654, 1987.

Cotton P: New approaches may aid patients with inflammatory bowel disease, *JAMA* 263:3121, 1990.

Craven PA and others: Actions of sulfasalazine and 5-aminosalicylic acid as reactive oxygen scavengers in the suppression of bile acid–induced increases in colonic epithelial cell loss and proliferative activity, *Gastroenterology* 92:1998, 1987.

Dallegri F and others: Cytoprotection against neutrophil derived hypochlorous acid: a potential mechanism for the therapeutic action of 5-aminosalicylic acid in ulcerative colitis, *Gut* 31:184, 1990.

Danovich SH: Fulminant colitis and toxic megacolon, *Gastroenterol Clin North Am* 18:73, 1989.

Das KM: Sulfasalazine therapy in inflammatory bowel disease, *Gastroenterol Clin N Am* 18:1, 1989.

DiSant'Agnes P and Davis P: Cystic fibrosis in adults, *Am J Med* 300:942, 1979.

Dissanayake AS and Truelove SC: A controlled therapeutic trial of long-term maintenance treatment of ulcerative colitis with sulphasulazine (salazopyrin), *Gut* 14:923, 1973.

Dorland's Illustrated Medical Dictionary, ed 26. Philadelphia, 1985, WB Saunders Co.

Duane T and Jager E: *Gastrointestinal and nutritional diseases.* In *Clinical ophthalmology,* Philadelphia, 1986, Harper and Rowe.

Duffy LF and others: Peripheral neuropathy in Crohn's disease patients treated with metronidazole, *Gastroenterology* 88:681, 1985.

Erlinger S and others: Hepatic handling of unconjugated dyes in the Dubin-Johnson syndrome, *Gastroenterology* 64:106, 1973.

Farmer RG: Infectious causes of diarrhea in the differential diagnosis of inflammatory bowel disease, *Med Clin North Am* 74:29, 1990.

Farmer RG and others: Long-term follow-up of patients with Crohn's disease, *Gastroenterology* 88:1818, 1985.

Farmer RG and others: Studies of family history among patients with inflammatory bowel disease, *Clin Gastroenterol* 9:271, 1980.

Feldman M: Southern internal medicine conference: Whipple's disease, *Am J Med Sci* 291:56, 1986.

Feldman M and Price G: Intestinal bleeding in patients with Whipple's disease, *Gastroenterology* 96:1207, 1989.

Feurle GE and others: Olsalazine versus placebo in the treatment of mild to moderate ulcerative colitis: a randomized double blind trial, *Gut* 1:1354, 1989.

Fiorentini MT and others: Acute pancreatitis during oral 5-aminosalicylic acid therapy, *Dig Dis Sci* 35:1180, 1990.

Franson TR and LaBrecque DR: Jaundice associated with bacteremias and extrahepatic infections, *Infect Surg* Mar:225, 1988.

Frezza M and others: High blood alcohol levels in women: the role of decreased gastric alcohol dehydrogenase activity and first-pass metabolism, *N Engl J Med* 322:95, 1990.

Gazzard B: Long-term prognosis of Crohn's disease with onset in childhood and adolescence, *Gut* 25:325, 1984.

Gibson PR and others: Ulcerative colitis — a disease characterized by the abnormal colonic epithelial cell? *Gut* 29:516, 1988.

Gilat T and others: Ulcerative colitis in the Jewish population of Tel-Aviv Jafo, *Gastroenterology* 66:335, 1974.

Ginsberg AL: Topical salicylate therapy (4-ASA and 5-ASA enemas), *Gastroenterol Clin North Am* 18:35, 1989.

Gitnick G: Is Crohn's disease a mycobacterial disease after all? *Dig Dis Sci* 29:1086, 1984.

Goldstein F: Immunosuppressant therapy of inflammatory bowel disease: pharmacologic and clinical aspects, *J Clin Gastroenterol* 9:654, 1987.

Goldstein F and others: Favorable effects of sulfasalazine on small bowel Crohn's disease: a long term study, *Am J Gastroenterol* 82:848, 1987.

Grant CS and Dozois RR: Toxic megacolon: ultimate fate of patients after successful medical management, *Am J Surg* 147:106, 1984.

Greenstein AJ and others: Cancer in universal and left-sided ulcerative colitis: factors determining risk, *Gastroenterology* 77:290, 1979.

Greenstein AJ and others: The extra-intestinal complications of Crohn's disease and ulcerative colitis: a study of 700 patients, *Medicine* 55:401, 1976.

Gueant JL and others: Malabsorption of vitamin B_{12} in pancreatic insufficiency of the adult and of the child, *Pancreas* 5:559, 1990.

Gyde SN and Allan RN: Cigarette smoking and ulcerative colitis, *N Engl J Med* 308:1476, 1983.

Hayreh MS and others: Methyl alcohol poisoning, III, ocular toxicity, *Arch Ophthalmol* 95:1851, 1977.

Hayward RS, Wensel RH, and Kibsey P: Relapsing *clostridium difficile* colitis and Reiter's syndrome. *Am J Gastroenterol* 85:752, 1990.

Heaton JM, McCormick AJ, and Freeman AG: Tobacco amblyopia: a clinical manifestation of vitamin B_{12} deficiency, *Lancet* 2:286, 1958.

Hedges TR: Consultation in ophthalmology, Philadelphia, 1987, BC Decker.

Hellers G and Bernell O: Genetic aspects of inflammatory bowel disease, *Med Clin North Am* 74:13, 1990.

Holick MF, Krane SM, and Potts JT: *Calcium phosphorus and bone metabolism: calcium regulating hormones.* In *Harrison's principles of internal medicine,* ed 12, New York, 1991, Wilson.

James SP and others: Crohn's disease: new concepts of pathogenesis and current approaches to treatment, *Dig Dis Sci* 2:1297, 1987.

Jarnerot G and others: Intensive intravenous treatment of ulcerative colitis, *Gastroenterology* 89:1005, 1985.

Jayanthi V and others: Current concepts of the etiopathogenesis of inflammatory bowel disease, *Am J Gastroenterol* 86:1566, 1991.

Jewell DP: Corticosteroids for the management of ulcerative colitis and Crohn's disease, *Gastroenterol Clin North Am* 18:21, 1989.

Jick H and Walker AM: Cigarette smoking and ulcerative colitis, *N Engl J Med* 308:261, 1983.

Kaplan MM: Primary biliary cirrhosis, *N Engl J Med* 316:521, 1987.

Kasahara Y and others: Intestinal involvement in Behçet's disease: review of 136 surgical cases in the Japanese literature, *Dis Colon Rectum* 24:103, 1981.

Katz KD and others: Intestinal permeability in patients with Crohn's disease and their healthy relatives, *Gastroenterology* 97:927, 1989.

Katzka I and others: Assessment of colorectal cancer risk in patients with ulcerative colitis: experience from a private practice, *Gastroenterology* 85:22, 1983.

Kawasaki H and others: Dye clearance studies in Rotor's syndrome, *Am J Gastroenterol* 71:380, 1979.

Keinath RD and others: Antibiotic treatment and relapse in Whipple's disease: long-term followup of 88 patients, *Gastroenterology* 88:1857, 1985.

Kirsner JB and others: Genetic aspects of inflammatory bowel disease, *Clin Gastroenterol* 2:557, 1973.

Korelitz BI: Carcinoma of the intestinal tract in Crohn's disease: results of a survey conducted by the National Foundation for Ileitis and Colitis, *Am J Gastroenterol* 78:44, 1983.

Kyle SM and others: Behçet's colitis: a differential diagnosis in inflammations of the large intestine, *Austrial NZ J Surg* 61:547, 1991.

Lanspa SJ and others: Pathogenesis of steatorrhea in primary biliary cirrhosis, *Hepatology* 5:837, 1985.

LaRusso NF and others: Primary sclerosing cholangitis, *N Engl J Med* 310:899, 1981.

Lashner BA: Recommendations for colorectal cancer screening in ulcerative colitis: a review of research from a single university-based surveillance program, *Am J Gastroenterol* 87:168, 1992.

Lashner BA and others: Colon cancer surveillance in chronic ulcerative colitis: historical cohort study, *Am J Gastroenterol* 85:1083, 1990.

Lashner BA and others: Dysplasia and cancer complicating structures in ulcerative colitis, *Dig Dis Sci* 35:349, 1990.

Lashner BA and others: Hazard rates for dysplasia and cancer in ulcerative colitis: results from a surveillance program, *Dig Dis Sci* 34:1536, 1989.

Lashner BA and others: Testing nicotine gum for ulcerative colitis patients: experience with single-patient trials, *Dig Dis Sci* 35:827, 1990.

Lawrence MAJ, McNiesh M, and Bova JG: Reiter's disease complicated by ulcerative colitis: a case report, *Milit Med* 151:550, 1986.

Lebwohl O and others: Ulcerative esophagitis and colitis in a pediatric patient with Behçet's syndrome: response to steroid therapy, *Am J Gastroenterol* 68:550, 1977.

Lennard-Jones JE and others: Prednisone as maintenance treatment for ulcerative colitis in remission, *Lancet* 1:188, 1965.

Lieber CS: Biochemical and molecular basis of alcohol-induced injury to liver and other tissues, *N Engl J Med* 319:1639, 1988.

Lindberg E and others: Smoking and inflammatory bowel disease. A case control study, *Gut* 29:352, 1988.

Lockhart JM, McIntyre W, and Caperton EM: Esophageal ulceration in Behçet's syndrome, *Ann Intern Med* 84:572, 1976.

Logan RFA and others: Smoking and ulcerative colitis, *Br Med J* 288:751, 1984.

Mahalanabis P: Breast feeding and vitamin A deficiency among children attending a diarrhoea treatment centre in Bangladesh: a case control study, *Br Med J* 303:493, 1991.

Malchow H and others: European cooperative Crohn's Disease Study (ECCDS): results of drug treatment, *Gastroenterology* 86:249, 1984.

Malins TJ, Wilson A, and Ward-Booth RP: Recurrent buccal space abscesses: a complication of Crohn's disease, *Oral Surg Oral Med Oral Pathol* 72:19, 1991.

Marbet UA, Stalder GA, and Gyr KE: Whipple's disease: a multisystemic disease with changing presentation, *Dig Dis* 4:119, 1986.

Matsuo T and others: Keratomalacia in a child with familial hypo-retinol-binding proteinemia, *Jpn J Ophthalmol* 32:249, 1988.

Matzen P and others: Ultrasonography, computed tomography, and cholescintigraphy in suspected obstructive jaundice—a prospective comparative study, *Gastroenterology* 84:1492, 1983.

Matzen P and others: Accuracy of direct cholangiography by endoscopic or transhepatic route in jaundice—a prospective study, *Gastroenterology* 81:237, 1981.

McInerney GT and others: Fulminating ulcerative colitis with marked colonic dilation: a clinicopathologic study, *Gastroenterology* 42:244, 1962.

Mekhjian HS and others: Clinical features and natural history of Crohn's disease, *Gastroenterology* 77:898, 1979.

Meyers S and others: Olsalazine sodium in the treatment of ulcerative colitis among patients intolerant of sulfasalazine, *Gastroenterology* 93:1255, 1987.

Meyers S and Janowitz HD: Systemic corticosteroid therapy of ulcerative colitis, *Gastroenterology* 89:1189, 1985.

Miller DJ and others: Jaundice in severe bacterial infection, *Gastroenterology* 71:94, 1976.

Mir-Madjlessi SH and others: Clinical course and evolution of erythema nodosum and pyoderma gangrenosum in chronic ulcerative colitis: a study of 42 patients, *Am J Gastroenterol* 80:615, 1985.

Muller DPR: Vitamin E—its role in neurological function, *Postgrad Med J* 62:107, 1986.

Nielsen OH and others: Abnormal metabolism of arachidonic acid in chronic inflammatory bowel disease: enhanced release of leucotriene B_4 from activated neutrophils, *Gut* 28:181, 1987.

O'Duffy JD: Behçet's syndrome, *N Engl J Med* 322:326, 1990.

Olaison G and others: Intestinal permeability to polyethyleneglycol 600 in Crohn's disease. Preoperative determination in a defined segment of the small intestine, *Gut* 29:196, 1988.

Orholm M and others: Familial occurrence of inflammatory bowel disease, *N Engl J Med* 324:84, 1991.

Palmucci L and others: Neuropathy secondary to vitamin E deficiency in acquired intestinal malabsorption, *Ital J Neurol Sci* 9:599, 1988.

Pepperlorn MA: Advances in drug therapy for inflammatory bowel disease, *Ann Intern Med* 112:50, 1990.

Podolsky DK: Inflammatory bowel disease (first of two parts), *N Engl J Med* 325:928, 1991.

Podolsky DK and Fournier DA: Alterations is mucosal content of colonic glycoconjugates. Inflammatory bowel disease defined by monoclonal antibodies, *Gastroenterology* 95:379, 1988.

Podolsky DK and Isselbacher KJ: Composition of human colonic mucin: selective alteration in inflammatory bowel disease, *J Clin Invest* 72:142, 1983.

Present DH: 6-Mercaptopurine and other immunosuppressive agents in the treatment of Crohn's disease and ulcerative colitis, *Gastroenterol Clin North Am* 18:57, 1989.

Present DH and others: 6-Mercaptopurine in the management of inflammatory bowel disease: short and long-term toxicity, *Ann Intern Med* 111:641, 1989.

Ramond MJ and others: A randomized trial of prednisolone in patients with severe alcoholic hepatitis, *N Engl J Med* 326:507, 1992.

Rankin GB: Extraintestinal and systemic manifestations of inflammatory bowel disease, *Med Clin North Am* 74:39, 1990.

Rankin GB and others: National Cooperative Crohn's Disease Study: extraintestinal manifestations and perianal complications, *Gastroenterology* 77:914, 1979.

Relman DA and others: Identification of the uncultured bacillus of Whipple's disease, *N Engl J Med* 327:293, 1992.

Rhodes JM: Colonic mucus and mucosal glycoproteins: the key to colitis and cancer? *Gut* 30:1660, 1989.

Robert JH and others: Management of severe hemorrhage in ulcerative colitis, *Am J Surg* 159:550, 1990.

Robinson MG: New oral salicylates in the therapy of chronic idiopathic inflammatory bowel disease, *Gastroenterol Clin North Am* 18:43, 1989.

Romano TJ and Dobbins JW: Evaluation of the patient with suspected malabsorption, *Gastroenterol Clin North Am* 18:467, 1989.

Roth R and others: Intestinal infection with *Mycobacterium avium* in acquired immune deficiency syndrome (AIDS): histological and clinical comparison with Whipple's disease, *Dig Dis Sci* 30:497, 1985.

Sandberg-Gertzen H and others: Azodisal sodium in the treatment of ulcerative colitis, *Gastroenterology* 90:1024, 1986.

Schulze K and others: Intestinal tuberculosis: experience at a Canadian teaching institution, *Am J Med* 83:735, 1977.

Scully RE and others: Case records of the Massachusetts General Hospital, *N Engl J Med* 306:1162, 1982.

Seeff LB and others: Acetaminophen hepatotoxicity in alcoholics: a therapeutic misadventure, *Ann Intern Med* 104:399, 1986.

Seidman EG: Nutritional management of inflammatory bowel disease, *Gastroenterol Clin North Am* 17:129, 1989.

Sharon P and Stenson WF: Enhanced synthesis of leukotriene B_4 by colonic mucosa in inflammatory bowel disease, *Gastroenterology* 86:453, 1984.

Shorb PE: Surgical therapy for Crohn's disease, *Gastroenterol Clin North Am* 18:111, 1989.

Siegel JH and Yatto RP: Approach to cholestasis: an update, *Arch Intern Med* 142:1877, 1982.

Singer HC and others: Familial aspects of inflammatory bowel disease, *Gastroenterology* 61:423, 1971.

Sitrin MD and others: Vitamin E deficiency and neurologic disease in adults with cystic fibrosis, *Ann Intern Med* 107:51, 1987.

Skelton WP and Skelton NK: Deficiency of vitamins A, B, and C: something to watch for, *Postgrad Med* 87:296, 1990.

Sleisenger MH and Fordtran JS: *Gastrointestinal disease: pathophysiology, diagnosis, management,* ed 4, Philadelphia, 1989, WB Saunders Co.

Smith LE: Surgical therapy in ulcerative colitis, *Gastroenterol Clin North Am* 18:99, 1989.

Smith MB and others: Smoking and inflammatory bowel disease in families, *Am J Gastroenterol* 83:407, 1988.

Sokol RJ: Vitamin E and neurological deficits, *Adv Pediatr* 37:119, 1990.

Sokol RJ and others: Vitamin E deficiency neuropathy in children with fat malabsorption: studies in cystic fibrosis and chronic cholestasis, *Ann NY Acad Sci* 570:156, 1989.

Somerville KW and others: Smoking and Crohn's disease, *Br Med J* 289:954, 1984.

Smiddy WE and Green WR: Nutritional amblyopia: a histopathological study with retrospective clinical correlation, *Grafe's Arch Clin Exp Ophthalmol* 225:321, 1987.

Stenson WF and Lobos E: Sulfasalazine inhibits the synthesis of chemotactic lipid by neutrophils, *J Clin Invest* 69:494, 1982.

Stowe SP and others: An epidemiologic study of inflammatory bowel disease in Rochester, New York: hospital incidence, *Gastroenterology* 98:104, 1990.

Stricker H and Malinverni R: Multiple, large aneurysms of pulmonary arteries in Behçet's disease: clinical remission and radiologic resolution after corticosteroid therapy, *Arch Intern Med* 149:925, 1989.

Stringer DA and others: Behçet's syndrome involving the gastrointestinal tract: a diagnostic dilemma in childhood, *Pediatr Radiol* 16:131, 1986.

Summers RW and others: National Cooperative Crohn's Disease Study: results of drug treatment, *Gastroenterology* 77:847, 1979.

Surawicz CM and Belic. Rectal biopsy helps to distinguish acute self-limited colitis from idiopathic inflammatory bowel disease, *Gastroenterology* 86:104, 1984.

Thayer WR and others: Possible role of mycobacteria in inflammatory bowel disease. II. Mycobacterial antibodies in Crohn's disease, *Dig Dis Sci* 29:1080, 1984.

Thommessen M and others: Nutrition and growth retardation in 10 children with congenital deaf-blindness, *J Am Diet Assoc* 89:69, 1989.

Tobin MV and others: Cigarette smoking and inflammatory bowel disease, *Gastroenterology* 93:316, 1987.

Truelove SC and others: Further experience in the treatment of severe attacks of ulcerative colitis, *Lancet* 2:1086, 1978.

Tysk C and others: Colonic glycoproteins in monozygotic twins with inflammatory bowel disease, *Gastroenterology* 100:419, 1991.

van Noort BA and others: Optic neuropathy from thiamine deficiency in a patient with ulcerative colitis, *Doc Ophthalmol* 67:45, 1987.

Vaughan D and Asbury T: *General ophthalmology,* ed 10, Los Altos, 1983, Lange.

Vilaseca J and others: Participation of thromboxane and other eicosanoid synthesis in the course of experimental inflammatory colitis, *Gastroenterology* 98:269, 1990.

Wall M, Hart WM Jr, and Burde RM: Visual field defects in idiopathic intracranial hypertension (pseudotumor cerebri), *Am J Ophthalmol* 96:654, 1983.

Whelan G: Epidemiology of inflammatory bowel disease. *Med Clin North Am* 74:1, 1990.

Williams JG and others: Toxic oxygen metabolite production by circulating phagocytic cells in inflammatory bowel disease, *Gut* 31:187, 1990.

Wokes F: Tobacco amblyopia, *Lancet* 2:526, 1958.

Yazici H and others: A controlled trial of azathioprine in Behçet's syndrome, *N Engl J Med* 322:281, 1990.

Zimmerman HJ: Intrahepatic cholestasis, *Arch Intern Med* 139:1038, 1979.

Zimmerman HJ and others: Jaundice due to bacterial infection, *Gastroenterology* 77:362, 1979.

Zinberg J and others: Double-blinded placebo-controlled study of olsalazine in the treatment of ulcerative colitis, *Am J Gastroenterol* 85:562, 1990.

13

Systemic Considerations and Ocular Manifestations of Diabetes Mellitus

BRIAN P. MAHONEY
JERRY CAVALLERANO

KEY TERMS

Hyperglycemia	*Diabetic Retinopathy*	*Neovascularization of the Disc (NVD)*
Protein Glycosylation	*Intraretinal Microvascular Abnormalities (IRMA)*	*Neovascularization Elsewhere (NVE)*
Glucose	*Panretinal Photocoagulation*	*Rubeosis Iridis*
Insulin	*Clinically Significant Macular Edema (CSME)*	*Diabetologist*
Ketoacidosis		
Diabetic Neuropathy		
Sulfonylurea Drugs		

---

*T*he sequelae of diabetes and diabetes-related conditions continue to be sources of signifi-cant morbidity and mortality despite advances in treatment. Diabetes and its related diseases consume a significant portion of each health care dollar spent in the United States. In 1980, 2% of total health care costs in the United States was consumed by diabetes and related conditions.[1] It is estimated that 10% of Americans over age 60 and 20% of Americans over age 80 have diabetes.[2] In 1987, diabetes was directly responsible for 1.8% of deaths and contributed to 8.4% of deaths in the United States.[1] Diabetic disease is also responsible for the greatest loss of potential years of life in the American population. The chronicity of this disease dictates the need for ophthalmic practitioners, as well as other health care workers, to be fully aware of the systemic and ophthalmic ramifications so that severe physical impairment and blindness can be minimized. Although diabetic oc-ulopathy develops as the disease progresses, it may be the presenting symptom that leads to the initial diagnosis. Eye care practitioners must actively par-ticipate on the health care team to avert blindness caused by this disease.

OVERVIEW OF DIABETIC DISEASE

Diabetes is a complex, multifaceted disease whose characteristic clinical feature is abnormally high fasting glucose levels and poor glucose metabo-lism. This elevation results from a disruption in the production or release of insulin and a decrease in the insulin response by the peripheral tissues as well as abnormalities in glucose utilization by the body. This occurs in various ways for both Type I, insulin-dependent diabetes mellitus (IDDM), and Type II, noninsulin-dependent diabetes melli-tus (NIDDM).

The mechanisms responsible for *hyperglycemia* in IDDM differ from those in NIDDM,[3] which has specific implications for treatment and manage-ment of patients in both classifications. Hypergly-cemia associated with pancreatic β-cell dysfunc-tion in IDDM patients results in decreased insulin production or release.[4] The presence of HLA sub-types may act as a genetic marker for the devel-opment of Type I diabetes.[5-7] Adequate insulin production and release occur in Type II diabetic patients, but poor tissue response (referred to as insulin resistance) results in the inability of periph-eral tissues to utilize available circulating glu-cose.[8] Obesity plays an important role in the de-velopment of insulin resistance associated with NIDDM. A strong genetic link for the develop-ment of Type II diabetes is suspected, considering a 90% concordance in identical twins and a high incidence in first-degree relatives of diabetic per-sons (approximately 43%).

The exact relationship between hyperglycemia and histopathologic responses in tissues through-out the body remains uncertain. Direct damage to tissues by sustained hyperglycemia has been well demonstrated (including loss of pericyte response to endothelin-1 and increased glomerular filtration

rate), but widespread tissue disease cannot be ex-plained by this single mechanism. Other mecha-nisms associated with tissue abnormalities include increased activity of the polyol pathway, increased *protein glycosylation*, and altered physiologic re-sponses in the affected tissues. Accumulation of sorbitol and fructose is associated with histopatho-logic changes in the lens as well as peripheral ner-vous tissues.[9-11] Protein glycosylation, a nonenzy-matic binding of glucose molecules to various pro-teins, alters their structural integrity and function (that is, red blood cells, lens proteins, and mye-lin). The various histopathologic manifestations associated with diabetes cannot be explained solely by these three mechanisms. Other factors must contribute to the development of chronic compli-cations (such as advanced systemic vasculopathy), so alternate mechanisms need to be considered.

Progression in the long-term changes can be slowed by controlling hyperglycemia, but reversal of advanced changes with good glycemic control has not been confirmed clinically.[12-15,34] This points to the indirect role hyperglycemia plays in their development and raises the issue of what con-stitutes good glycemic control and, more impor-tantly, what treatment modalities can achieve this goal. Tighter control of hyperglycemia is neces-sary to minimize the severity of chronic complica-tions from both Type I and Type II diabetes. These issues have changed the way diabetes is viewed. Diabetes can no longer be viewed as a disease of abnormal glucose metabolism only but rather it is considered a complex, multifaceted disease whose hallmark clinical feature is hyperglycemia.

EPIDEMIOLOGY

The prevalence of diabetes in the United States has dramatically increased over the past 40 years. This may have resulted from the increased life expect-ancy due to advances in medicine in addition to changes in the diagnostic criteria for diabetes. The prevalence of diabetes in the Caucasian race in the United States ranges from 0.05% in the young to approximately 4% in patients over 60 years old and is about 1.8% for black Americans.[16,17] IDDM is seen in about 0.1% to 0.2% of patients under age 20. Approximately 40% of IDDM patients manifest by the age 14, 30% between the ages of 15 and 34, and the remaining 30% over the age of 35. NIDDM is seen much more frequently than IDDM (93% versus 7%, respectively) in the United States.[16,17] The peak age for diagnosis of IDDM is between 10 and 15, with NIDDM diagnosed most frequently between the ages of 50 and 55. NIDDM is seen 50% more frequently in African Americans than Caucasian Americans in the United States. Other ethnic populations are at high risk for developing diabetes (for example, North Carolina Cherokee Indians at 25% of the population and 6.9% of the general population of Uruguay) which may be related to the increased body mass of these populations.

CAUSE OF HYPERGLYCEMIA

The circulating level of *glucose* at any given time depends on the person's diet and level of physical activity and is regulated by hormonal activity in an integrated manner. Hormonal influences, exerted primarily on the pancreas, liver, and adipose tissues, depend on *insulin* to initiate glucose transport into the cell for utilization, although some tissues use glucose independent of insulin (such as brain tissue). Interruption in the regulation of glucose levels frequently results in hyperglycemia and can decrease the viability of insulin-dependent tissues. Various situations are associated with hyperglycemia (see the box above, right).

The pathophysiology associated with hyperglycemia in diabetes has been described, although the cause of these changes is poorly understood. The presence of HLA-DR3 and DR4 complexes is associated with poor pancreatic β-cell regeneration in Type I diabetics. An immunologic response directed toward the islet of Langerhans cells (β-cells) is observed in these individuals.[17,18] The inciting event for the inflammation is unknown, but it decreases the level of insulin released into the circulation due to a loss of β-cell mass. Insufficient levels of endogenous insulin do not meet the

CONDITIONS ASSOCIATED WITH HYPERGLYCEMIA

Pancreatic disease (impaired β-cell function)
    Pancreatitis (viral/autoimmune)
    Pancreatic toxicity (drug)
    Hormonal
    Drug-induced (reversible with discontinuation)
    Poor proinsulin conversion

Poor insulin action
    Anti-insulin/antireceptor antibodies
    Excessive inhibitory hormones (glucagon)

Tissue defects
    Decreased number of insulin receptors
    Decreased cellular response to insulin (insulin resistance/elevated glucocorticoid levels)

demands of the body and hyperglycemia results. A genetic association with HLA-B8 and B15, in addition to DR3 and DR4, is commonly found in IDDM patients. Approximately 90% of Caucasian patients with diabetes onset prior to age 30 are HLA-DR3 or DR4 positive. The presence of these antigens may identify an individual at risk for developing IDDM but does not indicate inevitable disease development.

Altered insulin response in dependent tissues occurs despite adequate insulin levels in Type II diabetic patients. Inadequate binding of the insulin molecule to the cell receptor cannot initiate the normal cellular responses, which subsequently impairs the transport of glucose across the cell membrane. Insulin resistance causes hyperglycemia due to lack of glucose utilization despite excessive amounts of available glucose. Altered configuration and binding ability of the insulin receptor are attributed to increased body mass, which plays a major role in the development of insulin resistance. The relative insulin deficiency commonly observed as diabetes progresses in the NIDDM patient results in the eventual dependence on exogenous insulin for adequate control of hyperglycemia, at which time the patient is considered to have IDDM.

Patients' symptoms are frequently associated with hyperosmosis (related to hyperglycemia for Type II diabetes) and/or diabetic *ketoacidosis* (in Type I diabetes. Increased hyperosmolarity from hyperglycemia causes an imbalance in the intracellular and extracellular water. This imbalance is responsible for the symptoms of increased thirst and urination.[19] The body's energy demands cannot be met due to the lack of intracellular glucose. Increased food intake in an attempt to rectify this situation only increases the severity of the hyperglycemia. Increasing the intake of water and food fails to meet the physiologic or metabolic needs of the body. Altered lipid and protein metabolism resulting from hyperglycemia is life-threatening if ketoacidosis develops. The severity of all of these symptoms correlates with sustained levels of hyperglycemia. There is little doubt of the diagnosis of diabetes when these classic symptoms manifest, yet they may be ignored if they are mild.

Severe hyperglycemia (over 500 mg/dl) is associated with symptoms of dehydration, delirium, and focal neurologic deficits in diabetic patients who may not have been previously diagnosed. This situation is more commonly associated with Type II diabetes. Diabetic ketoacidosis is associated with glucose levels above 300 mg/dl, but elevated serum ketones and decreased serum pH (below 7.3) also accompany the hyperglycemia. Hepatic conversion of free fatty acids to ketone bodies results from severe insulin depletion, which is why this situation is more frequently associated with Type I than Type II diabetes.[18,19] Altered cognitive levels, dehydration, and hyperventilation develop with ketoacidosis, and can be a life-threatening situation requiring prompt medical intervention. Emergency care may be delayed if a patient has not been previously diagnosed with diabetes. Acute crisis, such as ketoacidosis, requiring emergency care often leads to the initial diagnosis for Type I diabetic patients but rarely precedes the initial diagnosis for Type II diabetic patients.

PATHOPHYSIOLOGY OF DIABETES

Other clinical features besides hyperglycemia have been implicated in the development of pathologic changes associated with diabetes. Glycosylation of tissue protein occurs with irreversibility and at a higher rate in the diabetic patient than in the nondiabetic patient. Nonenzymatic protein glycosylation involves various tissues, including the hemoglobin molecule, plasma proteins, lens proteins, vascular endothelium, and myelin sheath of nervous tissue. This process is associated with abnormalities in the structure and function of these tissues and is implicated in the development of vascular disease and neuropathy. The polyol pathway, which is utilized infrequently in nondiabetic individuals, is highly utilized in diabetic persons because of the sustained levels of hyperglycemia. The byproducts of this sequence of reactions are sorbitol and fructose, which act as strong osmotic agents similar to glucose. Accumulation of these products causes imbibition of water and tissue dysfunction. Loss of myoinositol concurrent with the accumulation of sorbitol is implicated in the development of peripheral neuropathy and diabetic cataract formation. The use of aldose reductase inhibitors in the therapy of diabetic patients has not proven effective in preventing these changes from occurring, but longer-term studies may demonstrate benefits.

Hypercoagulation plays a significant role in the development of microvascular disease (such as nephropathy), yet it plays an insignificant role in the development of macrovascular disease (such as coronary heart disease) associated with diabetes.[20-22] Microthrombus formation at sites of minimal endothelial damage results in increased platelet aggregation, decreased fibrinolysis, and decreased platelet life. Improved control of hyperglycemia has a positive effect on the development of these coagulation abnormalities, but a causal relationship has not been established. Hemodynamic abnormalities, primarily increased blood flow through the capillary beds, are caused by unknown mechanisms. These abnormalities are seen in the retina and kidney prior to any observation of significant vascular damage, capillary closure, or detection of other clinical signs or symptoms. Increased flow rate through these capillary beds does not allow for adequate perfusion of the capillary beds and contributes to the vessel wall damage. Glomerular hyperfiltration results in kidney malfunction and proteinuria with progressive renal damage.

CLINICAL FEATURES

Type I diabetes occurs most frequently prior to the age of 15, although it can manifest at any age. An acute onset of symptoms of polyuria, polyphagia, and polydipsia with fatigue and weight loss for weeks is typical. The severity of the symptoms progresses, which frequently results in diabetic ketoacidosis and possibly coma. These symptoms are directly related to the severity of insulin deficiency and ketosis. Supplemental exogenous insulin is necessary for the adequate control of these complications on an acute basis. Type I diabetes progresses with the development of long-term complications, with renal failure a frequent complication in Type I diabetes.[23,24]

A more gradual clinical course is seen in Type II diabetes, whose onset is most frequently seen after age 40. The mild nature and gradual progression of patient symptoms are frequently overlooked because serum glucose levels rarely rise acutely. Most Type II diabetic patients are diagnosed with hyperglycemia following routine work-up as part of a physical examination. Ketosis is rarely seen and does not result in acute hospital admission. Vasculopathy and neuropathy may be present at the time of diagnosis because these patients frequently have had diabetes for a considerable time prior to diagnosis. Myocardial infarction from severe coronary artery disease is a common complication in Type II diabetes.[23] A high rate of physical impairment is associated with peripheral neuropathy, peripheral vascular disease, and cerebrovascular disease, which compromise the quality of life for Type I and II diabetics.

COMPLICATIONS RELATED TO DIABETES

A relationship between sustained hyperglycemia and development of the long-term complications of diabetes exists, although the exact nature of this relationship is unclear.[14] Advanced vascular disease of the blood vessels of varying caliber is the most striking of these features. Macrovascular disease (cerebrovascular and coronary arteries) and microvascular disease (renal, retinal, and vasovasorum of peripheral nerves) is seen at a higher rate than in age-matched nondiabetic patients.[22,25-29] Lower extremity involvement of the large vessels manifests most frequently and contributes to claudication for many diabetic patients. It can contribute to decreased peripheral sensation and increased incidence of gangrene, frequently requiring amputation (Fig. 13-1). The development of large-vessel atherosclerotic disease, which is histopathologically identical to nondiabetic disease, occurs at an earlier age of onset and with greater severity than nondiabetic disease. Coronary artery disease accounts for 70% to 80% of mortality in Type II diabetic persons and may be associated with cerebrovascular disease and stroke (Fig. 13-2). Increased circulating low density lipoprotein levels contribute to vessel wall disease and the development of

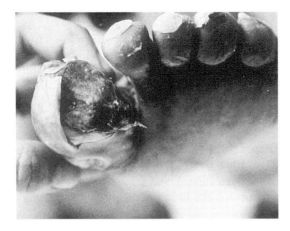

FIG. 13-1 Gangrenous toe. This diabetic patient presented with a gangrenous condition of his foot requiring amputation. This condition is usually associated with advanced vascular disease of the lower extremities. *(Courtesy of Robert Garber, DPM.)*

hypertension, which is seen 1.5 to 2 times more frequently in diabetic persons than nondiabetic persons. The mean systolic pressure is 10 to 12 mm Hg higher in these patients than in nondiabetic hypertensive patients, and the presence of hypertension increases the risk for development of diabetic retinopathy.

Clinical *diabetic neuropathy* is seen early in the course of the disease for both Type I and Type II diabetics, with most Type II diabetic persons manifesting some level of neuropathy at the time of diagnosis or shortly afterward. The frequency of neuropathy increases with the duration of the disease, with 89% of patients with retinopathy and 93% of patients with nephropathy having associated neuropathy. Elevated levels of nonenzymatic glycosylated tissue proteins with end product accumulation in vessel walls of the vasovasorum incite chronic insult. This results in vascular damage, decreased blood flow to the nerves, and clinical neuropathy. Mechanical, metabolic, and vascular factors all contribute to the development of

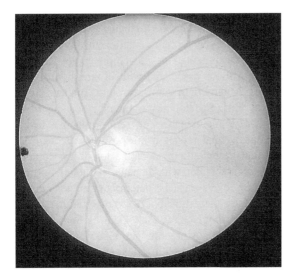

FIG. 13-2 Hollenhorst plaque in the left eye. Note the presence of the cholesterol plaque in the central cone of vessels on the disc. This 52-year-old NIDDM patient was diagnosed 5 years previous to this visit. He had early nephropathy and was experiencing episodes of transient ischemic attacks. This patient eventually had bilateral endarterectomies. Note the lack of diabetic retinopathy associated with this plaque.

the neuropathy in a cumulative way. Diabetic neuropathy can manifest as sensory, motor, or autonomic disturbance with focal or diffuse distribution (cranial nerve palsy versus ischemic pains in the legs). Conduction deficits of the heart (from vagal nerve involvement), loss of bladder control, impotence, decreased peristalsis, and tonic pupil are all variations of diabetic neuropathy. Diabetic neuropathy has an ischemic vascular component and can compensate with time (as in cranial nerve palsies) if it is caused by an acute, nonprogressive focal event. It can also be associated with decompensation (such as incontinence or impotence) when progressive insult occurs to the nerves or when complicated by metabolic abnormalities within the nerve itself.

Altered renal function is a complication for most IDDM patients and may be observed with lesser severity in NIDDM patients. Renal disease associated with hypertension, referred to as Kimmelstiel-Wilson disease, frequently manifests after 30 or more years of IDDM, and about 15% of patients with NIDDM present with proteinuria early in the course of their disease but do not progress to end-stage renal disease (ESRD) commonly encountered with IDDM patients. Elevated glomerular filtration rates are associated with microalbuminuria during periods of poor glycemic control, but this level of urinary protein is not indicative of advanced renal disease. Chronic hyperfiltration through the renal glomeruli is related to impaired renal function and hypertension (Fig. 13-3). Patients with ESRD require dialysis or renal transplant as part of their long-term treatment regimen.

DIAGNOSIS OF DIABETES

Many laboratory tests are used in both the diagnosis and monitoring of diabetic patients.[30-32] Laboratory tests are necessary when the ocular findings or systemic presentation is suggestive of diabetes. Numerous tests are available to the practitioner which yield specific information regarding various aspects of the diabetic condition (see box on p. 266). The fasting blood sugar (FBS) remains the most frequently ordered test to confirm the diag-

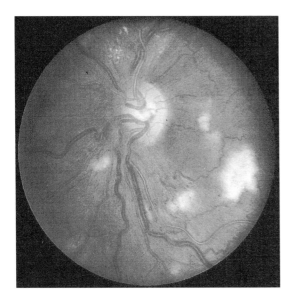

FIG. 13-3 Kimmelstiel-Wilson retinopathy. This 63-year-old diabetic patient had advanced renal disease with hypertension. Exacerbations in the severity of retinal microinfarction and vascular tortuosity were not associated with chronic capillary closure but did correlate with progressive renal impairment.

nosis of diabetes. Two successive readings above 140 mg/dl are diagnostic of diabetes. The results of the FBS play an instrumental role in the management of diabetes and are used to determine the efficacy of treatment (with optimal ranges determined on an individual basis). The oral glucose tolerance test, although not used as the primary test for the diagnosis of diabetes, aids in the diagnosis of impaired glucose tolerance and gestational diabetes.

Glycosylated hemoglobin levels are elevated above the normal levels of 5% to 7% in the diabetic patient whose serum glucose levels are sustained above normal fasting levels. These results confirm abnormal fasting serum glucose levels above 140 mg/dl. Practitioners should refrain from making inferences regarding glucose control based on isolated HbA_{1c} levels. Serial levels must be obtained and a comparison made over time to gain information regarding overall metabolic control using these results. Sustained values between 8% and 10% require strict glucose control and values above 10% may require aggressive therapy.

LABORATORY TESTING FOR DIABETES

Fasting serum glucose/fasting blood sugar (FBS)
Oral glucose tolerance test (OGTT)
Glycosylated hemoglobin (HbA_{1c})
Glycosylated serum proteins
Glycosuria
Urine/serum ketone levels
Proteinuria
Insulin and c-peptide levels

The remainder of the testing procedures listed in the box are used for obtaining information on patients in specific situations such as brittle or poorly controlled diabetic patients. Urinalysis and evaluation of serum or whole blood ketones are beneficial for patients prone to ketoacidosis or in poorly controlled Type II patients, but they play a minimal role in determining the overall or long-term efficacy of treatment.

TREATMENT OF DIABETES

The goal of therapy for diabetes is to control the levels of hyperglycemia (and acute symptoms), while minimizing the development of chronic complications associated with progression of diabetes. Much controversy surrounds diabetic treatment with respect to the "optimal" blood sugar levels. The maintenance of serum glucose levels within normal ranges has a positive effect in delaying the development of the long-term complications associated with diabetes. Although optimal glucose levels must be determined on an individual basis, there is support for maintaining levels in the normoglycemic ranges during both the preprandial and postprandial periods. Many problems are inherent in this philosophy, considering the impossibility of restoring physiologic responses to the prediabetic state.

The Diabetes Control and Complications Trial (DCCT), which achieved a mean blood glucose level of 155 mg/dl (outside the normoglycemic range), had a proven beneficial effect on the complications associated with diabetes.[33,34] Intensive treatment utilizing three to four insulin injections daily (or an insulin pump) in conjunction with multiple blood sugar readings (four or more) was compared with the conventional insulin regimen. Intensive therapy has demonstrated the beneficial effects of this level of control on the development of diabetic retinopathy, nephropathy, and neuropathy. Unfortunately, a higher incidence of hypoglycemia by a 2:1 or 3:1 margin was also associated with intensive therapy. Strict glycemic control in the DCCT did not have a beneficial effect for IDDM patients with severe hypoglycemia, hypoglycemic unawareness, or pre-existing advanced complications like ESRD, coronary artery disease, or cerebrovascular disease. Inferences regarding the effects of this same level of glycemic control and chronic complications for NIDDM patients could not be made at the conclusion of the study. The traditional concept of optimal glycemic control for IDDM as well as NIDDM patients is challenged by the results of the DCCT, and the impact of this study will be determined by future clinical experiences. Achievement of normoglycemic levels has not proven to be a cure for diabetic patients, but it now has proven efficacy in IDDM patients and remains the therapeutic goal for NIDDM patients.

The use of home monitoring devices is very helpful to patients and serves as a feedback device to help the patient relate any symptoms to their level of glycemic control. The health care practitioner also benefits from the use of home monitoring devices by using the patient's daily log to provide invaluable information concerning the efficacy of the treatment regimen.

A successful treatment regimen must be deeply rooted in patient education. Because patients play an important role in controlling their blood sugar, they need to understand the impact of diabetic control on the development of the acute and chronic complications related to diabetes. Life-style changes, including dietary restrictions and increased activity, are the patients' responsibility, and their understanding of the relationship between life-style changes and glycemic control is necessary. This is the first step in enhancing the body's

response to insulin without the use of pharmacologic agents. The American Diabetes Association (ADA) recommends a diet consisting of 30% fat, 20% protein, and 50% carbohydrates, with the total number of calories to be determined by the ideal body weight charts (related to age and height).[35,36] Physical activity increases the body's demand for glucose and enhances the effect of insulin. An increase in insulin-binding ability occurs with exercise, thereby utilizing available glucose more efficiently and decreasing the level of hyperglycemia by nonpharmacologic means.

Pharmacologic agents are necessary for control of hyperglycemia for Type I diabetes and for Type II diabetes when diet and exercise are inadequate for control of hyperglycemia. Exogenous insulin is essential for the treatment of Type I diabetes, with the type and dosage determined by the severity of hyperglycemia.[37,38] Insulin pumps have been very effective in regulating hyperglycemic events by both the open- and closed-loop devices.[39] These devices have not gained the favor of the medical community for routine use in diabetic therapy for numerous reasons, including the need for strict patient compliance, the risks of sepsis and local reactions at the subcutaneous infusion pump, and the poor portability of the units presently available.

Bedtime dosages of insulin (at low levels) decrease the overnight free fatty acid level, thereby reducing the severity of the early morning hyperglycemia in Type II diabetic patients.[40] Supplemental insulin is used in Type II diabetes patients when oral hypoglycemic agents fail to provide strict glycemic control. Exogenous insulin is also necessary for Type II diabetic patients during periods of emotional or physical stress when hyperglycemia exists. The Type II diabetic person is not considered insulin-dependent under these situations because the use of insulin is temporary. Oral hypoglycemic agents (*sulfonylurea drugs*) stimulate the release of insulin from the β-cells of the pancreas.[41,42] These agents are very effective in the treatment of Type II diabetes considering that a relative deficiency in the production and release of insulin exists which progresses with time. Controversy still exists regarding the mechanism of action of sulfonylurea medications and their effect on enhancing the receptor response to insulin in peripheral tissues. This mechanism is not proven clinically but could provide an adjunctive treatment modality for Type I diabetes.

Other systemic treatment modalities for diabetes have been explored in the hopes of minimizing the chronic complications if not finding a cure. Islet cell transplantation has proven beneficial in stabilizing or inhibiting the progression of retinopathy after a 5-year follow-up but is of little benefit for diabetic nephropathy after 1-year follow-up.[43] Patients with combined kidney and pancreatic transplants fared much better, with improved glomerular filtration rates compared with those of diabetic patients who received only one organ transplant (either kidney or pancreas). Any significant effect that transplantation has on the development of macrovascular disease is not confirmed, but hope remains in avoiding these complications. Type I diabetic patients account for most transplant recipients at this time.

Pharmaceutical agents whose primary action does not involve decreasing serum glucose levels have been used very effectively in the management of diabetic disease. The treatment of diabetes-associated coronary artery disease, congestive heart failure, cardiac arrhythmia, and cerebrovascular disease is by conventional means. Trental (pentoxyphylline) is beneficial for diabetic (as well as nondiabetic) claudication associated with peripheral vascular disease of the lower extremities.[44] Aldose reductase inhibitors decrease the accumulation of myoinositol in peripheral nerves of diabetic animals, thereby improving the nerve conduction to a limited degree, but nerve conduction and axonal flow may be only marginally improved. Aldose reductase inhibitors in conjunction with insulin can prevent the capillary basement membrane thickening in the deep capillary beds of the retina but have little effect on the vessel walls of the superficial retinal capillary beds.[45] It is not known if this combined therapy will prove beneficial for preventing long-term microvascular complications throughout the body. Enhanced insulin response in

the prediabetic state has been achieved in diabetic rats with the use of lithium salts and may prove to be beneficial in decreasing the insulin resistance seen with Type II diabetes. Further clinical research is needed.[46] Peripheral neuropathy (sensory) is currently improved with the use of low doses of Elavil for many Type I and Type II diabetic persons.

Present clinical research may reveal information regarding the exact pathogenic mechanisms and could provide a preventive treatment for diabetes. A decrease in the severity or prevention of long-term complications, which may result from future clinical trials, will enhance the quality of life for both Type I and Type II diabetic patients.

OCULAR COMPLICATIONS OF DIABETES MELLITUS*

Microvascular complications of diabetes mellitus generate significant health problems, principally related to neuropathy, nephropathy, and retinopathy. Although diabetic retinopathy is the ocular complication most commonly associated with diabetes mellitus, diabetic eye disease represents an end-organ response to a generalized medical condition; consequently, diabetes affects virtually all ocular structures (Table 13-1).

Patients with IDDM and NIDDM alike are at risk for diabetic retinopathy and diabetic ocular complications. Some ocular complications are of minor importance, such as premature presbyopia, and some, such as nerve palsies, are disconcerting and interfere with visual function but are usually self-limited. Vision loss, whether permanent or temporary, partial or complete, has more significant ramifications. The strategies for appropriate treatment of patients with diabetic retinopathy have been determined largely by three nationwide clinical trials—the Diabetic Retinopathy Study (DRS),[48-61] the Early Treatment Diabetic Retinop-

---

*This section was originally published in Cavallerano J: Ocular manifestations of diabetes mellitus, Optometry Clinics 2:2, 93-116, 1992. Reprinted by permission of Appleton & Lange, Inc.

TABLE 13-1 *Ocular Complications of Diabetes Mellitus*

Structure	Complication
Retina	Diabetic retinopathy
	Macular edema
	Optic disc pallor
	Optic disc swelling
Extraocular muscles	Nerve palsies
Cornea	Decreased sensitivity
	Corneal abrasion
	Recurrent erosion
Iris	Rubeosis iridis
	Ectropion uveae
Lens	Refractive changes
	Cataract

athy Study (ETDRS),[62-74] and the Diabetic Retinopathy Vitrectomy Study (DRVS).[75-79] As these studies have demonstrated, proper examination, monitoring, referral, and treatment can reduce the 5-year risk of severe visual loss from diabetic retinopathy to 5% or less.

Epidemiologic Factors

An estimated 14 to 15 million Americans have diabetes, but half of these cases are undiagnosed and the individuals are unaware of their condition. Diabetes is a leading cause of new blindness among working-age Americans, and any person with diabetes is at risk of ocular complications and visual loss. Vision loss from diabetes generally results from nonresolving vitreous hemorrhage; proliferative retinopathy leading to fibrous tissue formation and subsequent retinal or tractional retinal detachment; or diabetic macular edema.

Studies suggest that in the United States the prevalence of proliferative diabetic retinopathy (PDR) is 700,000 and the prevalence of macular edema (DME) is 500,000 cases. The annual projected incidence of new cases of PDR and DME is 65,000 and 75,000, respectively.[80-81] Persons

with PDR are at risk of severe visual loss, which is defined as best corrected vision of 5/200 or worse. Persons with DME are at risk of moderate visual loss, which is defined as a doubling of the visual angle (such as 20/40 reduced to 20/80).

Timely and appropriate laser surgery can reduce the 5-year risk of severe visual loss from PDR to 5% or less and can reduce the risk of moderate visual loss from DME by at least 50%, to 12% or less. Therefore, optometrists have a significant role in identifying patients at risk for visual loss that is amenable to surgical intervention; optometrists have an obligation to refer these patients for appropriate care.

Diabetic Retinopathy

Retinal complications of diabetes receive significant attention because these changes are usually the most sight-threatening. The processes by which diabetes result in retinopathy are not fully understood, but insulin deficiency and elevated blood glucose levels apparently are sufficient to cause diabetic retinopathy. Structural, physiologic, and hormonal changes cause the retinal capillaries to become functionally less competent, and the various lesions of diabetic retinopathy consequently develop (Table 13-2).

Classification and Stages of Diabetic Retinopathy. Diabetic changes in the retina have led to various classifications of the levels of diabetic retinopathy, most recently by the ETDRS[73] (see box on p. 271). The two broad categories of diabetic retinopathy are nonproliferative (NPDR) and proliferative (PDR) diabetic retinopathy. The ETDRS has established the risk of progression to PDR and high risk for PDR based on the level of NPDR.[73,80] Also, PDR less than high risk has significant risk of evolving to the high-risk stage. DME can be present at any level of NPDR or PDR and needs to be considered regardless of the level of retinopathy.

Nonproliferative diabetic retinopathy (NPDR). Diabetic retinopathy may be present at diagnosis of Type II diabetes and is usually present after 15 years of IDDM. In mild NPDR there is at least one retinal hemorrhage and/or microaneurysm (H/

TABLE 13-2 *Lesions of Diabetic Retinopathy*

Nonproliferative	Microaneurysms
	Hard exudates
	Intraretinal hemorrhages
	Dot/blot
	Flame-shaped
	Cotton-wool spots
	Intraretinal microvascular abnormalities (IRMA)
	Capillary and arteriolar occlusion
	Venous caliber abnormalities
Proliferative	Neovascularization on the disc and elsewhere
	Fibrous proliferation
	Vitreous hemorrhage
Macula	Macular edema
	Hard exudates
	Capillary nonperfusion

MA), but the degree of H/MA is less than depicted in standard photo 2A of the modified Airlie House Classification of Diabetic Retinopathy* (Fig. 13-4). No other diabetic retinal changes are present. If no macular edema is present and the H/MA is not in the macular area, mild NPDR does not present a threat to vision. Mild NPDR has a 5% risk of progression to PDR in 1 year and a 15% risk of progression to high-risk PDR within 5 years.[73] Annual examination with fundus photographs as indicated is generally sufficient if macular edema or other medical condition such as hypertension, renal disease, elevated lipid levels, or pregnancy is not present. The patient's medical doctor should be informed of examination results, even if minimal or no diabetic retinopathy is present.

In moderate NPDR, H/MA greater than standard photo 2A in four retinal photographic fields is present and no fields have greater severity, *or*

cotton-wool spots, venous beading, or *intraretinal microvascular abnormalities (IRMA)* of mild degree are present. Moderate NPDR has a 12% to 27% risk of progressing to PDR in 1 year and a 33% risk of progressing to high-risk PDR in 5 years.[73] Careful examination with an indirect ophthalmoscope, fundus contact lens, or fundus lens with the biomicroscope is necessary to establish the diagnosis. Fundus photography is strongly suggested, and repeat evaluation in 6 to 10 months is appropriate if no macular edema or complicating medical or risk factors are present. Although patients with mild or moderate NPDR generally are not candidates for scatter (panretinal) laser surgery, the presence of macular edema requires more frequent evaluation, consultation with a retinologist,* and, if *clinically significant macular edema (CSME)* is present, focal laser photocoagulation. Misdiagnosis at this level of retinopathy is hazardous and significantly underestimates a patient's risk of progression to PDR.

In severe NPDR H/MA greater than standard photo 2A is present in four retinal quadrants *or* moderate venous beading (greater than or equal to standard photo 6B) (Fig. 13-5) is present in at least one quadrant, *or* moderate IRMA (greater than or equal to standard photo 8A) (Fig. 13-6) is present in at least one retinal quadrant without frank neovascularization. Severe NPDR has a 52% risk of progressing to PDR in 1 year and a 60% risk of progressing to high-risk PDR in 5 years.[73] Follow-up every 2 to 3 months in consultation with a retinologist is advisable, and *scatter (panretinal) laser photocoagulation,* as determined by the clinical judgment of the retinologist, may be indicated. Focal laser treatment for CSME is strongly indicated because of the risk of development of PDR and high-risk PDR, and non-CSME may require focal treatment.

In very severe NPDR two or more criteria of severe NPDR are met. Very severe NPDR carries a substantial risk of progressing to PDR in 1 year

*In 1968 the Airlie House Symposium on Diabetic Retinopathy designated certain "standard photographs" to document levels and severity of diabetic retinopathy. These photographic standards were modified by the ETDRS research group.

*The term "retinologist" is used in this chapter to denote an ophthalmologist experienced in the management and treatment of diabetic retinopathy.

CLINICAL LEVELS OF RETINOPATHY

Nonproliferative diabetic retinopathy
    Mild stage
        At least one microaneurysm
        Definition not met for moderate NPDR or worse
    Moderate stage
        Hemorrhages and/or MA $\geq$ standard photo 2A (Fig. 13-4)
        Soft exudates, venous beading, and IRMA definitely present
        Definition not met for severe NPDR or worse
    Severe stage
        Soft exudates, venous beading, and IRMA all definitely present in at least two fields 4-7 (Fig. 13-5) or
        2 of 3 preceding lesions present in at least two fields 4-7 and H/MA in these four fields = 2A in at least
            one of them or
        IRMA present in fields 4-7 = standard photo 8A in two of them (Fig. 13-6)
        Definition not met for very severe NPDR or worse
    Very severe stage
        At least two of the criteria for severe stage not met for PDR

Proliferative diabetic retinopathy
    Composed of
        NVD or NVE
        Preretinal or vitreous hemorrhage
        Fibrous tissue proliferation
    Early PDR
        New vessels
        Definition not met for high-risk PDR
    High-risk PDR
        NVD $\geq$ 1/3-1/2 disc area (Fig. 13-7)
        NVD and vitreous or preretinal hemorrhage
        NVE $\geq$ 1/2 disc area and preretinal or vitreous hemorrhage

Clinically significant macular edema
    Thickening of the retina located 500 μ or less from the center of the macula
    Hard exudates with thickening of the adjacent retina located 500 μ or less from the center of the macula
    A zone of retinal thickening, one disc area or larger in size, located one disc diameter or less from the center
        of the macula

MA, microaneurysm; NPDR, nonproliferative diabetic retinopathy; IRMA, intraretinal microvascular abnormalities; H/MA, hemorrhage/microaneurysm; PDR, proliferative diabetic retinopathy; NVD, new vessel growth on the optic disc; NDE, new vessel growth elsewhere on the retina.

and high-risk PDR in 5 years. Follow-up evaluation every 2 to 3 months is suggested. Severe and very severe NPDR and PDR that is not high risk may require early scatter laser surgery, particularly if *neovascularization of the disc (NVD)* or elevated new vessels are present. Patients with moderate NPDR or worse are considered for focal treatment of macular edema whether the macular edema is

clinically significant or not, in preparation for the possible future need of scatter laser photocoagulation. Consultation with a retinologist is indicated.

Proliferative diabetic retinopathy (PDR). PDR is marked by NVD or *neovascularization elsewhere* on the retina *(NVE)* or by fibrous tissue proliferation. PDR that has not reached high-risk PDR has a 75% risk of progressing to high-risk PDR within

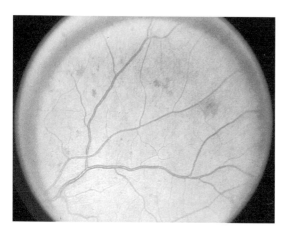

FIG. 13-4 Standard photograph 2A of the Modified Airlie House Classification of Diabetic Retinopathy demonstrating a moderate degree of hemorrhages and/or microaneurysms. *(Courtesy of the DRS Research Group.)*

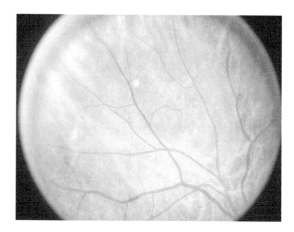

FIG. 13-6 Standard photograph 8A of the Modified Airlie House Classification of Diabetic Retinopathy demonstrating intraretinal microvascular abnormalities (IRMA). *(Courtesy of the DRS Research Group.)*

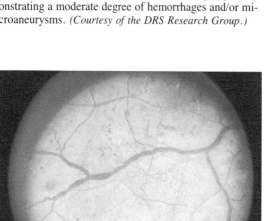

FIG. 13-5 Standard photograph 6B of the Modified Airlie House Classification of Diabetic Retinopathy demonstrating venous beading. *(Courtesy of the DRS Research Group.)*

a 5-year period.[73] Scatter laser photocoagulation may be indicated, and macular edema, even if not clinically significant, may benefit from treatment. Prompt referral to a retinologist is indicated.

The DRS conclusively demonstrated that scatter laser photocoagulation surgery significantly reduces the risk of severe visual loss from PDR.[55] Furthermore, this study identified specific retinal lesions that pose a significant threat of visual loss. The presence of any one of the following lesions constitutes high-risk PDR[55]:

Neovascularization on the disc or within one disc diameter of the nerve head (NVD) greater than approximately ¼ to ⅓ the disc area (that is, NVD equal to or greater than that pictured in standard photo 10A (Fig. 13-7); *or*

Neovascularization on the disc or within one disc diameter of the nerve head (NVD) less than approximately ¼ to ⅓ the disc area if fresh preretinal or vitreous hemorrhage is present; *or*

NVE on the retina if fresh preretinal or vitreous hemorrhage is present (Fig. 13-8).

To identify high-risk PDR, attention must be paid to the presence or absence of new vessels, the location of any new vessels, the severity of any new vessels, and the presence or absence of preretinal or vitreous hemorrhages. The risk of severe visual loss can be reduced by at least 50% if scatter laser surgery is initiated for eyes with high-risk PDR; consequently, all patients who demonstrate high-risk PDR should be referred immediately (within 24 hours) to a retinologist.

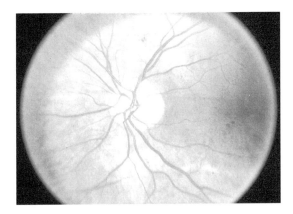

FIG. 13-7 Standard photograph 10A of the Modified Airlie House Classification of Diabetic Retinopathy demonstrating neovascularization of the optic disc covering approximately ¼ to ⅓ of the disc area. *(Courtesy of the DRS Research Group.)*

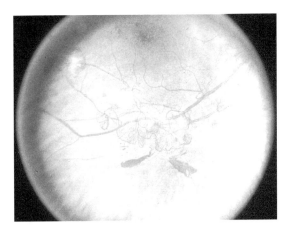

FIG. 13-8 Standard photograph 7 of the Modified Airlie House Classification of Diabetic Retinopathy demonstrating new vessels elsewhere (NVE) in the retina with fresh hemorrhage. *(Courtesy of the DRS Research Group.)*

Eyes with PDR which has not advanced to the high-risk stage should be considered similarly to eyes with high-risk PDR. Many retinologists consider scatter laser photocoagulation for eyes with PDR less than high risk, particularly if extenuating circumstances are present, such as poor patient compliance with examination regularity, the development of cataracts, or associated medical conditions such as difficulty in managing the diabetes, hypertension, nephropathy, or pregnancy. These same considerations pertain for patients with severe or very severe NPDR. The risk of severe visual loss from PDR may be as high as 60%, and the risk of moderate visual loss from DME may be as high as 25% to 30%. Timely and appropriate laser surgery, however, can reduce the 5-year risk of severe vision loss from PDR to 5% or less and the risk of moderate vision loss from DME by at least 50%.

The ETDRS investigated whether earlier scatter photocoagulation, performed before the development of high-risk retinopathy, further reduced the risk of severe vision loss. This investigation was necessary because the DRS did not provide a clear choice between prompt laser surgery and deferral of laser surgery unless there was progression to high-risk retinopathy. The ETDRS findings estab-

lished that early treatment, compared with deferral of photocoagulation until high-risk retinopathy develops, was associated with a small reduction in the incidence of severe visual loss, but 5-year rates were low for both the early treatment group and the group assigned to deferral of treatment (2.6% versus 3.7%).[70]

Scatter laser surgery generally is not recommended for eyes with mild or moderate NPDR. When retinopathy is more severe, scatter photocoagulation is considered and usually should not be delayed if the eye has reached the high-risk proliferative stage. Patients with signs of DME or severe NPDR or worse or with PDR that does not fulfill the definition of high-risk retinopathy should be referred to a retinologist for scatter laser photocoagulation. The goal of laser surgery is to induce regression of neovascularization without vitreous hemorrhage or fibrovascular proliferation resulting in retinal detachment or macular dragging.

Diabetic Macular Edema

Macular edema is the collection of intraretinal fluid in the macular area of the retina with or without lipid exudates or cystoid changes; it can occur at any stage of retinopathy. There may be nonper-

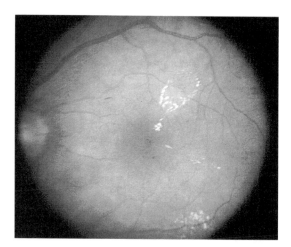

FIG. 13-9 Hard exudates in the macular area. There is adjacent retinal thickening, not appreciated without stereoscopic viewing.

fusion of the parafoveal capillaries or intraretinal or preretinal hemorrhages. Macular edema that threatens the center of the macula is considered "clinically significant."

Clinically significant macular edema as defined by the ETDRS includes any one of the following lesions[64]:

Thickening at or within 500 microns from the center of the macula; or

Hard exudates at or within 500 microns from the center of the macula, if there is thickening of the adjacent retina (Fig. 13-9); or

An area or areas of thickening at least one disc area in size, at least part of which is within one disc diameter of the center of the macula.

A person may have no ocular or visual symptoms in the early stages of DME, but as the process progresses the patient may notice a dramatic or subtle decrease in vision, a change in color perception, or a warping or bending of straight lines (such as the tile patterns on floors or bathroom walls). The ETDRS has conclusively demonstrated that treatment of DME reduces the risk of moderate visual loss by at least 50%. Because DME, like PDR, may cause no symptoms in the most treatable stages, all person with diabetes should be en-

couraged to have an annual comprehensive eye examination performed by an experienced and skilled examiner.

Clinical Considerations

Although there are no cures for diabetic retinopathy and DME, and no methods to prevent their occurrence, appropriate surgical modalities minimize the risk of visual loss and in some cases restore useful vision for those who have suffered visual loss.

For patients with CSME, focal laser surgery not only reduces the risk of moderate visual loss but also increases the chance of small improvements in visual acuity.[63] Because the principal benefit of treatment is the prevention of further decrease in visual acuity, focal laser surgery should be considered for all eyes with CSME, even if normal visual acuity is present. Both early scatter photocoagulation (before high-risk PDR) and deferral of treatment until high-risk retinopathy develops are effective in reducing the risk of severe visual loss from PDR. Although scatter laser photocoagulation generally is not indicated for mild to moderate NPDR, treatment can be considered as retinopathy approaches the high-risk stage and usually should not be delayed when the high-risk stage is present.

Minor errors in diagnosis of the severity of retinopathy significantly underestimate the risk of progression of retinopathy. Retinopathy levels are precisely defined by the ETDRS (on a scale up to level 90),[73] and the diagnosis of the precise level of retinopathy is not an easy task. Figure 13-10 demonstrates the risk of progression to high-risk PDR for eyes with varying levels of retinopathy at baseline.[70] Eyes with more severe retinopathy at baseline have a significantly greater risk of progressing to high-risk PDR within the follow-up period. Of equal importance, however, is the dramatic increase in rate of progression for eyes with retinopathy at the moderately severe NPDR level or worse. For example, at 1-year follow-up, the incidence rate of progression to high-risk PDR for a person with moderate NPDR is 33%, whereas the incidence rate for a person with severe NPDR

Rate of progression (%)

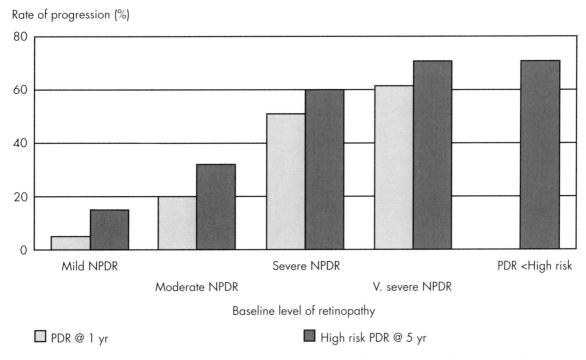

FIG. 13-10 Diagram indicating the risk of progression to high-risk proliferative diabetic retinopathy based on severity of retinopathy at time of entrance into the Early Treatment Diabetic Retinopathy Study. *(Adapted from ETDRS Report No. 12,[73] Ophthalmology, 98:823, 1991.)*

is 60%. The rate of progression to high-risk PDR for a person who already has some proliferative disease is 50% or more within a 1-year period and 75% within 5 years. Proper diagnosis of retinopathy level and of the risk of visual loss and prompt referral—particularly when macular edema is present or the retinopathy has reached or surpassed the moderate NPDR stage—are critical.

Clinically, patients with high-risk PDR should be referred immediately to a retinologist for laser surgery (usually within 24 hours); those with CSME should be referred for laser surgery in a timely fashion (usually within 2 weeks). Furthermore, eyes that are approaching PDR (that is, with severe or very severe NPDR or PDR that is not yet high risk) should be referred for consideration of laser surgery and certainly require careful observation by or consultation with a retinologist. Macular edema or retinal lesions that threaten the center of the macula also require specialist's care. Consultation with a retinologist should be obtained whenever thickening or hard exudates or hemorrhages in the macular area are seen or suspected. The closer the retinopathy status is to high-risk diabetic retinopathy, the more frequently examinations are needed. Patients should be advised that laser treatment does not cure retinopathy but merely reduces the risk of severe or moderate visual loss. The possible complications and side effects of laser photocoagulation should also be discussed (see box on p. 276).

Refractive Changes. Fluctuations in refractive error are common with diabetes. In general, elevated blood glucose levels increase myopia or decrease hyperopia in phakic eyes.[82-85] This shift in refraction can occur relatively quickly—within hours or less, but patients who consistently run elevated blood glucose levels find that their refrac-

POSSIBLE SIDE EFFECTS AND COMPLICATIONS OF SCATTER (PANRETINAL) LASER SURGERY

Constricted visual fields
Night blindness
Mild decrease in visual acuity
Macular edema
Serous and/or choroidal detachment
Angle-closure glaucoma
Decreased pupillary response
Decreased accommodation
Cornea and/or lens burns
Pain

tion or vision may not return to normal for several weeks or more after stabilization of glycemic control.

Symptomatically, a person with elevated blood glucose levels or with undiagnosed diabetes who is first experiencing elevated blood glucose levels may have blurred distance vision while the reading vision has cleared. Hyperopic persons may find that they no longer need their glasses to see clearly at a distance. Those who use glasses for reading only may find that their distance vision has become blurred but their reading vision seems clearer, even without their glasses.

The case history is useful in implicating blood glucose levels as a source of blurred or fluctuating vision in a patient who has or is suspected of having diabetes. In general, refractive changes that are not characteristic for a person's age are suspect. The patient should be questioned about blood glucose levels and the methods used for testing diabetic control. Testing with urine strips, although relatively inexpensive, depends heavily on an individual's renal threshold and is generally discouraged. Home self-monitoring meters can occasionally be unreliable. Also, hemoglobin A_{1c} (glycosylated hemoglobin) tests provide an *average* of blood glucose levels for the preceding few months, and even excellent readings may mask some elevations of blood glucose levels. Because blurred vision may be a presenting symptom of undiag-

nosed diabetes, patients without known diabetes should be questioned concerning a family history of diabetes and other medical conditions.

Discussions of refractive changes associated with diabetes frequently are directed to myopic shifts related to elevated blood glucose levels, but diabetes also affects accommodative ability.[82,86] Presbyopia may develop at an earlier age than normal, and transient accommodative paralysis accompanied by hyperopia may be associated with either a rise or fall in blood glucose levels, most frequently after insulin treatment has been started, and may be present even in young persons.

Reduced accommodative ability and diminished pupillary response sometimes follow scatter laser photocoagulation surgery.[87] This internal ophthalmoplegia is the result of direct injury to the parasympathetic motor fibers to the ciliary body and the iris, which enter the globe at the posterior pole and course forward between the sclera and the choroid. Anteriorly, the choroid becomes thinner, providing less protection to the underlying fibers against the heat generated in the retinal pigment epithelium from the photocoagulation. Unlike the paresis of accommodation associated with uncontrolled diabetes, internal ophthalmoplegia secondary to panretinal photocoagulation is generally irreversible because the laser burns cause permanent damage to the underlying parasympathetic nerve fibers.

Cataracts. Cataracts can cause fluctuating vision (particularly in varying light environments or with different tasks), a dimming of vision, a loss of contrast, or uncomfortable or disabling glare, especially for night driving or on bright, sunny days. Mild cataracts in conjunction with macular edema, vitreous hemorrhage, or prior laser treatments frequently cause visual symptoms disproportionate to the degree of cataract.

Age-related cataracts develop at a younger age and progress more rapidly in diabetic persons than in individuals who do not have diabetes.[82,88-92] Metabolic or "true" diabetic cataracts are relatively rare because they apparently result from prolonged periods of hyperglycemia. These cataracts, which are sometimes called "Christmas tree" cataracts because of their appearance, are sometimes partially reversible.[82,93-104]

Currently, the only treatment for cataracts is surgical removal of the clouded lens. Posterior chamber intraocular lens implantation is desirable, although the young age of a patient may be a mitigating factor in the type and timing of surgery. Because ocular surgery is a risk factor for the progression of retinopathy, a person with diabetes should have his or her retinal status evaluated as carefully as possible before cataract surgery.[105] Scatter laser photocoagulation before cataract extraction, or, if possible, waiting for PDR to enter a quiescent stage, may be appropriate. Laser surgery may need to be initiated soon after cataract surgery. A cataract that interferes with retinal examination or laser surgery may need to be removed, even if a patient does not complain of visual symptoms from the cataract, to provide clear media for focal or scatter laser photocoagulation.

Another consideration is the delayed wound healing that accompanies diabetes. Care must be taken in the postoperative period to monitor wound healing as well as retinal status. Recovery time following successful cataract extraction for a diabetic patient may be prolonged even if no complications arise.

Cornea. The cornea of a person with diabetes injures more easily and heals more slowly than the cornea of a person who does not have diabetes. This relative fragility of the cornea stems from a number of factors.[82,106-113] Corneal sensitivity, which may normally alert a person to either a dry-eye syndrome or a foreign body, may be reduced. Consequently, a minor problem may go unnoticed, resulting in corneal abrasion or ulceration. Reduced sensitivity is also significant because, structurally, the cornea of a diabetic person is more prone to injury. In a healthy eye, the basement membrane firmly attaches the corneal epithelium to the underlying corneal layers. This basement membrane is structurally altered by diabetes, and a cornea that is injured tends to heal more slowly and less completely.

Because of the increased risk of infection and the potential for harm to the cornea, diabetic patients fitted with contact lenses should be monitored closely. These patients need to be made fully aware of the potential complications and problems from lens wear. Generally, extended-wear contact lenses are contraindicated, and patients with unilateral visual loss should avoid contact lenses completely. Glasses with polycarbonate lenses provide an added level of protection for monocular patients.

A diabetic person with a corneal abrasion needs to be alerted to the risk of recurrent corneal erosions. Artificial tears may reduce this risk, especially in excessively dry environments. Some patients may need to add humidifiers to their homes. Other environmental situations, such as air-conditioned offices; air conditioners, heaters, or defrosters in cars; and dusty warehouses or stores, may contribute to a recurrence of the original abrasion, again indicating the need for lubricants. Iatrogenic abrasions can result from procedures such as applanation tonometry, gonioscopy, fundus contact lens examination, laser surgery, and vitrectomy.

Careful, aggressive treatment for corneal abrasions helps minimize complications. Topical antibiotics guard against infection, and a pressure patch or bandage contact lens may aid the healing process. When the abrasion has healed, an eye lubricant or ointment may be indicated. Recurrent erosions frequently occur upon awakening, caused by overnight corneal dehydration and the mechanical action of the eyelid opening for the first time in the morning.

Glaucoma. Although acute angle-closure glaucoma does not seem to be more common in diabetic individuals than in the general population, primary open-angle glaucoma is more common among diabetic individuals (4.0%) than among those without diabetes (1.8%).[82] Treatment of open-angle glaucoma in diabetic persons is influenced by a patient's general medical condition. Caution must be exercised with the use of topical beta-blockers, for they may mask hypoglycemic symptoms or adversely affect cardiovascular disease. Acetazolamide (Diamox) or other carbonic anhydrase inhibitors may cause electrolyte imbalance and may produce severe systemic side effects, and careful medical monitoring is essential. The presence of renal disease may influence the choice of medications.

Neovascular glaucoma is a serious complication of diabetes resulting from new vessel growth on the iris of the eye, similar to neovascularization on the retina.[82,114-119] This new vessel growth, *rubeosis iridis* or neovascularization on the iris, is most likely in response to relative retinal hypoxia. PDR is not necessarily present if iris neovascularization is observed, and new vessel growth can develop on the iris in the absence of diabetes mellitus. Usually, rubeosis begins near the pupillary border (Fig. 13-11). If the blood vessels extend over the iris and interfere with aqueous outflow, neovascular glaucoma may result. This type of glaucoma is frequently difficult to treat, and the retinologist may consult a glaucoma specialist to assist in the management. Laser treatments or other surgical modalities may be required, in addition to topical and systemic medications such as beta-adrenergic blocking agents or carbonic anhydrase inhibitors, which are used to depress aqueous formation and thereby lower intraocular pressure. Cycloplegic agents and topical steroid eye drops may be prescribed to reduce local ocular inflammation and relieve some of the associated pain. Frequently, pan-

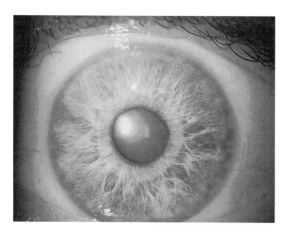

FIG. 13-11 Clinical appearance of rubeosis iridis at the pupil border.

retinal photocoagulation is effective in reducing rubeosis iridis.[120-123] If panretinal photocoagulation is impossible because of severe cataracts or vitreous hemorrhage, direct treatment of the new vessels in the filtration angle of the eye with goniophotocoagulation may be necessary.[124] When maximum laser and medical intervention fails, intractable neovascular glaucoma may be treated with filtration surgery or Molteno valve implants.

Patients with early rubeosis iridis are usually asymptomatic. In advanced stages patients may complain of redness of the eye or of pain, and sometimes they note decreased vision and light sensitivity. Routine eye examination should include evaluation of the iris with a biomicroscope slit lamp by an experienced observer. Gonioscopy is indicated for those with rubeosis to ensure that there is no threat of angle closure. In some cases, rubeosis can appear in the angle before presentation at the pupil border. Rubeosis iridis is a proliferative lesion, and referral to a retinologist is indicated even if intraocular pressures are within normal range and there is no angle involvement.

Nerve Palsies. Mononeuropathy of the third, fourth, or sixth cranial nerve is an uncommon but dramatic complication of diabetes, occurring in 4% of cases.[82,125-134] The third nerve (oculomotor) is most commonly affected, followed by the sixth (abducens) and, infrequently, the fourth (trochlear). The most common symptom caused by a cranial nerve palsy is double vision; headache or pain over the affected eye can also be present.

Third nerve palsies usually result in the affected eye being turned down and out. A full or partial ptosis or drooping of the upper lid of the affected eye may be present. These patients usually complain of double vision. Sparing of the pupillary fibers is usually considered a sign that a third nerve palsy is of diabetic origin, but as many as 20% of cases secondary to diabetes have pupillary involvement.[135-137] These cases pose a significant diagnostic challenge, especially if the diabetes or previous laser treatments have affected the pupillary response.

Patients with sixth nerve palsies usually have an esotropic posture. Because the sixth nerve controls abduction, patients with sixth nerve weaknesses have a weakness or inability to turn the affected eye temporally (past the midline in extreme cases). Some persons compensate for this problem by turning their heads in the direction of the affected eye to reduce the need to abduct the eye.

Fourth nerve palsies result in a combination of vertical and lateral diplopia. The patient may present with a head tilt or complain of a tilting image.

Care of patients with nerve palsies involves ruling out other causes for the palsy. Differential diagnosis includes Graves' disease, herpes zoster, cranial aneurysms, and mass lesions. Because other causes may be life-threatening, consultation with the patient's internist, *diabetologist,* and— frequently—a neurologist is in order. Ocular treatment for the palsies is palliative. Double vision can be eliminated by occluding one eye. In some cases, the unaffected eye may be occluded if the acuity in the other eye is better. Patients should be advised that diabetes-related palsies are usually self-limited and that they typically resolve within 6 weeks to 6 months or more.

Summary

Clinical care of the patient with diabetes requires annual, comprehensive examination through dilated pupils; both a full retinal evaluation and stereoscopic evaluation of the macula should be provided by an experienced examiner. Visual acuity, Amsler grid, color vision, or other adjunct tests are not diagnostic for macular edema or diabetic retinopathy, and no examination of vision or visual function can replace a stereoscopic evaluation of the posterior pole.

Additional specific examination criteria should be addressed to aid in the proper evaluation of patients. A patient's internist or diabetologist should be informed of the results of all eye examinations and advised of the patient's retinal status. Patients whose eyes that are not correctable to 20/20 or that exhibit abnormal Amsler grid testing should be referred to a retinal specialist or ophthalmologist experienced in the management and treatment of diabetic eye disease for evaluation.

Complete documentation of findings should be provided, including description of the presence or absence of rubeosis iridis; retinal hemorrhages and/or microaneurysms and, if present, whether they are greater or less than standard photo 2A; neovascularization at the disc and elsewhere; other retinal findings such as cotton-wool spots, intraretinal microvascular abnormalities, and venous beading; and macular hemorrhages, microaneurysms, and/or retinal thickening.

The goal of the examination is to identify patients with high-risk PDR and CSME who require laser surgery. A further goal is to identify patients who are approaching or reaching high-risk PDR (that is, patients with severe or very severe NPDR or PDR that is not quite high risk). Consultation with a retinologist should be initiated for all patients who are approaching or reaching high-risk PDR or who have macular edema, and those with high-risk PDR should be evaluated within 24 hours by a retinal specialist. Patients with CSME should be evaluated within 2 weeks. Careful examination, referral, and patient education by dedicated clinicians can preserve vision and virtually eliminate severe visual loss resulting from diabetes.

ACKNOWLEDGMENT

Special thanks to Lora Potter for her assistance in the preparation of this manuscript.

References

1. Trends in diabetes mellitus mortality, *MMWR* 37(50), December 23, 1988.
2. Geiss LS and others: Surveillance for diabetes mellitus—United States, 1980–1989, *MMWR* 42 (SS-2), June 4, 1993.
3. Himsworth HP: Diabetes mellitus: its differentiation into insulin-sensitive and insulin-insensitive types, *Lancet* 1936, p 117.
4. Gepts W: Pathologic anatomy of the pancreas in juvenile diabetes mellitus, *Diabetes* 4:619, 1965.
5. MacCuish AC and Irvine WJ: Autoimmune aspects of diabetes mellitus, *Clin Endocrinol Metab* 4:435, 1975.

6. Bottazzo GF and others: In situ characterization of autoimmune phenomenon and expression of HLA molecules in the pancreas of diabetic insulitis, *N Engl J Med* 313:353, 1985.

7. Friedlaender MH: Neurologic and endocrine diseases. In *Allergy and immunology of the eye,* ed 2, New York, 1993, Raven Press.

8. Salans LB and Cushman SW: *Relationship of adiposity and diet to the abnormalities of carbohydrate metabolism in obesity.* In Katzen HL and Mahler RJ, editors: *Advances in modern nutrition, vol 2, Diabetes, obesity and vascular disease,* New York, 1978, John Wiley & Sons.

9. Greene DA: Metabolic abnormalities in the diabetic peripheral nerve:relation to impaired function, *Metabolism* 32 (suppl 1):118, 1983.

10. Greene DA, Lattimer SA, and Sima AAF: Sorbitol, phospoinositides and potassium-ATPase in the pathogenesis of diabetic complications, *N Engl J Med* 316:599, 1985.

11. Clements RS Jr: Diabetic neuropathy—new concepts of its etiology, Diabetes 28:604, 1979.

12. Feldt-Rasmussen B, Mathisen E, and Deckert T: Effect of two years of strict metabolic control on progression of incipient nephropathy in IDDM, *Lancet* 2:1300, 1986.

13. Grunwald JE and others: Diabetic glycemic control and retinal blood flow, *Diabetes* 39:602, 1990.

14. Leicter SB: *Association between glycemic control and degenerative complications of diabetes mellitus: a brief review of current concepts.* In Kerstein MD, editor: *Diabetes and vascular disease,* Philadelphia, 1990, JB Lippincott.

15. Knatterud GL and others: Effects of hypoglycemic agents on vascular complications in patients with adult onset diabetes. VIII. Evaluation of insulin therapy: final report, *Diabetes* 31:1, 1982.

16. Davidson JK and DiGirolamo: *Non-insulin dependent diabetes.* In Davidson JK, editor: *Clinical diabetes mellitus: a problem oriented approach,* ed 2, New York, 1991, Thieme Medical Publishers.

17. Lernmark A: *Insulin-dependent diabetes mellitus.* In Davidson JK, editor: *Clinical diabetes mellitus: a problem-oriented approach,* ed 2, New York, 1991, Thieme Medical Publishers.

18. Lorenzi M: *Diabetes mellitus.* In Fitzgerald PA, editor: *Handbook of clinical endocrinology,* Norwalk, CT, 1992, Appleton & Lange.

19. Davidson JK: *Diabetic ketoacidosis and the hyperglycemic hyperosmolar state.* In Davidson JK, editor: *Clinical diabetes mellitus: a problem-oriented approach,* ed 2. New York, 1991, Thieme Medical Publishers.

20. Ambrus JL: *Microvascular changes in diabetes.* In Kerstein MD: *Diabetes and vascular disease,* Philadelphia, 1990, JB Lippincott.

21. Pugliese G and others: Effects of very mild versus overt diabetes on vascular hemodynamics and barrier function in rats, *Diabetologica* 2:845, 1989.

22. Beach KW and others: The correlation of arteriosclerosis obliterans with lipoproteins in insulin-dependent and non-insulin dependent diabetes, *Diabetes* 28:836, 1979.

23. Chronic disease reports: Deaths from diabetes—United States 1986, *MMWR* 38(31):543, 1989.

24. End-stage renal diasease associated with diabetes—United States 1988, *MMWR* 38(31):546, 1989.

25. Chan A and others: Carotid artery disease in NIDDM diabetes, *Diabetes* Care 6:562, 1983.

26. Strandess DE Jr and Stahler C: Arteriosclerosis obliterans. Manner and rate of progression, *JAMA* 196:1, 1966.

27. Cefalu WT and Clements RS Jr: *Diabetic neuropathy.* In Kerstein MD: *Diabetes and vascular disease,* Philadelphia, 1990, JB Lippincott.

28. Ballard DJ, Tancredi RG, and Palumbo PJ: *Coronary artery disease and other cardiac complications.* In Davidson JK, editor: *Clinical diabetes mellitus: a problem-oriented approach,* ed 2. New York, 1991, Thieme Medical Publishers.

29. WHO Multinational Study of Vascular Disease in Diabetics: Prevalence of small vessel and large vessel disease in diabetic patients from 14 centers, *Diabetologica* 28:615, 1985.

30. Harris MI: *Screening for undiagnosed non–insulin dependent diabetes.* In Alberti KGMM and Mazze RS, editors: *Current trends in non–insulin dependent diabetes mellitus,* New York, 1989, Elsevier.

31. Seltzer HS: *Diagnosis of diabetes.* In Ellenberg

M and Rifkin H, editors: *Diabetes mellitus: theory and practice,* New York, 1970, McGraw-Hill.

32. Dunn PJ and others: Reproducibility of hemoglbin A$_{1c}$ and sensitivity to various degrees of glucose intolerance, *Ann Intern Med* 91:390, 1979.

33. The Diabetes Control and Complications Trial Research Group: The effect of intensive treatment of diabetes on the development and progression of long-term complications in insulin-dependent diabetes mellitus, *N Engl J Med* 329:977, 1993.

34. American Diabetes Association: Implications of the diabetes control and complicaitons trial: position statement (approved by the Executive Committee of the Board of Directors, June 1993), *Clin Diabetes,* July/August 1993, p 91.

35. National Institutes of Health: Concensus development conference on diet and exercise on non–insulin dependent diabetes mellitus, *Diabetes Care* 10:639, 1987.

36. Rabkin SW and others: A randomized clinical trial comparing behavior modificaiton and individual counseling in the nutritional therapy of non–insulin dependent diabetes mellitus: comparison of the effect on blood sugar, body weight, and serum lipids, *Diabetes Care* 6:50, 1983.

37. Nathan DM: Modern management of insulin-dependent diabetes mellitus, *Med Clin North Am* 72:1365, 1988.

38. Campbell PJ and others: Pathogenesis of the dawn phenomenon in patients with insulin-dependent diabetes mellitus, *N Engl J Med* 312:1473, 1985.

39. Westphal SA and Goetz FC: Current approaches to continuous insulin replacement for insulin-dependent diabetes: pancreas transplantation and pumps, *Adv Intern Med* 35:107, 1990.

40. Taskinen MR and others: Bedtime insulin for suppression of overnight free-fatty acid, blood glucose and glucose production in NIDDM, *Diabetes* 38:580, 1989.

41. Katterman OG and Olefsky JM: The impact of sulfonylurea treatment on the mechanisms responsible for the insulin resistance in Type II diabetes, *Diabetes Care* 17(suppl 1):86, 1984.

42. Berger M: *Oral agents in the treatment of diabetes mellitus*. In Davidson JK, editor: *Clinical diabetes mellitus: a problem-oriented approach,* ed 2, New York, 1991, Thieme Medical Publishers.

43. Ramsey RC and others: Progression of diabetic retinopathy after pancreas transplantation for insulin-dependent diabetes mellitus, *N Engl J Med* 318:208, 1988.

44. Schwartz RW and others: Pentoxifylline increases extremity blood flow in diabetic atherosclerotic patients, *Arch Surg* 124:434, 1989.

45. Chakrrabarti S and Sima AAF: Effect of aldose reductase inhibition and insulin treatment on retinal capillary basement membrane thickening in BB rats, *Diabetes* 38:1181, 1989.

46. Rosetti L: Normalization of insulin sensitivity with lithium in diabetic rats, *Diabetes* 38:648, 1989.

47. Corbett JA and others: Aminoguanidine, a novel inhibitor of nitric oxide formation, prevents diabetic vascular dysfunction, *Diabetes* 41:552, 1992.

48. The Diabetic Retinopathy Study Research Group: Preliminary report on effects of photocoagulation therapy, *Am J Ophthalmol* 81:383, 1976.

49. The Diabetic Retinopathy Study Research Group: Photocoagulation treatment of proliferative diabetic retinopathy: the second report of Diabetic Retinopathy Study findings, *Am J Ophthalmol* 85:82, 1978.

50. The Diabetic Retinopathy Study Research Group: Four risk factors for severe visual loss in diabetic retinopathy: the third report from the Diabetic Retinopathy Study, *Arch Ophthalmol* 97:654, 1979.

51. The Diabetic Retinopathy Study Research Group: Photocoagulation treatment of proliferative diabetic retinopathy: a short report of long range results. Diabetic Retinopathy Study (DRS) Report Number 4, Amsterdam, 1980, Excerpta Medica.

52. The Diabetic Retinopathy Study Research Group: Photocoagulation of proliferative diabetic retinopathy: relationship of adverse treatment effects to retinopathy severity. Diabetic Retinopathy Study Report Number 5, *Dev Ophthalmol* 2:248, 1981.

53. The Diabetic Retinopathy Study Research Group: Design, methods, and baseline results. Diabetic Retinopathy Study Report Number 6, *Invest Ophthalmol Vis Sci* 21:149, 1981.

54. The Diabetic Retinopathy Study Research Group: A modification of the Airlee House classification of diabetic retinopathy. Diabetic Retinopathy Study Report Number 7, *Invest Ophthalmol Vis Sci* 21:210, 1981.

55. The Diabetic Retinopathy Study Research Group: Photocoagulation treatment of proliferative diabetic retinopathy: clinical application of Diabetic Retinopathy Study (DRS) findings. Diabetic Retinopathy Study Report Number 8, *Ophthalmology* 88:583, 1981.

56. Ederer F and others: Assessing possible late treatment effects in stopping a clinical trial early: a case study. Diabetic Retinopathy Study Report Number 9, *Controlled Clin Trials* 5:373, 1984.

57. Rand LI and others: Factors influencing the development of visual loss in advanced diabetic retinopathy. Diabetic Retinopathy Study Report Number 10, *Invest Ophthalmol Vis Sci* 26:983, 1985.

58. Kaufman SC and others: Intraocular pressure following panretinal photocoagulation for diabetic retinopathy. Diabetic Retinopathy Study Report Number 11, *Arch Ophthalmol* 105:807, 1987.

59. Ferris FL and others: Macular edema in Diabetic Retinopathy Study patients. Diabetic Retinopathy Study Report Number 12, *Ophthalmology* 94:754, 1987.

60. Kaufman SC and others: Factors associated with visual outcome after photocoagulation in the Diabetic Retinopathy Study, *Invest Ophthalmol Vis Sci* 30:23, 1989.

61. The Diabetic Retinopathy Study Research Group: Indications for photocoagulation treatment of diabetic retinopathy. Diabetic Retinopathy Study Report Number 14, *Int Ophthalmol Clin* 27:239, 1987.

62. The Early Treatment Diabetic Retinopathy Study Research Group: Photocoagulation for diabetic macular edema. ETDRS Report Number 1, *Arch Ophthalmol* 103:1796, 1985.

63. The Early Treatment Diabetic Retinopathy Study Research Group: Treatment techniques and clinical guidelines for photocoagulation of diabetic macular edema. ETDRS Report Number 2, *Ophthalmology* 94:761, 1987.

64. The Early Treatment Diabetic Retinopathy Study Research Group: Techniques for scatter and local photocoagulation treatment of diabetic retinopathy. ETDRS Report Number 3, *Int Ophthalmol Clin* 27:254, 1987.

65. The Early Treatment Diabetic Retinopathy Study Research Group: Photocoagulation for diabetic macular edema. ETDRS Report Number 4, *Int Ophthalmol Clin* 27:265, 1987.

66. The Early Treatment Diabetic Retinopathy Study Research Group: Case reports to accompany Early Treatment Diabetic Retinopathy Study Reports 3 and 4, *Int Ophthalmol Clin* 27:273, 1987.

67. The Early Treatment Diabetic Retinopathy Study Research Group: Detection of diabetic macular edema. Ophthalmoscopy versus photography. ETDRS Report Number 5, *Ophthalmology* 96:746, 1989.

68. The Early Treatment Diabetic Retinopathy Study Research Group: Early Treatment Diabetic Retinopathy Study design and baseline patient characteristics. ETDRS Report Number 7, *Ophthalmology* 98:741, 1991.

69. The Early Treatment Diabetic Retinopathy Study Research Group: Effects of aspirin treatment on diabetic retinopathy. ETDRS Report Number 8, *Ophthalmology* 98:757, 1991.

70. The Early Treatment Diabetic Retinopathy Study Research Group: Early photocoagulation for diabetic retinopathy. ETDRS Report Number 9, *Ophthalmology* 98:766, 1991.

71. The Early Treatment Diabetic Retinopathy Study Research Group: Grading diabetic retinopathy from stereoscopic color fundus photographs—an extension of the modified Airlee House classification. ETDRS Report Number 10, *Ophthalmology* 98:786, 1991.

72. The Early Treatment Diabetic Retinopathy Study Research Group: Classification of diabetic retinopathy from fluorescein angiograms. ETDRS Report Number 11, *Ophthalmology* 98:807, 1991.

73. The Early Treatment Diabetic Retinopathy Study Research Group: Fundus photographic risk factors for progression of diabetic retinopathy. ETDRS Report Number 12, *Ophthalmology* 98:823, 1991.

74. The Early Treatment Diabetic Retinopathy Study Research Group: Fluorescein angiographic risk factors for progression of diabetic retinopathy. ETDRS Report Number 13, *Ophthalmology* 98:834, 1991.

75. The Diabetic Retinopathy Study Research Group: Two-year course of visual acuity in severe proliferative diabetic retinopathy with conventional management. Diabetic Retinopathy Study Report Number 1, *Ophthalmology* 92:492, 1985.

76. The Diabetic Retinopathy Vitrectomy Study Research Group: Early vitrectomy for severe vitreous hemorrhage in diabetic retinopathy. Two-year results of a randomized trial. Diabetic Retinopathy Vitrectomy Study Report Number 2, *Arch Ophthalmol* 103:1644, 1985.

77. The Diabetic Retinopathy Vitrectomy Study Research Group: Early vitrectomy for severe proliferative retinopathy in eyes with useful vision. Results of a randomized trial. Diabetic Retinopathy Vitrectomy Study Report Number 3, *Ophthalmology* 95:1307, 1988.

78. The Diabetic Retinopathy Vitrectomy Study Research Group: Early vitrectomy for severe proliferative diabetic retinopathy in eyes with useful vision. Clinical application of results of a randomized trial. Diabetic Retinopathy Vitrectomy Study Report Number 4, *Ophthalmology* 95:1321, 1988.

79. The Diabetic Retinopathy Vitrectomy Study Research Group: Early treatment for severe vitreous hemorrhage in diabetic retinopathy. Four-year results of a randomized clinical trial. Diabetic Retinopathy Study Report Number 5, *Arch Ophthalmol* 108:958, 1990.

80. Klein R and others: The Wisconsin Epidemiologic Study of Diabetic Retinopathy. II. Prevalence and risk of diabetic retinopathy when age at diagnosis is less than 30 years, *Arch Ophthalmol* 102:250, 1984.

81. Klein R and others: The Wisconsin Epidemiologic Study of Diabetic Retinopathy. III. Prevalence and risk of diabetic retinopathy when age at diagnosis is 30 or more years, *Arch Ophthalmol* 102:527, 1984.

82. Waite JH and Beetham WP: The visual mechanism in diabetes mellitus: a comparative study of 2002 diabetics and 457 nondiabetics for control, *N Engl J Med* 212:367, 429, 1935.

83. Gwinup G and Villarreal A: Relationship of serum glucose concentration to changes in refraction. *Diabetes* 25:29, 1976.

84. Duke-Elder WS: Changes in refraction in diabetes mellitus, *Br J Ophthalmol* 9:167, 1925.

85. Kinoshita JH and others: Osmotic changes caused by the accumulation of dulcitol in the lenses of rats fed with galactose, *Nature* 194:1085, 1962.

86. Marmor MF: Transient accommodative paralysis and hyperopia in diabetes, *Arch Ophthalmol* 89:419, 1973.

87. Rogell GD: Internal ophthalmoplegia after argon laser panretinal photocoagulation, *Arch Ophthalmol* 97:904, 1979.

88. Klein BEk, Klein R, and Moss SE: Prevalence of cataracts in a population-based study of persons with diabetes mellitus, *Ophthalmology* 92:1191, 1985.

89. Ederer F, Hiller R, and Taylor RH: Senile lens changes and diabetes in two population studies, *Am J Ophthalmol* 91:381, 1981.

90. O'Brien CS, Molsberrry JM, and Allen JH: Diabetic cataract, *JAMA* 103:892, 1934.

91. Kinoshita JH: Mechanisms initiating cataract formation, *Invest Ophthalmol Vis Sci* 17:713, 1974.

92. Chylack LT and Kinoshita JH: A biochemical evaluation of a cataract induced in a high glucose medium, *Invest Ophthalmol Vis Sci* 8:401, 1963.

93. Harding RH, Chylack LT, and Tung WH: The sorbitol pathway as a protector of the lens against glucose-generated osmotic stress, *Invest Ophthalmol Vis Sci* 20(Suppl):34, 1981.

94. Bursell S-E, Karalekas DP, and Craig MS: The effect of acute changes in blood glucose on lenses in diabetic and non-diabetic subjects using quasi-elastic light scattering spectroscope, *Curr Eye Res* 8:821, 1989.

95. Bursell S-E and others: Clinical photon correlation spectroscopy evaluation of human diabetic lenses, *Exp Eye Res* 49:241, 1989.

96. Epstein DL: Reversible unilateral lens opacities in a diabetic patient, *Arch Ophthalmol* 94:461, 1976.

97. Lawrence RD, Oakley W, and Barre IC: Temporary lens changes in diabetic coma and other dehydrations, *Lancet* 2:63, 1942.

98. Lawrence RD: Temporary cataracts in diabetes, *Br J Ophthalmol* 30:70, 1946.

99. Roberts W: Rapid lens changes in diabetes mellitus, *Am J Ophthalmol* 33:1283, 1950.

100. Neuberg HW, Griscom JH, and Burns RP: Acute development of diabetic cataracts and their reversal: a case report, *Diabetes* 7:21, 1958.

101. Jackson RC: Temporary cataracts in diabetes mellitus, *Br J Ophthalmol* 39:629, 1955.

102. Turtz CA and Turtz AI: Reversal of lens changes in early diabetes, *Am J Ophthalmol* 46:219, 1959.

103. Brown CA and Burman D: Transient cataracts in a diabetic child with hyperosmotic coma, *Br J Ophthalmol* 57:429, 1973.

104. Rosen E: Diabetic needles, *Br J Ophthalmol* 29:645, 1945.

105. Aiello LM, Wand M, and Liang G: Neovascular glaucoma and vitreous hemorrhage following cataract surgery in patients with diabetes mellitus, *Ophthalmology* 90:814, 1983.

106. Ishida N and others: Corneal nerve alterations in diabetes mellitus, *Arch Ophthalmol* 102:1380, 1984.

107. MacRae SM and others: Corneal sensitivity and control of diabetes, *Cornea* 1:223, 1982.

108. Schwartz DE: Corneal sensitivity in diabetics, *Arch Ophthalmol* 91:174, 1974.

109. Rogell GD: Corneal hypesthesia and retinopathy in diabetes mellitus, *Ophthalmology* 87:229, 1980.

110. Hyndiuk RA and others: Neurotrophic corneal ulcers in diabetes mellitus, *Arch Ophthalmol* 95:2193, 1977.

111. Hatchell DL, Pederson HJ, and Faculjak ML: Susceptibility of the corneal epithelial basement membrane to injury in diabetic rabbits, *Cornea* 1:227, 1982.

112. Kenyon K and others: Corneal basement membrane abnormality in diabetes mellitus, *Invest Ophthalmol Vis Sci* 17(Suppl):245, 1978.

113. Khodadoust AA and others: Adhesion of regenerating corneal epithelium, *Am J Ophthalmol* 65:339, 1968.

114. Gartner S and Henkind P: Neovascularization of the iris (rubeosis iridis), *Surv Ophthalmol* 22:291, 1978.

115. Zirm M: Protein glaucoma—overtaxing of flow mechanisms? Preliminary report, *Ophthalmologica* 184:155, 1982.

116. Brown GC and others: Neovascular glaucoma: etiologic considerations, *Ophthalmology* 91:315, 1984.

117. Pavan PR and Folk JC: Anterior neovascularization, *Int Ophthalmol Clin* 24:61, 1984.

118. Madsden PH: Rubeosis of the iris and hemorrhagic glaucoma in patients with proliferative diabetic retinopathy, *Br J Ophthalmol* 55:368, 1971.

119. Ohrt V: The frequency of rubeosis iridis in diabetic patients, *Acta Ophthalmol* (Copenh) 49:301, 1971.

120. Krill AE, Archer D, and Newell FW: Photocoagulation in complications secondary to branch vein occlusion, *Arch Ophthalmol* 85:48, 1971.

121. Aiello LM and others: *Ruby laser photocoagulation and treatment of diabetic proliferating retinopathy.* In Goldberg MF and Fine SL, editors: *Symposium on the treatment of diabetic retinopathy,* US Public Health Service Publication No. 1890, Washington, DC, 1969.

122. Wand M and others: Effects of panretinal photocoagulation on rubeosis iridis, angle neovascularization, and neovascular glaucoma, *Am J Ophthalmol* 86:332, 1978.

123. Pavan PR and others: Diabetic rubeosis and panretinal photocoagulation: a prospective, controlled, masked trial using iris fluorescein angiography, *Arch Ophthalmol* 101:882, 1983.

124. Simmons RJ and others: Goniophotocoagulation for neovascular glaucoma, *Trans Am Acad Ophthalmol Otol* 83:80, 1977.

125. Zorrilla E and Kozak GP: Ophthalmoplegia in diabetes mellitus, *Ann Intern Med* 67:968, 1967.

126. Rucker CW: Paralysis of the third, fourth, and sixth cranial nerves, *Am J Ophthalmol* 46:787, 1958.

127. Rush JA and Younge BR: Paralysis of cranial nerves III, IV, and VI, *Arch Ophthalmol* 99:76, 1981.

128. Rucker CW: The causes of paralysis of the third, fourth, and sixth cranial nerves, *Am J Ophthalmol* 61:1293, 1966.

129. Asbury AK and others: Oculomotor palsy in diabetes mellitus: a clinico-pathological study, *Brain* 93:555, 1970.

130. Weber RB, Daroff RB, and Mackey EA: Pathology of oculomotor nerve palsy in diabetics, *Neurology* 20:835, 1970.

131. Jackson WPU: Ocular nerve palsy with severe headache in diabetics, *Br Med J* 2:408, 1955.

132. Waind APB: Ocular nerve palsy associated with severe headache, *Br Med J* 1:901, 1956.

133. Lincoff HA and Cogan DG: Unilateral headache and oculomotor paralysis not caused by aneurysm, *Arch Ophthalmol* 57:181, 1957.

134. King FP: Paralyses of the extraocular muscle in diabetes, *Arch Intern Med* 104:318, 1959.

135. Goldstein JE and Cogan DG: Diabetic ophthalmoplegia with special reference to the pupil, *Arch Ophthalmol* 64:592, 1960.

136. Eareckson VO and Miller JM: Third-nerve palsy with sparing of pupil in diabetes mellitus, *Arch Ophthalmol* 47:607, 1952.

137. Green WR, Hackett ER, and Schlezinger NS: Neuro-ophthalmologic evaluation of oculomotor nerve paralysis, *Arch Ophthalmol* 72:154, 1964.

14

Endocrine Ophthalmopathy

BRUCE G. MUCHNICK

*E*ndocrine ophthalmopathy, or Graves' disease, comprises the characteristics of hyperthyroidism, toxic diffuse *goiter,* and ophthalmopathy.[1] The ophthalmopathy, however, may occur independently of the thyrotoxic goiter.[2] Therefore, for endocrine ophthalmopathy to be considered a multisystem disorder of endocrine origin, it must be associated with one or more of the following clinical features: thyroid disease (that is autoimmune in nature), an ophthalmopathy that is characterized by infiltrates, and pretibial myxedema (or dermopathy).[2]

Because clinical investigations have traditionally concentrated on the thyrotoxic goiter, little progress has been made in identifying the pathogenesis and evolution of the *orbitopathy*.[1] Only recently has Graves' ophthalmopathy received the concentrated attention of researchers and clinicians alike.[1] For this reason no consensus exists yet on the terminology to be used in describing this disorder[1] (see box on p. 287).

Traditionally the term "Graves' eye disease" or "Graves' ophthalmopathy" has been widely used but remains unsatisfactory because the orbitopathy includes Hashimoto's thyroiditis.[1] In 1987, Volpe suggested the term "autoimmune ophthalmopathy" or "autoimmune orbitopathy," which at least identifies the physiologic underpinning of the disorder but sacrifices its relationship with thyroid disease.[3] In 1990 Wall and How suggested that the term "thyroid-associated ophthalmopathy" be adopted to encompass all the characteristics associated with Graves' disease.[1] Kahaly, writing in 1993, used the term "endocrine ophthalmopathy" to describe

NAMES SYNONYMOUS WITH ENDOCRINE OPHTHALMOPATHY

Graves' eye disease
Graves' ophthalmopathy
Graves' orbitopathy
Dysthyroid eye disease
Dysthyroid orbitopathy
Exophthalmic goiter
Immune exophthalmos
Thyroid-associated ophthalmopathy
Autoimmune orbitopathy
Autoimmune ophthalmopathy

the autoimmune origin, histologic cell infiltration of the orbital tissues, and classic signs and symptoms historically ascribed to Graves' eye disease.[2] Likewise, this chapter refers to thyroid-associated ophthalmopathy as endocrine ophthalmopathy, or EO.

That there is so much ambivalence concerning nomenclature suggests the larger and more complex problems facing researchers: What causes EO and how is it related to thyroid disease?[1] In addition, clinicians are still faced with the issues of how best to diagnose and treat EO.[1]

Optometry can readily serve in this new focus on EO by acting in coordinated effort with endocrine researchers and clinicians to identify the at-risk group of patients before they show any manifestations of the orbitopathy. These patients may then be closely monitored by all the involved disciplines as signs and symptoms develop. Through such a rational approach, the true biochemical, immunologic, and pathologic basis for EO may at last be discovered.

This chapter presents the latest thoughts on the autoimmune nature of this disease. Also described are the diagnostic strategies available to the optometrist when evaluating a patient with, or suspected of having, EO. Finally, the medical and surgical management of EO is presented, including the use of novel drugs, plasmapheresis, radiation therapy, orbital decompression, and corrective eye surgery.

THYROID DISEASE

EO may occur independently of thyroid disease (so-called Graves' euthyroid orbitopathy), but the ophthalmopathy occurs mostly in patients with hyperthyroidism.[4] It is clear, therefore, that these two conditions share some pathophysiologic relationship and that an understanding of thyroid disease is necessary to study the pathogenic mechanism behind EO.

Thyroid Physiology

A sensitive feedback loop exists to regulate the level of serum thyroid hormones.[5] This modulating system is known as the hypothalamic-pituitary-thyroid axis.[5] The basal *hypothalamus* located in the lateral wall of the third ventricle contains nerve endings that release *thyroid-releasing hormone* (TRH), a tripeptide.[6] TRH stimulates thyroid-stimulating hormone (TSH) secretion from the pituitary gland.[5] TSH is a polypeptide that is the primary agent stimulating the thyroid gland to produce two metabolically active hormones: *triiodothyronine* (T_3) and *thyroxine* (T_4).[5] Elevated levels of T_3 (three iodide atoms) and T_4 (four iodide atoms) in turn exert a negative feedback at the level of the *pituitary gland,* thus reducing TSH production. Therefore, TSH is controlled by both the hypothalamic hormone TRH and the thyroid hormones T_3 and T_4.

Thyroid Function Tests (see box on p. 288)

There are three types of thyroid function tests: serum thyroid hormone tests, hypothalamic-pituitary-thyroid axis tests, and direct thyroid functions tests.[7] The serum thyroid hormone tests include serum T_4, serum T_3, serum free T_4 and T_3, T_3 resin uptake, and free T_4 index.

The serum thyroid hormone tests analyze T_4 and T_3 by radioimmunoassay, which measures the total bound and unbound fractions of each.[7] The unbound (free) levels more accurately reflect the metabolic state than do the bound levels. The normal T_4 level is 4 to 12 μg/dl, and the normal T_3 level is 75 to 195 μg/dl.[5] Hyperthyroidism and hypothyroidism produce changes in serum levels of T_3 and T_4 detected in these tests.[5] The T_4 is the stan-

---

THYROID FUNCTION TESTS

Serum thyroid hormones
    Serum T_4
    Serum T_3
    Serum free T_4 and T_3
    T_3 resin uptake
    Free T_4 index

Hypothalamic-pituitary-thyroid axis tests
    Serum TSH
    TRH stimulation test
    T_3 suppression test (Cytomel)
    TSH immunoradiometric assay (TSH-IRMA)

Direct thyroid function tests
    Radioactive iodine uptake (RAIU)

---

dard screening procedure for diagnosing hyperthyroidism and hypothyroidism.[7]

Another serum thyroid hormone test is serum free T_4 and T_3, but it is difficult to perform and expensive to measure these free hormones directly.[7] The serum thyroid hormone test that is most commonly used to evaluate thyroid binding is the T_3 resin uptake (T_3RU).[7] This test does not measure circulating T_3. Instead, the patient's serum is incubated with a T_3 tracer (radioiodine-labeled T_3) and an insoluble resin to bind the remaining free T_3.[7] The T_3 tracer has a greater affinity for the available serum binding sites, so after incubation the fraction of the labeled T_3 absorbed on the resin is determined.[5] What is actually measured is the amount of radioactivity bound on the resin.[5] The T_3RU is low in hypothyroidism and high in hyperthyroidism.[5] The normal T_3RU is 25% to 35%.[7] The free T_4 index is a mathematical computation involving the total serum T_4 and T_3RU, and it provides a good approximation of free T_4 (normal free T_4 index = 1 to 4).[7]

The hypothalamic-pituitary-thyroid axis tests include the serum TSH, the TRH test, and T_3 suppression test.[7] The serum *thyrotropin* (TSH) level is measured by radioimmunoassay, and normal is less than 7 μU/ml. If elevated, hypothyroidism is suspected. Serum TSH is not of value in determin-

ing hyperthyroidism because most assays are not sensitive enough to distinguish normal from low levels.[5] However, a new and very sensitive double-antibody technique for measuring below-normal TSH levels has been developed. The TSH immunoradiometric assay (TSH-IRMA) can detect low TSH levels, indicating mild hyperthyroidism.[7]

The TRH stimulation test determines how well the pituitary can secrete TSH in response to an intravenous injection of 200 to 500 mg of TRH. A normal TSH response to TRH excludes hyperthyroidism. An abnormally low response of TSH to TRH indicates hyperthyroidism, and an exaggerated TSH response reflects hypothyroidism.[7]

The *T_3 suppression test* (Cytomel) is a radioactive iodine-uptake (RAIU) test preceding and following injection of T_3 three times daily for 10 days. A comparison is then made of the two RAIU readings. Normally, the RAIU is reduced to less than half over the 10-day period. If this occurs, then hyperthyroidism is ruled out.[7] The T_3 suppression test has been largely supplanted by the TRH stimulation test.[5]

A direct test of thyroid function is the radioactive iodine uptake (RAIU) test. Radioisotope is injected and competes with stable iodine. This test is limited in its diagnostic uses and is now of primary value in the T_3 suppression test.[7]

The eye care specialist who encounters a suspected EO should have T_3 and T_4 levels run. If T_3 and T_4 are normal, then the hypothalamic-pituitary-thyroid axis should be tested by a TRH stimulation test or by the more sensitive TSH-IRMA test. The TSH-IRMA may be more sensitive in diagnosing the so-called Graves' euthyroid patient.[7] The optometrist should consult with an endocrinologist who specializes in thyroid disease for any patient suspected of having EO.

Abnormal Thyroid Function

Hyperthyroidism. This term, first used in 1907 by Mayo, describes an abnormal state produced by elevated serum thyroid hormone levels.[5] The most common cause of hyperthyroidism is Graves' disease, which was first recognized and described by Parry in 1825. The cause of the hyperthyroidism

SYMPTOMS OF HYPERTHYROIDISM

Major symptoms
  Nervousness
  Hyperactivity
  Insomnia
  Swings of emotion

Common symptoms
  Heat intolerance
  Excessive perspiration
  Palpitations
  Increased appetite
  Weight loss
  Diminished menstrual flow
  Muscle weakness

Occasional symptoms
  Anorexia
  Nausea
  Vomiting
  Dyspnea

PREDISPOSITIONS OF GRAVES' DISEASE

Familial predisposition
Most frequent ages: 25 to 50
Ten times more common in women than men

in Graves' disease is an autoimmune disorder that results in the formation of thyroid-stimulating immunoglobulins. These immunoglobulins are antibodies most likely directed against the thyroid cell receptor, where they mimic TSH and cause the thyroid to overproduce and release thyroid hormones. The result of Graves' disease is a diffuse goiter with infiltrative ophthalmopathy and, on occasion, an infiltrative dermopathy of flesh-colored papules on the shin known as *pretibial myxedema*.

The most common symptom of hyperthyroidism (see box above) is excessive nervousness, accompanied by insomnia, hyperactivity, and palpitations. Patients usually note that they have lost weight despite an increase in appetite. There may be a cessation of menstrual flow. The patient may notice tremors of the digits, heat intolerance, fatigue, and weakness.

Significant clinical signs of hyperthyroidism include a prominant stare secondary to retraction of the upper lid, sinus tachycardia, goiter, thyroid bruit, hyperactive deep tendon reflexes, and vitiligo in 10% of patients. The course of the disease

is varied, and the goiter may remit and spontaneously reoccur years after treatment.

The diagnosis of hyperthyroidism (see box above) is made based on clinical suspicion of patients exhibiting any of the above signs and symptoms, a significant history, physical examination, and laboratory testing. In most cases of hyperthyroidism the free T_4 index is elevated and establishes the diagnosis in a likely suspect. If a patient is suspected of having a hyperthyroid state but the free T_4 index is normal, then a serum T_3 measurement should be obtained. If abnormal, this condition is called T_3 thyrotoxicosis.[5]

Three therapeutic strategies are available at present for the treatment of hyperthyroidism: drug treatment, radioiodine therapy, and surgery. Methimazole *(Tapazole)* and propylthiouracil *(PTU)* act to block the synthesis of thyroid hormones and have immunosuppressive effects. Neither causes permanent hypothyroidism, and treatment usually lasts a total of 12 to 18 months. Usually in the first 3 months the serum thyroid hormone levels drop to a euthyroid level. These medications have some significant side effects. Antithyroid medications are advised for children and young adults or patients with small goiters and mild symptoms.[5]

Potassium iodine has been used as a valuable adjunct to radiation therapy by blocking release of hormone from the thyroid gland. Beta-blockers have been used to reduce the hyperactive states associated with hyperthyroidism.[7]

Adults over the age of 40 with hyperthyroidism should receive radioactive iodine therapy.[5] Full amelioration of the symptoms and signs and a return to a euthyroid state occur in 75% of patients 2 to 6 months after administration of radioactive iodine.[7] Fifteen percent to 20% of all patients develop hypothyroidism within the first year of treatment.[5] Therefore, all patients undergoing radioactive iodine treatment should be made aware of the signs and symptoms of hypothyroidism.

Surgery is considered only rarely in the management of hyperthyroidism. Children and young adults should have antithyroid drug therapy before inadequate control forces a surgical decision.[5] Patients who decline radiation therapy or who have large goiters may be candidates for surgery.[7] There has been some evidence that *thyroidectomy* (near-total removal of the thyroid gland) has a positive effect on EO, but not enough studies have been done to confirm this.[8]

Hypothyroidism. If an insufficient amount of thyroid hormone results in a reduced metabolic state, then a state of hypothyroidism exists. The most common cause of hypothyroidism is Hashimoto's thyroiditis.[7] As mentioned previously, treatment of hyperthyroidism by radioactive iodine or thyroidectomy may result in hypothyroidism.

Hypothyroidism has few early symptoms and may exist as a subclinical entity for many years before being diagnosed. Patients have few symptoms beyond cold intolerance, peripheral paresthesias, and complaints of bloating.[5] Diagnosis of hypothyroidism is made on a suspicious patient on the laboratory finding of a low free T_4 index. Unfortunately the free T_4 index may be normal in mild hypothyroidism. The most sensitive laboratory indicator for hypothyroidism is an elevated serum TSH level (in spite of a normal T_4 index). Serum T_3 is not a sensitive indicator of hypothyroidism.[5]

Hypothyroidism is readily treated by restoring normal circulating thyroid hormones by use of *L-thyroxine*.[7] The serum TSH assay can be used to precisely adjust thyroid replacement therapy in order to optimize the level of circulating hormones.[7]

Hashimoto's Thyroiditis. Thyroiditis is an inflammation of the thyroid gland, and there are several forms based on cause and pathology. Hashimoto's thyroiditis is the most common thyroid disease and most common cause of goiter in the United States, as well as the most common of all autoimmune diseases.[7]

Patients usually experience the subtle signs and symptoms of hypothyroidism with a diffuse, non-painful, firm, and asymmetric goiter.[5] Laboratory testing confirms the diagnosis of Hashimoto's thyroiditis. Treatment is the same as hypothyroidism in that administration of L-thyroxine inhibits TSH secretion, causing goiter regression. Therapy may last the life of the patient.[5]

ENDOCRINE OPHTHALMOPATHY

Pathogenesis

For as-yet-unknown reasons, antibodies called thyroid-stimulating immunoglobulins are directed against the TSH receptor on the thyroid gland. HLA-DR antigens on certain cells of the thyroid may facilitate the action of these antibodies.[4] Some evidence indicates that perhaps a bacterial or viral infection stimulates antibody production against the invading organism but that these immunoglobulins cross-react with the thyroid TSH receptor.[9] These antibodies mimic TSH activity, causing hormonal overproduction that yields a hyperthyroid state.

Less clear are the autoimmune aspects of EO.[10] The thyroid has been established as the target site of thyroid-stimulating antibodies, and EO has been established as an autoimmune disease most frequently associated with hyperthyroidism, but the biochemical and immunologic links between the two remain largely unexplored. This is because the retro-orbital tissues of patients with EO are not readily available for study.[11] Many laboratory approaches are currently used to study the established fact that autoantibodies (T lymphocytes) are reacting against retro-orbital tissues.[11] Such studies indicate that the eye muscles and surrounding connective tissue are the target of the autoimmune response, but the antigen for this reaction and the immunopathologic processes occurring in the orbit have not been established.

One theory linking the autoimmune nature of thyroid disease with the histologic changes in the swollen extraocular muscles would be a cross-reactive antigen within the thyroid and the orbit. One study suggests that T cells (autoantibodies) are sensitized to orbital antigens in patients with EO.[12] If this is the case, autoantibodies could become sensitized to orbital tissues and these T cells could infiltrate the muscle, releasing cytokines that activate *fibroblasts*. It has been firmly established that these autoantibodies react with fibroblasts.[13] The fibroblasts produce *glycosaminoglycans* (GAGs), which cause swelling and fibrosis of the

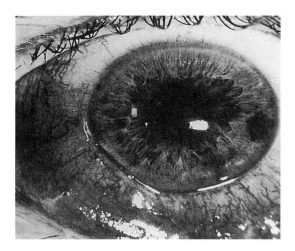

FIG. 14-1 Acute inflammatory endocrine ophthalmopathy with minimal exophthalmos and dramatic conjunctival chemosis and exposure keratopathy. *(From Kahaly G: Endocrine ophthalmopathy: molecular, immunological and clinical aspects, Dev Ophthalmol 25:7, 1993.)*

extraocular muscles.[12] GAGs are molecules that induce edema.[14] This muscular edema is rich in mucopolysaccharides, and so research efforts are focusing on autoantibodies with cell-stimulating properties.[15] The autoantibodies to eye muscles in patients with EO can be detected by enzyme-linked immunosorbent assay testing (ELISA), but the detection rate is less than 60%.[16]

Diagnostic Tests and Clinical Techniques

Clinical Signs and Symptoms. In endocrine ophthalmopathy an infiltration of the extraocular muscles with chronic inflammatory cells, associated with edema and fibrosis of the connective and adipose tissue of the orbit, causes an enlargement of the retrobulbar contents leading to proptosis.[17-21] The lacrimal gland may also become inflamed.[22] Many patients with endocrine ophthalmopathy complain of a gritty foreign body sensation. Exposure keratoconjunctivitis, nocturnal lagophthalmos, lacrimal gland involvement, reduced amplitude of blinking (Pochin's sign), and a reduced blink rate (Stellwag's sign) all contribute to the symptoms of dry eye (Fig. 14-1).

The exophthalmos of EO appears to be due to an increase in extraocular muscle volume displacing the globe forward (Fig. 14-2). The lid retraction (Dalrymple's sign) and lid lag (von Graefe's sign) result in a "thyroid stare" and are most likely

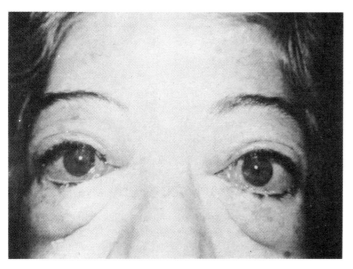

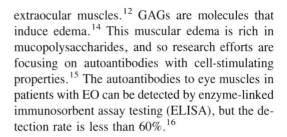

FIG. 14-2 Rapidly developing exophthalmos with marked chemosis. *(From Newell FW:* Ophthalmology: principles and concepts, *St. Louis, 1992, Mosby-Year Book.)*

due to inflammatory adhesions between the levator aponeurosis and other fixed orbital tissues[23,24] (Fig. 14-3). The white bulbar conjunctiva above the upper limbus, usually hidden under the upper lid, is revealed. This is known a "baring of the sclera" (Fig. 14-4).

An early sign of EO is periorbital swelling above the upper lids that is worse in the morning. It may be due to anterior displacement of orbital fat secondary to extraocular muscle enlargement or subcutaneous inflammation[24] (Fig. 14-5). Patients with more advanced EO may exhibit ocular motility restrictions (Ballet's sign) (see Fig. 14-6) with or without diplopia. This is invariably due to the enlargement and fibrosis of the extraocular mus-

cles. The most common muscle involved in EO is the inferior rectus, which causes vertical diplopia increasing on upward gaze.[25] A weakness of convergence may also be present (Moebius' sign).

Visual acuity reduction in EO may occur secondary to corneal drying and induced astigmatism or from direct compression of the optic nerve by enlarged extraocular muscles.[26] There appears to be no inflammatory process causing an optic neuritis, so the optic neuropathy is the result of increase orbital volume.[24] The greater the extraocular muscle volume, the more frequent is the optic neuropathy. Loss of color vision is also a result of this optic nerve compression. Visual field loss can

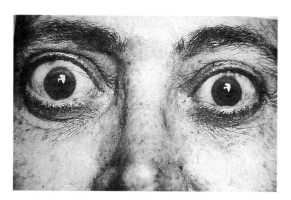

FIG. 14-3 Severe bilateral upper lid retraction in endocrine ophthalmopathy. *(From Kahaly G: Endocrine ophthalmopathy: molecular, immunological and clinical aspects, Dev Ophthalmol 25:7, 1993.)*

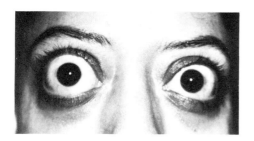

FIG. 14-4 Extreme bilateral lid retraction. Note "baring of the sclera" with no signs of conjunctival chemosis. *(From Newell FW: Ophthalmology: principles and concepts, St. Louis, 1992, Mosby-Year Book.)*

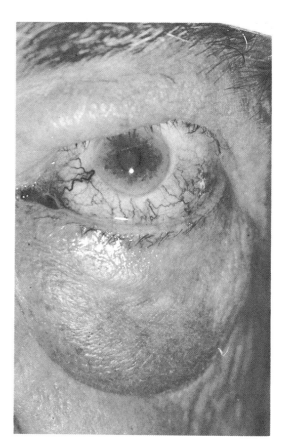

FIG. 14-5 Note periorbital swelling of upper and lower lids, with chemosis and exposure keratopathy. *(From Arffa R: Grayson's diseases of the cornea, St. Louis, 1991, Mosby-Year Book.)*

occur in EO but in no specific or predictable pattern.

Eye Signs. When diagnosing a patient with EO, it is important to look for the following signs[27,28]:

1. Extraocular muscle signs:

   Ballet's sign: a palsy of one or more extraocular muscles.

   Möbius' sign: a weakness of convergence.

   Suker's sign: poor fixation on lateral gaze.

   Wilder's sign: jerking of eyes on horizontal versional movements.

2. Lid signs:

   Boston's sign: jerking of the upper lid as the patient looks down.

   Dalrymple's sign: lid retraction in primary gaze (elevation of upper lid margin above its normal resting level in primary gaze).[24]

   Enroth's sign: edema of the lower lid.

   Gifford's sign: difficulty in everting the upper lid.

   Griffith's sign: lower lid lag on upward gaze.

   Jellinek's sign: increased pigmentation of lids (Fig. 14-7).

   Joffroy's sign: absence of forehead wrinkling on upward gaze.

   Rosenbach's sign: tremor of closed lids.

   Vigouroux's sign: puffiness of lids.

   von Graefe's sign: lid lag (additional lid retraction apparent in downgaze).[24]

3. Proptosis involvement:

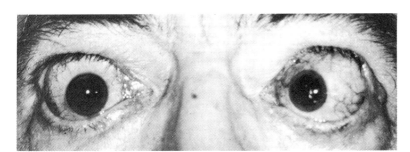

FIG. 14-6 Severe exophthalmos and eyelid retraction with fibrosis of extraocular muscles. *(From Newell FW: Ophthalmology: principles and concepts, St. Louis, 1992, Mosby-Year Book.)*

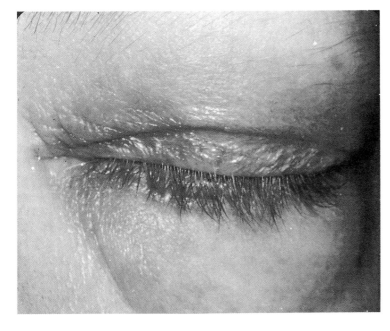

FIG. 14-7 Pigmentation of eyelids in a patient with endocrine ophthalmopathy (Jellinek's sign). *(From Arffa R: Grayson's diseases of the cornea, St. Louis, 1991, Mosby-Year Book.)*

Payne-Trousseau sign: dislocation of the globe.

Mean's sign: increased superior sclera visible on upgaze.

4. Pupil involvement:
Cowen's sign: jerky pupillary contraction to consensual light.

5. Blink involvement:
Stellwag's sign: infrequent blinking.
Pochin's sign: reduced blink amplitude.

Differential Diagnosis. The differential diagnosis of EO includes orbital tumors causing proptosis, vascular abnormalities such as hemangiomas, and orbital pseudotumors, and cavernous sinus disease with orbital sequelae.[29]

Diagnostic Testing (see box). It is important to quantitate the clinical signs of EO by careful and appropriate testing and documentation.

DIAGNOSTIC TESTING IN ENDOCRINE OPHTHALMOPATHY

Basic ocular testing
  Exophthalmometry
  Measurement of lid retraction
  Measurement of periorbital swelling
  Measurement of horizontal exclusions

Visual analysis
  Visual acuity
  Slit-lamp examination
  Stereoscopic analysis of optic nerve head
  Color testing
  Visual field testing
  Pupil testing

Diagnostic imaging
  Ultrasonography
  Computed axial tomography
  Magnetic resonance imaging

Laboratory testing
  TRH
  T_3
  T_4
  Thyroid scan
  ELISA (for thyroid antibodies)

---

1. Proptosis measurement: Exophthalmometry, either by a Hertel or Luedde *exophthalmometer,* measures the amount of proptosis, with readings up to 22.4 mm being normal.[30] This technique is best suited for measuring increases in exophthalmos over time.

2. Lid retraction measurement: To measure lid retraction in primary gaze, hold a millimeter rule in front of the open eye and measure the amount of sclera that shows above the superior limbus. Then repeat the measurement as the patient looks down. Baring of the sclera and lid lag may be the first signs of EO because they are due to inflammatory lesions of the levator aponeurosis or fibrosis of the levator muscle.[23,24]

3. Periorbital swelling measurement: Periorbital swelling of the upper lid can likewise be measured with a ruler by positioning the straightedge within the upper lid fold and allowing the swollen tissue to rest on the rule. A measurement is recorded as the amount of periorbital swelling.[24]

4. Horizontal excursion measurement: In horizontal excursions, the normal patient should be able to fully bury the lateral limbus under the lateral canthus. Limitation of horizontal excursions is demonstrated by sclera being exposed between the lateral canthus and lateral limbus in a fully abducted eye. This amount of exposed sclera is measured by a millimeter rule. The limitation of ductions is the best indicator of the severity of the disease.[24,31]

5. Visual loss measurement: A loss of visual acuity should be assessed by visual acuity testing, slit-lamp examination of the cornea, refraction and keratometry to rule out induced astigmatism, fluorescein dye testing, and Schirmer tear analysis. Tonometry readings should be taken in primary gaze and superior gaze.

If it appears that visual loss is due to optic neuropathy, then color vision testing using the Farnsworth Munsel-100 hue test or pseudoisochromatic plates is necessary.[2] Automated, threshold, static visual fields are necessary to follow peripheral field losses in EO[24] (Figs. 14-8 and 14-9). Optic

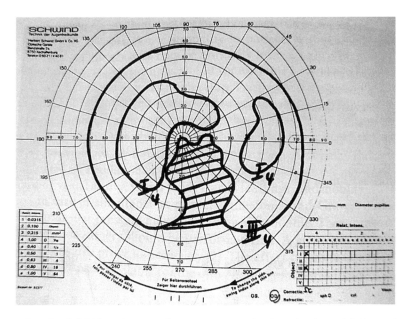

FIG. 14-8 Preoperative visual field loss due to optic nerve compression in endocrine ophthalmopathy. *(From Pickardt CR and Boergen KP, editors: Graves' ophthalmopathy. Developments in diagnostic methods and therapeutical procedures. Dev Ophthalmol, vol 20, 1989.)*

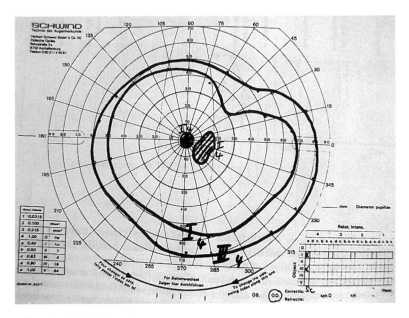

FIG. 14-9 Postoperative visual fields showing marked improvement following orbital decompression. *(From Pickardt CR and Boergen KP, editors: Graves' ophthalmopathy. Developments in diagnostic methods and therapeutical procedures, Dev Ophthalmol, vol 20, 1989.)*

disc edema accompanied by an afferent pupillary defect may occur secondary to optic nerve compression.[32]

Diagnostic Imaging Techniques. *Ultrasonography.* A-scan ultrasonography can measure the cross-sectional diameter of the extraocular muscle in question (Fig. 14-10).[33] B-scan ultrasonography produces a two-dimensional image of the muscle, and an experienced ultrasonographer is able to detect an enlarged diameter[34] (Fig. 14-11). Ultrasonography is performed without risk of radiation, in the office, and at a modest cost. It does require expertise and may miss muscle enlargement at the muscle apex.[24]

Ossoinig has pointed out that standardized ophthalmic echography serves three functions in evaluating an EO patient: It diagnoses, confirms, or rules out EO, it follows its course and the effectiveness of therapy, and it detects possible optic nerve compression.[35] Echography confirms the presence of EO when three criteria are met: no mass lesion is detected, the orbital tissues are enlarged, and at least two extraocular muscles are thickened.[35]

Computed axial tomography (CT). High-res-

olution two-dimensional images of the extraocular muscles, optic nerves, lacrimal glands, and orbits can be achieved with CT scans.[24] It is possible to demonstrate specific characteristics of EO, such as extraocular muscle enlargement, proptosis, periorbital swelling, lacrimal gland swelling, and orbital apex crowding (Figs. 14-12 and 14-13). The CT scan yields highly detailed anatomic studies and is commonplace, but the test uses radiation and continues to be expensive.[24]

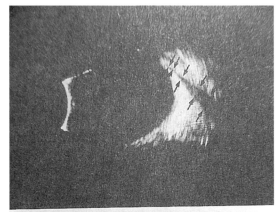
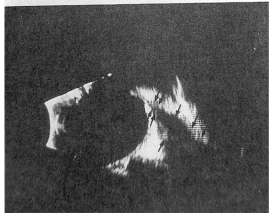

FIG. 14-11 **Top,** Patient with EO. Arrows pinpoint a dark region, which is a longitudinal section of muscle surrounded by fat (lighter zone). Notice the thinness of muscle insertions. **Bottom,** Patient with myositis. Notice thickened muscle insertions. *(From Wall JR and How J, editors: Graves' ophthalmopathy, Boston, 1990, Blackwell Scientific Publications.)*

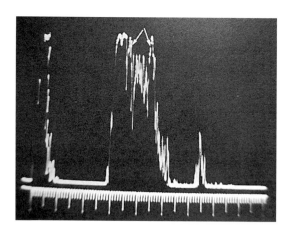

FIG. 14-10 Transocular A scan with cross-section of thickened inferior rectus muscle in endocrine ophthalmopathy. *(From Pickardt CR and Boergen KP, editors: Graves' ophthalmopathy. Developments in diagnostic methods and therapeutical procedures, Dev Ophthalmol, vol 20, 1989.)*

A CT scan of the orbits in a patient with severe EO can readily detect massive enlargement of the extraocular muscles along with the thin muscle insertions. In addition, compression of the optic nerve by muscles at the orbital apex can be visualized. The location of the equator of the globe can be compared with that of the lateral orbital rim in order to document the exophthalmos[24] (Fig. 14-14). CT sections in two planes, the axial and coronal, should be ordered when evaluating a patient with EO.[29] The coronal sections best reveal the enlargement of the extraocular muscles and measurements are possible[36] (Fig. 14-15).

Magnetic resonance imaging (MRI). The MRI improves on the CT scan by allowing for even finer differentiation of soft tissue structure without

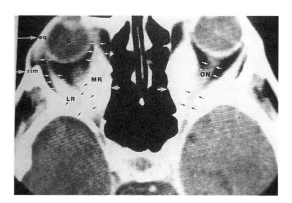

FIG. 14-14 CT scan of patient with EO. Small arrows on left denote massive enlargement of medial and lateral rectus muscles. Small arrows on the right show compression of the optic nerve. The large arrows point to the medial walls bowing inward secondary to increased pressure. Notice that the equator (eq) is forward of the orbital rim (rim). *(From Wall JR and How J, editors: Graves' ophthalmopathy, Boston, 1990, Blackwell Scientific Publications.)*

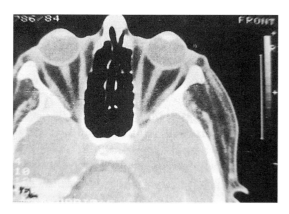

FIG. 14-12 CT scan image showing normal orbit. *(From Pickardt CR and Boergen KP, editors: Graves' ophthalmopathy. Developments in diagnostic methods and therapeutical procedures, Dev Ophthalmol, vol 20, 1989.)*

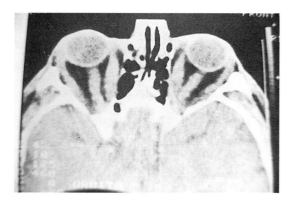

FIG. 14-13 CT scan image showing increased density of extraocular muscles in a patient with EO. *(From Pickardt CR and Boergen KP, editors: Graves' ophthalmopathy. Developments in diagnostic methods and therapeutical procedures, Dev Ophthalmol, vol 20, 1989.)*

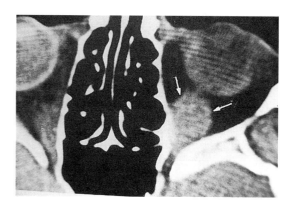

FIG. 14-15 Coronal view of enlarged right inferior rectus *(arrows)*. *(From Pickardt CR and Boergen KP, editors: Graves' ophthalmopathy. Developments in diagnostic methods and therapeutical procedures, Dev Ophthalmol, vol 20, 1989.)*

requiring the use of ionizing radiation. However, it is not readily available and is very expensive. Recently studies have shown that the T2-weighted image during MRI can accurately assess the acute inflammatory reaction within the orbital tissue.[37] MRI sections in two planes, the axial and coronal, should be used in evaluating EO.[29] The use of a paramagnetic contrast medium (gadolinium-DTPA) has been advocated to help differentiate fibrotic extraocular muscle changes from edema.[36]

Laboratory Testing. The ELISA may reveal antibodies to eye muscle, but the test is not specific to EO and positive results occur in patients with other autoimmune disorders.[38] In a patient with EO but no evidence of thyroid disease, detailed thyroid tests (TRH, T_4, T_3, and thyroid scan), thyroid antibody tests (including ELISA), and orbital scans help confirm the diagnosis.[38] To confirm EO in a patient with hypothyroidism, ocular assessment includes exophthalmometry, measurement of lid signs, elevated intraocular pressure on superior gaze, and orbital scans.[39]

Management (see the box above, right)

Amelioration of Risk Factor. Cigarette smoking has been shown to be a significant environmental risk factor in the development of EO.[39] It has been postulated, but not proven, that cessation of smoking may prevent the onset of EO in genetically susceptible individuals.[40]

Medical Management. Because of our poor understanding of the pathophysiology and evolution of EO and the lack of controlled clinical trials, managing this disorder remains difficult and controversial. The goals of medical management of EO are met if the EO is halted or reversed by antithyroid drugs and if the patient's ocular signs and symptoms are largely controlled by various local therapeutic strategies, thus avoiding significant orbital complications. Some studies point to a beneficial effect on EO with use of antithyroid medications such as methimazole.[41] But there is as yet no clear evidence for the mitigation of EO with antithyroid medication.[42]

Local Therapy. Local measures to provide symptomatic relief of the ocular sequelae of EO, such as exposure keratopathy, provide significant

---

THERAPEUTIC MANAGEMENT OF ENDOCRINE OPHTHALMOPATHY

Local symptomatic therapy
    Artificial tear solutions
    Artificial tear ointment
    Nocturnal lid taping
    Therapeutic and collagen contact lenses
    Sleep with head elevated
    Corrective prisms (for diplopia)

Medical management
    Antithyroid drugs
        Methimazole (Tapazole)
        Propylthiouracil (PTU)
        Potassium iodide
        Beta-blockers
    Immunomodulatory drugs
        Systemic steroids
        Cyclosporine
        Methotrexate
        Cyclophosphamide
        Azathioprine

Plasmapheresis

Orbital radiation therapy

Orbital decompression

---

relief for the patient but do not modify or ameliorate the disease process. These local maneuvers include the use of artificial tear solutions by day and lubricating ointment at night. The new viscous products (such as Celluvisc) provide good relief from asthenopia for many hours. If nocturnal lagophthalmos is present, taping the lids shut at night helps prevent exposure keratitis. Even dark sunglasses during the day help reduce the epiphora associated with EO. If exposure keratopathy worsens in spite of application of tear substitutes, the appropriate use of a therapeutic bandage soft contact lens may be helpful. A collagen corneal contact lens may be of value in particularly tenacious keratopathies. The patient who experiences periorbital edema that is worse in the morning should be advised to sleep with his head in a mildly elevated position.

Corrective prisms have limited use in patients complaining of diplopia secondary to EO. At best, the prisms allow for binocularity in only one particular position of gaze because the restrictive nature of EO does not produce any consistent pattern of extraocular motility palsy. The prism correction may have to be repeatedly revised as the motility pattern changes over time. Stabilization of the diplopia may never occur, and this creates a frustrating experience for the patient.

Systemic Therapy. The goal of the medical treatment of EO is to slow or stop the inflammatory reaction in order to permit, if necessary, corrective eye surgery at an earlier stage.[42] Medical therapy to ameliorate the actual disease process should be attempted when vision is threatened by corneal disease or optic neuropathy.[43] Therapy consists of immunosuppressive agents given very early in the disease process when edema is causing extraocular muscle problems but no fibrosis has occurred. The oral or intravenous use of large doses of glucocorticoids has been shown to reduce soft tissue edema.[44-47] Many patients have responded favorably to ACTH and cortisone,[48] and high-dose steroids are effective in 66% of patients.[49]

Unfortunately, large doses of steroids produce the well-known side effects in most patients. Some investigators have pointed to the potential of retrobulbar injections of steroids to reduce potential systemic side effects, but the technique has found only limited use in the routine therapy of EO.[50,51] Other studies point to cytotoxic and immunosuppressive drugs such as methotrexate, cyclophosphamide, and azathioprine (which inhibits T-cell proliferation) as possibly effective in the treatment of EO, but more research is needed.[39,52,53]

The vast majority of the literature supports the finding that two of every three patients benefit from immunosuppressive therapy.[39] The most favorable response to immunosuppression is a reduction in soft tissue signs, with moderate improvement in motility and vision loss. The least improvement is seen in the exophthalmos, which reduces on average by only 1 mm.[39] Immunosuppressive therapy rarely cures the eye disease and most patients need eye surgery, albeit at an earlier time, following immunosuppression.[54]

Plasmapheresis. Plasmapheresis, or plasma-exchange therapy, is a technique to extract antibodies from the blood,[54] which, in autoimmune disorders such as EO, should theoretically be of benefit. A typical treatment plan has the patient undergo four plasmapheresis treatments in a 1-week period, followed by steroid (prednisolone) and azathioprine given for 3 months to reduce recurrences of EO.[54] The amount of blood that is removed is replaced by solutions of plasma proteins. Clinical trials have shown that plasmapheresis is ineffective in chronic, nonprogressive EO but is very effective in early, acute, rapidly progressive EO. One third of the patients studied had recurrence of EO after 6 months following cessation of immunosuppressive therapy. All patients were stabilized by another course of plasmapheresis and a shorter course of immunosuppressive agents.[55]

Orbital Radiation. Radiation therapy makes use of well-collimated megavoltage irradiation generated by a linear accelerator and directed at retro-orbital structures, where there is a predominance of radiation-sensitive lymphocytes in the infiltrate.[56] Irradiation affects inflamed tissues in three ways. First, it corrects a state of acidosis by inducing ionization, thus converting the inflamed retrobulbar tissue to an alkylotic state.[55] Second, lymphocytic activity is suppressed, thus mitigating this component of the inflammatory response. Third, fibroblasts are suppressed by radiation effects, with a consequent reduction of GAG production.

Orbital radiation therapy is well tolerated,[57] with no long-term complications found in clinical studies (Fig. 14-16). No cataract formation, radiation retinopathy, or radiation-induced tumors have been reported on treated patients.[55] Many patients have nearly complete resolution of signs and symptoms, and only one third of radiated subjects need to proceed to surgical treatment.[55] Studies have shown that orbital radiation therapy in most cases halts progression of the disease, and in some cases improvement of signs and symptoms occurs. Orbital radiation therapy is recommended prior to surgical intervention to stabilize the ocular manifestations of EO.[57] Like plasmapheresis, it is most

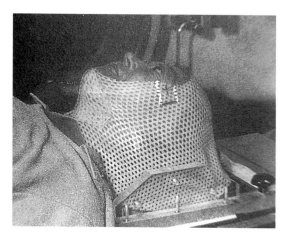

FIG. 14-16 Stable fixation of head for orbital radiation therapy (European approach). *(From Wall JR and How J, editors:* Graves' ophthalmopathy, *Boston, 1990, Blackwell Scientific Publications.)*

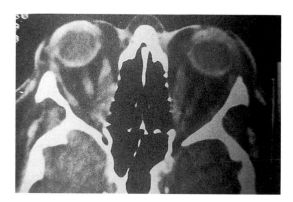

FIG. 14-17 Compression of the optic nerve by enlarged medial rectus muscle, preoperative axial CT scan. *(From Wall JR and How J, editors:* Graves' ophthalmopathy, *Boston, 1990, Blackwell Scientific Publications.)*

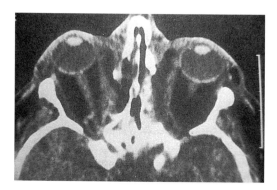

FIG. 14-18 Postoperative view of orbital decompression showing deviation of medial rectus muscles medially into ethmoidal air spaces with relief of optic nerve compression. *(From Wall JR and How J, editors:* Graves' ophthalmopathy, *Boston, 1990, Blackwell Scientific Publications.)*

effective in severe, progressive EO of recent onset.[58]

Orbital Decompression. For almost a century surgical removal of one or more of the bones comprising the bony orbit has been performed for EO.[59] This decompression procedure allows for expansion of the enlarged orbital contents and attempts to ameliorate many of the signs of dysthyroid orbitopathy, including proptosis. An otolaryngologist usually chooses the surgical procedure, and an ophthalmologist is present to assess the operation.[60]

The surgical approach is usually tailored to the individual patient. For example, if the patient has posterior optic nerve compression due to an enlarged medial rectus muscle but little proptosis, the medial wall is removed all the way back to the sphenoid sinus. This allows the medial rectus to expand into the ethmoidal air sinus, thus reducing pressure on the optic nerve[60] (Figs. 14-17 and 14-18). If the medial rectus and inferior rectus are involved with mild proptosis, the medial wall and medial portion of the orbital floor are removed.[60] With significant proptosis, three- or four-wall decompression with lateral wall or orbital roof removal can help reduce the exophthalmos.[60]

Indications for orbital decompression include marked proptosis, corneal exposure with possible keratopathy, cosmetic disfigurement, or compression of the optic nerve which threatens vision.[61] Other indications include orbital pain and orbital congestion resistant to steroids.[60]

Before orbital decompression is attempted, the patent should have immunosuppressive therapy in an attempt to reduce the orbital disease. If steroid toxicity develops, radiation therapy is a valuable alternative. Only after these therapies have been tried and the ocular condition has been stabilized

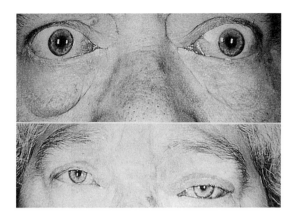

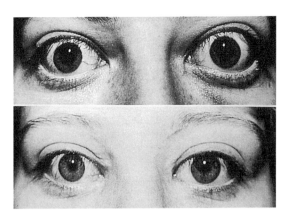

FIG. 14-19 Top, Preoperative appearance demonstrating exophthalmos following radiation and corticosteroid treatment. Bottom, Two months following orbital decompression. *(From Pickardt CR and Boergen KP, editors: Graves' ophthalmopathy: Developments in diagnostic methods and therapeutical procedures, Dev Ophthalmol, vol 20, 1989.)*

FIG. 14-20 Top, Preoperative appearance following steroid therapy. Bottom, Two and one-half years following orbital decompression. *(From Pickardt CR and Boergen KP, editors: Graves' ophthalmopathy. Developments in diagnostic methods and therapeutical procedures, Dev Ophthalmol, vol 20, 1989.)*

should orbital decompression be considered[60] (Fig. 14-19).

Orbital decompression may have serious complications. It has been noticed that in some cases the lid retraction actually worsens following surgery.[60] In some cases the cornea may be abraded or the optic nerve injured (causing visual loss) during surgery.[60] The most common complication of orbital decompression surgery is contraction of the rectus muscles, which causes postoperative diplopia. Only surgical recession improves this condition, and this should be attempted after swelling has subsided (about 3 months).[62]

The expected results of orbital decompression surgery include improvement of visual acuity, resolution of visual field defects, recession of the proptosis, and amelioration of the diplopia (Fig. 14-20). Unfortunately, the correction of diplopia, one of the most troubling symptoms of EO, has a low postoperative success rate.[63] This usually necessitates strabismic surgery to recess the involved muscles.

Corrective Eye Surgery. Patients with lid retraction are usually disturbed by the angry or surprised look that their eyes convey. In addition, they lose some of their ability to communicate

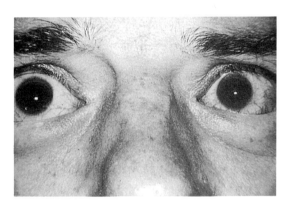

FIG. 14-21 Preoperative appearance following orbital decompression. *(From Pickardt CR and Boergen KP, editors: Graves' ophthalmopathy. Developments in diagnostic methods and therapeutical procedures, Dev Ophthalmol, vol 20, 1989.)*

nonverbally.[63] For this reason most surgeons believe that eyelid correction is not cosmetic but functional surgery to restore facial expression[64] and prevent corneal exposure.

Lid surgery is performed following decompression and strabismus surgery, which reduces proptosis and stabilizes the ocular condition. The surgery, which is modified for each individual case,

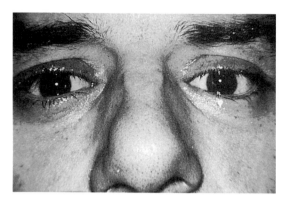

FIG. 14-22 Postoperative appearance following corrective lid surgery. *(From Pickardt CR and Boergen KP, editors: Graves' ophthalmopathy. Developments in diagnostic methods and therapeutical procedures, Dev Ophthalmol, vol 20, 1989.)*

can be performed under intravenously assisted local anesthesia[65] (Figs. 14-21 and 14-22).

SUMMARY

EO may begin with an accumulation of activated T lymphocytes (autoantibodies) that have become sensitized to cross-reactive antigens of both eye muscle and thyroid gland tissue.[66,67] The antibodies release cytokines, which stimulate the synthesis of glysoaminoglycans from fibroblasts. The glyco-aminoglycans produce inflammation in the extraocular muscles. The edema itself induces the expression of autoantigens on the muscle cells, thus further heightening the orbital immune reaction.[67] The orbital tissues become infiltrated with lymphocytes, mast cells, macrophages, and fibroblasts. Muscle, connective, and adipose tissues all become pathologically altered.[68] The extraocular muscles hypertrophy and degenerate as fat accumulates, inducing the proptosis, extraocular muscle dysfunction, and periorbital edema that is seen clinically.

Some EO patients do not require therapy of any kind. If a mild orbitopathy is present, patients may be treated with local supportive efforts (artificial tears) or corticosteroids. Severe EO should be treated as soon as possible with immunosuppressants, such as cyclosporine and/or retro-orbital radiation. Unfortunately, the combination of irradiation therapy and glucocorticoids has little effect on the proptosis or diplopia.

Orbital decompression surgery is performed if medical management does not effectively halt the progress of the disease and vision continues to be threatened.

No optimal therapeutic regimen is available to reverse the orbital disorder associated with EO. This will come with a greater understanding of the pathogenesis of endocrine ophthalmopathy.

References

1. Wall JR and How J: *Graves' ophthalmopathy: current issues and future prospects*. In *Graves' ophthalmopathy,* Boston, 1990, Blackwell Scientific Publications.

2. Kahaly G, editor: *Endocrine ophthalmopathy: molecular, immunological and clinical aspects,* Basal, 1993 Karger.

3. Volpe R: Endocrine ophthalmopathy, *Dev Ophthalmol.* 20:213, 1989.

4. Gorman AG and Bahn RS: Pathogenesis of Graves' ophthalmopathy, *Dev Ophthalmol* 20:1, 1989.

5. Sofianides T: *Thyroid gland disorders.* In Noble J, editor: *Textbook of general medicine and primary care,* Boston, 1987, Little, Brown & Co.

6. Jackson IMP: Thyrotropin releasing hormone, *N Engl J Med* 306:145, 1982.

7. Hyman BN and others: *Thyroid disease.* In *Update on general medicine,* San Francisco, 1992, American Academy of Ophthalmology.

8. Grussendorf M and others: Effect of near total thyroidectomy on ophthalmopathy in patients with Graves' disease, *Dev Ophthalmol* 20:89, 1989.

9. Wenzel BE and others: Thyroid autoantigens and plasmid encoded proteins of enteropathogenic Yersinia show antigenic homologies, *Endocrinology* 120(Suppl):31, 1987.

10. Todd JA, Bell JI, and McDevitt HO: HLA-DQ beta gene contributes to susceptibility and

resistance to insulin-dependent diabetes mellitus, *Nature* 329:599, 1987.

11. How J, Bernard N, and Wall JR: Cell-mediated immunity in Graves' ophthalmopathy, *Dev Ophthalmol* 20:38, 1989.

12. Weetman AP, Tandon N, and Metcalf RA: T-cell reactivity in endocrine ophthalmology, *Dev Ophthalmol* 20:20, 1989.

13. Westermark K, Lilja K, and Karlsson FA: Effects of sera and immunoglobulin preparations from patients with endocrine ophthalmology on the production of hyaluronate and the incorporation of titrated thymidine in fibroblasts, *Acta Endocrinol* 121:85, 1989.

14. Winand RJ and Wadeleux P: Orbital connective tissue antibodies, *Dev Ophthalmol* 20:29, 1989.

15. Rotella CM and others: Ability of monoclonal antibodies to the thyrotropin receptor to increase collagen synthesis in human fibroblasts: an assay which appears to measure exophthalmogenic immunoglobulins in Graves' sera, *J Clin Endocrinol Metab* 62:357, 1986.

16. Kendall-Taylor P and others: The nature and role of eye muscle antibodies, *Dev Ophthalmol* 20:17, 1989.

17. Gorman CA: The presentation and management of endocrine ophthalmopathy, *Clin Endocrinol Metab* 7:67, 1978.

18. Volpé R: The pathogenesis of Graves' disease: an overview, *Clin Endocrinol Metab* 7:3, 1978.

19. Sergott RC and Glaser JS: Graves' ophthalmopathy. A clinical and immunologic review, *Surv Ophthalmol* 26:1, 1981.

20. Kroll AJ and Kuwabara T: Dysthyroid ocular myopathy: anatomy, histology, and electron microscopy, *Arch Ophthalmol* 76:244, 1966.

21. Riley FC: Orbital pathology in Graves' disease, *Mayo Clin Proc* 47:975, 1922.

22. Campbell RJ: Pathology of Graves' ophthalmopathy. In Gorman CA, Waller RR, and Dyer JA, editors: *The eye and orbit in thyroid disease,* New York, 1984, Haven Press.

23. Grove AS Jr: Upper eyelid retraction and Graves' disease, *Ophthalmology* 88:499, 1981.

24. Feldon SE: *Diagnostic tests and clinical techniques in evaluation of Graves' ophthalmopathy.* In Gorman CA, Waller RR, and Dyer JA, editors: *The eye and orbit in thyroid disease,* New York, 1984, Haven Press.

25. Feldon SE and Weiner JM: Clinical significance of extraocular muscle volumes in Graves' ophthalmopathy: a quantitative computed tomography study, *Arch Ophthalmol* 100:1266, 1982.

26. Trokel SL and Jakobiec FA: Correlation of CT scanning and pathological features of ophthalmic Graves' disease, *Ophthalmology* 88:553, 1981.

27. Volpé R: Autoimmunity in the endocrine system, *Monogr Endocrinol* 17:20, 1981.

28. O'Brien JF: *Glycosaminoclycans and exophthalmos.* In Gorman CA, Waller RR, and Dyer JA, editors: *The eye and orbit in thyroid disease,* New York, 1984, Haven Press.

29. Lieb WE: Autoimmune endocrine ophthalmology—an ophthalmologist's view. In Gorman CA, Waller RR, and Dyer JA, editors: *The eye and orbit in thyroid disease,* New York, 1984, Haven Press.

30. Knudzton K: On exophthalmometry: the result of 724 measurements with Hertel's exophthalmometer on normal adult individuals, *Acta Psychiatr Neurol* 24:523, 1949.

31. Hallin ES and Feldon SE: Graves' ophthalmopathy. Section II. Correlation of clinical signs with measures derived from computed tomography, *Br J Ophtalmol* 72:678, 1988.

32. Garritt JA and others: Orbital decompression: long term results. In Gorman CA, Waller RR, and Dyer JA, editors: *The eye and orbit in thyroid disease,* New York, 1984, Haven Press.

33. Shammas HJF, Minkler DS, and Ogden C: Ultrasound in early thyroid orbitopathy, *Arch Ophthalmol* 98:277, 1980.

34. Ossoinig KC: Ultrasonic diagnosis of Graves' ophthalmopathy. In Gorman CA, Waller RR, and Dyer JA, editors: *The eye and orbit in thyroid disease,* New York, 1984, Raven Press.

35. Ossoinig KC: The role of standardized ophthalmic echography in the management of Graves' ophthalmopathy, *Dev Ophthalmol* 20:29, 1989.

36. Markl AF, Hilbertz TH, and Mann K: Graves' ophthalmopathy: standardized evaluation of computed tomography examinations, magnetic resonance imaging, *Dev Ophthalmol* 20:48, 1989.

37. Pedrosa P and others: Ergebnisse kernspintomographischer Untersuchungen bei endokriner Orbitopathie, *Klin Monatsbl Augenhelkd* 193:169, 1988.

38. Kendall-Taylor P and others: The diagnostic value of antibody tests in Graves' ophthalmopathy, *Dev Ophthalmol* 20:55, 1989.

39. Wierskinga WM: Immunosuppression in endocrine ophthalmology: why and when? *Dev Ophthalmol* 20:128, 1989.

40. Barbosa J, Wong E, and Doe RP: Ophthalmopathy of Graves' disease. Outcome after treatment with radioactive iodine, surgery and antithyroid drugs, *Arch Intern Med* 130:11, 1972.

41. Pope RM and McGregor AM. Medical management of Graves' ophthalmopathy, *Dev Ophthalmol* 20:98, 1989.

42. Wiersirga WM: Novel drugs for treatment of Graves' ophthalmopathy, *Dev Ophthalmol* 20:124, 1989.

43. Kahaly G and others: Cyclosporin and prednisone. V. Prednisone in treatment of Graves' ophthalmopathy: a controlled, randomized and prospective study, *Eur J Clin Invest* 16:415, 1986.

44. Apers RC, Oosterhuis JA, and Bierlaagn JJM: Indications and results of prednisone treatment in thyroid ophthalmopathy, *Ophthalmologica* 173:163, 1976.

45. Mulherin JL JR; Temple TE JR, and Cudney DW: Glucocorticoid treatment of progressive infiltrative ophthalmopathy, *South Med J* 65:77, 1972.

46. Kendall-Taylor P and others: Intravenous methyl-prednisolone in the treatment of Graves' ophthalmopathy, *Br Med J* 297:1574, 1988.

47. Kinsell LW, Partridge JW, and Foreman N: The use of ACTH and cortisone in the treatment and in the differential diagnosis of malignant exophthalmos: a preliminary report, *Ann Intern Med* 38:913, 1953.

48. Brain R: Cortisone in exophthalmos: report on a therapeutic trial of cortisone and corticotrophin (ACTH) in exophthalmos and exophthalmic ophthalmoplegia by a panel appointed by the Medical Research Council, *Lancet* 1:6, 1955.

49. Garber MI: Methylprednisolone in the treatment of exophthalmos, *Lancet* 1:958, 1966.

50. Bartalena L and others: Orbital cobalt irradiation combined with systemic corticosteroids for Graves' ophthalmopathy: comparison with systemic corticosteroids alone, *J Clin Endocrinol Metab* 56:1139, 1983.

51. Bigos ST and others: Cyclophosphamide in the management of advanced Graves' ophthalmopathy, *Ann Intern Med* 90:921, 1979.

52. Burrow GN and others: Immunosuppressive therapy for the eye changes of Graves' disease, *J Clin Endocrinol Metab* 31:307, 1970.

53. Wall JR and others: Thyroid binding antibodies and other immunological abnormalities in patients with Graves' ophthalmopathy: effect of treatment with cyclophosphamide. *Clin Endocrinol (Oxf)* 10:79, 1979.

54. Glinder D, Schrooyen M, and Winand RJ: The role of plasmapheresis in Graves' ophthalmopathy, *Dev Ophthalmol* 20:127, 1989.

55. Peterson IA, Donaldson SS, and Driss JP: Orbital radiotherapy: the standard experience, *Dev Ophthalmol* 20:135, 1989.

56. Sauiter-Bihl ML: Orbital radiotherapy: recent experience in Europe, *Dev Ophthalmol* 20:145, 1989.

57. Marcocci C and others: Orbital radiotherapy in the treatment of endocrine ophthalmopathy. when and why? *Dev Ophthalmol* 20:134, 1989.

58. Dollinger J: Die druckerentlastund der augenhohle durch erthgerring der ausseren orbitalwand bei hochgradigem exophthalmus (morbus base dowii) und konsekutiuer hornhauterkkrankung, *Dtsch Med Wochenschr* 37:1888, 1911.

59. Scherer H: Orbital decompression surgery, *Dev Ophthalmol* 20:169, 1989.

60. Kennerrdell JS: Orbital decompression: an overview, *Dev Ophthalmol* 20:160, 1989.

61. Mann W and others: Orbital decompression for endocrine ophthalmopathy: the endonasal approach, *Dev Ophthalmol* 20:142, 1989.

62. Garritt JA and others: Orbital decompression: an overview, *Dev Ophthalmol* 20:176, 1989.

63. Code're FC: Cosmetic and corrective eye surgery, *Dev Ophthalmol* 20:183, 1989.

64. Beyer-Machule CK: Surgical treatment of eyelid retractions, *Dev Ophthalmol* 20:211, 1989.

65. Weetman AP: Thyroid associated eye disorder: pathophysiology, *Lancet* 338:25, 1991.

66. Wall JR, Salvi M, and Bernard N: Eye disease and autoimmune thyroid disorders: mechanisms for the association, *Dev Ophthalmol* 20:72, 1989.

67. Naumann JA: Biological activity of antibodies circulating in endocrine ophthalmopathy, *Dev Ophthalmol* 20:34, 1989.

68. Harsen C and others: Adipose tissue in endocrine ophthalmopathy, *Dev Ophthalmol* 20:68, 1989.

15

Hematology and Oncology

ELOIS ROGERS-PHILIPS
AL PHILIPS

HEMATOLOGIC DISORDERS

*H*ematology is the branch of medicine that involves disorders of the blood and blood-forming tissues. These conditions include but are not limited to anemia, polycythemia, leukemia, and the coagulopathies.

Anemia

Anemia can be due to several factors, including a decrease in the number of circulating erythrocytes, or a reduced hemoglobin amount. Whatever its cause, anemia is one of the most common disorders presenting to the primary care physician.

Whenever the clinical sign of the anemia is established, it is important to determine the underlying cause. Possible causes include blood loss (for instance, from gastrointestinal cancer), iron deficiency, nutritional deficiencies, chronic disease states (such as end-stage renal failure), and drugs.

Symptoms. The symptoms of anemia vary depending on cause. Acute anemia, such as from blood loss, produces postural hypotension, overall weakness, and shock, whereas chronic anemia produces feelings of fatigue, dyspnea, palpitations, and angina. Some mild anemias produce no symptoms and are found only on laboratory testing.

Classification. Anemia is best classified by the underlying pathophysiologic mechanism combined with red blood cell (RBC) morphology and survival. Therefore, anemias may be due to decreased production of RBCs (secondary to nutritional deficiency or chronic disease) or increased destruction of RBCs (secondary to drugs, trauma, or instrinc hereditary defects). The morphologic classification of anemia involves cell size and color.

Therefore, macrocytic anemia is characterized by large RBCs, whereas normocytic and microcytic anemias reveal normal and small RBCs, respectively. Normochromic anemia has normal-colored RBCs, whereas the erythrocytes of hypochromic anemia are pale.

Diagnosis and Therapy. Once anemia is clinically suspected, it can be confirmed by laboratory testing, including a complete blood count (CBC): hemoglobin and hematocrit (H & H), RBC count, white blood cell (WBC) count, a differential, and RBC indices. A reticulocyte count helps determine the bone marrow's capacity to respond to anemia by increasing erythrocyte production. To detect morphologic changes of the erythrocyte, a peripheral blood smear is examined.

Anemia due to iron deficiency (the most common form) is characterized by a reduced hemoglobin with hypochromic, microcytic (pale, small) erythrocytes. Iron therapy is instituted while further investigation of the cause is done. Anemia due to a deficiency of vitamin B_{12} is known as pernicious anemia. Therapy is directed at vitamin B_{12} administration. Anemias due to chronic disease states (second most common form) are characterized by normochromic, normocytic RBCs and are hypoproliferative in origin. They are commonly caused by chronic renal failure, chronic liver disease, and endocrine dysfunction. Specific therapy for anemia of chronic disease is not necessary because it resolves with successful treatment of the associated disorder.

Aplastic anemia. Aplastic anemia is typically devastating owing to inability of the bone marrow to produce some or all peripheral blood elements. It is difficult to treat and may be unresponsive to any therapy. It is characterized by normocytic or macrocytic RBCs combined with a very low reticulocyte count. Therapy includes bone marrow transplant (from a suitable donor), immunosuppressive therapy, and blood transfusions (Fig. 15-1).

Thalassemias. This group of syndromes results from genetic defects that produce unstable globin chains causing damage to the RBC membrane. This problem leads to hemolysis. There are two

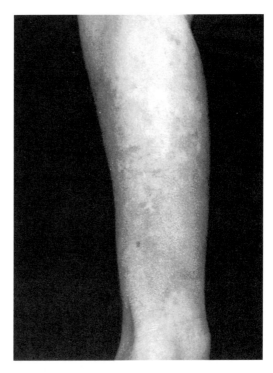

FIG. 15-1 This patient with aplastic anemia has spontaneous bleeding into the skin of the leg. *(From Habif TB:* Clinical dermatology, *St. Louis, 1990, Mosby–Year Book.)*

forms of thalassemia; β-thalassemia major (Cooley's anemia) and α-thalassemia.

β-Thalassemia is a severe form of the disease and is usually fatal in childhood. It is diagnosed by the findings of microcytic, hypochromic RBCs combined with other specific test results. The disease may present as a homozygous β-thalassemia or a heterozygous form. This type of patient has β-thalassemia trait, which is usually free of symptoms. Genetic counseling is of utmost importance to these individuals. Therapy for β-thalassemia major includes frequent transfusions and iron chelation (to remove excess iron).

Homozygous α-thalassemia results in intrauterine demise. The heterozygous form should be suspected in Asians with hypochromic, microcytic anemia without iron deficiency. Special testing is necessary in these individuals.

Polycythemia. An increase in the absolute number of circulating erythrocytes is termed polycythemia. This is reflected in the laboratory test known as the hematocrit. This erthrocytosis is due to chronic hypertension and stress or secondary causes such as high altitude, chronic lung disease, tumors, and kidney disease. Primary polycythemia (polycythemia vera) is treated with phlebotomy and, possibly, with radioactive phosphorus and alkylating agents.

Leukemia. Leukemia is a malignancy of the blood-forming organs which may cause changes in the WBC count. Leukemia may be classified as acute or chronic, and its description is based on the type of cell involved and the presence of abnormal WBCs in the blood.

HEMATOLOGY AND THE EYE

The ophthalmic consequences of hematologic diseases can be easily divided into congenital and acquired categories. The importance of an adequate history with regard to the ophthalmic complaint as well as antecedent medical problems is paramount to the effectiveness of the ophthalmic evaluation and appropriate triage.

Congenital Hematologic Disease

There are many congenital hematologic diseases; however, few express ophthalmic consequences at birth.

Fanconi Syndrome. Fanconi syndrome is congenital aplastic anemia. The disease can best be described as severe pancytopenia—depression of the hemoglobin, WBC count, and platelets, or any combination thereof, within the first 6 weeks of life. In addition to retinal findings of flame-shaped hemorrhages associated with thrombocytopenia, there is usually a platelet count of less than 20,000/dl. Patients may also present with congenital cataracts.

Retinopathy of Prematurity. Retinopathy of prematurity is a rare cause of progressive visual loss and is associated with birth weights of 1000 g or less. Approximately 1300 children born each year have some visual loss due to retinopathy of prematurity. A severe visual loss occurs in 250 to 500 of these children. The pathophysiology is produced by ischemia-induced retinal neovascularization. These changes can be severe enough to cause blindness 8% of the time.

Rh Factor Incompatibility. Rh factor incompatibility may present in a live fetus with microphthalmos. The overall syndrome is caused by a major red blood cell antigen incompatibility, resulting in severe hemolytic anemia at birth. Although this syndrome is incompatible with prolonged survival, ophthalmic evaluations may be necessary.

The remaining congenital problems express their abnormalities at a later time in the patient's life; however, the congenital abnormality is the underlying prerequisite for their expression.

Sickle-cell Anemia. The frequency of the sickle cell gene is approximately 12% in the American population. It encompasses individuals of African American, mediterranean, Middle Eastern, and South East Asian ancestry in descending order of frequency. Normal adults inherit two genes that code for normal adult hemoglobin (AA). The abnormal hemoglobins arc inherited as autosomal dominants; consequently, individuals who have at least one gene coding for normal adult hemoglobin (A) therefore have the trait (AS) only and rarely have complications. When the sickled hemoglobin is combined with other abnormal hemoglobins (thalassemia, sickle hemoglobin C, hemoglobin E), ophthalmic pathology may be expected in the second decade of life.

The diagnosis of abnormal hemoglobin may be suggested by abnormal red cell morphology (sickle cells, target cells, hemoglobin crystals in the cytoplasm). The diagnostic clinical test is hemoglobin electrophoresis, which not only confirms the presence of abnormal hemoglobin but also quantitates the specific amounts. This quantitation can frequently aid in the clinical and prognostic decisions in this disease.

The origin of the sickled gene can be traced to the African continent. Data suggest that this mutation of the hemoglobin chain protected those affected from malaria infestation. Genetically, valine is substituted for glutamic acid, causing a structural deformity of the hemoglobin chain. This structural abnormality causes the hemoglobin chain to form crystals, accounting for the sickle-shape red blood cell that leads to intravascular clotting (Fig. 15-2). The resulting ophthalmic pathologic changes can be divided as follows: (1) superficial, as evidenced by comma-shaped vessels seen in the conjunctiva; (2) nonproliferative retinal hemorrhages that may be preretinal, intraretinal, or subretinal in position. As these hemorrhages resolve, various signs occur depending on the depth of retinal invasion. These findings include salmon patches, refractile deposits, and black sunbursts. The nonproliferative findings rarely affect vision and consequently require no treatment. (3) A proliferative retinopathy usually affects the retinal periphery and because of its progressive nature is associated with visual loss.

Photocoagulation as well as retinal surgery has been used to stabilize these lesions. Peripheral neovascularization (seafans) has been reported to regress spontaneously 50% of the time. The proliferative findings have been most consistently associated with individuals having hemoglobin C (AC, SC, CC).

Acquired Hematologic Disease

The acquired hematologic manifestations occur primarily in the adult population. They can be categorized by evaluations of the red blood cells, the white blood cells, coagulation disorders, and abnormalities of the blood viscosity.

Basic to an understanding of acquired disorders is the integrity of the blood system. Blood is the fluid by which the body creates, destroys, utilizes, and stores all elements essential to survival. Because this fluid traverses every organ and space of the body, the eye presents a unique avenue to visualize its deficiencies. The cardinal symptom of conjunctival pallor, usually expressed when the red blood cell count is 50% of normal, is a variable clinical finding. A CBC, consisting of a WBC count, RBC count, hematocrit (packed red cell mass), quantitative hemoglobin, mean corpuscular volume, total platelet count, and WBC differential, is rarely unavailable today and would be the minimum laboratory studies necessary for evaluating ocular problems associated with acquired anemia. The normal values may vary depending on the laboratory, but general guidelines are listed in Table 15-1.

The clinical findings of retinal hemorrhage, usually flame-shaped, may also be of the dot and blot variety as well as white-centered intraretinal hemorrhages (Roth spots), depending on the level of anemia. When the anemia has occurred rapidly or is extremely severe, cotton-wool retinal exudates (nerve fiber layer infarcts) may also be seen. The tortuosity of the retinal vessels varies inversely with the level of anemia. Rarely, papilledema oc-

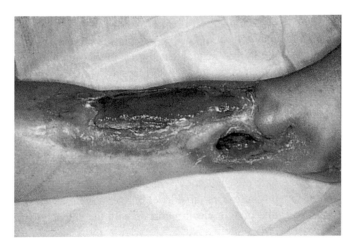

FIG. 15-2 This patient with sickle-cell anemia shows associated leg ulcers. *(From Lawrence CM and Cox NH: Physical signs in dermatology: color atlas and text, London, 1993, Wolfe Medical Publishers, Ltd.)*

TABLE 15-1 *Blood Cell Values in a Normal Population*

	Men		Women
White cell count, $\times 10^9$/L blood		7.8 (4.4-11.3)	
Red cell count, $\times 10^{12}$/L blood	5.21 (4.52-5.90)		4.60 (4.10-5.10)
Hemoglobin, g/dl blood	15.7 (14.0-17.5)		13.8 (12.3-15.3)
Hematocrit, ratio	0.46 (0.42-0.50)		0.46 (0.36-0.45)
Mean corpuscular volume, fl/red cell		88.0 (80.0-96.1)	
Mean corpuscular hemoglobin, pg/red cell		30.4 (27.5-33.2)	
Mean corpuscular hemoglobin concentrations, g/dl RBC		34.4 (33.4-35.5)	
Red cell distribution width, CV (%)		13.1 (11.5-14.5)	
Platelet count, $\times 10^9$/L blood		311 (172-450)	

curs associated with a type of pseudotumor cerebri precipitated by cerebral anoxia.

The causes of the acquired anemias are varied. The pathophysiology lies in the failure of the bone marrow to produce RBCs because of deficiencies such as iron or vitamin B_{12}, hemolysis secondary to drugs, and or antibody formation.

Leukemia. Ophthalmic pathology may be present in both acute and chronic leukemias. As mentioned earlier, WBCs are one of the formed elements of blood. Malignant proliferation of WBCs or any of their developmental forms is called leukemia. The CBC and bone marrow tests are the basis of such a diagnosis. Important in the understanding of this disease process is that the initial presentation may relate to a visual complaint. Emergent triage to a subspecialist conversant in the management of these disorders is paramount to the patient's survival. In short, leukemia is an ocular emergency until proven otherwise.

Leukemia can be of the acute or chronic variety, depending on the rapidity of onset. The French, American and British (FAB) presented a classification of acute leukemia (1976) which correlates the morphologic cell type, clinical course, and prognostic implications for the lymphoid (L1, L2, L1) and nonlymphoid (ANLL) (M1-M7) varieties (Table 15-2). Chronic leukemia affecting the lymphoid or myeloid cells is much more insidious

in onset. Ophthalmic findings are seen in 50% to 70% of patients with leukemia. Leukemic infiltrates of the optic nerve can be seen.

Polycythemia. Blood viscosity can affect the appearance of the eye in various ways. Polycythemia, or excessive numbers of RBCs, has been associated with transient blindness (amaurosis fugax), generalized blurring, and vascular congestion. Although the excess RBCs are the major problem, white cell and platelet counts may be elevated. The unifying pathophysiology is tissue hypoxia of a primary (idiopathic) or secondary (pulmonary, cardiac, renal, or vascular) origin. The retinal pathology is usually associated with red cell counts in excess of 6 million/mm^3.

Serum Protein Abnormalities. Blood viscosity may also be influenced by plasma proteins. There are three general categories of plasma proteins which circulate with the liquid fraction of blood: (1) albumin, (2) several types of globulins, (3) and fibrinogen. Again, diseases associated with protein abnormalities can be primary or secondary (Table 15-3). The ophthalmic pathology is that of a congestive retinopathy. Waldenstrom's macroglobulinemia as well as myeloma has been associated with this pathology. The laboratory findings, in addition to a variable level of anemia, are an abnormal protein electrophoresis with the characteristic "M" protein spike.

TABLE 15-2 *Classification of Acute Leukemia*

Type	FAB* Classification	Frequency (%)	Cases/Year (US Children <age 15)
ALL			1,500-2,000
AML	L1	85	
	L2	14	
	L3	1	
AML			
AML	M1	20	400-500
AML with differentiation	M2	20	
APML	M3	3	
MMMol	M4	25	
AMOL	M5	26	
Erythroid leukemia	M6	4	
Acute megakaryocytic leukemia	M7	2	

*French-American-British

ALL = acute lymphoblastic leukemia; AML = acute myelogenous leukemia; APML = acute promyelocytic leukemia; MMMol = acute myelomonocytic leukemia.

TABLE 15-3 *Electrophoresis of Serum and Urine Proteins in Diseases Associated with Protein Abnormalities*

Clinical Indications	Abnormality and Interpretation
Unexplained edema or ascites	Hypoalbuminemia
Suspected liver disease	Hypoalbuminemia frequent; hyperglobulinemia suggests cirrhosis or chronic active hepatitis
Collagen diseases, sarcoidosis	Polyclonal hyperglobulinemia
Unusual susceptibility to infections	Hypogammaglobulinemia or agammaglobulinemia
CLL, malignant lymphoma	Hypogammaglobulinemia or, rarely, IgG or IgM M components
Unexplained proteinuria	Albumin or a mixture of all serum proteins is found with urinary tract infections or the nephrotic syndrome; homogeneous urine proteins that migrate in the globulin region are usually indicative of plasma cell neoplasms secreting free light or heavy chains.
Evidence of plasma cell neoplasms, e.g., bone pain, frequent infections, elevated sedimentation rate, rouleaux formation, proteinuria, or osteolytic skeletal lesions	Serum or urinary monoclonal protein, with reduced normal immunoglobulins and hypoalbuminemia
Amyloidosis	Monoclonal serum or urinary proteins frequent

Coagulopathies. The flow of blood has a regulatory mechanism to retard or stop the egress of the precious fluid. This system is called the coagulation or clotting system. The production, destruction, and quality of its components as well as the number and quality of the circulating platelets regulate bleeding. The clotting cascade is a complex scheme explaining the sequential steps in the intrinsic and extrinsic clotting system. A disorder at any point in this system is called a *coagulopathy*.

Hemophilia. The more severe coagulopathies are usually sex-linked and therefore have their greatest expression in males (hemophilia A and B). The more frequent bleeding diatheses are associated with deficiencies of those factors made by the liver. Accurate diagnosis requires the interpretation of the prothrombin time, activated partial thromboplastin time, platelet count, and specific assays where indicated. Treatment is with specific replacement of the factor by human blood products or synthetic derivatives. Intraocular or extraocular hemorrhage may occur spontaneously, by trauma, or during surgery.

Hypercoagulable syndromes. In the past 5 to 10 years clinical presentation of hypercoagulable syndromes has been better described. The circulation of activated clotting factors could result in uninhibited intravascular clotting (usually venous). The critical inhibitors of this coagulation are antithrombin III, protein C, and protein S. Congenital deficiency states have been associated with ophthalmic thrombotic complications (1 in 500,000 live births).

Disseminated intravascular coagulation. Disseminated intravascular coagulation is a dynamic hematologic state in which, because of the underlying processes, clotting occurs throughout the body, with consumption of clotting substances in excess of the body's ability to replenish the consumed substances. This is usually an acute emergent process associated with thrombocytopenia, prolonged prothrombin time, prolonged activated partial thromboplastin time, low fibrinogen level, and fragmented RBCs on the peripheral smear. No test is available to confirm the diagnosis. However, with a rapidly evolving clinical picture and generalized bleeding, a high index of suspicion is the single most important factor in proper diagnosis and treatment. Although the recommendations for treatment are varied, none is successful unless the underlying mechanism is controlled.

ONCOLOGIC DISORDERS

With 25% of American deaths each year caused by cancer, it is important for the eye-care practitioner to remain vigilant for primary ocular tumors, involvement of the eye or adnexa by direct extension, and metastasis from another site.

Diagnosis of the Cancer Patient

Cancer is diagnosed in patients who are asymptomatic by a thorough history, physical examination, and testing. The history includes risk factors such as smoking, alcohol, radiation, and environmental toxic exposure. Depending on the patient, the physical examination should include a systemic head, neck, and breast examination, digital rectal examination, and pelvic examination for women. A dermatologic examination should be performed with a magnifier to help detect basal cell carcinomas, particularly on exposed skin surfaces (see Chapter 8). Laboratory testing should include mammography in women, a Pap test, a stool occult blood test, and sigmoidoscopy in patients over the age of 50 years.

Further testing to localize the involved area may use radiologic imaging such as plain radiography, computed tomography, and magnetic resonance imaging. Pathologic confirmation is obtained by biopsy as quickly as possible.

ONCOLOGY AND THE EYE

Only approximately 5% of ocular tumors are considered primary to the eye. The remaining 95% occur by metastasis or direct extension. The remainder of this discussion deals only with ophthalmologic consequences of metastatic disease or its treatment.

Ocular Metastases

The incidence of ocular metastases is approximately 300,000 per year. The single most important reason for this figure is the prolonged survival of the cancer patient. The pathophysiology may be directly associated with metastases or the consequence of internal malignancy (see box below). Breast cancer has been shown to be the most frequent causative primary cancer in choroidal metastases (Table 15-4). Treatment of the primary tumor is usually associated with regression of the ocular metastases.

The nonmetastatic ocular pathophysiology is that of infection. Host immunosuppression caused by the underlying malignancy predisposes the host to opportunistic infections that are primarily viral, fungal, or protozoan (see box below, right). These infections are extremely difficult to treat and invariably need the recommendations of an infectious disease specialist to avoid catastrophic blindness.

OPHTHALMIC MANIFESTATIONS OF SYSTEMIC CANCER

Metastatic
   Orbit
   Ocular
      Anterior segment
      Posterior segment

Nonmetastatic
   Infections
   Treatment-related complications
   Remote effects (paraneoplastic)

TABLE 15-4 *Most Common Primary Cancers in Choroidal Metastases*

Primary Cancer	Percent of Choroidal Metastases
Breast	71.8
Lung	8.9
Genitourinary	3.2
Gastrointestinal	2.4
Gynecologic	1.6
Sarcoma	1.6
Other	10.0

Ocular Tumor Detection

Intraocular tumors, whether primary or the result of metastatic extension, may be suspected on the basis of six characteristics (see Figs. 15-3 and 15-4):

1. Increase in size: suspicious lesions of the eye or adnexa may be visualized grossly or require diagnostic techniques. These approaches include direct ophthalmoscopy, indirect ophthalmoscopy, stereoscopic ophthalmoscopy (with 60, 75, or 90 diopter lens and biomicroscope), and gonioscopy. Tumors of the ciliary body may be visualized by retroilluminating the sclera with a bright penlight placed near or on the limbus 180 degrees away from the suspected lesion.

   Whatever technique is used, the lesion must be described as well as possible, drawn, measured accurately, and, if possible, photographed. Photographic alternatives include standard slit-lamp or retinal cameras, stereoscopic cameras, and videography. The suspicious lesion should be remeasured at regular intervals. Growth raises the possibility that the lesion is malignant.

2. Discoloration: In general, a lesion is more suspicious for malignancy if it reveals a discoloration compared with the normal surrounding

---

COMMON OCULAR INFECTIONS IN CANCER PATIENTS

Anterior segment
   Herpes zoster (iritis, keratitis)
   Herpes simplex (iritis, keratitis)

Posterior segment
   Toxoplasmosis (retinitis)
   Cytomegalovirus (retinitis)
   Herpes simplex (retinitis)
   Fungal infections
      Candida species (retinitis)
      Mucormycoses (vasculitis)

Endogenous endophthalmitis
   Bacterial
   Fungal

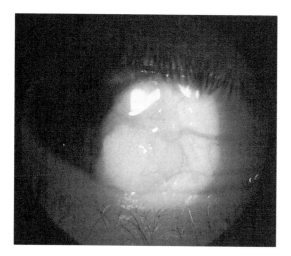

FIG. 15-3 A preoperative view of a conjunctival tumor which was suspicious due to increasing size, discoloration (from normal conjunctival tissue), surrounding engorged blood supply, indistinct margins, distortion of surrounding conjunctiva and induced astigmatism causing a loss of visual function.

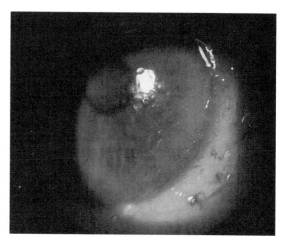

FIG. 15-4 The postoperative appearance of the same patient as in Fig. 15-3. Biopsy revealed a primary conjunctival malignancy.

tissue. This is just one small piece of evidence suggesting a serious disorder; of course, many discolored ocular lesions are benign.

3. Neovascular growth: Vascular changes may occur to a greater degree within or overlying intraorbital tumors than in benign lesions. Any lesion that is associated with a dilation of surrounding normal vasculature (for example, on the conjunctiva) or is associated with neovascular growth should be evaluated for possible malignancy.

   Intraocular tumors may produce vascular abnormalities as visualized on fluorescein angiography. They may hyperfluoresce, hypofluoresce, or be "invisible" to the test, depending on the nature of the choroidal tumor.

4. Indistinct margins: In general, benign ocular tumors tend to have distinct margins, whereas malignant lesions have indistinct margins. This is because the malignancy is growing and spreading through the surrounding tissue. The tumor border may reveal both lateral spread and deep tissue invasion.

5. Distortion of surrounding tissue: A malignant tumor has a greater tendency to distort the normal tissue surrounding it than does a benign growth. Again, this is due to lateral and deep spread of the malignancy through the tissues around it. Also, metastatic islands of spread may be detected visually around the main lesion.

6. Loss of function: In general, benign lesions cause little or no loss of normal organ function. Malignant tumors have a greater potential for interfering with ocular function. Therefore, an iris melanoma may cause a pupillary anomaly; a ciliary body tumor may alter aqueous production and hence intraocular pressure; and a choroidal malignancy may be associated with a serous detachment and possible loss of vision.

Management of Ocular Malignancy

The management of both ocular metastases and primary ocular malignancies may include irradiation of the eye or surrounding tissue. Ophthalmic consequences may be immediate: dry eye, corneal

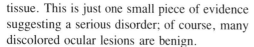

REMOTE EFFECTS OF CANCER IN THE VISUAL SYSTEM: VISUAL PARANEOPLASTIC SYNDROMES

Ocular
  Optic neuritis
  Photoreceptor (retinal) degeneration (melanoma, oat cell carcinoma)

Oculomotor
  Opsoclonus (breast cancer, lung cancer)
  Opsoclonus-myoclonus syndrome (neuroblastoma, thyroid, breast)
  Lambert-Eaton myasthenic syndrome

TABLE 15-5 *Ocular Complications of Systemic Chemotherapy*

Lids	Lacrimal system
5-Fluorouracil (entropion)	5-Fluorouracil (ductal fibrosis)
Vincristine (ptosis)	Cornea (keratitis)
Vinblastine (ptosis)	Busulfan
	Chlorambucil
Conjunctiva (conjunctivitis)	Cytarabine
5-Fluorouracil	
Methotrexate	Uvea
Melphalan	BCG
Cyclophosphamide	Thiotepa
	Retina
Lens (cataract)	Mitotane
Busulfan	Tamoxifen (refractile deposits)
Corticosteroids	
Mitotane	Chlorambucil (hemorrhage)
	Cisplatin
Optic nerve (optic neuritis)	Nitrosourea (BCNU)
Vincristine	
Cisplatin	
Nitrosourea (BCNU)	

OCULAR SIDE EFFECTS OF INTRA-ARTERIAL CHEMOTHERAPY

Intracarotid nitrosurea
  Local pain (eye, orbit)
  Conjunctivitis
  Keratitis
  Disc edema
  Optic neuritis
  Ocular ischemia and neovascularization
  Retinal degeneration (vasculitis)

Intracarotid cisplatin
  Optic neuritis
  Transient visual loss
  Retinal degeneration, with characteristic photopic electroretinographic changes
  Toxic neuroretinitis
  Pigmentary changes in retina, constricted arterioles, pale nerve

ulceration, delayed cataract, neovascularization, ischemic ocular syndrome, neovascular glaucoma, and optic neuropathy secondary to radionecrosis.

The prolonged survival of the cancer patient can also be associated with neuroendocrine syndromes related to tumor kinetics, toxins, antibodies, nutritional deprivation, or tumor hormone elaboration (see box above, left). These are extremely unusual syndromes, and the occurrence of this pathology indicates a need for further evaluation for a primary cancer.

The ocular complications from systemic or local (regional) chemotherapy are constantly increasing (Table 15-5 and box above). Complete medical history is the single most important factor in minimizing the impact of these drugs.

The ophthalmic consequences of systemic cancer require continuing dialogue and early referrals of the eye-care professional and the practicing oncologist. When they work together, the life and vision of the patient may be significantly prolonged.

Bibliography

Allen RA and Straatsma BR: Ocular involvement in leukemia and allied disorders. *Arch Ophthalmol* 66:68, 1961.

Bedford MA: *Color atlas of ocular tumors,* Chicago, 1979, Mosby–Year Book.

Char DH: *Clinical Ocular Oncology,* New York, 1989, Churchill Livingston.

Doxanas MT, Green UR: Sebacious gland carcinoma: review of 40 cases, *Arch Ophthalmol* 102:245, 1984.

Doxanas MT, Green UR, Iliff CE: Factors in the successful surgical management of basal cell carcinoma of the eyelids, *AMJ Ophthalmol* 91:726, 1981.

Shields CL, Shields JA, Peggs M: Metastatic tumors to the orbit. *Ophthalmic Reconstr Plast Surg* 4:73, 1988.

Shields JA: *Intraocular tumors: A text and atlas,* Philadelphia, 1992, WB Saunders.

Shields A, editor: *Update on malignant ocular tumors,* Boston, 1992 Little, Brown and Co.

Yanoff M, and Fine BS: *Ocular pathology: A text and atlas,* ed 3, Philadelphia, 1989, JB Lippincott.

16

Neurology and Psychiatry

ALEXANDER S. ZWIL

KEY TERMS

Pneumoencephalogram

Contrast Myelography

Positron Emission
Tomography (PET)

Single Photon Emission
Computed Tomography
(SPECT)

Regional Cerebral Blood
Flow (rCBF)

Electroencephalography
(EEG)

Visual Evoked Responses
(VERs)

Brainstem Auditory Evoked
Responses (BAERs)

Somatosensory Evoked
Responses (SERs)

Electromyography (EMG)

Nerve Conduction Studies
(NCS)

Meningitis

Encephalitis

Parkinsonism

Seizure

Epilepsy

Myopathy

Psychosis

Neurosis

Schizophrenia

Hallucination

Delirium

Dementia

Depression

Mania

Anxiety

Migraine

Photopsia

Alexia

Suicide

Somatization

Hypochondriasis

---

*T*his chapter describes the evaluation and treatment of diseases that primarily affect the nervous system, including the brain, spinal cord, peripheral nerves, and neuromuscular junction. Historically, diseases that produce identifiable anatomic, physiologic, electrical, or chemical changes in nervous tissue have been called "neurologic," whereas those that result in changes in thought, mood, intellect, or behavior have been called "psychiatric." Although this is an arbitrary distinction scientifically, it remains a useful distinction in clinical practice.

CLINICAL SPECIALTIES

The two specialties of modern medicine which are most concerned with diseases of the nervous system are neurology and psychiatry. Neurologists deal primarily with physical diseases of the nervous system, including those resulting in strokes, paralyses, sensory loss, seizures, and involuntary movements. Behavioral neurologists subspecialize in diseases of the cerebral cortex, which result in disturbances of complex functions such as language and memory. Psychiatrists deal primarily with disorders of mental processes such as depression, anxiety, and disturbances of thought and behavior. Neuropsychiatrists are psychiatrists who specialize in the treatment of behavioral or emotional complications of organic brain disease or in the evaluation of the neurologic substrates of mental illness.

In addition to neurology and psychiatry, members of other medical specialties are involved with the diagnosis and treatment of neurologic and mental illness. Neurologic surgeons (neurosurgeons) specialize in surgery involving the brain and spinal cord. Neuroradiologists have special proficiency in interpreting neurologic imaging studies. Neuro-ophthalmologists deal with the neurologic aspects of vision.

Although not trained as physicians, some psychologists are also engaged in clinical work. Clinical psychologists are trained in psychiatric diagnosis and in the practice of psychotherapy. Neuropsychologists are proficient in the evaluation of higher cognitive functions and in the administration of psychometric tests.

DEFINITIONS

Although the reader of this book is expected to be familiar with basic neuroanatomy and neurophysiology, a brief review of terminology may be helpful. The central nervous system (CNS) consists of the brain and spinal cord; the peripheral nervous system encompasses neural elements outside of the CNS, including nerves, organs of sensation, and the neuromuscular junction. The brain and spinal cord are enclosed in the skull and vertebral column, where they float suspended in the cerebrospinal fluid (CSF), which fills the subarachnoid space and the ventricles of the brain. Cranial nerves exit the CNS directly from the brain. There are twelve pairs of cranial nerves, conventionally labeled with Roman numerals I through XII; they innervate the skin and muscles of the face, as well as the organs of sight, hearing, smell, taste, and balance. Spinal nerves leave the CNS from the spinal cord and innervate the muscles of movement and posture, the skin of the body surface, and the internal organs. Nerve impulses are conducted electrically along the axons of individual neurons and transmitted to the next neuron in the pathway by chemical messengers, called neurotransmitters, which are released into a space between the membranes of the two neurons, called a synapse. Sequential pathways of neurons are called tracts in the CNS and nerves in the peripheral nervous system. Motor nerves make chemical contact with muscles at the neuromuscular junction.

NEUROLOGY

Neurologic Diagnosis

Diagnosis in neurology, as in other branches of medicine, entails a complete history, a physical examination, and ancillary studies as indicated.

The Neurologic Examination. The neurologic examination is that portion of the physician's physical examination which deals with the nervous system. It provides information about function and dysfunction and can pinpoint the anatomic location of the lesion, although it usually does not reveal the cause of the disease. A differential diagnosis is generated, and ancillary studies are necessary to establish the exact diagnosis.

The nervous system is organized topographically. Nuclei in the CNS receive sensory information from specific sense organs or areas of the body and transmit directions to specific muscles or effector organs along specific tracts and nerves. Thus, a localized lesion in the CNS usually produces a predictable pattern of sensory loss and dysfunction in the body parts under its control. By observing known patterns of neurologic dysfunction during the physical examination, a physician may often deduce the location of the lesion responsible for the deficits. This is called topographic diagnosis.

An example of topographic diagnosis is provided by the examination of visual fields in an optometrist's office. A lesion somewhere in the visual pathways interrupts the transmission of information from the retina to the occipital cortex and produces a characteristic visual field defect, depending upon its location and which fibers or tracts are damaged. An optometrist can deduce the location of the lesion using his knowledge of the anatomy of the visual pathways. For instance, a lesion compressing the optic chiasm from above can destroy the decussating fibers, originating in the nasal half of the retina, while sparing the nondecussating temporal fibers. Because the damaged fibers carry information about the temporal visual fields, this lesion results in a bitemporal hemianopsia; this is the only location in the visual pathway where a single lesion can produce this particular field defect. By a similar process, a neurologist may often localize lesions anywhere in the nervous system, including those causing muscular paralysis, sensory loss, loss of coordination, involuntary movements, language or memory deficits, and certain psychic phenomena. However, knowing *where* the lesion is does not tell the physician *what* the lesion is because a variety of disease processes, including infarctions, hemorrhages, tumors, and demyelination, can produce the same pattern of dysfunction if they occur at the same location. To discover the cause of the lesion, the physician must use his knowledge of differential diagnosis or use ancillary studies if any are available.

The major portions of the neurologic examination are the following:

1. The mental status examination (MSE): Usually briefer than that used in psychiatry, this evaluates functions of the cerebral cortex such as language, memory, calculating ability, fine motor dexterity, complex sensory processing, and the capacity for insight and judgment.
2. Cranial nerves: This examination localizes lesions involving the cranial nerves or their nuclei; this is especially helpful for localizing lesions in the brainstem.
3. Motor examination: This entails the evaluation of muscle strength to localize lesions of the motor cortex and tracts, anterior horns of the spinal cord, and peripheral nerves.
4. Sensory examination: Like the motor examination, this evaluates lesions in the brain, spinal cord, or nerves causing loss of somatic sensation.
5. Cerebellar examination: This examines the pattern of muscular incoordination caused by lesions of the cerebellum or its descending tracts.
6. Deep tendon reflexes: This examines the deep tendon reflex arc between the muscles and spinal cord, as well as the influence of higher nervous centers.
7. Pathologic reflexes: This takes note of reflexes, like the Babinski's response and frontal release signs, which are not present in the healthy nervous system but appear as a result of specific diseases.

For further details, see Chapter 2.

Lumbar Puncture. Lumbar puncture (also known as LP, or spinal tap) allows direct measurement of intracranial pressure (ICP) and examination of the CSF. The CSF is analyzed for blood cell count, glucose and protein content, and presence of antibodies or cultured for bacteria, fungi, or viruses.

Anatomic Imaging. Diagnostic imaging in neurology has recently been enormously expanded by the development of new contrast media and sophisticated computerized techniques, which allow the detailed examination of neuroanatomy in living patients.

Roentgenograms (X-rays, radiographs, or plain films) are produced when an x-ray beam passes through the human body and exposes a photographic film. They can image bony structures such as the skull and vertebral column but cannot image neural structures or CSF spaces. Fig. 16-1 illustrates roentgenograms of the head.

A *pneumoencephalogram*, produced by injecting air into the CSF spaces via lumbar puncture, outlines the cerebral ventricles on a plain roentgen-

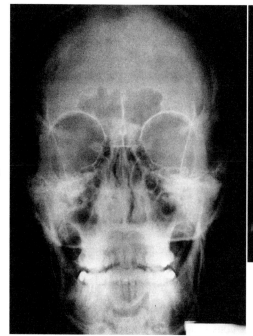
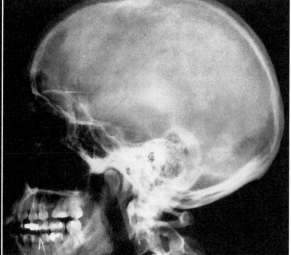

FIG. 16-1 Cranial roentgenograms, in anteroposterior (**A**) and lateral (**B**) projections. *(Courtesy of Barry B. Goldberg, M.D., and Daniel A. Merton, B.S., R.D.M.S., Department of Radiology, Jefferson Medical College, Philadelphia, PA.)*

ogram. This technique is seldom used today owing to the availability of more sophisticated techniques for imaging soft tissues and fluid spaces within the body.

Computed tomography (CAT scan or CT scan) uses an array of x-ray cameras to construct a matrix of tissue densities in three dimensions, from which a gray-scale or color-coded image is reconstructed by computer. Unlike plain roentgenography, it can discriminate CSF and several levels of tissue density. The images are usually displayed as serial sections through the brain, from which three-dimensional anatomy can be appreciated by visual inspection. The sections may be oriented to any plane, most commonly the axial. Fig. 16-2 illustrates the use of CT images in neurologic diagnosis.

Magnetic resonance imaging (MRI) uses the energy emitted by spinning protons in an imposed magnetic field to produce computer-reconstructed

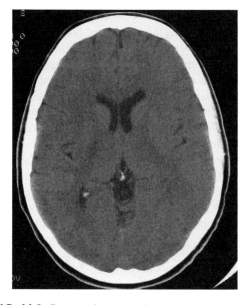

FIG. 16-2 Computed tomography scan of the brain of a normal subject in axial projection. *(Courtesy of Barry B. Goldberg, M.D., and Daniel A. Merton, B.S., R.D.M.S., Department of Radiology, Jefferson Medical College, Philadelphia, PA.)*

images, which are commonly displayed in the sagittal, coronal, and axial planes. Unlike CT, this technique does not expose the patient to x-rays. Variations in technique allow very high resolution imaging of anatomic structures and pathologic pro-

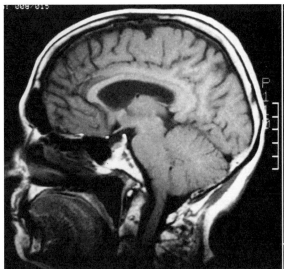

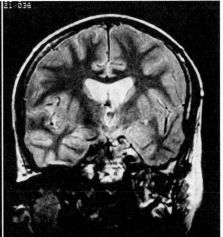

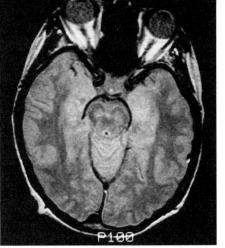

FIG. 16-3 MRI scan of the brain in a normal subject: sagittal section (**A**), coronal section (**B**), axial section (**C**). *(Courtesy of Barry B. Goldberg, M.D., and Daniel A. Merton, B.S., R.D.M.S., Department of Radiology, Jefferson Medical College, Philadelphia, PA.)*

cesses. Fig. 16-3 shows an example of a MRI scan of the brain.

In contrast arteriography, radiopaque dye is injected into the bloodstream, allowing the direct radiographic visualization of cerebral blood vessels.

Contrast myelography entails injection of contrast dye into the CSF via lumbar puncture, for imaging of the spinal canal.

Physiologic Imaging. Physiologic (or "functional") imaging techniques display, in pictorial form, the active physiologic properties of brain regions, as opposed to the static anatomic representations obtained from radiographs, CT, and MRI. The recent development of these techniques has started a revolution in medicine and radiology which may soon allow the dynamic evaluation of physiologic and pathologic processes in the living patient.

Several physiologic imaging techniques are nearing or entering the stage of clinical application, including positron emission tomography (PET), single photon emission computed tomography (SPECT), and regional cerebral blood flow (rCBF). They all use radioactive isotopes, usually attached to physiologically active carrier molecules, to image areas or structures of interest.

Positron emission tomography (PET) detects the pair of photons, emitted in opposite directions, produced by the mutual annihilation of a positron and an electron. It has the potential to produce images of very high resolution but requires the use of short-lived isotopes that must be produced by a cyclotron or particle accelerator located close to the scanner. This requirement has made PET scanning very expensive and has limited its clinical use. At present, it is used primarily as a research tool. Fig. 16-4 is an example of a PET scan.

Single photon emission computed tomography (SPECT) theoretically has a lower resolution than

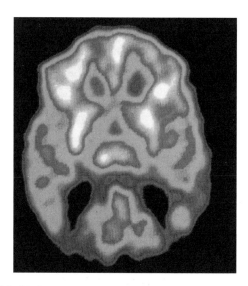

FIG. 16-4 Positron emission tomography (PET) scan of the brain of a normal subject, recorded following the administration of radioactive fluorodeoxyglucose. The lighter areas are the most active metabolically and the darker areas the least active. *(Courtesy of P. David Mozley, M.D., Division of Nuclear Medicine, University of Pennsylvania, Philadelphia, PA.)*

PET, but the applicability of longer-lived isotopes has made it cheaper, more easily administered, and more widely available. At present, SPECT technology is available for routine clinical use at most university hospitals in the United States.

The *regional cerebral blood flow (rCBF)* technique produces topographic (two-dimensional) maps of blood flow distribution across the surface of the brain. It allows quantitative measurements of flow rates and repetitive studies during a single recording session. Although it has been used in research for many years, it has not yet found wide clinical applicability.

Each of these techniques can be applied to the study of various brain functions. Regional brain metabolism is usually studied with PET, using radioactive fluorodeoxyglucose. This carrier molecule is injected into the bloodstream and is preferentially extracted by actively metabolizing neurons in the brain. These active areas produce bright spots on the computer-reconstructed image, revealing which parts of the brain were physiologi-

cally active at the time of injection (Fig. 16-4). This technique can be adapted to investigate how the brain functions in health and in disease. For instance, if the patient has his eyes open and is actively engaged in visual examination of a target, intense activity appears on the image in the visual areas of the occipital cortex. Damage to a portion of the visual cortex, rendering it nonfunctional, would be visualized as a blank spot on the image.

Relative blood flow to specific brain structures or areas can be studied in two dimensions with rCBF and in three dimensions with SPECT or PET. Because the volume of blood flow to a particular region of the brain is proportional to its metabolism, these techniques can also be used to investigate which parts of the brain are more active during some mental task or are damaged by a disease process.

Receptor imaging studies identify regions of the brain which are rich in receptor sites for specific drugs or neurotransmitters. Receptors are molecules on neuronal cell membranes which serve as sites of action for neurotransmitters and drugs. These receptors can be labeled with radioactively tagged analogues of their natural ligands and then visualized using PET and SPECT.

Cerebral Electrophysiology. *Electroencephalography (EEG)* measures the spontaneous electrical activity of the brain, using an array of electrodes pasted to the scalp. Fluctuations in electrical potentials in the cerebral cortex are recorded as deflections of a pen over a continuously moving roll of paper. EEG is the definitive diagnostic study for epileptic seizures and can contribute to the diagnosis of a wide variety of brain diseases, including metabolic derangements and structural lesions.

A variety of methods for the computer-assisted analysis of EEG data have been devised. Evoked potential studies use an adaptation of the EEG to measure conduction and response latencies in the CNS. Computer-averaging techniques are used to detect electrical responses evoked in the brain or spinal cord by sensory stimuli. *Visual evoked responses (VERs)* test the visual system including the occipital cortex; *brainstem auditory evoked responses (BAERs)* test the auditory pathways in the ear and brainstem; *somatosensory evoked responses (SERs)* test the sensory pathways of the spinal cord and thalamus. Topographical mapping techniques, which display the distribution of specific waveforms or frequencies over the cerebral cortex, are used in research but have not yet been found to be clinically helpful.

Peripheral Electrophysiology. Several techniques are available to study electrical conduction in the peripheral nervous system. *Electromyography (EMG)* and *nerve conduction studies (NCS)* are used to measure the transmission of electrical impulses along nerve fibers and to evaluate the integrity of sensory organs, muscles, and the neuromuscular junction.

Biopsy. Biopsy involves the surgical removal of a small sample of tissue for histopathologic study. It is the definitive diagnostic procedure for tumors and is also used for the diagnosis of non-neoplastic conditions. Although biopsy of the brain requires a neurosurgical procedure to obtain the tissue sample, it is frequently performed prior to the removal of brain tumors and is occasionally used to diagnose other life-threatening neurologic conditions.

Overview of Neurologic Disease

Disease in the nervous system, as elsewhere in the body, can result from inflammatory, neoplastic, and infectious processes. Frequently, genetic influences play a large part. Although the causes of some diseases are known, those of many neurologic illnesses are not. Diseases whose causes are not known are referred to as idiopathic. Diseases or defects that are present at birth, usually as a result of genetic causes or intrauterine events, are referred to as congenital.

The science of identifying and classifying individual disease entities is referred to as nosology. There are many different ways to classify the known neurologic diseases. The method adopted here divides them into large, easily distinguishable groups to orient the beginning student. Only the most common and important diseases are described individually.

Cerebrovascular Disease. Disease of the blood vessels, in the nervous system as elsewhere, re-

sults from atherosclerosis, from vasculitis, or from congenital defects in blood vessel walls.

Atherosclerosis is a process by which plaques composed of proteins and cholesterol are gradually deposited along the inner lining of blood vessels, narrowing their lumina and weakening their walls. Although the process begins in adolescence, it usually does not become advanced enough to cause clinical disease until the sixth or seventh decade of life. It is greatly accelerated by uncontrolled hypertension, diabetes mellitus, cigarette smoking, and hereditary hyperlipidosis. The first two of these are the major risk factors for atherosclerotic disease of the central nervous system.

Atherosclerosis of the large- and medium-sized cerebral vessels can result in hemorrhages and infarctions, which are collectively referred to as strokes, or cerebral vascular accidents (CVAs). A hemorrhage results from the bursting of a diseased vessel. An infarction results when a vessel becomes occluded, blocking the flow of blood. The tissue that was supplied by the vessel then dies, or becomes necrotic. With time, the necrotic tissue is reabsorbed, leaving empty spaces or areas of softened brain tissue, referred to as encephalomalacia, which may be visible on CT or MRI scans. Infarctions may be thrombotic, occurring when a blood clot forms acutely at a narrowed point of the diseased vessel, or they may be embolic, resulting when a clot in a distant vessel, often one of the carotid arteries, breaks off and travels to the brain, where it becomes jammed in a narrow cerebral vessel.

Strokes become evident clinically by the sudden onset of focal neurologic deficits, resulting from dysfunction of the neurons in the field supplied by the vessel which has burst or become occluded. These deficits may include paralysis, sensory loss, loss of language ability, visual field loss, or other impairments. Transient ischemic attacks (TIAs) are sudden, brief episodes of focal neurologic dysfunction which resemble strokes but resolve within 24 hours and leave no permanent impairment. They are caused by brief, temporary occlusions of blood vessels, resulting from the same disease processes that cause strokes. Often, the occurrence of

TIAs represents a warning sign of an impending stroke. Amaurosis fugax, or transient monocular visual loss, results from TIAs affecting the central retinal artery.

Vasculitis, or inflammation of the blood vessel walls and surrounding tissues, occurs most often in the CNS in association with systemic inflammatory diseases like systemic lupus erythematosus and sarcoidosis. Vasculitis limited to the nervous system occurs rarely. Vasculitis, systemic or local, is usually treated with anti-inflammatory agents, including nonsteroidal anti-inflammatory drugs (NSAIDs) and corticosteroids.

Aneurysms of cerebral vessels are usually due to idiopathic, probably congenital, weakening of isolated portions of the vessel wall, resulting in a saclike outpouching. They are often referred to as berry aneurysms because of their appearance on cerebral angiograms and pathologic specimens. They occur most frequently in the large vessels at or near the circle of Willis at the base of the brain. Arteriovenous malformations (AVMs) are nests of small abnormal vessels which can occur along any blood vessel in the brain and are also probably congenital in origin. The spontaneous bursting of a cerebral aneurysm or AVM can result in a stroke or subarachnoid hemorrhage. Aneurysms may be surgically clipped to prevent further bleeding after they have burst. AVMs may sometimes be surgically removed or occluded by embolizing them with inert gluelike substances introduced through catheters threaded into the vessels supplying them with blood.

Neoplasms. Neoplastic tumors occurring in the CNS can be primary, originating from cells within the nervous system, or secondary, resulting from metastases from primary tumors in other parts of the body. Primary tumors may arise from any of the cell types found within the CNS. Table 16-1 shows a classification of tumors originating in the CNS and the cells from which they arise.

Tumors in the CNS can present clinically with signs of increased ICP (headache, vomiting, papilledema), obstruction of CSF circulation (hydrocephalus), or neurologic deficits due to compression or destruction of neural structures. The clini-

TABLE 16-1 *Common Tumors of the Central Nervous System and Their Probable Cells of Origin*

Tumor	Cell of Origin
Nerve cell tumors	
Ganglioneuroma, ganglioglioma	Neurons
Medulloblastoma	Immature neurons
Glial cell tumors	
Astrocytoma (benign)	Astrocytes
Glioblastoma (malignant)	Astrocytes
Oligodendroglioma	Oligodendroglia
Ependymomas	Ependymal cells (lining of ventricles)
Meningioma	Arachnoid mater
Pituitary gland tumors	
Craniopharyngioma	Rathke's pouch remnants
Pituitary adenoma	Pituitary gland cells
Tumors on non-neural elements	
Hemangioblastoma	Endothelial cells (lining of blood vessels)
Lymphoma	White blood cells
Melanoma	Pigment cells
Teratomas	Germ cells

cal diagnosis is made by CT or MRI scan. The treatment of choice is surgical removal, if possible. Radiation therapy can be used to reduce the tumor mass and may occasionally be curative. High-dose corticosteroids are used to relieve intracranial compression by reducing vasogenic edema associated with the tumor.

Infections. Infections of the CNS can involve bacteria, fungi, or viruses, as well as atypical microorganisms and "slow viruses." *Meningitis* is an infection of the membranes enclosing the brain and of the subarachnoid space, which contains the CSF. Acute meningitides are usually the result of bacterial infections, whereas more chronic, gradual-onset meningitides are caused by fungal or tuberculous infections. Clinically, meningitis presents with fever, headache, and stiffness of the neck and back muscles. Definitive diagnosis is by lumbar puncture and examination of the CSF. CSF protein is usually high, whereas glucose can be low, especially in bacterial meningitis. White blood cells are present in the CSF, predominantly polymorphonuclear leukocytes in bacterial meningitis and mononuclear cells in fungal and viral meningitides. Microorganisms may be cultured from the CSF. Bacterial meningitis is treated by the intravenous administration of antimicrobial agents. Viral meningitis, a more benign disease that usually runs its course in 10 to 14 days and rarely causes permanent impairment or death, usually requires no specific treatment.

Encephalitis is an infection of the brain parenchyma, usually by viruses. It presents with somnolence, disorientation, and confusion. Focal neurologic signs may be present, especially in encephalitis secondary to herpes simplex virus infection. Treatment with antiviral agents like acyclovir is indicated, but the prognosis is guarded.

An unusual group of infectious agents, which appear to be unique to the nervous system, are referred to as "slow viruses," "unconventional agents," or "prions." They are not true viruses and are so poorly understood by science that they have not yet been classified and given an appropriate name. Unlike any other known living organisms, they do not contain any detectable nucleic acid (DNA or RNA) and appear to be composed entirely of protein. They are the only known "organisms" that can reproduce themselves without nucleic acids to serve as genetic templates, and they appear able to do so only by infecting nervous tissue. Kuru, a now-extinct disease that was formerly prevalent among a tribe of New Guinea villagers who practiced ritual cannibalism, was transmitted by direct ingestion of infected nervous tissue. Creutzfeldt-Jakob disease, which occurs sporadically throughout the world, causes a rapidly progressive dementia that inevitably leads to death. Although its usual method of transmission is unknown, some cases appear to have been acquired through corneal transplants and through direct contact of brain tissue with infected instruments during neurosurgery. Because it is known to be present in the cornea of infected individuals, can be transmitted by contact with instruments, and is not destroyed by routine clinical sterilization procedures, it may be transmissible by ocular tonometry probes, although this has never been systematically investigated or proven to occur. The disease has a very long incubation period, and as many as 20 years may elapse between infection and the first appearance of clinical disease.

Acquired immunodeficiency syndrome (AIDS) is a disorder in which systemic infection by human immunodeficiency virus type 1 (HIV-1) causes suppression of the body's immune defense mechanisms, leaving the patient vulnerable to repeated infections by other microorganisms and to the development of certain malignant tumors. Patients with AIDS have a high incidence of neurologic and psychiatric symptoms. These include dementia, delirium, focal neurologic deficits, depression, mania, and psychosis. These complications may result from direct invasion of the CNS by HIV-1 or by opportunistic pathogens, from the effects of septicemia and systemic metabolic disturbances, or from emotional reactions to the presence of a life-threatening illness. The incidence of neuropsychiatric impairment in individuals infected with HIV-1 who have not yet developed the signs and symptoms of AIDS is small.

Central Demyelinating Diseases. This group of diseases is marked by the primary destruction of myelin, leading to abnormalities in nerve impulse conduction. Myelin, composed of proteins and complex lipids, forms a protective sheath around the axons of certain neurons, increasing the speed with which electrical impulses are conducted. Destruction of myelin sheaths results in the slowed and disordered conduction of nerve signals. Myelin is formed by oligodendroglial cells in the CNS and by Schwann cells in peripheral nerves. Because central and peripheral myelin are anatomically, biochemically, genetically, and immunologically distinct, they are affected by different disease processes. This section deals with diseases affecting the myelin of the CNS; diseases of peripheral myelin are considered in the section on peripheral neuropathies.

The most common of the central demyelinating diseases is multiple sclerosis (MS). MS is an autoimmune disease in which the immune system, which normally protects the body against invasion by foreign substances, recognizes a normal body constituent, in this case a myelin protein, as being foreign and produces antibodies and immune cells directed against it. As a result, focal areas of deteriorating myelin, called MS plaques, form in scattered locations throughout the CNS. MS afflicts whites more often than blacks or Orientals and women more often than men (2 : 1). Its incidence increases with distance from the equator. Onset usually occurs in early adulthood, with 65% of cases occurring between 20 and 40 years of age.

Clinically, MS is defined by the occurrence of multiple central demyelinating plaques, separated by space or time. These lesions may occur in the optic nerves (optic neuritis), in the spinal cord (transverse myelitis), or in the brain. Plaques can be seen on CT or MRI scan or demonstrated by abnormalities in evoked responses. Polyclonal banding of gammaglobulins is seen on electropheresis of the CSF. Treatment with adrenocorticotrophic hormone (ACTH) or high-dose steroids is used to alleviate severe symptoms during the acute phases of the disease. The clinical course is variable, marked by recurrent exacerbations and remissions.

Devic's disease, a variant of MS, presents with bilateral optic neuritis and spinal cord involvement. It has a progressive downhill course and a poor prognosis.

Degenerative Diseases. Degenerative diseases are marked by progressive deterioration of (usually) several neural systems. The causes are usually unknown, and the disease processes cannot usually be halted or reversed with present technology.

Alzheimer's disease is marked by progressive global deterioration of intellectual function. In the early stages it presents with loss of recent memory and disorientation for familiar surroundings and progresses to complete social and intellectual debility requiring custodial care. Severe cerebral atrophy is seen on CT or MRI scan.

Parkinsonism, a clinical syndrome marked by tremor, rigidity, and bradykinesia, results from loss of dopaminergic neurons in the substantia nigra of the midbrain. Although it can result from CVAs, follow CNS infection (epidemic encephalitis lethargica), or occur as a component of a multisystem degenerative disease, its most common occurrence today is in the isolated, idiopathic form, called Parkinson's disease.

Parkinson's disease occurs in persons above the age of 50 and can be accompanied by psychiatric symptoms, chiefly depression. Symptoms can be ameliorated with dopamine replacement therapy (L-dopa) or dopamine agonists (bromocriptine or amantadine) none of these drugs can halt progression of the disease.

Huntingdon's disease ("Woody Guthrie's disease") results from degeneration in the corpus striatum. It is marked by involuntary choreoathetoid movements and intellectual deterioration. It is transmitted as an autosomal dominant mendelian trait, with onset of symptoms after the age of 40 years.

Amytrophic lateral sclerosis (ALS or "Lou Gehrig's disease") is characterized by degeneration in the motor tracts of the spinal cord, with preservation of sensory and intellectual function.

Seizure Disorders (Epilepsy). A *seizure* is defined as a distinct episode of excessive, uncontrolled electrical activity occurring in the brain. During a seizure (called the ictus), while neurons are firing indiscriminately, various parts of the brain may be overactivated, resulting in a variety of acute neurologic manifestations. Most seizures are brief, lasting only a few seconds. When the seizure has passed, the abnormal electrical activity subsides and the patient returns to his previous, normal state. A seizure is often followed by a period of decreased cerebral electrical activity, during which the patient may be lethargic or confused and during which signs and symptoms of focal neurologic dysfunction may be present; this is called the postictal state. Rarely, a seizure may continue without interruption for a long or indefinite period of time; this is referred to as status epilepticus.

Seizures may be primary (or idiopathic), or they may be secondary to another known illness or process, such as a brain injury, infection, or toxic agent. A seizure may be generalized, involving the entire brain simultaneously, or focal (or partial), initially involving only one part of the brain, and perhaps spreading to involve other contiguous structures later in its course. Focal seizures may be preceded by an aura or premonition, caused by the activation of a small piece of brain tissue by the initial localized discharge from which the abnormal electrical activity spreads outward. Common seizure types include:

Grand mal epilepsy. This is an idiopathic (of unknown cause) disorder marked by generalized seizures, usually occurring without warning. Loss of consciousness occurs early in the attack, and loss of bowel and bladder control may also occur. The characteristic muscle activity consists of a tonic phase of sustained contraction of all muscle groups, followed by a clonic phase of jerking, symmetric limb movements, and sometimes followed by a second tonic phase. The postictal state is frequently marked by somnolence, fatigue, or confusion.

Petit mal epilepsy. This is a disorder of childhood, characterized by 3 cycle-per-second spike-and-wave activity, appearing simultaneously in all channels of the EEG. During an attack, the patient loses consciousness momentarily but usually does not fall down or lose control of bowel or bladder; onlookers and the patient himself may not be aware of the occurrence of a seizure. Petit mal seizures frequently stop in adolescence, although a proportion of patients subsequently develop grand mal epilepsy.

Simple motor (Jacksonian) seizures. These are partial seizures beginning in the primary motor area of the cerebral cortex. Jerking muscle movements begin in an isolated limb or area of the body and spread to contiguous muscle groups as the abnormal electrical activity travels across the motor cortex. In the later stages, the seizure may cross the corpus callosum to involve the contralateral

hemisphere as well, resulting in a generalized (tonic-clonic) seizure.

Complex partial seizures. These are focal seizures beginning in the limbic-connected association areas of the temporal or frontal lobes. They are characterized by loss or alteration of consciousness, complex stereotypic movements (automatisms), and complex psychic or emotional experiences, including hallucinations, feelings of dissociation from one's own body, *deja vu,* and fear, anger, or joy. Because they occur in brain structures concerned with the modulation of emotions and autonomic functions, they may be preceded by auras composed of emotional experiences, gastrointestinal sensations, and psychic phenomena.

The diagnosis of *epilepsy* is based upon the clinical presentation and upon the presence of characteristic electrical activity patterns on the EEG. The treatment is usually pharmacologic, and the great majority of patients achieve remission or adequate reduction in seizure frequency through the use of medications now available. Focal epilepsies that are refractory to pharmacologic treatment may be treated by the surgical removal of the seizure focus.

Disorders of Involuntary Movement. These disorders, as the name implies, are marked by the appearance of uncontrollable movements of the limbs or trunk, which the patient is unable to suppress or direct. The form of the involuntary movement is characteristic of each disorder.

Tics are sudden, rapid, stereotyped movements of the face or limbs. They can be suppressed voluntarily for short periods of time but soon recur when the patient's concentration fatigues. In Tourette's disorder, motor tics occur conjointly with vocal and verbal tics, sudden vocalizations or exclamations that are similarly under the patient's incomplete control.

Tremor refers to a pattern of rhythmic, repetitive, reciprocal movement of the limbs or trunk. A tremor may be present at rest and decrease during movement (resting tremor) or may appear or be exacerbated during movement (intention tremor). In Parkinson's disease, a resting tremor is present in conjunction with muscle rigidity and bradykinesia. Damage to the lateral cerebellar hemispheres, which function to coordinate the movements of the limbs, results in dysmetria, an intention tremor, when the patient attempts to reach for an object.

Several forms of involuntary movement may result from damage to various portions of the basal ganglia. Chorea consists of jerky, random movements, whereas athetosis consists of rhythmic, snakelike, twisting movements. Choreoathetoid movements occur in Huntingdon's disease, in Sydenham's chorea (a transitory movement disorder occurring as a complication of rheumatic fever), and in Wilson's disease, a heritable metabolic disorder that results in the excessive accumulation of copper in the brain and other tissues. Ballismus, which occurs following strokes or damage to the subthalamic nucleus, consists of sudden, high-amplitude flailing movements of the limbs contralateral to the lesion.

Ataxia refers to a loss of trunkal balance, with a staggering, wide-based gait and a tendency to fall in either direction. It occurs with damage to the midline portion of the cerebellum, with loss of proprioceptive sense due to injury to peripheral nerves or to the posterior white columns of the spinal cord, and in alcohol intoxication.

Obsessive-compulsive disorder is an illness in which the patient experiences repetitive obsessional thoughts and compulsive, ritualistic behaviors, such as repeated hand washing or checking of doors and locks, which he cannot suppress. Although it has traditionally been considered a neurosis by psychiatrists, some cases have been associated with radiologic evidence of basal ganglia injury and may represent a movement disorder in which the involuntary movements consist of complex thoughts and behaviors.

Neuromuscular Disorders. Neuromuscular diseases affect transmission of nerve impulses from motor neurons to muscle membranes across the neuromuscular junction (NMJ, or motor endplate). The most common neuromuscular disorder is myasthenia gravis.

Myasthenia gravis (MG) is an autoimmune disease in which antibodies to acetylcholine receptor proteins circulate in the blood, bind to acetylcholine receptors on muscle membranes, and block synaptic transmission at the NMJ. MG affects young adults (ages 20 to 40), with a higher incidence in women; many cases are associated with thymomas or thymic hyperplasia.

Clinically, MG presents with weakness and fatigability of voluntary muscles, most often the muscles of the eyes, face, throat, and palate. The weakness increases with exercise, recovers with rest, and becomes aggravated later in the day. The diagnosis is made by observation of transient improvement in signs and symptoms following injection of a cholinesterase inhibitor (Tensilon test) or by decreasing muscle potentials by repetitive stimulation on EMG. Treatment consists of long-acting cholinesterase inhibitors such as pyridostigmine (Mestinon) and thymectomy (even in the absence of a thymoma or thymic hyperplasia). Plasmapheresis is used during myasthenic crises; such crises may be severe enough to require ventilatory support.

Peripheral Neuropathies. Neuropathies can result from damage to peripheral nerves by a variety of agents and disease processes. They frequently begin in the distal extremities and progress proximally (ascending neuropathy). Diabetic neuropathy results from diffuse microvascular disease and affects mainly sensory nerve fibers. Toxic neuropathies can result from exposure to chemical toxins or from the prolonged abuse of ethanol. They also mainly involve sensory nerve fibers. Bell's palsy is an isolated, unilateral paralysis of the facial nerve. It is usually sudden in onset and clears spontaneously within weeks or months. Treatment with steroids is controversial. Bell's palsy must be differentiated from other more serious diseases that can present with facial nerve palsies, including strokes, tumors, and the Guillain-Barré syndrome.

The Guillain-Barré syndrome (GBS) is an immune-mediated, demyelinating neuropathy affecting predominantly motor fibers. It is marked by ascending muscle weakness that may progress to total paralysis, followed by full and spontaneous recovery in most cases. In severe cases, ventilatory support for weeks or months may be nec-

TABLE 16-2 *Classification of the Muscular Dystrophies*

Type	Inheritance	Age at Onset	Progression
Duchenne's	X-linked, recessive	Early childhood	Rapid, fatal
Becker's	X-linked, recessive	Second decade	Slow, nonfatal
Limb-girdle	Autosomal, recessive	Variable, first to sixth decades	Variable, disability usual
Facioscapulohumeral	Autosomal, dominant	Variable, childhood to late adulthood	Benign, not progressive
Oculopharyngeal	Autosomal, dominant	Fifth decade	Slowly progressive
Ocular	Autosomal, dominant	Fifth decade	Slowly progressive
Distal	Autosomal, dominant	Middle to late adulthood	Slowly progressive
Myotonic	Autosomal, dominant	Variable	Slowly progressive

essary. Plasmapheresis may be used during the acute phase to minimize the level of debility. Onset is frequently preceded by a viral infection, which presumably triggers an autoimmune reaction to peripheral nerve myelin. Thus, GBS is a pathophysiologic analogue of multiple sclerosis but involves peripheral, instead of central, myelin.

Myopathy. The term *myopathy* refers to a heterogeneous group of diseases that affect primarily muscle cells. Although they are not, strictly speaking, neurologic disorders, they must be considered in the differential diagnosis of patients presenting with neurologic complaints.

Inflammatory myopathies result from inflammation of muscles fibers and membranes, resulting in weakness and muscle tenderness. Polymyositis and dermatomyositis are characterized by symmetric limb girdle weakness, often accompanied by compromise of the swallowing or respiratory muscles. In dermatomyositis, a red, edematous rash is also present on the face and dorsal surfaces of the fingers. These disorders may result from viral infections, systemic autoimmune disease, or immunologic reactions to malignant tumors elsewhere in the body. Serum creatine kinase levels are elevated, characteristic findings are present on EMG, and muscle biopsy reveals signs of inflammation and necrosis. Treatment consists of the use of im-

munosuppressive agents and treatment of the underlying immune disorder, if possible.

Noninflammatory myopathies result from genetic errors of carbohydrate or lipid metabolism or from long-term treatment with high doses of steroid medications.

The muscular dystrophies (MD) are a group of hereditary diseases characterized by progressive, noninflammatory, and usually untreatable degeneration of muscle fibers. Of several distinct syndromes currently recognized, three frequently present with prominent ocular or facial muscle signs. The facioscapulohumeral form involves face and shoulder girdle as well as the extraocular muscles. The oculopharyngeal and ocular forms present with ptosis and extraocular muscle weakness and may progress to involve the face and the muscles used in swallowing. Table 16-2 summarizes the muscular dystrophies.

PSYCHIATRY

The medical specialty of psychiatry is concerned with diseases whose primary signs and symptoms consist of alterations in mood, emotion, thought processes, and behavior. Although these illnesses result from pathophysiologic processes occurring in the brain and are not fundamentally different in this regard from the neurologic illnesses discussed in the previous section, they have traditionally been referred to as diseases of the mind. The historical roots of the brain versus mind dichotomy arise in religious doctrines, which assume the viewpoint that "body" and "soul" are distinct and separable entities. During the nineteenth century, when medicine began to assume its modern form, diseases whose neural substrates were identifiable were relegated to neurology and labeled "organic," whereas those whose neural substrate was unknown were relegated to psychiatry and labeled "functional."

In modern usage (and as defined in the current edition of *The Diagnostic and Statistical Manual of Mental Disorders* of the American Psychiatric Association), the terms "organic" and "functional" are no longer used literally. They now refer to arbitrary groupings of disorders which are not fundamentally different but are distinguishable in everyday clinical usage. The terms remain useful, just as the terms "organic" and "inorganic" chemistry remain useful today, although their original literal meaning is no longer valid. "Organic" disorders are marked by prominent disturbances in orientation, attention, concentration, and memory. In "functional" disorders these faculties are mainly intact, but disturbances in mood, perception, and thought patterns are prominent.

Historically, the development of psychiatric diagnosis and nosology has been dominated by two alternate, although not necessarily conflicting, viewpoints: the phenomenologic and the psychodynamic. The phenomenologic viewpoint assumes that specific diseases can be diagnosed by the observation of characteristic signs and symptoms (Karl Jaspers' "first-rank symptoms"). This is similar to the diagnostic process used in other branches of medicine; in psychiatry, however, laboratory, radiologic, and pathologic validation of the clinical diagnosis is mostly lacking. For this reason, phenomenologic diagnosis in psychiatry consists mainly of identifying clinical syndromes, without the ability to identify the underlying cause. The psychodynamic viewpoint sees the development of the mind to be a dynamic process, beginning at birth and strongly influenced by important persons and events encountered during childhood

and adolescence. It emphasizes environmental, rather than genetic or physiologic, contributions to the development of mental illness. Although it has the potential to identify the causative factors of an individual's illness, these interpretations are highly individual and subjective, difficult to validate objectively, and difficult to relate to biologic processes like the patient's genetic endowment and the influence of drugs or brain injury. A modern synthesis of these two concepts views genetic and physiologic factors, as reflected in the phenomenology of an illness, to be contributory to the process of mental illness, whereas psychodynamic factors frequently determine the content of the patient's symptoms. In current practice, it is most helpful to use phenomenologic (descriptive or categorical) diagnoses for statistical reporting purposes and when treating patients with major psychiatric disturbances such as depression, mania, and psychosis, which have a strong biologic influence. Psychodynamic diagnoses are most helpful in the psychotherapeutic treatment of patients with neurotic or personality disorders.

The Diagnostic and Statistical Manual of Mental Disorders, Third Edition, Revised *(DSM-III-R)* of the American Psychiatric Association, contains the diagnostic criteria for all of the psychiatric disorders recognized in the United States. It strongly emphasizes the phenomenologic perspective. Its chief purpose is to standardize the diagnosis and reporting of mental illness. It is continually being revised. Publication of the next edition, DSM-IV, is planned for 1994.

Terms and Definitions

In this section, some frequently used (and abused) terms in psychiatry are defined, and some common misconceptions about psychiatric terminology are clarified.

Psychosis does not refer to any specific illness. It is an inexact term, referring to an extreme level of impairment in which a patient begins to lose touch with reality; it is often marked by the presence of hallucinations and delusions.

Neurosis is a psychodynamic term, referring to an intrapsychic process in which unresolved conflicts, repressed from consciousness during childhood and adolescence, re-emerge during later life, causing a variety of symptoms. Overused and abused in the past, the term is no longer used in *DSM-III-R* but remains useful in psychotherapy with certain patients.

"Split personality" is popularly believed to refer to *schizophrenia*. "Schizophrenia" was coined by Eugene Bleuler to refer to a "splitting of different psychic functions," which he believed to be a cardinal manifestation of that disease. Patients who behave as though they possess more than one personality at different times are diagnosed as having multiple personality disorder, not schizophrenia.

Catatonia is not a specific disease, but a clinical syndrome that can occur in a variety of diseases, including bipolar disorder, schizophrenia, and a variety of organic and neurologic conditions. It is marked by a constellation of unusual motor behaviors, including stereotypy, bizarre gaits and postures, stupor or excitement, and echo phenomena. Common before the introduction of psychotropic medications, it is rarely seen today.

Electroconvulsive therapy (ECT, "shock treatments") is the most effective, and probably the safest, treatment available today for severe depression. An electric shock applied to the scalp induces a generalized seizure, which results in alleviation of depression in most patients following a course of seven to ten treatments. Today, the procedure is performed using general anesthesia and other technical refinements, making it a much less traumatic experience than it was in the past. The procedure and its benefits are widely misunderstood by the general public.

Affect refers to the outward, observable expression of a patient's emotional state; mood refers to the patient's subjective report of his inner emotional state. These two qualities are usually congruent in healthy persons but are frequently discordant in psychiatric patients. "Affective disorders" is an inexact term, used collectively for disorders with prominent disturbances of mood and affect, including depression, bipolar disorders, and anxiety disorders.

The mental status examination (MSE) is that portion of the physician's physical examination which evaluates the patient's mental faculties and probes for signs and symptoms of psychiatric disease. It includes assessments of the patient's level of awareness, orientation, attention span, speech and language formation, motor activity and behavior, mood and its expression (affect), form and content of thought, capacity for abstraction and aperception, cognitive abilities, judgment, and capacity for insight. It is the psychiatrist's cross-sectional view of the patient's present mental status, whereas the history provides the longitudinal view (analogous to the physical examination and history, respectively, in other branches of medicine, including optometry).

"Insanity" and "insane" have no meaning in modern psychiatry. However, they are used by courts and lawyers in reference to defendants who are claiming diminished responsibility based upon mental illness. As such, they are legally defined terms, the definitions of which vary depending upon the legal jurisdiction. When giving expert testimony at a trial involving a plea of insanity, a psychiatrist or psychologist can provide information as to the patient's mental state but cannot decide whether a patient is "insane"; only the judge or jury can make that decision.

"Nervous breakdown" is not a psychiatric term. It is used by laymen indiscriminately to describe a variety of acute psychiatric illnesses and crises, including depression, psychosis, anxiety attacks, suicide attempts, and numerous others.

A *hallucination* is a false sensory perception, such as seeing something that is not there. An illusion is a distorted sensory perception, such as perceiving a bedpost to be a person. (Hallucinations and illusions can occur in all sensory modalities, including visual, auditory, olfactory, tactile, gustatory, vestibular, and somatosensory.) A delusion is an untrue belief that does not respond to reason, logic, or reasonable evidence to the contrary; delusional thinking was formerly referred to as "paranoia."

Overview of Psychiatric Disease

A brief overview of psychiatric disorders, as recognized by psychiatrists in the United States, is presented.

Organic Disorders. *DSM-III-R* defines as "organic" those mental disorders that are known or presumed to be secondary to an identifiable brain disease or neurologic process. Although this may be an arbitrary distinction (as discussed above), it remains useful for clinical purposes. Organic mental disorders are frequently marked by prominent disturbances of orientation, attention, concentration, and memory.

Delirium is an acute syndrome characterized by a transient disorganization of a wide range of cognitive functions due to widespread derangement of cerebral metabolism ("acute brain failure"). It is usually the result of a significant medical, metabolic, or neurologic disturbance (such as sepsis, uremia, cerebral hypoxia). Its presence constitutes a medical emergency, often requiring intensive life support. Treatment consists of treating the underlying medical disturbance.

Dementia is a chronic, progressive deterioration in global intellectual functioning. Although it is often seen as irreversible and progressive, some cases can be reversed or arrested if the cause is identified. Causes include degenerative neurologic diseases (for example, Alzheimer's disease), vascular diseases, infections (for example, neurosyphilis, Creutzfeld-Jakob disease), vitamin deficiencies, and endocrine/metabolic disturbances (for example, hypothyroidism).

Schizophrenia. The historical development of concepts of severe mental illness emphasized the progressively deteriorating longitudinal course of patients with schizophrenia (originally called "dementia praecox" by Emile Kraepelin) as opposed to the better prognosis and cyclicly recurring and remitting course of patients with affective disorders. Although many attempts were made to define schizophrenia upon the basis of a characteristic set of clinical signs and symptoms, no single sign or set of signs was found to be diagnostic. Today, the diagnosis must be based upon a variety of criteria, including duration of illness, positive symptoms (including hallucinations and delusions), and negative symptoms (such as social withdrawal and poor capacity for social interactions).

The dopamine hypothesis, originally framed during the 1950s, stated that schizophreniform symptoms were the result of an overabundance of dopamine in the forebrain. This was based upon the observations that (1) the use of stimulant drugs (such as amphetamine and cocaine), which cause the release of dopamine, can produce schizophrenia-like psychoses; (2) *Rauwolfia* alkaloids (such as reserpine), which deplete catecholamines, including dopamine, in the forebrain, alleviate schizophrenic symptoms; and (3) treatment of parkinsonism with L-dopa (which increases dopamine in the forebrain) can precipitate schizophreniform symptoms. Although the hypothesis has been much modified since then, variants continue to be the best neurochemical explanations for this disease today.

All antipsychotic drugs in clinical use today are dopamine D_2 receptor blockers, although several new drugs being investigated may soon disprove this rule. The terms "antipsychotics" and "neuroleptics" are often used interchangeably to describe these drugs. "Neuroleptic" properly refers to the sedative and neurologic side effects of these drugs, as distinct from their specific antipsychotic effects. Most patients with schizophrenia require long-term treatment with antipsychotic medications to alleviate distressing hallucinations and delusional thinking and to allow them to focus their thoughts coherently.

Delusional Disorders. Delusional disorders (formerly called "paranoid disorders") are characterized by fixed, nonbizarre, plausible but untrue, well-encapsulated delusion(s), in the absence of other symptoms (such as hallucinations and flattened affect) characteristic of schizophrenia. Common variants include:
1. Erotomanic type: the belief that some famous person is in love with the subject.
2. Grandiose type: the delusion of inflated worth, power, knowledge, or station.
3. Jealous type: the fixed belief that the subject's spouse or sexual partner is unfaithful.
4. Persecutory type: the delusion of being followed, mistreated, or abused by some person or agency.

5. Somatic type: the unfounded belief of having some physical illness or deformity.

Depression. The term unipolar *depression* refers to depression in patients who have never experienced a manic episode. In epidemiologic studies, unipolar depression is distinct from the bipolar disorders, has a strong familial and genetic predisposition, and occurs more often in women than in men. The disorder follows a recurring and remitting course, with distinct episodes of depression, between which the patient enjoys a normal mood and personality. Although some depressions (reactive) occur in response to stressful events and others (endogenous) appear to result from disturbances in brain chemistry, this is not a clear distinction, and many patients show features of both types simultaneously. Dysthymia is a pattern of mild, chronic depression that may last throughout life.

The observation that all known antidepressant drugs increase the concentrations of norepinephrine and/or serotonin at nerve synapses led to the biogenic amine hypothesis, which originally postulated that depression was the result of decreased secretion at norepinephrine and serotonin nerve terminals in the limbic forebrain. Modern hypotheses of depression continue to postulate dysfunction in noradrenergic and serotoninergic pathways or receptor sites.

Antidepressant medications fall into two large classes. Tricyclics and related compounds inhibit reuptake of norepinephrine and/or serotonin at nerve terminals. Their major adverse effects are orthostatic hypotension and cardiac arrhythmias, especially in the elderly. Monoamine oxidase inhibitors (MAOIs) prevent the breakdown of norepinephrine and serotonin and prolong their effects at nerve terminals. Tyramine-rich foods (such as ripe cheeses and red wines) must be avoided during the use of these drugs, to avoid hypertensive crises.

Electroconvulsive therapy (see above) is the most effective and probably also the safest available treatment for severe, life-threatening depression. Owing to misunderstanding by the general public, it is usually reserved for use, when all else has failed, in medication-refractory or acutely suicidal patients.

Bipolar Disorder. Bipolar disorder is defined by the presence of alternating periods of mania and depression, usually interspersed with periods of euthymia (that is, normal mood). *Mania* is a state characterized by elated or irritable mood, hyperactive behavior, inflated self-esteem, pressured speech, flight of ideas or racing thoughts, and a tendency toward socially indiscrete and disruptive behavior. Hypomania is a similar, quantitatively lesser, state. It has recently been recognized that there is a spectrum of bipolar disorders, characterized by mood swings of variable amplitude and duration; they are collectively referred to as bipolar spectrum disorders.

Lithium carbonate is the mainstay of pharmacologic treatment for bipolar disorders, but because of its delayed onset of action, neuroleptics or sedatives are usually required during acute manic episodes. Carbamazepine and valproic acid may be used as alternatives in patients who cannot tolerate lithium therapy.

Anxiety Disorders. *Anxiety* is an adaptive psychophysiologic reaction to acutely stressful situations. If excessive or chronic, however, it constitutes an illness and must be treated as such. Pathologic anxiety can be generalized, can occur in discrete panic attacks, and can be associated with avoidant (phobic) behavior.

TOPICS OF SPECIAL INTEREST TO OPTOMETRISTS

Headache and Facial Pain

Headache and facial pain are common complaints in medical, neurologic, and optometric practice. They are very nonspecific complaints and can result from a variety of causes, ranging from trivial to life-threatening. Chronic headaches can result from eye strain due to poor vision and resolve with correction of the refractive error. Although facial pain usually has extraocular causes, it can be localized in the area of the eye and often causes patients to seek optometric or ophthalmologic care.

Headache. *Migraine* headaches are of vascular origin. They are frequently unilateral but may be bilateral, are sudden in onset, and may have a throbbing quality. There is frequently a family history of migraine and a history of motion sickness since childhood. They are treated by prophylaxis with beta-blockers or tricyclic antidepressants, by intervention with ergot alkaloids and/or caffeine, or symptomatically with analgesics.

The mechanism leading to a migraine headache is a complex process involving several stages. In the early (preheadache) stage, vasoconstriction, triggered by unknown causes, occurs in the large arteries on the surface of the brain. Constriction of distal branches of the internal carotid artery, which supplies important areas of brain tissue, results in localized, transient ischemia, giving rise to focal signs of neurologic dysfunction, called the migraine aura. These focal signs may include sensory changes, language dysfunction, vertigo, or mental status abnormalities. Constriction of branches of the ophthalmic artery during the aura phase of a migraine results in scotomas or visual field defects, which usually resolve prior to onset of the headache. During the later (headache) stage, reflex vasodilation in the branches of the external carotid artery results in severe, throbbing pain. Later still, edema of the vessel walls results in muscular contraction and an aching pain that lingers after the vascular events have subsided.

There are many variants of migraine headache. Classic migraine is usually frontal and unilateral, preceded by visual or vestibular auras, and may be accompanied by gastrointestinal symptoms. Common migraine is often bilateral, may have a dull, aching quality, and is not accompanied by auras or gastrointestinal symptoms. It is frequently misdiagnosed as tension or sinus headache. Complicated migraine is accompanied by gross neurologic deficits, due to persistent auras, which may overshadow the headache and may linger for hours or days after onset. Cluster headaches are unilateral, localized behind the eye, and accompanied by lacrimation and conjunctival injection. They are frequently nocturnal and occur daily in "clusters"

of 6 to 12 weeks, which may occur at the same time each year.

Tension headaches are related to tightness of the neck, jaw, and facial muscles and are associated with anxiety and environmental stressors. They frequently begin in the neck muscles below the occiput and spread forward around the entire head. They respond to acetaminophen, aspirin, anti-inflammatory drugs, stress relaxation biofeedback techniques, massage, tranquilizers, and holidays.

Sinus headache is usually associated with overt sinus congestion, is centered in the maxillary region, and responds to decongestants with or without analgesics.

Temporal arteritis is a systemic inflammatory disease whose major manifestations are localized to the tissues surrounding the superficial temporal arteries. It occurs in elderly persons, may be accompanied by swelling over one or both temples, and is accompanied by an elevated erythrocyte sedimentation rate. Definitive diagnosis is by temporal artery biopsy, and immediate treatment with high doses of steroid medications is necessary to prevent blindness.

Increased ICP, due to tumors or hydrocephalus, can cause headaches that are worst in the morning; increase with position changes, coughing, straining, and Valsalva's maneuver; and are accompanied by vomiting, sometimes without nausea. They are without localizing value and are usually accompanied by other signs of increased ICP (such as papilledema, visual field loss). Management consists of treating the underlying disease.

Subarachnoid hemorrhage usually results from rupture of congenital "berry" aneurysms at or near the circle of Willis and constitutes an acute neurosurgical emergency. The headache is abrupt in onset; has a sharp, burning quality; and is described as "the worst headache of my life." Definitive diagnosis is by CT of the brain, and surgical intervention is frequently necessary.

Meningitis is usually accompanied by headache, stiffness of the neck and back muscles, and fever. Definitive diagnosis is examination of the CSF (increased protein, decreased glucose, pleocytosis).

Table 16-3 shows the characteristic features of the different types of headache.

Facial Pain. Trigeminal neuralgia (also known as tic douloureux) is a burning, tingling pain that occurs within the sensory field of one of the branches of the trigeminal nerve. It is unilateral, lasts for seconds at a time with multiple recurrences and variable periods of remission, and is sometimes provoked by touching "trigger points" on the mouth or lips. Its cause is unknown, although vascular, viral, inflammatory, and rheumatic causes have been proposed. Most cases respond to treatment with carbamazepine (Tegretol), clonazepam (Klonopin), or phenytoin (Dilantin).

Postherpetic neuralgia is confined to the dermatomal distribution of herpes zoster. It can begin several days before the pustular eruption and linger for weeks or months following its resolution. There is no good treatment, although local and systemic analgesics can be used.

Facial migraine is a variant of migraine involving various branches of the external carotid artery. Its pathophysiology and treatment are similar to those described above for migraine headache. Occasionally, migrainous phenomena may occur in other parts of the body, including the abdominal organs.

Dental dysfunction, including malocclusion, temporomandibular joint dysfunction, and a variety of diseases of the teeth, jaws, and gums, can result in facial pain or headache.

Table 16-4 shows the characteristic features of the different types of facial pain.

Disorders of Complex Visual Processing

The cerebral cortex is the area of the brain where sensory information, passed up from the sense organs through several levels of neural processing, is integrated to form complex perceptions, thoughts, and emotions. Disorders of complex visual processing occur as a result of lesions in cortical areas subserving the processing of visual stimuli.

Visual Processing in the Cerebral Cortex. Visual information, originating in the retinas, is transmitted via the optic nerves, chiasm, optic tracts, lateral geniculate nuclei, and optic radiations to the primary visual cortices (also known as striate cortex, V1, and Brodmann's area 17), located along the lips of the calcarine fissures in the occipital lobes. A lesion anywhere along this pathway results in simple visual loss, the shape of the visual field defect depending upon which tracts or nuclei are damaged. Damage to the primary visual cortex results in homonymous field defects. Stimulation of the primary visual cortex, by an irritable seizure focus or by electrodes during surgery, results in simple visual hallucinations called *photopsias,* often described as flames or tongues of light.

From the primary visual cortex, visual information is transmitted forward to the unimodal visual association cortex (also known as peristriate cortex or V2), located in Brodmann's areas 18 and 19 in the occipital lobes, and areas 20, 21, and 37 on the middle and inferior temporal gyri. Here, complex visual images are formed and stored in memory. Lesions in these areas cause impairments in the perception of colors, forms, and complex motions and the inability to match percepts with the appropriate memory templates. Stimulation of these areas causes complex, well-formed visual hallucinations.

Subsequently, visual information is transmitted to more anterior and dorsal areas of the cortex, where further processing occurs. In the multimodal association areas, located in the frontal, temporal, and parietal lobes, visual information is integrated with auditory, somatosensory, gustatory, and olfactory information, resulting in complex sensory associations. Lesions here cause visual-spatial disorientation, eye-tracking and eye-scanning abnormalities, and disorders of visual orientation. In the language association areas, located in the frontal and temporal cortex around the sylvian fissure in the dominant hemisphere, sensory information is converted into verbal form, allowing the brain to describe what it sees in words or in writing. In the limbic and paralimbic areas of the inferior frontal and medial temporal lobes, sensory information acquires an emotional color-

TABLE 16-3 *Characteristics of Headache Syndromes*

	Classic Migraine	Common Migraine	Cluster Headache	Tension Headache
Age at onset	Adolescence	Adolescence or young adulthood	Age 20-50	Any age
Gender	F > M	F > M	M > F	Both
Quality of pain	Throbbing, pulsatile	Dull, aching	Sharp, stabbing	Pressure
Location of pain	Unilateral, frontal	Unilateral or bilateral	Behind one eye	Sides and back of head
Diurnal pattern	Variable	Variable	Daily, nocturnal, seasonal	Late in day
Aggravating factors	Bright light, noise	Bright light, noise	Alcohol	Stress, overwork
Relieving factors	Dark room, rest, sleep	Dark room, rest, sleep	None	Rest, sleep
Associated features	Visual, vestibular, or gastrointestinal auras	No aura	Lacrimation, conjunctival injection	Muscle stiffness
Treatment	Ergotamine, methysergide, caffeine	Amitryptiline, betablockers, analgesics	Ergotamine, methysergide	Analgesics, anti-inflammatory drugs

Key: > = Greater than; M = male; F = female.   *Continued.*

ing and is integrated with memories of significant past experiences. Lesions here cause disturbances in visual memory and the inability to match percepts with memory templates.

Clinical Syndromes. When the cortical substrates of complex visual processing are injured by disease, a variety of syndromes may be observed clinically. The evaluation of patients with such disorders makes use of specialized techniques and knowledge and may require consultation with a neuro-ophthalmologist or behavioral neurologist.

Cortical visual loss. Cortical blindness occurs when the entire primary visual cortices of both hemispheres are destroyed, leading to the inability of the cortex to encode visual information transmitted to it from the retina. The combination of cortical blindness and anosagnosia (see below) is referred to as Anton's syndrome. Patients with this unusual disorder deny that they are blind, although the visual examination easily demonstrates the lack

of any useful vision. Anton's syndrome sometimes occurs after extensive bilateral posterior strokes and usually resolves within days or weeks of onset, although the blindness may remain and be permanent.

The visual agnosias. Lesions that damage the ventral portions of the cortical visual processing system give rise to a series of disorders called the visual agnosias. An agnosia is a disorder in which stimuli are perceived normally and accurately but without the ability to identify them or to grasp their significance. Patients with agnosia may fail to recognize previously familiar objects while retaining the ability to describe them accurately or to match them with similar objects. In visual agnosia, the impairment is limited to the visual realm, although primary vision is preserved, as is the ability to recognize nonvisual stimuli. For instance, patients with visual agnosia may be unable to recognize a key on visual confrontation but may be able to

TABLE 16-3 *Characteristics of Headache Syndromes—cont'd*

Sinus Headache	Temporal Arteritis	Intracranial Pressure	Subarachnoid Hemorrhage	Meningitis
Any age	Over 60	Any age	Any age	Any age
Both	Both	Both	Both	Both
Pressure	Burning	Dull ache	Sharp, stabbing	Dull soreness
Frontal, maxillary regions	Temporal scalp	Entire head	Entire head	Entire head
None	Worse at night	Worse in morning	None	None
None	Touching, combing hair	Coughing, sneezing, bending	None	Flexing neck, extending legs
None	None	Standing	None	None
Sinus congestion	Malaise, weight loss	Vomiting, blurred vision, papilledema	Sudden, abrupt onset	Fever, neck stiffness
Decongestants, analgesics	High-dose steroids	Neurosurgery	Neurosurgical emergency	Intravenous antibiotics

TABLE 16-4 *Characteristics of Facial Pain Syndromes*

	Trigeminal Neuralgia	Herpetic Neuralgia	Facial Migraine	Dental Origin
Age at onset	Over 50	Elderly	Any age	Any age
Gender	F > M	F > M	M > F	Both
Quality of pain	Burning, tingling	Continuous burning	Pulsatile, throbbing	Aching, soreness
Location of pain	Unilateral, one branch of CN V	Unilateral, one branch of CN V	Anywhere on face	Radiating from jaw
Temporal pattern	Sporadic, isolated attacks	Continuous	Sporadic, isolated attacks	Continuous, worse when chewing
Aggravating factors	Hot/cold, facial movement	Touch, cold	Alcohol	Chewing, yawning, pressure
Treatment	Carbamazepine, phenytoin, clonazepam	Analgesics	Ergotamine, methysergide	Bite correction, dental surgery

Key: > = Greater than; M = male; F = female; CN V = cranial nerve V.

match it with another key from an array of objects displayed on a table or to recognize the sound of keys jingling. Several forms of visual agnosia have been described.

Patients with apperceptive visual agnosia (also known as visual form agnosia) have lost their ability to perceive forms visually while retaining normal perception through other sensory modalities (touch, hearing, smell) and the perception of color and motion. Although it is included in this discussion of the visual agnosias, it is not a true agnosia because visual perception is not normal, and the patient is unable to perceive objects normally. This disorder is rare and occurs with extensive bilateral damage to the visual association cortices.

Associative visual agnosia (also known as visual object agnosia) is a true agnosia in which a patient is unable to recognize objects visually, despite normal perception of form, color, and motion and preservation of the abilities to match objects and to copy figures. This disorder results from bilateral damage to the ventral (occipitotemporal) visual association cortices, obstructing the flow of visual information to the multimodal temporal association cortices and paralimbic areas.

Prosopagnosia is the inability to discriminate faces. It occurs following bilateral damage to ventral (occipitotemporal) visual association cortices, usually less extensive than those causing visual object agnosia. Patients with prosopagnosia, in addition to being unable to recognize familiar faces, are usually impaired in their ability to discriminate between individual members of a set of objects, for example, to differentiate specific models of automobiles or specific breeds of farm animals. Their understanding of the group is preserved, but they are unable to distinguish individual members of the group.

Central achromatopsia is the decreased or absent ability to perceive colors, resulting from an isolated lesion in the ventral occipitotemporal cortex. It is described by patients as seeing everything in shades of grey (in severe cases) or in "washed-out colors" in milder cases. The defect may involve only one hemifield (as in homonymous hemiachromatopsia) when the lesion is unilateral. All colors are equally affected. The ability to perceive forms is completely preserved. This disorder is different from retinal color blindness, in which specific colors are confused or perceived as other colors.

Color agnosia (also known as color anomia) is the inability to name colors, with preserved ability to match colors. The appearance of this deficit requires the destruction of the left visual cortex, radiations, or geniculate body *and* a lesion in the left subsplenial occipitotemporal white matter, that is, loss of the right visual field and disconnection of the right visual cortex from language association areas of the left hemisphere. Thus, the patient is able to perceive color perfectly well in the preserved left hemifield but is unable to generate the word used to describe it.

Alexia (also known as pure alexia or alexia without agraphia) is the loss of the ability to read, with preservation of normal speech and writing ability. This results from destruction of the left visual cortex, radiations, or geniculate body *and* a lesion of the forceps major (the section of the corpus callosum which interconnects the two visual cortices) *or* a single lesion in the left paraventricular white matter disconnecting both occipital lobes from the left hemispheric language areas. Thus, the patient is able to produce normal speech and to write normally because the language-generating areas are intact. Although these patients often have a right homonymous hemianopsia, they are able to perceive and copy the form of written text using their preserved left visual field; however, this information cannot reach the language-processing area in the left hemisphere, where the linguistic meaning of the text is deciphered. This leads to the seemingly paradoxical situation in which a patient is unable to read what he himself has written several minutes previously.

Visual-spatial syndromes. Damage to the dorsal portions of the cortical visual processing system results in a group of disorders marked by disturbances in visual-spatial orientation. In these disorders, vision may be preserved, but the patient's ability to control his gaze or to scan the visual environment and to direct his visual attention appropriately may be impaired.

Isolated simultanagnosia is the inability to simultaneously perceive more than one or two isolated elements of a complex visual field. It is caused by bilateral lesions confined to the superior occipital cortex (unimodal visual association area), sparing the parietal lobes. A patient with this disorder can describe small regions of a complex picture or table accurately but cannot grasp it in its entirety. This deficit may rarely occur as an isolated disorder but more frequently is seen as a component of other, more extensive syndromes.

Balint's syndrome is characterized by a triad of findings: (1) simultanagnosia, as described above; (2) optic ataxia, an inability to execute visually guided movements; and (3) ocular apraxia (also known as "psychic gaze paralysis," or spasm of fixation), a visual scanning deficit in which the patient is unable to volitionally shift gaze from one object to another and in which intentional saccades are absent or inaccurate, although random saccades and smooth pursuit movements are normal. A patient with this disorder is able to perceive a small segment of the visual field, where his gaze has fixated randomly, but is unable to direct his fixation at will. As a result, he is unable to reach for objects in three-dimensional space under visual guidance, although he can do so by guidance from other sensory modalities, such as reaching for a ringing bell or following an examiner's arm down to the outstretched fingertip with his own fingers. Because these patients may spontaneously fixate their gaze upon a talking examiner but are unable to comply when asked to reach for objects, they are frequently misdiagnosed as malingerers or hysterics following a cursory examination. Balint's syndrome results from bilateral dorsal occipitoparietal lesions.

Topographic agnosia is the inability to use maps or to orient oneself geographically. It results from right parietooccipital lesions.

Anosagnosia is a denial of illness or disability which results from damage to cortical processing systems rather than to psychological processes or to willful denial. It can occur with lesions in a variety of cortical locations, most prominently with right parietal lobe involvement. When associated with cortical blindness, the combination is referred to as Anton's syndrome (see above).

Constructional impairment (also known as "con-structional apraxia," although this term is a misnomer) is the inability to accurately draw or copy figures. Although this deficit may occur with lesions almost anywhere in the cortex, the most severe constructional impairments accompany right parietal lesions owing to a loss of eye-hand coordination and of the ability to accurately perceive objects in space.

The dementias. The dementias are disorders leading to global and progressive intellectual decline owing to neuronal loss throughout the cerebral cortex. Although the cognitive impairment is global in nature, meaning that deficits are observable in all cerebral functions, including visual processing, the decline is often uneven, and visual complaints may predominate during one phase of the disease.

Vascular dementias result from the effects of cerebrovascular disease. Multi-infarct dementia (MID) results from the cumulative neuronal loss due to multiple infarctions scattered throughout the brain. Multiple lacunes, or small infarctions deep in the white matter of the cerebral hemispheres, result from long periods of uncontrolled hypertension or diabetes mellitus and are a common cause of MID. Binswanger's disease results from diffuse cerebrovascular disease in the small arterioles of the periventricular and deep white matter regions, leading to perivascular demyelination and subsequent cognitive impairment. The progression of a vascular dementia can be halted by scrupulous control of blood pressure, treatment of diabetes mellitus, and cessation of cigarette smoking, although the damage due to previous loss of brain cells cannot be undone.

Infectious dementias may result from chronic infections, including tuberculosis, syphilis, and some viruses. They may be reversible with early diagnosis and treatment. Creutzfeldt-Jakob disease, caused by a "slow virus" infection, is not reversible and follows a rapidly progressive deteriorating course.

Metabolic dementias may result from hormonal disturbances of pituitary, thyroid, or parathyroid origin; chronic deficiencies of vitamins B_1, B_{12}, or folic acid; or genetic errors of metabolism, such as Wilson's disease. They may often be reversed if the metabolic disturbance is diagnosed and treated early in its course.

Primary degenerative dementias are those whose cause is either genetic or unknown and which usually follow an inexorable deteriorating course. Although some symptoms can be palliated with medications or psychological treatments, the progression of the disease cannot be halted. Some of these disorders are discussed above, in the section on degenerative neurologic diseases. This category includes Alzheimer's disease, Parkinson's disease, Huntingdon's disease, progressive supranuclear palsy, and others. Although the visual system, like the rest of the cortex, is affected by these diseases, visual complaints are usually not prominent.

Although progressive dementias usually present with global impairment, some cases begin with focal involvement of one area and progress to involve the entire cortex in the later stages. Collectively, these diseases are called focal progressive cortical atrophies. Frontal lobe dementia begins with degeneration confined to the frontal regions, whereas Pick's disease involves the frontal lobes and anterior temporal lobes bilaterally, sparing the rest of the cortex until late in its course. Posterior

cortical atrophy (also referred to as Alzheimer's disease with Balint's syndrome, or the visual-spatial form of Alzheimer's disease) is a variant of Alzheimer's disease which begins with severe degeneration in the parietal and occipital lobes. In its early stages, it presents with prominent impairments of visual-spatial abilities, resembling Balint's syndrome or visual agnosia, and relatively mild signs of dysfunction referable to other lobes of the brain. In the later stages of the disease, degeneration progresses throughout the brain, and the clinical picture becomes indistinguishable from the late stages of typical Alzheimer's disease. The box below shows the typical findings on the optometric examination in a patient with posterior cortical atrophy in an early stage.

Psychiatric Problems in Optometric Practice

The management of patients with serious psychiatric conditions in an optometric (or any nonpsychiatric) practice can be difficult and frustrating because patients often cooperate poorly with examinations and instructions and may require large investments of a physician's time and patience.

Several principles should be kept in mind when

SIGNS AND SYMPTOMS OF POSTERIOR CORTICAL ATROPHY (VISUAL-SPATIAL FORMS OF ALZHEIMER'S DISEASE)

Complaints: Blurred vision, reading difficulty, difficulty walking up and down stairs and inclines, difficulty reaching for objects, confusion when presented with an array of objects, objects "pop in and out of view."

Acuity: Rarely completely normal, usually approximately 20/30 until the disease is far advanced.

Visual fields: Testing is labored and inconsistent, especially to multiple simultaneous stimuli. Formal kinetic testing usually reveals constricted fields. Automated static testing is hopeless as a result of impersistence and inattention.

Color vision to plain squares is normal. The patient is unable to perform the Ishihara test owing to visual-spatial inability.

Ocular apraxia: Visually guided saccades and pursuit movements are abnormal. Saccades to nonvisual commands are slowly initiated. Random saccades are of normal amplitude and velocity.

Optic ataxia: Misreaching for external targets (such as the examiner's fingertip). Reaching for the patient's own clothing or body parts (under somesthetic guidance) is normal.

Bilateral visual inattention: spotty piecemeal performance on line cancellation test.

Simultanagnosia: Identification of pictures of single objects is relatively preserved; performance on complex scenes or pictures of multiple objects is dramatically poorer.

Visual memory for familiar or famous faces is intact, although testing may be difficult owing to inability to fix gaze.

one is dealing with such patients:

1. Severely impaired patients should have nonessential examinations or treatments deferred until their mental conditions have been stabilized.
2. Trained assistants and family members, who are experienced in handling the patient and with whom the patient is comfortable, should be used when available.
3. Potentially violent or unstable patients should be examined or treated only in the presence of sufficient safeguards (such as security officers, physical restraints, medications) to ensure the safety of all persons present.

In the event of a psychiatric crisis or emergency in an optometric office, it is helpful to know what psychiatric resources are available in the area.

For mental health purposes, the United States is divided into catchment areas, the size of which varies depending upon the population density. Typically, each catchment area has a medical facility, designated as its crisis center, which functions as a "psychiatric emergency room," with 24-hour psychiatric and social work services for patients needing immediate psychiatric attention. Patients may present there voluntarily for assistance, individually or accompanied by friends or relatives. State laws provide for the involuntary transport by police, and evaluation in the crisis center, of patients who are a danger to themselves or others as a result of mental illness. Such procedures may be activated, in response to a dire psychiatric crisis in a doctor's or optometrist's office, by dialing the Police and Fire emergency telephone number ("911" in many municipalities in the United States). Most crisis centers have telephone lines to call for advice or direction in less emergent circumstances; the telephone number may be obtained from police, a local hospital, or a telephone directory.

Optometric practices located at hospitals, medical facilities, and multidisciplinary group practice locations often have access to on-campus psychiatric consultation services on an urgent or emergent basis. It should be remembered that most chronic psychiatric patients have a regular psychiatrist, psychologist, or social worker who can be called for advice or telephone consultation in the event of need.

Management of Psychiatric Emergencies. The principles of managing emergency situations in the optometric office are:

1. Have a plan.
2. Rehearse the plan with the office staff.
3. When a real emergency arises, follow the plan without deviation.

Guidelines for managing common psychiatric emergency situations in the optometrist's office follow:

The suicidal patient. Most patients who are planning or contemplating *suicide* make it known to others and accept help if it is properly offered. If a patient in your office tells you that he is contemplating suicide:

1. Take the threat seriously. Let him know that you want to help him prevent it. Do not fear that your talking about it will "put ideas into his head."
2. Do not try to assess the level of danger beyond what is obvious from the patient's statements; this must be done by a psychiatrist.
3. Your efforts should aim at transferring the patient to professional care with as much expediency and under as good security as is reasonably possible, and your stated recommendations should make this clear to the patient and/or to his family.
4. If the danger seems immediate, have the patient transferred to psychiatric care via ambulance or police. If appropriate, have available family members, family physicians, friends, or others take charge of getting the needed assistance.
5. Do not put yourself in the position of excusing or condoning inadequate treatment or attention, even if you cannot prevent it. For instance, if you suggest that the patient's spouse take him immediately to the nearest emergency room and he or she declines, make it clear that your recommendation stands.
6. If an actual suicide attempt occurs in your office (for example, a patient ingests pills or tells you that he ingested pills just before coming in), assume that the attempt is potentially le-

thal and handle it as a medical emergency; call an ambulance immediately without waiting for the patient's permission.

7. If the severity of the situation is not clear (as is commonly the case during an emergency), err on the side of safety. If the threat seems real and quick action will avert potential death or harm to your patient, do what appears to be necessary. Do not fear that you will be sued for forcing emergency care upon an unwilling patient, as long as you are acting in his best interests. You are more likely to be sued if you ignore the danger and harm comes to your patient.

Threatened violence. If the threat is due to a psychiatric condition (as opposed to premeditated criminality), physical violence is usually preceded by signs of escalating anxiety and fear. When you notice this, or when overt threats have been made:

1. Give the patient a wide space; do not stand close to him.
2. Do not be confrontational; this is sure to cause the behavior to escalate.
3. If possible, leave the room. Usually, the patient is relieved and does not object.
4. Once the immediate threat has been defused, call for the appropriate assistance (such as security officers, police, 911, or "panic buttons").
5. Do not attempt to restrain or physically evict violent patients yourself. Let trained staff, security guards, or police do so.

Emergent side effects of psychotropic medications. For example, dystonic reactions, hypotension, dizziness). Handle as you would any other medical emergency.

Psychogenic Disease

When examining a patient who presents with physical symptoms, a modern physician is trained to search for, identify, and treat the underlying disease. In clinical practice, however, a sizable minority of patients present with symptoms whose pathophysiologic basis cannot be identified, despite the thorough application of tests that should be capable of detecting it. These symptoms, which commonly include pain, neurologic deficits, and gastrointestinal complaints, may be due to physical disease that is beyond the resolution of medical knowledge or may be the reflection of psychologic distress. Patients with somatic complaints of psychologic origin are common in clinical practice because they consult physicians frequently and consume a disproportionately high percentage of health care resources. These patients are often not recognized by nonpsychiatric physicians until exhaustive testing has failed to reveal a cause for the complaint.

Somatization. *Somatization* is a process by which mental symptoms, such as anxiety, depression, or psychic conflict, are transformed into physical complaints instead of being expressed psychologically. A psychogenic somatic symptom is defined as a physical symptom that is not accompanied by any (or by sufficient) objective evidence of a pathophysiologic process to explain it. Rather, it represents the outward clinical expression of a psychologic illness or conflict. Once this is recognized, the underlying psychologic process should become the focus of the physician's evaluation and treatment.

Differential Diagnosis. Psychogenic somatic symptoms can occur in a wide variety of psychiatric conditions.

Anxiety is often accompanied by autonomic (sympathetic) arousal, with its resultant signs and symptoms, including tachycardia (heart palpitations), tremulousness, tachypnea (hyperventilation), blurred vision, dry mouth, chest pain, abdominal discomfort, and urinary urgency. These symptoms may overshadow the subjective feeling of anxiety per se. The patient may focus on these complaints and even deny subjective anxiety.

Depression is often accompanied by a negative self-image, including somatic preoccupation and symptoms; sometimes the patient may focus on these symptoms ("depressive equivalents") and deny the subjective feelings of depression. In patients with psychotic depression, the somatic symptoms may have the strength of delusions, often of fantastic proportions. An example of this is Cotard's delusion, in which the patient asserts that he is dead or decomposed. The somatic symptoms resolve with effective treatment of depression.

Schizophrenia may be accompanied by somatic delusions, often of a bizarre and fantastic nature. They are usually associated with other manifestations of schizophrenia, such as auditory hallucinations, flattened affect, and disorganization of thought processes.

Monosymptomatic hypochondriacal delusional syndrome is classified in *DSM-III-R* as a primary delusional (paranoid) disorder. Common variants involving somatic delusions include:

Olfactory reference syndrome: the delusion of having an offensive and unpleasant body odor.

Dysmorphophobia: the delusional belief of physical, usually facial, disfigurement.

Parasitosis: the delusional belief of cutaneous parasitic infestation.

Cancerophobia: the belief that one has, or is very susceptible to, cancer.

Malingering describes the situation in which a person, consciously and intentionally, pretends to be sick in order to achieve an ulterior gain, such as financial compensation or evasion of work.

Factitious disorder is a very baffling psychiatric condition in which a patient willfully, and often very cleverly, produces objective pathophysiologic signs of some known physical illness. Examples include thyrotoxicosis secondary to self-injection of thyroid hormones and chronic skin ulcers secondary to excoriation. It should be noted that factitious disorder is an exception to the definition of a psychogenic somatic symptom because the patient's actions actually produce objective physical signs and lesions. Munchausen syndrome is a particularly dramatic form of factitious illness in which a patient wanders from hospital to hospital, cleverly tricking physicians into performing unnecessary surgical procedures on himself. Factitious disorder differs from malingering in that ulterior motives, other than the pathologic desire to obtain medical or surgical treatment, are not apparent in patients with factitious disorders.

The somatoform disorders are a group of illnesses characterized primarily by prominent so-matic symptoms and preoccupation. Somatization disorder, formerly known as Briquet's syndrome or "chronic hysteria," is a chronic disorder characterized by multiple, recurring, subjective somatic complaints. Conversion disorder, formerly known as hysterical conversion or hysterical neurosis, is an acute, monosymptomatic complaint, usually loss of a function mediated by the voluntary, sensory, or autonomic nervous systems, such as blindness or limb paralysis. In the classic psychodynamic formulation, a conversion symptom allows the patient to avoid or temporarily resolve an unconscious conflict that would otherwise cause unbearable anxiety. Examples include sudden muteness during an argument with a spouse and paraparesis in a soldier on the eve of battle. Somatoform pain disorder, also known as "psychogenic pain syndrome," is characterized by preoccupation with pain in the absence of adequate physical findings to account for the pain or its intensity. This disorder occurs in acute and chronic forms.

Hypochondriasis is the persistent and pervasive fear or preoccupation that one has a serious physical illness. The preoccupation is with the presence of disease, instead of with the symptom itself, as is the case in somatization disorder. Typically, patients with hypochondriasis are very focused on bodily sensations and often misinterpret transient or innocuous sensations to be indicative of serious diseases.

Psychogenic Visual Loss. Psychogenic visual loss occurs in conversion disorder, malingering, and somatization disorder. Ruling out organic blindness due to intraocular disease is usually easy and straightforward, but differentiating visual loss of psychogenic origin from that resulting from neurologic disease in the cerebral cortex can be very difficult. Because patients with damage to the posterior regions of the cerebral cortex frequently have preservation of some spontaneous visual function but complain that they cannot see, it is easy to assume that they are not telling the truth or have a psychiatric disorder. A very careful and knowledgeable examination is required to differentiate psychogenic visual loss from cortical blindness, visual agnosia, Balint's syndrome, and other disorders of complex visual processing. It is difficult or impossible to be absolutely certain that an individual symptom is psychogenic in origin, and the clinician must always be ready to change his opinion if new evidence warrants an organic diagnosis. Because psychogenic and organically based symptoms frequently co-exist, even the presence of definite nonorganic visual symptoms does not exclude the possibility of ocular or neurologic disease and does not excuse the optometrist from performing a careful and thorough examination.

The presence of psychogenic illness should be suspected, however, when the patient's complaints do not conform to any known ocular or neurologic illness and when they are not consistent with known anatomy and physiology. Because patients are usually not knowledgeable about the details of anatomy and physiology, psychogenic symptoms frequently do not conform to patterns observed in physical disease. For instance, the cutaneous sensory fields of spinal nerves overlap along the ventral midline of the chest and abdomen, resulting in preservation of sensation near the midline when a spinal nerve is severed or damaged; sensory loss stopping exactly at the midline cannot be neurologic in origin. Common psychogenic visual complaints may often be suspected because of inconsistent or unexplainable findings on the optometric examination.

Psychogenic blindness occurs in conversion disorder ("hysterical blindness"), usually as the result of an unconscious conflict that the patient is unable to resolve without experiencing extreme anxiety. It is typically abrupt in onset and occurs as an isolated complaint, without other neurologic symptoms. Because it helps to allay anxiety, it is often accompanied by an air of detached unconcern, called *la belle indifference,* which is in marked contrast to the obvious distress usually seen in patients with new-onset blindness. Ocular reflexes and optokinetic nystagmus are always preserved in psychogenic blindness; however, they may also be preserved in some cases of near-total retinal or cortical blindness, even when little functionally useful vision remains. Sometimes patients

with psychogenic blindness may be tricked into responding to unexpected visual stimuli of a threatening or exciting nature. They may be observed to avoid obstacles in their path, to reach for objects without groping, or to find their way through unfamiliar surroundings without guidance.

Monocular psychogenic visual loss must be differentiated from optic neuritis. In optic neuritis, there is a loss or decrease of the direct pupillary response to light, with preservation of the consensual response, while both reflexes are normal in psychogenic visual loss. The diagnosis can also be made by holding a red lens over the "good" eye and asking the patient to read a string of alternating red and black letters on a screen. Because the patient is usually unaware that red letters are invisible when viewed through a lens of the same color, preserved vision in the "affected" eye is demonstrated if the patient reads the letters correctly.

Psychogenic visual field loss manifests as "tunnel vision," in which the patient complains of constricted vision but perimetry demonstrates fields of equal diameter at all test distances. In peripheral field loss due to retinal pathology or to bilateral hemianopsia of cortical origin with macular sparing, more distant fields become progressively larger, as the cone of preserved vision expands with distance. It must be remembered, however, that drug intoxication and other organic conditions can occasionally give rise to the phenomenon of tunnel vision. Homonymous field defects and central scotomas are almost never reported in psychogenic conditions.

Diplopia and blurred vision are frequently reported in somatization disorder, hypochondriasis, and malingering. When binocular, complaints of psychogenic and organic origin are very difficult to distinguish. Monocular complaints, however, are usually of psychogenic origin if intraocular disease and optic neuritis can be excluded.

Treatment of Patients with a Psychogenic Somatic Symptom in Optometric Practice. The management of patients with psychogenic somatic symptoms is a difficult task in a nonpsychiatric practice. Efforts by an optometrist or other practitioner to refer patients for psychiatric treatment are usually met with hostility. However, attempts to treat the symptoms by conventional medical techniques are futile and wasteful and do not result in any lasting improvement in the patient's condition. The principles of management are as follows:

1. Rule out all possible organic causes, even if this requires an extensive work-up.
2. Refer the patient for psychiatric evaluation. Do not be surprised if he reacts negatively to this suggestion.
3. Acknowledge the reality and importance of the symptom to the patient, without necessarily colluding with the patient's interpretation of it. Do not insinuate that he is "lying" or "crazy."
4. Once all possible organic causes have been ruled out by an examination and adequate ancillary studies, resist the temptation to repeat the work-up or to order tests that would not ordinarily be indicated, although the patient may urge you to do so.

For example, if a patient states that he cannot see and your examination shows that he can, do not confront him with this. Acknowledge that he cannot see, and tell him that you cannot find a reason for it. If he proposes a plausible cause, such as, "I think I have a tumor in my eye," tell him that your examination has ruled this out, and explain why. If he states that you must be missing something, do not display anger, but say in a matter-of-fact manner that you are confident about your diagnosis. Refer him for further studies or professional consultations, if these are indicated. If not, diplomatically suggest that a psychiatrist may be able to help him. If the patient is not willing to consider this option, family members or friends may help to persuade him. Remember that the patient perceives the symptom to be real and obvious and perceives a denial by the doctor to be either absurd or insulting. By acknowledging the symptom to be real but not to be the result of an organic cause, the optometrist is setting the stage for the next step, in which the psychiatrist proposes that the symptom is secondary to a psychologic problem such as anxiety, depression, or an unconscious conflict.

Visual Hallucinations

Although auditory hallucinations are commonly encountered in psychiatric disease and olfactory hallucinations frequently occur during seizure auras, visual hallucinations occur most commonly as symptoms of neurologic disease in the eye or the visual pathways or of psychoactive drug use. In the clinical setting, visual hallucinations are defined by a patient reporting, or acting as though he sees, objects or events that are not visible to the examiner. Visual hallucinations can be simple shapes or lights (phosphenes) or complex scenes; static or dynamic; in color or shades of grey; repetitive in content or different from one occasion to the next. The nature and content of the hallucination give the clinician clues to its origin.

Although most visual hallucinations are pathologic, some occur in normal individuals without visual or psychiatric disease. Pressure applied to the globe, or quick eye movements, may produce sudden flashes of light, called flick phosphenes. Hypnogogic hallucinations, often of people, animals, or complex scenes, occur during the process of falling asleep in many normal individuals. Sensory deprivation, as can occur in prolonged imprisonment or hospital confinement, or in blindness, often gives rise to visual hallucinations in otherwise normal people.

Ocular and Optic Nerve Disease. Individuals with dense cataracts or advanced macular degeneration often experience complex, well-formed visual hallucinations, perhaps on the basis of sensory deprivation. Traction on the retina, from scarring or from age-related shrinkage of the vitreous body, may give rise of vertical flashes of light, known as Moore's lightning streaks, during eye movements. Retinal ischemia, from retinal migraine or vascular disease, may produce visual hallucinations having the appearance of scintillating colored lights. Phosphenes induced by ocular movement or sudden loud sounds may occur in the early stages of optic neuritis secondary to multiple sclerosis or inflammation of the optic nerve.

Brain Lesions. Vascular or neoplastic lesions in the midbrain give rise to the syndrome of peduncular hallucinosis. This consists of vivid, moving visual hallucinations of complex scenes, which may be of normal or lilliputian proportions, accompanied by the subjective feeling of pleasant entertainment. This is usually associated with other signs and symptoms of focal midbrain disease, including cranial nerve palsies and deficits due to damage to the traversing motor and sensory tracts.

Paroxysmal focal alterations in cerebral electrical activity, occurring during localized seizures, can give rise to ictal hallucinations. Focal seizures originating in the primary visual cortex produce simple phosphenes, often described as flashing lights or tongues of flame. Seizure activity in the visual association areas of the ventral, occipital and temporal lobes produces hallucinations of complex, dynamic, panoramic scenes; these hallucinations can include intense emotional experiences if the seizure involves the limbic-connected cortex of the medial temporal lobe.

Visual hallucinations may occur during the aura preceding a migraine headache. They usually take the form of scintillating scotomas or fortification spectra composed of concentric wavy or zig-zag lines. In addition, visual illusions, including micropsia, macropsia, and distortion of images, are common during migrainous auras.

Visual hallucinations secondary to focal cerebral lesions, in the absence of ictal or migrainous events, are referred to as release hallucinations. They are believed to occur as a result of the release from inhibition of one brain area when another is damaged. Following injury to the occipital, occipitoparietal, and posterior temporal regions, release hallucinations usually occur in the visual field contralateral to the lesion, frequently confined to the resulting visual field defect. They may be simple or complex.

The Charles Bonnet Syndrome. This eponym is used to describe the occurrence of complex, well-formed visual hallucinations in elderly patients with chronically diminished vision. The hallucinations are usually vivid, dynamic scenes with strong emotional content. In addition to visual loss due to ocular or neurologic disease, many cases are associated with systemic metabolic disturbances or psychoactive medication use.

Drug-Induced Hallucinations. A variety of medications and drugs of abuse can cause visual hallucinations. Prescription medications reported to cause this side effect in some patients include beta-blockers, digitalis preparations, antiarrhythmics, tricyclic antidepressants, anticholinergics, dopamine agonists, and sympathomimetic decongestants.

Hallucinogenic drugs, including lysergic acid diethylamide (LSD), mescaline, and psilocybin produce intense, dynamic, visual hallucinations in which the user often experiences a melding of sensory impressions from the visual, auditory, olfactory, and somatosensory spheres. Other drugs used for their hallucinatory, including visual, potential include phencyclidine, cannabis, and volatile solvents. In addition, visual hallucinations can occur during withdrawal syndromes that follow the abrupt discontinuation of alcohol, sedatives, and numerous other drugs after a prolonged period of use.

ACKNOWLEDGMENT

The author is grateful to Chrystyna Zwil, OD, for reviewing the manuscript and offering many helpful suggestions.

Bibliography

Adams RD and Victor M: *Principles of neurology*, New York, 1993, McGraw-Hill.

Arana GW and Hyman SE: *Handbook of psychiatric drug therapy*, ed 2, Boston, 1991, Little, Brown & Co.

Cassem NH, editor: *Massachusetts general hospital handbook of general hospital psychiatry*, ed 3, Mosby Year Book.

Cummings JL: *Clinical neuropsychiatry*, Boston, 1985, Allyn and Bacon.

Escourolle R and Poirier J: *Manual of basic neuropathology*, ed 2, Philadelphia, 1978, WB Saunders.

Kaplan HI and Sadock BJ, editors: *Comprehensive textbook of psychiatry/V*, Baltimore, 1989, Williams & Wilkins.

Mesulam M-M: *Textbook of behavioral neurology,* Philadelphia, 1985, FA Davis.

Patten J: *Neurological differential diagnosis,* New York, 1977, Springer-Verlag.

Stinnett JL: The functional somatic symptom. *Psychiatr Clin North Am* 10:19-33, 1987.

Stoudemire A: *Clinical psychiatry for medical students,* Philadelphia, 1990, JB Lippincott.

Tomb DA: *Psychiatry for the house officer,* ed 4, Baltimore, 1992, Williams & Wilkins.

Weiner HL and Levitt LP: *Neurology for the house officer,* ed 4, Baltimore, 1989, Williams & Wilkins.

Weintraub MI: *Hysteria.* Clinical Symposia, Ciba-Geigy, 1977.

17

Emergency Medicine

DAVID P. SENDROWSKI
JOHN F. MAHER

---

*T*he purpose of this chapter is to familiarize the practitioner with common emergencies that may occur in practice. When dealt with in a calm, methodical manner, these emergencies have a more successful outcome. The practitioner should always be prepared for the unexpected in an office, home, or public place.

SYNCOPE (FAINTING)

Syncope is a common emergency faced by many practitioners. The practitioner confronted with a patient who has fainted or reports fainting spells must decide whether the patient has a serious underlying vascular or cardiovascular condition or a less threatening problem. Syncope occurs more frequently in older men, patients with known heart disease, and young women who are prone to vasovagal episodes, although stressful, painful, and claustrophobic conditions can be precipitating factors for a syncopal episode. In the author's experience there have been several occasions where contact lens application and applanation tonometry have also precipitated a syncopal episode.

Pathophysiology

The underlying cause of a syncopal episode is inadequate cerebral perfusion causing a loss of consciousness. The flow of blood to the cerebral area fails to meet the metabolic needs of the tissues in the brain. A marked peripheral arterial dilation takes place, especially in the larger muscular beds. This dilation results in an overall reduced peripheral resistance with no associated increase in cardiac output to compensate for the peripheral dilation. The result is an overall blood pressure decrease over the course of seconds to minutes. During this time lightheadedness and peripheral field constriction occur prior to the loss of consciousness.

Clinically, the patient may complain of lightheadedness, nausea, dizziness, and sweating. Pallor of the skin may also be noted. The heart rate rapidly increases prior to loss of consciousness. At the onset of the syncope, the pulse rate slows down owing to the influence of the vagus nerve. The episode usually lasts for several minutes, at the end of which time the patient regains consciousness. No loss of bowel or bladder control occurs during the episode.

Syncope has many causes (see box above, right), but the vasodepressor type is by far the most common.

Work-Up/Clinical Evaluation

The history and physical examination usually define the need for a work-up. The history should include such factors as relationship to posture and

---

CAUSES OF SYNCOPE

Vasodepressor
Orthostatic hypotensive
Cardiogenic
    Cardiac arrhythmias
    Aortic stenosis, hypertrophic cardiomyopathy
    Myocardial infarction
    Subclavian steal syndrome
    Sick sinus syndrome
Cough
Micturition
Cerebrovascular disease
Metabolic
    Hypoxia
    Hyperventilation
    Hypoglycemia

---

physical activity prior to the syncope. The medical history should be evaluated for heart disease, drug therapy (antihypertensive medications, diuretics, vasodilators), pulmonary symptoms, associated diseases, and evidence of precipitating features.

The physical examination may provide valuable clues to the cause. The patient should have his or her blood pressure and heart rate assessed and checked for postural changes. The carotid pulse should be evaluated for bruit or diminished amplitude, which may suggest cerebrovascular disease. The heart beat should be assessed with a stethoscope for evidence of arrhythmia or murmur.

Laboratory studies are not indicated for a first episode of syncope. A history of several attacks, especially those that occur suddenly and end abruptly, may be referred for an electrocardiogram (ECG). If the cause of the syncope cannot be found and if the patient has not had a physical examination for several years, referral to an internist for a physical examination is warranted.

Treatment

It is important for the practitioner to realize that the immediate risk for the patient is the loss of consciousness and injury that may be sustained during a fall. The practitioner can prevent the syncope by having the patient lie down or by lowering the patient's head below the level of the heart, usually below the patient's knees. The syncopal episode with an unknown cause in a young patient without cardiovascular disease has a good prognosis.

HYPERVENTILATION

The action of *hyperventilation* may be an inappropriate response to an anxiety state or an appropriate response to an underlying abnormality. The causes of hyperventilation syndrome include emotional upset, respiratory compensation for acidosis, and respiratory alkalosis. Hyperventilation is rarely observed in children, men, or women over the age of 40 years. The typical person who experiences hyperventilation is an overly anxious female between the ages of 14 and 40 years. Hyperventilation usually results in impaired consciousness, with unconsciousness being rare.

Pathophysiology

Hyperventilation leads to respiratory alkalosis, a primary decrease in carbon dioxide pressure resulting in an elevation of the pH of the blood and a decrease in the carbon dioxide content. The Pa_{CO_2} and the cerebral tissue Pa_{CO_2} fall, and at the same time the plasma and cerebral tissue pH rises. The combination of these two events results in cerebral vasoconstriction and hypoxia.

Clinically, the patient presents with a ventilation pattern of frequent, deep, sighing respirations or sustained rapid, deep respirations. The latter may result in the patient complaining that she "can't catch her breath."

The pH change causes a change in the ionic balance that results in nerve irritability. This becomes apparent, clinically, if the patient starts to complain of tingling or numbness in the hands, fingers, or feet. The feet are more often affected than the other extremities. Some other clinical entities that the practitioner may note are tetany, acroparesthesia, lightheadedness, giddiness, and syncope. The

area surrounding the mouth is sometimes affected as well.

Treatment

The main cause for the patient's symptoms is low carbon dioxide pressure. Therefore, having the patient rebreathe her own carbon dioxide helps to relieve the symptoms.

It is beneficial for the practitioner to find the stimulus of the hyperventilation. For example, if the patient is experiencing anxiety hyperventilation about an optometric test, removing the equipment and reassuring the patient may cause the hyperventilation episode to subside. On the other hand, if the patient is anxious, putting a paper bag over the patient's nose and mouth may increase the anxiety and exacerbate the hyperventilation. A paper bag over the mouth and nose does help the patient to rebreathe her CO_2 and reverses the pathophysiologic process. Use of a plastic bag is not recommended and may cause accidental suffocation. The technique of rebreathing exhaled CO_2 is contraindicated in patients with central nervous system disturbances, as the procedure may exacerbate the underlying problem. If patient reassurance and rebreathing techniques are not successful, it is prudent to call for emergency assistance and transportation to a medical facility.

ORTHOSTATIC (POSTURAL) HYPOTENSION

The autonomic nervous system is responsible for regulating blood pressure when a person changes from a recumbent to a sitting or standing position. *Orthostatic hypotension* may occur in persons who have an inadequate responding autonomic nervous system, or it may be secondary to a medication or disease that affects the volume of blood or regulation of blood flow.

The person usually has a history of syncope or lightheadedness upon postural change. The syncope is not associated with the normal sweating, pallor, and other signs. Consciousness is regained promptly when the person assumes a recumbent position. The most frequent causes are excessive doses of diuretic medications and protracted bed rest from a prolonged sickness or injury.

Pathophysiology

When a patient with orthostatic hypotension stands up, the sudden stress of the stance causes blood to pool in the venous capacitance vessels of the leg. The volume of blood returning to the heart is diminished, and the blood pressure and cardiac output decrease. In a normal patient, the baroreceptors in the aortic and carotid plexus region cause an increase in heart rate to restore the blood pressure. A patient with orthostatic hypotension has an abnormality in the afferent, efferent, or central portions of the reflex arc caused by disease, drugs, or autonomic nervous system abnormality. This break in the reflex arc does not allow the compensatory increase in heart rate, and the blood perfusion to the cerebral tissue falls and unconsciousness ensues.

Clinically, no predisposing symptoms normally occur in a patient with syncope. The patient regains consciousness upon reassuming the recumbent position. The syncope is caused by the act of postural change.

Treatment

As with normal syncope, care should be taken to make sure that the patient sustains no bodily damage during the loss of consciousness. When the orthostatic hypotension is due to hypovolemia or drug excess, it is rapidly reversed by correcting these problems. The orthostasis of protracted bed rest is best handled by having the patient sit up in bed each day.

If the patient has an underlying neurogenic problem, it is usual to treat the symptoms rather than the neurogenic cause. In essence, an oral medication is given to maintain an increased blood pressure by peripheral assistance (e.g., ephedrine, 25 to 50 mg orally) so that postural changes do not affect cerebral perfusion. Increasing dietary sodium intake may increase fluid volume in the body and reduce the risk of hypovolemic hypotension.

SEIZURES

A *seizure* is a peripheral manifestation of an irritative focus at some location in the brain. The type of seizure of which most people are aware is the major motor seizure. This type of seizure produces jerking of body parts, loss of consciousness, and incontinence in the afflicted patient. Focal seizures may involve only a single body part, whereas other seizures present as repetitive, automatic acts of behavior, an example being lip smacking or chewing.

The two most important points a practitioner should keep in mind in aiding a patient having a seizure is to keep the patient's airway open and to prevent bodily damage during the seizure. Also important is a careful description of the seizure episode. This can be very helpful to the medical diagnostician. The aforementioned lip smacking and chewing strongly suggest a temporal lobe cause for the seizure.

Pathophysiology

A seizure episode is caused by an abnormal neural discharge from an area in the brain. The normal inhibitory mechanisms in the brain are eluded, allowing the discharge to spread. The mechanism of this event is not completely understood at this time. Given a sufficient stimulus (such as convulsant drugs or hypoglycemia), even the normal brain can discharge in an abnormal fashion and induce a seizure episode in susceptible individuals. Seizures can be precipitated by exogenous stimuli such as sound or light.

Major motor seizures, the bilateral tonic-clonic type of convulsions, can be without focal onset, in which the seizure occurs suddenly in the patient. The seizure can also have a focal onset, such as in the fingers or toes, and follow in cortical representation of body parts. There is a greater likelihood of finding an underlying cause for the focal type of seizure than for the nonfocal type.

Seizures are rare in adults with a febrile disease, even those with body temperature greater than 102°F. It is also rare for patients with an initial embolic stroke to the brain to have a seizure. Seizures are more likely after the embolic stroke rather than during the event. Alcohol withdrawal seizures usually occur 7 to 48 hours after cessation of alcohol, with the peak incidence between 13 and 24 hours. Finally, head trauma of a severe nature (open head trauma) can cause seizures any time after the incident, whereas closed head trauma is not associated with seizures. A variety of cerebral or systemic disorders may cause a seizure episode (see box).

Treatment

During a seizure episode, the most important things that the practitioner can do are to keep the patient's airway open and to prevent injury during the convulsions. A firm but reasonably soft object should be inserted between the patient's teeth (e.g., a handkerchief). The handkerchief protects the tongue from being bitten, although at no time should the practitioner put fingers in, around, or near the patient's mouth during the convulsive stage, as amputation or severe damage of the digits can occur. The practitioner should not attempt to put anything in the mouth that could damage teeth or be swallowed by the patient. The patient should be moved away from instruments or furniture that could cause bodily injury during the convulsive seizure. Clothing around the neck should be loosened and a pillow should be placed under the head if available. At no time should the patient be restrained or held during the convulsive seizure.

After the seizure has abated, the patient should be transported to a medical facility where a thorough examination can be done. A complete description of the episode should be relayed to the medical personnel in order to facilitate the diagnosis of the disorder.

The prognosis is good for most patients. If the examination and imaging series reveal no evidence of localized disorders, then drug therapy can completely control seizures in 50% of cases and greatly reduce the frequency in another 35% of cases.

SHOCK

Shock is a condition in which there is a severe reduction of tissue perfusion of blood. If this con-

---

CONVULSIVE SEIZURES

Cerebral hypoxia
   Anesthesia
   Carbon monoxide poisoning
   Breath holding

Brain defects
   Congenital
   Developmental

Space-occupying lesions
   Intracranial neoplasm
   Intracranial hemorrhage
   Subdural hematoma

Severe cerebral trauma
   Skull fracture (open head wound)
   Birth injury

Cerebral infarction (after the initial event)

Cerebral edema
   Hypertensive encephalopathy

Central nervous system infections
   Meningitis   Tetanus
   Encephalitis   Toxoplasmosis
   Neurosyphilis Cysticercosis
   Brain abscess Rabies

Toxic agents
   Lead   Camphor
   Alcohol   Strychnine
   Pentylenetrazol

Metabolic disorders
   Hypoglycemia
   Phenylketonuria
   Hyperparathyroidism

Withdrawal periods
   Alcohol
   Tranquilizers
   Hypnotics

tinues, impaired cellular function and ultimately cell death occur. The cause of shock usually lies in a failure of the circulatory system. The layman's idea of shock is lethargy and confusion. The actual condition is much more serious.

"Shock" itself is never a diagnosis. It is always precipitated by something else. A heart attack, a bee sting, or a lacerated artery could all cause the condition termed shock, which if untreated often results in death of the patient.

There are three categories of shock: (1) hypovolemic shock, (2) cardiogenic shock, and (3) low-resistance shock.

Hypovolemic Shock

This is a state in which the circulating blood volume is not great enough for the size of the circulatory system.

Pathophysiology. Hypovolemic shock is usually caused by bleeding, either externally or internally into a body cavity such as the peritoneum. Blood volume can also be decreased by loss of large quantities of bodily fluids such as in sweating, burns, vomiting, and severe diarrhea. Persistent diarrhea in an infant or child can result in an electrolyte imbalance and a decrease in blood volume, which can lead to hypovolemic shock.

When the blood volume is not adequate to perfuse the tissues, then tissue hypoxia can lead to metabolic acidosis and a progressive impairment of myocardial performance. This leads to a decrease in blood pressure and tissue perfusion, and the vicious circle continues. Unchecked, it leads to patient death.

Cardiogenic Shock

The patient's circulation is inadequate as a result of poor pumping action of the heart. This leads to poor perfusion of the tissues even though the blood volume is normal.

Pathophysiology. The mechanism is the same as for hypovolemic shock. The cause may be an acute myocardial infarction or heart failure from valvular disease such as mitral stenosis. There may be such extracardiac causes as pericardial tamponade or pulmonary embolism.

Low-resistance Shock

In this condition the blood volume and cardiac performance may be normal but the vascular space is enlarged.

Pathophysiology. Blood vessels supplying the skin or the gut become dilated. Blood is pooled in abnormally large amounts in these vessels, causing a drop in tissue perfusion elsewhere. These blood vessels may be in the gut or in the skin or both.

The cause of this condition is usually neurologic or chemical changes that have resulted in the opening of these large-capacitance vessels. The bacteria or bacterial toxins of septic shock can result in dilation of vessels. Acidosis, adrenal insufficiency, and some drugs may all cause or contribute to the above process. Damage to the central nervous system from trauma or stroke may result in neurologic reflexes causing vascular dilatation and low-resistance shock.

Clinical Evaluation

The clinical appearance of all three types of shock is similar. The skin is cool, clammy, and pale. With low-resistance shock the skin may also appear somewhat red and warm. Tachycardia is usually present as the body attempts to increase cardiac output and tissue oxygenation. In the early stages of shock the patient may be restless and complain of thirst. As the syndrome progresses there may be weakness, confusion, disorientation, and ultimately coma. Blood pressure is low even if the patient is in a reclining position. Mucous membranes of the lid and mouth appear dry and can be cyanotic. Neck veins may be flat and urine output diminished. With low-resistance shock secondary to sepsis, the patient may evidence fever and chills.

Treatment

Treatment must start with the correct diagnosis. One should suspect shock in a patient who has had prolonged vomiting or diarrhea. The nausea and vomiting that can occur with angle-closure glaucoma may result in dehydration and shock by the above mechanisms.

After the appropriate history has been taken, the status of the patient's pulse, blood pressure, and respirations should be rapidly assessed. An adequate airway should be maintained. If respiration is inadequate or the carotid pulse is absent, then CPR should be instituted immediately. Otherwise the patient should be in the supine position with the head lower than the body and to one side so that vomitus is not aspirated.

If there is evidence of pulmonary edema, placing the patient in a sitting position allows the patient to breath easier. When the patient is cool and clammy, as in hypovolemic and cardiogenic shock, the patient should be kept warm with blankets or clothing until help arrives.

MYOCARDIAL INFARCTION

Although heart attacks are more common in the middle or later years, they may occur in a younger, seemingly healthy patient who lacks obvious risk factors. However, patients having the following risk factors have an increased chance of myocardial infarction:

1. Increasing age (50s to 70s)
2. Family history of heart trouble
3. Cigarette smoking
4. Hypertension
5. Diabetes mellitus
6. Elevated blood cholesterol
7. Sedentary life style

Pathophysiology

Although the heart is responsible for pumping blood to the rest of the body, the heart muscle itself must receive an adequate blood supply. If the heart's own blood supply is deficient, then the heart muscle does not receive an adequate amount of oxygen and begins to die. Some of the heart muscle may die and be replaced by scar tissue. The heart may still be able to pump an adequate amount of blood to itself and the rest of the body. However, when enough heart muscle is lost, the heart's function as an effective pump is severely compromised and death may occur. In addition, the heart's pumping ability may be maintained, but other lethal events may occur.

The inciting cause of a myocardial infarction is an occluded artery. Blockage may be caused by a clot, an embolus, or a cholesterol plaque in the wall of the artery that gradually occludes the lumen of the vessel. If a large amount of heart muscle dies, then cardiogenic shock occurs. The heart's pumping ability is compromised and death results.

If the heart is able to keep pumping, the dead heart muscle is replaced by scar tissue. However, the heart may rupture in the area of the scar tissue. This condition is fatal. If the heart muscle containing the heart's conduction system is damaged, then life-threatening cardiac arrhythmias may occur.

Finally, the heart muscle that supplies the cardiac valves may be involved, resulting in valvular insufficiency. An example of this is mitral regurgitation.

Clinical Evaluation

The patient may complain of excruciating pain. It is often substernal but may radiate to one or both arms or to the back. It is most commonly crushing but may sometimes be mild and centered in the epigastrium. The pain is usually not transitory. It is rather prolonged, lasting between 15 minutes and several hours or longer. Some patients, strangely, do not complain of pain. Rather they may have malaise, weakness, difficulty breathing, vague nausea, or a sense that something is not right.

When examined, the patient may be agitated or may simply appear tired or quiet. Some patients may be afraid to move about for fear that their pain will increase. Cyanosis, sweating, and vomiting may be observed.

On examination the rales of pulmonary edema may be heard. The pulses on palpation may be weak and thready. It may be impossible to palpate the brachial or radial pulses. However, the carotid pulse is usually present if the heart is still pumping.

The mental status of the patient should be checked. If the patient is alert and able to respond to simple questions, then the brain is probably receiving adequate blood flow. However, if the patient begins to become lethargic or confused, then central nervous system perfusion is likely to be depressed and the condition is even more serious.

Treatment

Although the medical treatment of a myocardial infarction is beyond the scope of this chapter, the following principles should be kept in mind. An adequate airway should be established if the patient is not conscious. If breathing or perfusion is inadequate, then *cardiopulmonary respiration (CPR)* should be instituted. If the patient is conscious, he should be kept warm and at rest to minimize oxygen consumption. If oxygen is present, it should be administered. The patient should be kept in a supine position unless pulmonary edema and breathing difficulties occur. He should then be placed in the sitting position. The prompt recognition of this life-threatening emergency enables the practitioner to summon the appropriate help quickly.

HYMENOPTERA STINGS

The stings of the *Hymenoptera*, which include bees, wasps, hornets, and fire ants, are common medical emergencies. In the unrecognized sensitive individual, a sting represents a life-threatening situation. Twice as many people die in the United States of these stings as of snake bites. If a patient has been stung by a bumblebee, honeybee, hornet, or yellow-jacket, emergency measures must be taken immediately to arrest the serious anaphylaxis that occurs in 1% of the population.

Pathophysiology

Bee venom contains vasoactive substances such as histamine which are hemolytic and neurotoxic agents. In addition, the venom is a powerful hypersensitizing agent, such that repeated stings in sensitive individuals cause a serious systemic re-action. Reactions in sensitive individuals tend to get worse with repeated stings.

Work-up and Clinical Evaluation

The patient presents with a history of acute pain, usually recognizing that a sting has occurred within the past few minutes. The area stung is usually erythematous and itchy, with a local wheal. You must try to ascertain if the patient is hypersensitive to bee sting. If he does not know, treat him as if he is hypersensitive.

Hypersensitive individuals may develop body-wide itching and edema within minutes, accompanied by a deep-seated feeling that something is seriously wrong. This may be associated with nausea, abdominal pain, shortness of breath, and hypertension. Eventual coma and death may occur following respiratory distress and failure if treatment is not instituted in these patients.

Immediate Treatment

Immediate treatment of bee sting begins with removal of the venom sac with forceps. Try not to squeeze the sac, as this forces more venom into the patient. Following removal of the sac, the area should be cleansed with cool water and soap. Cool compresses can then be applied to the area.

Allergic patients require a subcutaneous injection of 0.3 to 0.5 ml of epinephrine (1:1000). The patient should also swallow an oral antihistamine agent such as Chlortrimeton.

Hypersensitive individuals should be rushed to an emergency room even if injected with epinephrine. They may go into respiratory distress and require oxygen and Benadryl injection.

The Insect-sting Kit

Several kits are available which may be purchased by prescription for the patient to self-administer an injection of epinephrine. These kits contain preloaded epinephrine syringes, antihistamine tablets, and a tourniquet.

The tourniquet is placed proximal to the site of the sting if it is on an extremity. The patient should be instructed on the proper self-injection technique. The patient should swallow the antihistamine tablet and head for the nearest emergency room.

Long-term Prophylaxis

The patient with a severe, acute reaction to bee sting should be tested (1 month later) with venom extracts by an allergy specialist. For those highly sensitive individuals, long-term immunotherapy, with sensitizing injections of venom over a period of years or for life, may reduce the risk of life-threatening anaphylaxis.

DIABETIC EMERGENCIES

Diabetes mellitus is discussed in Chapter 13. In-office diabetic emergencies may occur when a diabetic patient becomes hyperglycemic (for example, from too little insulin) or hypoglycemic (from too much insulin or not enough nutritional intake). It is important to recognize the warning signs of an impending diabetic emergency. Early action may prevent the patient from slipping into diabetic shock or coma.

In an emergency situation it is really not important to differentiate diabetic shock from diabetic coma. The emergency care remains the same until the patient reaches the hospital.

The Hyperglycemic Patient

The hyperglycemic patient is at risk for *diabetic coma*. Hyperglycemia is due to a decrease in insulin supply or to overeating. The patient develops an elevated serum glucose level and begins to use fats for energy. This produces blood that is acidotic.

The symptoms of hyperglycemia usually come on slowly. Patients may feel dry and thirsty and experience pain and vomiting. They are not hungry, may breath heavily, and have a distinctive sickly sweet smell to their breath.

The Hypoglycemic Patient

The hypoglycemic patient is at risk for *diabetic shock*. Hypoglycemia is due to an increase in insulin supply or to insufficient nutritional intake.

Serum glucose level is decreased; with reduced sugar available to the brain the patient may fall unconscious and ultimately experience brain damage.

The symptoms of hypoglycemia come on suddenly; they include headache, dizziness, fainting, extreme hunger, salivation, and weakness.

Treatment

The treatment of both hypoglycemia and hyperglycemia is sugar. Orange juice or sublingual sugar tablets do not harm the hyperglycemic patient and certainly help the hypoglycemic patient.

One should arrange for immediate transportation to the nearest hospital for emergency care. One should not attempt to inject insulin because this may worsen the situation if the wrong amount of insulin is injected or if insulin is not required for treatment.

LID TRAUMA

Lids cover and protect the globe. If the nature and extent of injury are not determined and corrected soon after its occurrence, there could be long-term implications for the function and health of both the globe and the lids.

Pathophysiology

A comprehensive review of lid anatomy and function is too extensive to present here. However, mention of these subjects is made as they are encountered in the discussion of lid trauma.

Clinical Evaluation

In cases of lid trauma, attention must first be directed to the eye itself. Eyelid trauma is secondary in importance to injury of the globe. Monocular vision should be assessed and ocular health determined. If the globe is lacerated, the examination is over. Preparations are made to repair a lacerated cornea or sclera immediately. Only when the condition of the eye has been stabilized can full attention be directed to the eyelids.

One must first determine the extent of the injury. Small lacerations must be probed. Large lacerations of the lids must be laid open and explored for foreign bodies. After one is reasonably sure that the wounds are clean, they may receive a primary repair. Because of the great vascularity of the face and lids, an excellent surgical result is frequently obtained.

If the wound is "dirty," as in a construction nail injury or dog bite, it is frequently left unsutured and allowed to heal by primary intention. Suturing a possibly contaminated wound is believed to increase the chance of anaerobic infection. Patients experiencing any penetrating injury should be administered human tetanus immune globulin (human TIG) as prophylaxis.

A blow to the periocular area can result in rupture of facial blood vessels. There can be ecchymosis of one lid with occasional spreading of the subcutaneous blood to the other periocular area. This extravasation of blood into the loose areolar tissue of the lid can give a marked reddish blue discoloration to the skin. It usually resolves spontaneously over the course of a few weeks.

Palpation of the bony orbital rim should be undertaken in an effort to locate a rim fracture. Orbital skull films or computed tomography (CT) or magnetic resonance imaging (MRI) is invaluable here. Examination of the globe with particular attention to forced duction testing is helpful in identifying a *blow-out fracture*.

Traumatic ptosis may be observed. After trauma has occurred, the lid fissure may be narrowed and there may be apparent ptosis. If the lid does not elevate itself once the lid edema has resolved, then trauma must be presumed to be the cause of the ptosis. The cause may be damage of the levator palpebral superioris tendon or muscle or a partial or complete third cranial nerve paresis. The patient should be observed for at least 3 months before any surgical intervention or revision is contemplated.

Treatment

As mentioned above, an eyelid wound should be probed and explored for foreign bodies and the wound débrided. Human TIG should be administered. Appropriate topical and oral antibiotics should be administered, including coverage for anaerobes if a human or dog bite or other "dirty" wound is encountered. With dog or other animal bites, prophylaxis against rabies should also be considered. Bleeding should be controlled. When a periocular fracture is suspected, skull films should be taken. The lacrimal drainage apparatus should be inspected and its integrity tested if necessary.

Surgical repair of the eyelids should be done by separate layer closure. The lid may be thought of as being constructed in three layers: skin, orbicularis muscle, and tarsus/conjunctiva. By closing each of these individually with fine suture material, one is able to effect a more pleasing cosmetic and functional result.

If a large portion of the upper or lower eyelid is missing, it may still undergo a primary repair by a variety of techniques. With up to one quarter of the lid gone, the defect may be sutured in a layered closure, usually with little difficulty. If the lid defect is between one quarter and one half of the lid, then lateral cantholysis and the surgical technique of sliding skin flaps may be used. With greater than one half of the lid missing, full- or split-thickness skin grafts must be used, as well as possible mucous membrane grafts.

Injuries to the medial area of the lids may result in lacrimal drainage system damage. If the upper canaliculus is damaged and the lower is intact, nothing more need be done because the lower canaliculus alone can probably handle the tears. If the lacrimal drainage system is damaged and tearing is present, surgical treatment must be instituted.

The patient is administered local anesthetic, and an operating microscope is used. The punctum is dilated and punctal probes are inserted into the upper and lower canaliculi. Alternately, the canaliculus may be intubated with silicone tubing. Fine 9-0 nylon suture material can then be used to repair the canaliculus.

Treatment of thermal or chemical burns of the lids depends on the degree of injury. One should remove foreign material and débride burned tissue. With first- and second-degree burns, only wet dressings and antibiotic ointment need be used on the skin. With third-degree burns most of the epidermal elements of the skin have been destroyed. This can lead to scarring of the lid, along with retraction and ectropion. When this occurs then moist chambers and lubricants must be used in an effort to protect the globe. If this is not enough, then a lateral and/or a medial tarsorrhaphy must be done. Eventually, with severe burns and eyelid retraction, it is likely that the patient will have to undergo full-thickness skin grafts and full-scale lid reconstruction.

Early recognition and attention to eyelid injuries can have favorable consequences not only on the eventual function and cosmetic appearance of the lid but also on the eye itself.

ORBITAL TRAUMA

Blunt trauma to the orbital area can result in damage to the bony walls. This may occur even without significant injury to the globe. Treatment of orbital wall fractures is subordinate to treatment of the globe. However, early suspicion and prompt diagnosis of these injuries aid in management.

Pathophysiology

The globe and extraocular muscles are surrounded by fat and connective tissue. This in turn is surrounded by the bony walls of the orbit and anteriorly by the orbital septum. When a blunt force is exerted on the anterior orbital surface, the intraorbital contents are compressed. The pressure within the orbit increases and the orbital wall may fracture at its weakest point, often the orbital floor. When the floor fractures alone or in combination with other fractures, this is termed a *blow-out fracture*.

Clinical Evaluation

There usually is lid edema, ecchymosis, and erythema. If there is periocular hemorrhage, then proptosis may be present. If fracture of the medial wall has occurred, there may be subcutaneous emphysema with air under the skin causing crepitance on palpation. With severe fractures of the orbital floor, the globe may assume the sunken appearance of enophthalmos. There may be an inward and downward displacement of the globe with an increase in the supratarsal sulcus. Damage to the infraorbital nerve can lead to anesthesia of the lower lid and side of the nose (see Chapter 2). On palpation, defects of the orbital rim can sometimes be palpated despite considerable edema. With a blow-out fracture, diplopia is usually the result of prolapse of the inferior rectus and inferior oblique through the floor into the antrum of the maxillary sinus below. These muscles may become entrapped there, causing double vision on both downward and upward gaze.

Forced duction testing should be done whenever a blow-out fracture with diplopia occurs. This need not be done immediately after the injury, as ocular and other injuries take precedence; however, it may be attempted several days after the injury. The eye is anesthetized with topical anesthesia. A small toothed forceps is used to grasp the globe at the limbus and gently drag it up and down to see if it moves freely. If there is resistance, then entrapment of the extraocular muscles is likely and the diplopia is not simply a result of a muscle contusion, edema, hemorrhage, or nerve damage.

Radiologic examination should be undertaken with periocular trauma and suspected orbital fractures. Tomography and intraorbital radiopaque techniques have been used in the past, and plain films are still commonly ordered. However, for precise localization and delineation of the problem, CT and MRI scans are best. If the roof of the orbit is fractured, there may be damage to the superior rectus or levator palpebrae superioris muscles with limitation on up-gaze or ptosis, respectively. There can also be pulsating exophthalmos and cerebrospinal fluid leak, which usually emanates from the nose. With damage to the medial wall, the patient may have the aforementioned lid emphysema. Patients may also have epistaxis and a limitation of abduction because of damage to the medial rectus muscle. Damage to the lateral orbit can result in multiple zygomatic bone fractures, often called tripod fractures. These usually involve the inferior orbital rim and can frequently be palpated.

Treatment

Tripod and other fractures involving the orbital rim require surgical wiring of the rim. Inferior and medial wall fractures may safely be observed for 2 weeks or more without scarring and fibrosis of the extraocular muscles. Entrapped medial or inferior rectus or oblique muscles often reduce themselves spontaneously. If, however, significant enophthalmos or diplopia is present, then surgical repair of the bony walls of the orbit must be undertaken and the orbital contents released from entrapment. It is wise to obtain a neurosurgical consultation in the case of a superior wall fracture.

Above all, immediate attention to and monitoring of the ocular status take precedence over treatment of the orbit.

ORBITAL CELLULITIS

Orbital *cellulitis* requires immediate attention. Left untreated, it can result in damage to the optic nerve and blindness in a matter of a few hours. Prior to the emergence of antibiotics, blindness and even fatalities from septic meningitis and cavernous sinus thrombosis were common. However, with prompt intravenous antibiotic treatment, blindness from septic optic neuritis can usually be avoided.

Pathophysiology

Orbital cellulitis usually results from an infection in the paranasal sinuses, most often the ethmoids. Because the walls of these sinuses are thin and are adjacent to the orbit, infections can spread from them into the orbit. Also, the blood flows freely between the ethmoidal and ophthalmic veins. Infections may spread through the vascular channels that connect one compartment with another.

Clinical Evaluation

Patients usually have lid edema and erythema associated with pain. This may be accompanied by facial cellulitis and conjunctival injection. The globe may be displaced, often in the "down-and-out" position. An ominous sign is pupillary involvement with a dilated, poorly responsive pupil. Decreased vision is the most serious sign, as it indicates involvement of the optic nerve.

Work-up of the patient should be directed toward finding the source of the infection. The nose should be inspected for hyperemia, swelling, or pus. Examination of the lids and periocular area for evidence of abscess formation should be undertaken. Radiologic studies including CT and MRI are invaluable and are mandatory in an effort to determine the location of the infection. A consultation with an ear, nose, and throat specialist is wise to aid in evaluation of the paranasal sinuses.

Treatment

Orbital cellulitis is an urgent situation requiring hospitalization and broad-spectrum intravenous antibiotics. The patient should be frequently examined by physicians and nurses to evaluate the ocular status, most importantly vision, and vital signs. A white blood cell count, blood cultures, and if possible culture of the periocular abscess should be undertaken.

Any abscess that is found should undergo incision and drainage by a surgeon. Prompt diagnosis and treatment help avert blindness.

INTRAORBITAL AND INTRAOCULAR FOREIGN BODIES

A high index of suspicion must be maintained for the presence of an intraorbital foreign body. If the patient gives a history of working around machinery or metallic objects and suffers decreased vision or a red, painful eye, the possibility of a foreign body must be entertained. Whenever periorbital tissues are lacerated or punctured, the doctor must also consider the presence of a foreign body.

Pathophysiology

Although some foreign bodies may be composed of glass or vegetable matter, the majority of them are metallic. They are small but strike the lids or globe with sufficient force to penetrate the tissues. Their entrance wound, however, may be trivial and go unnoticed. Foreign bodies in the orbit may cause little harm, whereas those in the eye can sometimes be disastrous. Iron- and copper-containing foreign bodies can cause chronic degenerative processes in the eye and should usually be removed surgically.

Clinical Evaluation

A painful, red eye following a history of trauma should start the clinician on a search for a possible foreign body. The lids and globe should be inspected with proper illumination and magnification. Double eversion of the eyelid is helpful in inspecting the superior fornix. Fluorescein can be used to find discontinuities in the ocular surface. By performing gonioscopy, one can determine the presence of a foreign body in the angle. Transillumination of the iris and globe can sometimes localize a foreign body on the iris or ciliary body.

Indirect ophthalmoscopy with maximum pupillary dilation is by far the best technique for examining the posterior segment. If the patient later develops a cataract or vitreous hemorrhage that obscures the view, the chance for this important examination is lost.

A variety of radiologic techniques have been used in the past to find foreign bodies and assess their size and shape. This can be difficult, as the structure and contents of the orbit are complex and it is often extremely difficult to determine whether, for instance, the foreign body is within the wall of the globe or in the orbit. In addition to radiologic techniques, A- and B-scan ultrasonography and electronic foreign body locators have been used with some success. However, these techniques have in recent years been superseded by CT and MRI scans. These scans are readily available in most areas and provide superb imaging and localization.

Treatment

Most foreign bodies are sterile and so infection is not usually present. Intraorbital foreign bodies may usually be observed and do not cause further problems. Intraocular foreign bodies, on the other hand, may cause a great deal of injury. Immediately there is the mechanical injury, which can cause a cataract or other serious problem. Mechanical retinal damage may lead to a retinal detachment.

Practitioners must weigh the risks and benefits in deciding whether to remove a retained intraocular foreign body. Although materials such as glass may be retained in the eye without further problem, others such as copper or iron may lead to glaucoma or chronic retinal pigmentary degeneration. Copper and wood foreign bodies may lead to a sterile endophthalmitis that can mimic infection. These foreign bodies must usually be removed.

Foreign bodies in the anterior chamber may usually be removed with a forceps under the direct visualization of the operating microscope. Metallic foreign bodies in the posterior chamber may sometimes be removed by a magnetic device in the operating room. Rarely an intrascleral foreign body is removed with orbital surgery. The majority of posterior segment foreign bodies are removed with vitreous surgical techniques. The surgeon is usually better able to visualize and manipulate the foreign body with less trauma with these methods than with the foreign body magnet.

The management of intraorbital and intraocular foreign bodies is difficult. It requires a high index of suspicion, good clinical skills, and judgment in knowing when and when not to intervene.

Bibliography

Adams RD and Victor M: *Principles of neurology,* ed 4, New York, 1989, McGraw-Hill.

Annegens JF, and others: Seizures after head trauma: a population study, *Neurology* 30:683, 1980.

Bates B: *A guide to physical examination and history taking,* ed 4, Philadelphia, 1987, JB Lippincott.

Eagle KA and others: Evaluation of prognostic classification of patients with syncope, *Am J Med* 79:455, 1985.

Harrison TR and others: *Principles of internal medicine,* ed 8, New York, 1977, McGraw-Hill Book Company.

Hauser WA and others: Seizure recurrence after a first unprovoked seizure, *N Engl J Med* 307:522, 1982.

Hornblass A: *Oculoplastic, orbital and reconstructive surgery*, vols 1 & 2, Baltimore, 1990, Williams & Wilkins.

Lipsitz LA and others: Post-prandial reduction in blood pressure in the elderly, *N Engl J Med* 309:81, 1983.

Pavan-Langston D: *Manual of ocular diagnosis and therapy*, Boston, 1980, Little, Brown & Co.

Peyman G, Sanders D, and Goldberg M: *Principles and practice of ophthalmology*, vol 3, Philadelphia, 1980, WB Saunders Co.

Reeh MJ and others: *Ophthalmic anatomy*, 1981, American Academy of Ophthalmology.

Russ LS: The diagnostic assessment of single seizures, *Arch Neurol* 40:744, 1983.

Schatz IJ: Orthostatic hypotension, Arch Intern Med 144:773, 1984.

Spittel JA Jr: Vasoplastic disorders *Cardiovasc Clin* 13(2):78 1983.

Stephenson HE Jr: *Immediate care of the acutely ill and injured*, St. Louis, 1974, The CV Mosby Co.

Tasman W, Jaeger E: *Duane's clinical ophthalmology*, vols 2 & 5, Philadelphia, 1991, Lippincott Co.

Walton JN: Brain's diseases of the nervous system, ed 9. Oxford, 1985.

Weissler A and others: Vasodepressor syncope: factors influencing cardiac output, *Circulation* 15:875, 1957.

Wyngaarden JB and others: *Textbook of medicine*, ed 19; Philadelphia, 1993, WB Saunders Co.

PART III

The Eye in Systemic Disease

18

The Anterior Segment in Systemic Disease

RONALD E. SERFOSS
ANGELO M. ANACLERIO

KEY TERMS

Keratitic Precipitates	*Koeppe Nodules*	*Spondyloarthropathies*
Hypopyon	*Arlt's Triangle*	*Treponema Pallidium*
Posterior Synechiae	*Luetic Infection*	*Rapid Plasma Reagin (RPR)*
Circumcorneal Flush	*Gallium Scan*	*MHA-TP*
Busacca Nodules	*HLA-B27*	*Borrelia Burgdorferi*

---

*T*his chapter highlights the anterior segment ocular disorders and their possible relationship to systemic disease. Although the discovery of ocular pathology may sometimes be straightforward, it is important to uncover any relationship to an underlying systemic disorder. Understanding the ocular finding as it may relate to an underlying systemic disease allows the optometrist to provide clinically significant advice to a patient and meaningful consultation with the patient's primary care physician. Although the emphasis of this chapter is on systemic relationships, the optometrist's primary responsibility is to treat the ocular condition. This should be done in the context of preventing blindness and co-managing the patient with the primary care physician to treat the whole patient.

ANTERIOR UVEITIS

The discovery of anterior uveitis is usually uncomplicated. The patient may complain of unilateral or bilateral pain, photophobia, redness, tearing, and diminished vision. Examination of the anterior segment reveals the hallmark ocular signs of anterior chamber cells and flare, a slightly miotic pupil, perilimbal ciliary injections, and in some cases a lowered intraocular pressure. *Keratitic precipitates* (KPs) may be present on the corneal endothelium. The more severe and rare findings are mutton-fat KPs, cells in the vitreous, and *hypopyon*. Chronic anterior uveitis may be entirely asymptomatic with no external signs of ocular inflammation. The only indication of inflammation may be cells and flare in the anterior chamber. The severity of each of the signs and symptoms varies from the subtle to the obvious, and therefore a careful clinical examination with the slit lamp is of utmost importance. This is especially true for asymptomatic patients.

The treatment of a typical anterior uveitis consists of a protocol of appropriate mydriatic/cycloplegic agents to reduce pain, photophobia, and the possibility of *posterior synechiae* and topical corticosteroids to provide nonspecific inhibition of the ocular inflammatory reaction. This usually provides a successful therapeutic and clinical outcome. The intensity of the treatment is obviously related to the severity of the disease. Topical agents may not always be sufficient, and systemic and periocular medication may be necessary.

The successful ocular treatment of uveitis is one goal of patient care. Another, sometimes more important, goal is the discovery of the cause of the uveitis. Anterior uveitis should be viewed as a possible ocular sign of an underlying systemic disease. A causally related systemic illness is present in approximately 50% of all anterior uveitic conditions, most commonly a spondyloarthropathy.[14] However, patients do not present with a label that says "ankylosing spondylitis" or "sarcoid." It behooves the clinician to have a systematic approach to the evaluation of the whole patient in order to arrive at an ocular and perhaps a systemic diagnosis, and then with this information to counsel the patient and to communicate with other health care providers.

Definitions

In order for there to be a general understanding of the meaning of the various terms used to describe

anterior uveitis, this chapter adheres to the following definitions:

Acute uveitis: An episode of rapid symptomatic onset which lasts for 6 weeks or less. If it recurs after the initial attack, it is acute recurrent uveitis.

Anterior uveitis: Uveal inflammation of the iris (iritis), the ciliary body (cyclitis), or the iris and ciliary body (iridocyclitis). Although the terms "iritis" and "iridocyclitis" are sometimes interchanged, only iridocyclitis has cells in the vitreous.[2]

Band keratopathy: Calcium deposits seen in Bowman's layer of the cornea. The gray-white band, sometimes with clear holes in it, starts at the nasal or temporal limbus and curves gradually across the cornea (Fig. 18-1).

Busacca nodules: White or yellowish nodules found on the stroma of the iris but not at the pupillary margin. They are reliable indicators of a granulomatous anterior uveitis.

Chronic uveitis: The episode persists for months or years. Its onset is insidious and often asymptomatic. It may not clear completely between exacerbations.[1]

Endogenous uveitis: Uveitis caused by invasion of the uvea by microorganisms, antigens, or irritants from within the body. This chapter deals mostly with endogenous uveitis, such as

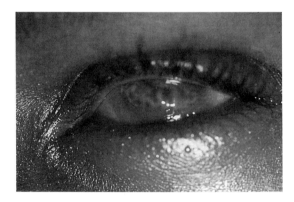

FIG. 18-1 Band keratopathy. Calcium deposits in Bowman's layer of the cornea in juvenile rheumatoid arthritis. *(Courtesy of Jane Stein.)*

that secondary to systemic disease.

Exogenous uveitis: Uveitis caused by external injury of the globe and by invasion of the uvea by microorganisms, antigens, or irritants from outside the body.

Granulomatous uveitis: Uveitis characterized by a tendency to form Koeppe or Busacca iris nodules and mutton-fat KPs.[2]

Koeppe nodules: Whitish yellow nodules found at the pupillary margin of the iris. They are indicators of granulomatous anterior uveitis.

Nongranulomatous uveitis: Uveitis characterized by fine KPs and no tendency to form iris nodules or mutton-fat KPs.[2]

Vitritis: Inflammatory cells in the vitreous.

The Uveitis Work-up

The Clinical Picture. A history of the patient's symptoms should be followed by an initial evaluation of the affected eye. The best visual acuity by pin hole or refraction should be recorded in standard notation. The use of the ETDRS chart (see Chapter 13) has been suggested by Nussenblatt and Patestine[3] because the chart includes lines for 20/100, 20/125, 20/160, and 20/200. Each line has five letters, and every three lines is a doubling of the visual angle. This allows a more precise

evaluation of any relative change in acuity to assess the effectiveness of therapy.

The evaluation of the pupillary response can be difficult. Irritation of the iris causes the release of prostaglandins and miosis.[12] Additionally, because several conditions that involve the anterior and posterior uvea may cause damage to the optic nerve and because some of the related systemic disorders may affect the optic nerve, assessment of the pupillary responses may be difficult owing to an underlying afferent pupillary defect. The presence of posterior synechiae inhibits the pupillary responses.

Conjunctival injection secondary to uveitis is different from conjunctivitis because it is more intense circumlimbally and not in the periphery (Fig. 18-2). The cornea may have KPs on the endothelial surface. These accumulations of lymphocytes and neutrophils are usually on the lower half of the cornea in a base-down triangular distribution called *Arlt's triangle* and are seen with slit-lamp examination in either direct or indirect retroillumination. Small KPs are called nongranulomatous (Fig. 18-3) and large are called mutton-fat or granulomatous KPs (Fig. 18-4). These usually disappear after resolution of the inflammation. It is of interest to note here that several conditions do not

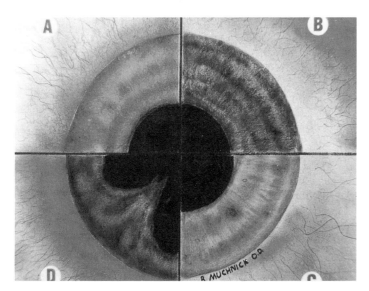

FIG. 18-2 Conjunctival injection patterns in conjunctivitis and uveitis. **A,** Acute uveitis demonstrates *circumcorneal flush*. **B,** Bacterial conjunctivitis demonstrates greatest injection in the fornices. **C,** Allergic and viral demonstrates an overall pink injection pattern. **D,** Chronic uveitis demonstrates either a white and quiet conjunctiva (as in juvenile rheumatoid arthritis) or the profuse circumcorneal injection seen here.

create the Arlt's triangle of KPs but have a more generalized distribution. This characteristic is seen in Fuch's heterochromic iridocyclitis and herpes simplex keratouveitis.[4]

Slit-lamp examination of the anterior chamber with a narrow and small aperture typically show flare and cells. The flare is caused by an increase in the aqueous protein content because of an alteration in the blood-aqueous barrier. When one views an oblique beam across the anterior chamber, the increased protein content produces the Tyndall effect, that is, the ability to see the beam

as it traverses the aqueous (Fig. 18-5). The amount of light scattering in the beam is directly related to the concentration of protein in the aqueous. The presence of flare alone is not an indication for treatment with steroids because it represents the results of damaged blood vessels and is not necessarily an indication of active inflammation.

The specks seen in the slit-lamp beam are not flare but are cells. These are primarily lymphocytes and neutrophils. The number of cells and the degree of flare are an indication of inflammatory activity in the iris and ciliary body and can be used to judge the severity of the episode and the effectiveness of therapy (Fig. 18-6). A plastic iritis occurs in a severe acute nongranulomatous uveitis with a high fibrin content in the aqueous (Fig. 18-7).

The severity of flare and cells is often graded on a scale of 0 to 4. The following scales (using a 1×1 mm beam) are widely accepted as adopted from Schlaegel[8] and Hogan and others.[9]

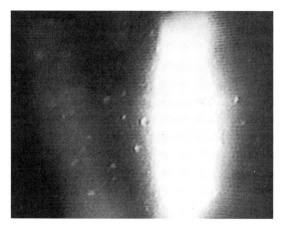

FIG. 18-3 Keratitic precipitates on the corneal endothelium. These small KPs are usually the result of nongranulomatous disease.

	Flare	*Cells*
0	Absence	No cells
1	Very slight	Occasional cell
2	Mild to moderate	16-25
3	Moderate	26-60
4	Severe	>60
4.5		Too many to count

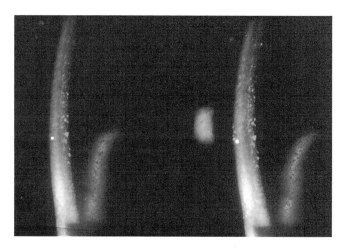

FIG. 18-4 Keratitic precipitates. These larger KPs are likely the result of granulomatous disease processes. *(Courtesy of Jane Stein.)*

In severe granulomatous episodes the inflammatory process invades the iris, and accumulations of inflammatory cells may be found within the iris itself. Busacca nodules, found almost exclusively in granulomatous iritis, are located on the iris away from the pupillary border, whereas Koeppe nodules are smaller and are located on the pupillary border. Because of their location at the pupillary border where synechiae form, the Koeppe nodules are very easy to miss if the clinician is not looking for them.

The release of mediators for clotting and fibrin deposition during inflammation relates to the formation of synechiae. Posterior synechiae usually form between the pupillary border and the anterior lens capsule, whereas peripheral anterior synechiae form between the anterior peripheral iris and the cornea. Peripheral anterior synechiae can obstruct the flow of aqueous through the trabecular meshwork, causing an increase in intraocular pressure, whereas the posterior synechiae can cause pupillary block glaucoma (Fig. 18-8).

Hypopyon (Fig. 18-9) is obviously a sign of a severe ocular condition. It can be infectious as in endophthalmitis and infectious keratouveitis from herpes simplex or herpes zoster, or it can be non-

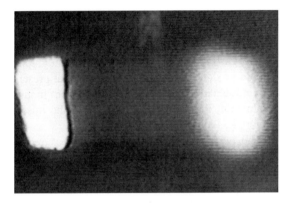

FIG. 18-5 Flare in the anterior chamber. The bright light reflex on the left is the cornea and on the right is the iris. The normally invisible aqueous is visible as a hazy band extending through the anterior chamber.

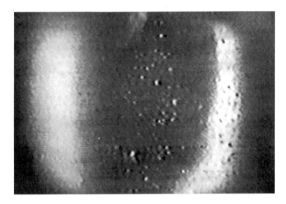

FIG. 18-7 Plastic iritis. This severe, acute, nongranulomatous uveitis has flare due to a high fibrin content in the aqueous with Grade 4 cells.

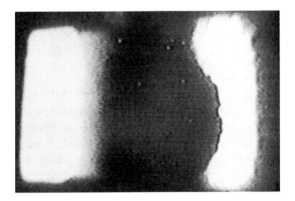

FIG. 18-6 Cells in the anterior chamber. Grade 2 cells represent a moderate uveitic reaction.

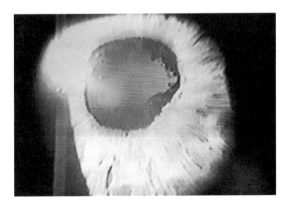

FIG. 18-8 Posterior synechiae. These adhesions between the iris and anterior lens surface can cause pupil distortion and block aqueous flow into the anterior chamber.

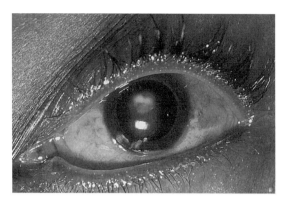

FIG. 18-9 Hypopyon. Note the subtle area of hypopyon at the most inferior aspect of the anterior chamber. *(Courtesy of Jane Stein.)*

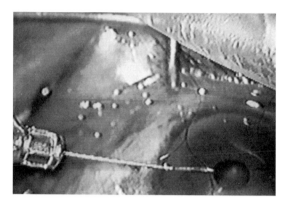

FIG. 18-10 Fine-needle aspiration (paracentesis) of a hypopyon for culturing and pathologic evaluation.

infectious, as in inflammatory uveitis (Behçet's syndrome) or in a masquerade syndrome. It can also be present in any uveitis that is acute and severe. In infectious hypopyon the anterior chamber cells are polymorphonuclear leukocytes and the infectious organisms. In inflammatory conditions polymorphonuclear neutrophils are found but no organisms. In masquerade syndromes such as retinoblastoma, tumor cells can be found. The diagnosis can be relatively direct; for example, the presence of a corneal pathology is strongly suggestive of an infectious cause. However, hypopyon in a quiet eye suggests a masquerade syndrome. Behçet's syndrome is often identified as a noninfectious condition associated with hypopyon. In many cases a more definitive diagnosis requires fine-needle aspiration to determine the cell type (Fig. 18-10).

It is possible to find cells and flare in the anterior chamber which are the result of a primarily posterior pole condition. Several conditions, notably choroiditis, pars planitis (an intermediate uveitis), Vogt-Koyanagi-Harada's syndrome, toxocariasis, toxoplasmosis, and masquerade syndromes, can have anterior chamber inflammation accompanying the primary posterior condition.[2] In any anterior chamber inflammation, it is important to evaluate the fundus with indirect ophthalmoscopy. Dilation may be difficult, and it may take intensive treatment before the inflammation has sub-

sided enough to conduct a good examination. When the fundus is not visible, ultrasonography should be done to rule out conditions that present as masquerade syndromes. Without the fundus evaluation, the primary condition may be misdiagnosed as an anterior inflammation.

The intraocular pressure must be measured at the outset and then monitored throughout the course of treatment. The pressure can be lower in the beginning of an anterior uveitis because the inflammation of the ciliary body may cause a reduction in the production of aqueous. However, inflammation in the area of the trabecular meshwork or the accumulation of inflammatory cells and debris in the trabecular meshwork may cause an increase in the intraocular pressure. Posterior synechiae or peripheral anterior synechiae may cause an increased intraocular pressure, as in pupillary block glaucoma. When doing tonometry, one should choose a method that does not use fluorescein or do applanation tonometry at the end of the examination. NaFl can penetrate an intact cornea and its introduction can stain the aqueous and prevent evaluation of the anterior chamber flare. Tonometry should be done routinely during the course of treatment because of the use of corticosteroids. Patients may respond to the steroids and, over the course of the disease treatment, develop an increase in intraocular pressure.

Once the presence of an anterior uveitis is documented and confirmed by physical examination, a careful history must be taken and then selected laboratory testing done as needed for differential diagnosis. Often, treatment of the ocular condition must be initiated before a thorough diagnostic evaluation can be completed. The skillful clinician does not presumptively label the anterior uveitis and the cause before gathering as many facts as possible. The history itself may provide evidence suggesting a particular systemic condition and may lead to a more directed series of laboratory tests. For example, an asymptomatic 8-year-old girl is discovered to have bilateral cells and flare during a routine eye examination. The history reveals the presence of joint stiffness and pain in the right knee. The laboratory studies should be narrowed to confirm the probable diagnosis of juvenile rheumatoid arthritis (JRA). An across-the-board series of tests would not be warranted because of the high likelihood of JRA. One should not be in a hurry to make a diagnosis; one should complete the clinical picture with a thorough physical examination and a detailed history and then choose laboratory tests selectively.

A frame of reference is helpful to describe the clinical picture. The following scheme of clinical classification of anterior uveitic conditions has been modified from Smith and Nozik[2] and Muchnick.[7]

1. Laterality: Uniocular or binocular
2. Onset: Insidious or sudden
3. Severity: Mild (nongranulomatous) or severe (granulomatous)
4. Pattern: Single episode or repeated episodes (nonrecurrent or recurrent)
5. Duration: Acute or chronic (The International Uveitis Study Group (IUSG) has recommended that any episode lasting longer than 3 months be considered long or chronic and under 3 months as being short.[10])
6. Anatomic: Location of the primary inflammation, that is, iritis, vitritis
7. Systemic signs and symptoms
8. Demographics: Age, race, gender, residence, etc.
9. Response to therapy

For example, a case might be described as "a sudden, uniocular, acute, granulomatous, recurrent iritis in a 30-year-old African-American woman with a chronic cough." Use of the above scheme when describing an episode of anterior uveitis ensures a consistent basis for an inclusive description of each case.

The Clinical History

Ocular history. One should take a detailed history of the current episode as early in the presentation as possible. This is when the patient more easily remembers details. If there have been previous episodes, the clinical scheme above is used for classification of the uveitis and then the history is directed toward systemic factors. If there have been no previous episodes, the history is directed toward a general medical background. As the clinician becomes more familiar with the various uveitic entities, the questioning becomes more directed.

Medical history. If the episode is nonrecurrent, have there been any preceding systemic symptoms? Consider antecedent flu or systemic infection, such as measles, mumps, varicella, or allergic reaction. These may be the causative agent in an endogenous uveitis.[6] General symptoms of cough, fever, malaise, joint pain, lower back pain, knee pain, pain on urination, skin lesions, and chancre formation may relate to specific systemic conditions. Each of these is explained in more detail in the section on characteristics of systemic diseases associated with anterior uveitis.

Although inheritance is rare, some families have specific human leukocyte antigens (HLA), and family members may develop related conditions such as ankylosing spondylitis, Reiter's syndrome, acute recurrent nongranulomatous iridocyclitis, and inflammatory bowel disease.[2] There may be exposure to tuberculosis if someone in the family has had infectious tuberculosis. Racial characteristics can be diagnostic. Caucasians have more of the HLA-B27 arthritides such as ankylosing spondylitis and Reiter's syndrome. African Americans have a higher incidence of sarcoid, and those of Asian background may have a higher prevalence or Vogt-Koyanagi-Harada and Behçet's syndromes. Persons of Mediterranean ancestry have more Behçet's syndrome.[2]

Demographic information can be of great assistance. It is unusual for a primary uveitis to appear as an acute single episode for the first time in old age.[11] However, the patient's age can be generally used to assist in narrowing a diagnosis. JRA, Kawasaki's syndrome (mucocutaneous lymph node syndrome), and retinoblastoma are often discovered in childhood, whereas ankylosing spondylitis and Reiter's syndrome are usually first seen in young adulthood and middle age. Sarcoidosis and toxoplasmosis may appear through middle age, and a uveitis of tuberculosis or of luetic origin can be found at any age.[11] The gender of a patient can be diagnostic. The uveitis of JRA is found more often in girls than boys and that of ankylosing spondylitis and Reiter's syndrome is more often found in males. HLA-B27–related conditions such as ankylosing spondylitis and Reiter's syndrome are found more often in Caucasians, whereas sarcoid is more common in African Americans.

Luetic infections, Reiter's syndrome, or acquired immunodeficiency syndrome (AIDS) can have anterior uveitis as one of the presenting signs of the disease. It is important that any history exploring the sexual and social background of a patient be done very carefully. It may be important for the primary physician to explore the areas of sexual activity and social behavior.

Diagnostic Laboratory Testing. Requesting laboratory tests that will be of clinical diagnostic significance requires each of the following: (1) an understanding that some uveitic conditions require no further testing; (2) a clear clinical picture of the current ocular presentation; (3) a complete ocular and systemic patient history; and (4) an understanding of the signs and the symptoms of the systemic conditions that can cause an anterior uveitis.

Traumatic uveitis, glaucomatocyclitic crisis (Posner-Schlossman syndrome), disease-related iritis such as herpes zoster or herpes simplex keratouveitis, Fuch's heterochromic iridocyclitis, or a first unilateral uncomplicated episode in an adult requires no further testing because it has a probable definitive clinical diagnosis. However, an anterior uveitis with any of the following characteristics should have more investigative testing for differential diagnosis: bilateral (or having occurred in either eye), recurring, asymptomatic in juveniles, granulomatous, or with systemic signs or symptoms.[13] The paradox is deciding whether to employ a broad battery of tests or to use tests selectively. The selective approach makes clinical and fiscal sense. Utilizing all the information gathered from the history and clinical examination with the descriptive classification mentioned previously should allow a selective approach to corroborate the clinical impression.

The following tests are often used in the differential diagnosis of systemic conditions related to anterior uveitis (see Chapter 3):

Hematologic testing. A complete blood cell count and a chemistry series such as SMA12 are usually obtained as part of the patient's general health status evaluation rather than as part of a specific diagnostic evaluation. These tests are indicated if there is evidence of a systemic process. They are also obtained prior to starting medications for baseline findings, especially if toxicity from a medication is a possibility.

Erythrocyte sedimentation rate (ESR). The ESR is a measure of the speed at which red blood cells settle in 1 hour in well-mixed venous blood. Although it is a nonspecific test, it is useful to indicate the presence or absence of systemic inflammatory activity in a patient. Inflammatory conditions cause an increase in electrostatic forces on the erythrocytes, causing them to aggregate, and the aggregates settle more rapidly.[57]

The ESR is increased in Reiter's syndrome, scleroderma, rheumatoid arthritis, temporal arteritis, ankylosing spondylitis, diabetes, and age.

Borrelia titers in lyme disease. The enzyme-linked immunosorbent assay (ELISA) and the immunofluorescent assay (IFA) are sensitive techniques utilizing enzyme and fluorochrome labeling to detect the presence of antigens and/or antibodies. These tests are used to detect IgG and IgM directed against the tick-borne *Borrelia burgdorferi* spirochete in Lyme disease. Many patients in stage 1 with erythema chronicum migrans have elevated IgM responses. Some patients are ill for several weeks before the levels of IgG and IgM become elevated.[56] However, after 5 or 6 weeks of the illness, most patients have elevated IgG and IgM titers, as do almost all patients with Lyme disease who manifest arthritis.[11]

Radiology. There are several conditions for which a radiologic consultation and roentgenograms should be obtained. A chest roentgenogram is helpful in patients suspected of having sarcoid, tuberculosis, and histoplasmosis. Patients with a profile that would typify sarcoidosis who have an anterior uveitis should obtain a chest roentgenogram. Chest roentgenographic changes are found in 80% of patients with ocular sarcoid.[11] Active pulmonary sarcoidosis usually shows bilateral hilar adenopathy preceding the peripheral pulmonary infiltration.[11] A chest roentgenogram can provide evidence of the presence of active or prior granulomatous disease in tuberculosis.

When any of the seronegative spondyloarthropathies, such as ankylosing spondylitis, Reiter's syndrome, and psoriatic arthritis, are suspected, a sacroiliac series radiologic study should be obtained. Marginal sclerosis, erosions, and fusion of the sacroiliac joints are often the earliest changes found.[58] The sacroiliac joints become blurred, sclerotic, and then undecipherable as the disease progresses over the years.[3] The radiographic evidence may precede any symptoms, such as lower back pain, and an iridocyclitis may even precede the clinical joint disease. Therefore, it may be prudent to obtain sacroiliac radiographs of all males with recurrent iridocyclitis regardless of systemic complaints.

When a child presents with iridocyclitis, a routine knee roentgenogram should be obtained because the pauciarticular presentation of JRA often develops the worst iridocyclitis.[11]

Skin testing. The most useful test antigen is the purified protein derivative (PPD) for tuberculosis. This test, however, is relatively nonspecific if used to screen all patients with uveitis and may have more false-positive than true-positive results. Today the disease is considered to be a very rare cause of uveitis.[14] Tuberculosis should be considered when a granulomatous uveitis does not respond to systemic corticosteroids. A chest roentgenogram should be obtained for evidence of active or prior granulomatous disease.

Some patients are often anergic to all skin tests, as in sarcoidosis, AIDS, Hodgkin's disease, rheumatoid diseases, and chronic lymphocytic leukemia. A positive reaction to skin testing requires an immune response and confirms the positive functioning of cell-mediated immunity. It should be noted that corticosteroids can cause a reduction or elimination of skin test reactions. Some authors conservatively recommend the testing of a patient's ability to react to a new antigen as confirmation of cell-mediated immunity.[11]

The Kveim antigen test has limited utility in testing for sarcoid because it is difficult to obtain and is not absolutely specific for sarcoid. Sarcoid patients are sometimes anergic to skin testing, indicating the lack of a delayed hypersensitivity reaction.[2,59]

Rheumatoid factor (RF). Rheumatoid arthritis and related conditions produce globulins that are known as rheumatoid factors, notably autoantibodies IgG and IgM.[57] They are produced by lymphocytes in the synovial joints and directed against the patient's own IgG and IgM. Once this occurs, it is followed by complement fixation and the subsequent destruction of leukocytes and platelets. This contributes to the rheumatoid nodule formation and other manifestations of rheumatoid arthritis.[11] Within 6 months after the onset of the disease, RF is produced by 50% of the affected population, and 75% produce it within 10 months. The RF is also found in patients with disseminated lupus erythematosus, chronic active hepatitis, and chronic infections. The test detects the presence of these autoantibodies in rheumatoid serum.[58]

The RF is not useful in testing for systemic disease in patients with uveitis. Rheumatoid arthritis is associated with scleritis, episcleritis, and keratitis sicca from secondary Sjögren's syndrome[60] and is not a consideration in the differential diagnosis of uveitis.[14] *RF is negative* in the pauciarticular JRA patients who develop uveitis and in the seronegative spondyloarthropathies—ankylosing spondylitis, Reiter's syndrome, psoriatic arthritis, and arthritis with ulcerative colitis.

Angiotensin-converting enzyme (ACE). ACE is produced by the endothelial cells of the lung and by the cells of the proximal renal tubules. The level of serum ACE is a function of total body granulomatous activity. Serum ACE levels are elevated in about 75% of patients with active untreated systemic sarcoidosis and about 40% of chronic untreated patients.[11]

ACE levels reflect activity of the disease and thus the effect of therapy because the use of systemic steroids reduces the level of ACE. The test is usually negative in patients with proven sarcoidosis that is in remission but rises with relapse.[61] Granulomatous uveitis in the presence of an elevated serum ACE level is suggestive of sarcoid uveitis.[24] However, the sensitivity of these tests for sarcoid that is confined to the eye is not established. The ACE and a *gallium scan* are considered to be the procedures of choice to establish the diagnosis of sarcoid.[62] Consideration must be given to the cost, lack of therapeutic implications, and limited and uncertain sensitivity before routinely obtaining serum ACE and gallium scans.

Antinuclear antibodies (ANA). ANA are produced in response to the nuclear DNA component of leukocytes perceived to be abnormal.[57] In conditions such as lupus erythematosus, Raynaud's disease, scleroderma, and Sjögren's syndrome, the ANA have a pathogenic role because the antigen-antibody complexes are directed against their own tissue, causing damage.[2] The ANA are detected by the IFA method, which is a nonspecific assay for several different ANA. The results are reported by titer and by the pattern of fluorescence in the nuclei. The test is considered positive if the titer is greater than 1:10.[2]

Greater than 95% of the patients with systemic lupus erythematosus (SLE) have a positive titer for ANA.[65] If the ANA screen is negative for SLE, the chance of the disease being present is low.[57] However, even though SLE is a potential cause of uveitis,[63] testing all patients with uveitis for ANA is not good clinical practice. Rosenbaum and Wernick[14] have calculated that in this instance there will be 100 false-positive tests for each positive

test that actually is SLE. They conclude that the ANA test should be used only if a patient with uveitis has other signs and symptoms of SLE, such as rash, arthritis, and nephritis.

The ANA is reported to be positive in up to 80% of the JRA patients who develop chronic bilateral nongranulomatous iridocyclitis.[64] JRA children with a negative test rarely develop uveitis. A subset of ANA-negative HLA-B27–positive boys develop the spondylarthropathic type of acute unilateral, alternating, recurrent iridocyclitis.[26]

Human leukocyte antigen (HLA). The DNA located on chromosome 6 comprises the major histocompatibility complex, which contains the HLA. The HLA genes define antigenic differences among humans. Class I HLA molecules have three different loci labeled A, B, and C that are found on the surface of almost every cell.[11] The Class I molecules, found on virtually every cell, provide a recognition target for lymphocytes responsible for cell-mediated immunity. Class II HLA molecules include the D and DR loci and are restricted to lymphocytes, macrophages, and immunocompetent cells, essential for normal antigen presentation and interaction. Five hundred and thirty diseases have been linked to certain specific HLA antigens. No one antigen is specific for a particular disease; rather, the presence of an HLA antigen is suggestive of an associated disease.[11] In uveitis, HLA-B27 is one of the most important antigens.

Several HLA locations are important in uveitis:

HLA-B27. Six to eight percent of Caucasian persons are positive. About 70% of patients with unilateral, acute onset anterior uveitis are positive.[4] An HLA-B27–positive Caucasian person is 69% more likely to develop ankylosing spondylitis than a person who is not B-27 positive.[2]

HLA-B27 patients with acute anterior uveitis are more likely to be younger at the age of onset, to be male, to show frequent unilateral alternating eye involvement, to have severe symptoms with each episode, to have a higher incidence of ocular complications, to lack mutton-fat KPs, and to have an associated seronegative spondyloarthropathy.[11] HLA is positive in 75% of patients with Reiter's syndrome, 75% of patients with psoriatic spondylitis, and 40% to 45% of patients with acute iridocyclitis without rheumatoid involvement.[2]

HLA-DR5. This antigen is associated with the early-onset pauciarticular form of JRA characterized by patients who are more likely to develop chronic bilateral uveitis associated with a band keratopathy. This form of JRA is more often found in female patients who have a positive ANA titer. Uveitis occurs in 53% of the patients with HLA-DR5–related early-onset JRA, found mostly in females.[11]

HLA-B27 is associated with the later-onset form of pauciarticular JRA and acute recurrent inflammation.[21] Uveitis occurs in 25% of patients with the HLA-B27 late-onset form, usually found in males.[11]

HLA-B5. This antigen is often associated with Behçet's disease, which is found most often in people of the Mediterranean and Far East, especially Japan. HLA-B5 is positive in 30% of the Japanese control population and 70% of the Japanese population with diagnosed Behçet's disease.[2] The most common ocular manifestation of the disease is recurrent iridocyclitis with transient hypopyon.[2]

HLA-BW22. This antigen is often associated with Vogt-Koyanagi-Harada disease. HLA-BW22 is positive in 13% of the Japanese control population and 45% of the population with Vogt-Koyanagi-Harada disease.[2]

HLA tests are not ordered on a routine basis. Complete typing is never ordered as part of an evaluation for uveitis.

SYSTEMIC DISORDERS ASSOCIATED WITH ANTERIOR UVEITIS

A number of clinically significant disorders are associated with anterior uveitis. The ocular findings are listed in Table 18-1.

Juvenile Rheumatoid Arthritis

JRA should be suspected in any child with iridocyclitis. JRA is an arthritic inflammation of unknown origin that usually occurs in children before the age of 16 (see Chapter 7).[17] It is an important cause of crippling in children. The ocular complications are significant because of the possi-

bility of serious visual disability if the condition goes undiscovered or does not respond to treatment. Approximately 20% of the patients with JRA develop anterior uveitis.[21]

JRA has three distinct presentations:

Still's Disease. This is the systemic form, highlighted by an onset in early childhood, a high spiking fever, and an erythematous rash and often accompanied by lymphadenopathy or hepatosplenomegaly. The joint disease is often late appearing and may be overshadowed by the febrile illness, erythematous rash, pleuropericarditis, splenomegaly, and generalized lymphadenopathy.[66] There is rare ocular involvement. The ANA and RF are usually negative.

Polyarticular Juvenile Rheumatoid Arthritis. This condition is highlighted by involvement at the outset of five or more joints. This group is the most common and has an onset between the ages of 9 and 15 years. The disease may be variable and causes deformity in the knees and wrists and often symmetrically affects the small joints of the hand. There are two subgroups: (a) RF positive and associated with HLA-DR4, occurring more often in girls than boys. Ocular involvement is rare.[18] (b) RF negative and HLA-B27 positive. Sacroilitis and spondylitis are common. Ocular involvement is an acute recurrent iridocyclitis in 25% of the affected patients.[19]

Pauciarticular or Oligoarticular Juvenile Rheumatoid Arthritis. This condition is highlighted by the involvement of four or fewer joints. Although the systemic features may be mild, this group is most commonly associated with iridocyclitis, often estimated at 25%. There are two subgroups.

The early-onset group, 8 years or younger, is (1) usually RF negative and ANA positive (80%)[21]; (2) HLA-DR5 and HLA-DR8 associated[19]; (3) occurs more often in girls than boys.[19] The arthritis is usually lower extremity and involves the knee. The condition exacerbates and remits, rarely leaving a deformity. *A chronic bilateral nongranulomatous iridocyclitis occurs most frequently in this group.* In fact, Glass and others[20] found that 53% of the patients that are ANA and HLA-DR5 positive have a chance of developing an anterior uveitis. Of the patients with JRA

TABLE 18-1 *Ocular Findings*

Systemic Disease Causing Uveitis	Class	Primary System Affected	Path	ET	Age
Ankylosing spondylitis	Collagen Vascular	Lower vertebrae	Bony fusion	Possible genetic infection association	Young adult
Reiter's syndrome	Collagen Vascular	Bone joints	Arthritis	Possible genetic infection association	Young adult
Juvenile rheumatoid arthritis	Collagen Vascular	Joints (knee)	Arthritis	Unknown auto-immune	<16 yr
Crohn's disease	Inflammatory	GI	Ulcers and granulomas	Possible genetic association	20-40 yr
Sarcoidosis	Inflammatory	Pulmonary	Granulomas	Immune response to airborne antigen	20-50
Lyme disease	Infectious	Multi Derm Cardiac Arthritis	Inflammatory, infection, and immune	*Borrelia burgdorferi* (spirocheta)	Any age
Syphilis	Infectious	Multi Derm Neuro	Inflammatory and infection	*Treponema pallidum* (spirochete)	Any age
Tuberculosis	Infectious	Pulmonary	Bacterial infection	Tubercle bacilli	Any age
Herpetic disease	Infectious	Multi (derm)	Viral infection	DNA virus	Any age

Sex	Race	Key Symptoms	Key Lab Tests	Systemic Treatment	Possible Sequellae
M > F	W > B	Lower back pain	HLA-B27 X-ray back RF (−) ESR (+)	Steroids NSAID Physical therapy Self limits in 2 years or more	Limited motility of back and legs
M > F	W > B	Arthritis Urethritis Conjunctivitis	HLA-B27 ESR (+) ANA (−) RF (−) Urethral swab	Steroids NSAID Self limiting	Advanced arthritis: corneal "melt-down"
M < F	W = B	Knee pain	X-ray knee RF (−) ANA (+)	Steroids NSAID Immunosuppres-sants	Phthisis bulbi: knee joint immo-bility
M = F	W = B	Gut pain	GI workup Endoscopy Rectal biopsy Barium enema HLA-B27	Steroids Diet Surgery Stress reduction	Severe GI compli-cations
M < F	W < B	Cough	Biopsy lung. Biopsy conj. nod-ule ACE-elevated Galium scan of lung (chest x-ray)	Steroid therapy	5% mortality (death rate); respi-ratory distress
M = F	W = B	Rash Fever Arthritis	ELISA (+) for antispirochetal Antibody titer	Antibiotics: tetra-cycline or doxycy-cline or amoxicillin	Advanced cardiop-athy and neuropa-thy
M = F	W = B	Rash Fever Chancre	FTA-ABS or MHA-TP VDRL or RPR	Systemic antibod-ies	Tertiary stage with neuropathy
M = F	W = B	Cough	PPD Mantoux X-ray chest Sputum culture	INH-isoniazid	Lung excavations and cavaties
M = F	W = B	Skin vesicles	Skin biopsy Skin culture Consider HIV test-ing	Oral acyclovir	Postherpetic neu-ralgia: cataract

GI = gastrointestinal; RF = rheumatoid factor; ESR = erythrocyte sedimentation rate; ANA = antinuclear antibody; ACE = angiotensin converting enzyme; ELISA = enzyme-linked immunosorbent assay; FTA-ABS = fluorescent treponemal absorbed; MHA-TP = microhemagglutination-*Treponema pallidum;* VDRL = Venereal Disease Research Laboratory; RPR = rapid plasmin reagin; PPD = pu-rified protein derivation; HIV = human immunodeficiency virus; NSAID = nonsteroidal anti-inflammatory drug; INH = isoniazid.

who develop iritis, 80% have a positive ANA and those who do not develop iritis are ANA negative.[2] Seventy-five percent of all patients with JRA and uveitis are girls.[1]

The first indication of any change may be the reduced vision that brings the child in for examination. Patients may have no overt systemic signs and symptoms other than reduced visual acuity or a "white" pupil (cataract). The eyes may appear quiet with no pain, photophobia, or redness. For this reason the iridocyclitis may go unnoticed until the vision is reduced. On examination, patients can have essentially a nongranulomatous iridocyclitis, early band keratopathy, anterior or posterior synechiae, secondary cataract, and secondary glaucoma. The condition is usually bilateral and chronic, and untreated it can progress to severe visual loss (Fig. 18-11).

The late-onset group with a mean onset age of 12 years is (1) ANA negative[26]; (2) HLA-B27 positive in 90% of the children[19]; (3) male by an incidence of 5:1.[19] The important differentiation in this group is that *the iridocyclitis is an acute, recurring, unilateral, alternating inflammation* similar to that occurring in the adult HLA-B27– related conditions, rather than a chronic bilateral iridocyclitis as seen in early-onset JRA.[26] The ar-

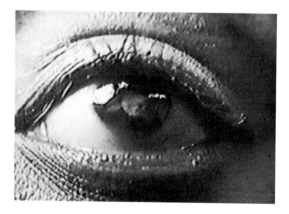

FIG. 18-11 Iridocyclitis in a patient with juvenile rheumatoid arthritis revealing a "white" pupil due to a cataract and a distorted pupil secondary to posterior synechiae.

thritis is the large-joint, lower-extremity type, often sacroilitis progressing to ankylosing spondylitis. Approximately 25% of the patients develop the acute recurrent iritis.[26]

Because of the risk of uveitis in JRA, Kanski[17] has recommended the following schedule of ocular examinations:

Systemic onset	Annual examination
Polyarticular onset	Every 6 months
Pauciarticular onset	Every 3 months
Positive ANA	Every 3 months

The recommendation is to follow the patient for 7 years from the onset of JRA.

Several key differential diagnoses must be made in uveitis occurring in children. Toxocariasis, pars planitis, and toxoplasmosis can cause an anterior uveitis that accompanies the primarily posterior condition. Sarcoid iridocyclitis patients can mimic JRA, although it is rare in children and is usually granulomatous. Sarcoid iridocyclitis patients develop arthritis and skin lesions. JRA patients who develop uveitis most likely have a positive ANA and lack systemic symptoms. The evaluation should include chest and knee radiographs to rule out sarcoid and systemic rheumatoid arthritis. Comanagement with a pediatrician and rheumatologist is warranted.

Sarcoidosis

Sarcoidosis is a granulomatous disease of unknown origin (see Chapter 11). The clinical picture can vary from the radiographic finding of hilar adenopathy with erythema nodosum or sarcoid nodules of the skin (Fig. 18-12) to debilitating febrile systemic illness with severe cough and dyspnea. Fatigue is frequently the only symptom of low-grade systemic involvement.[42] The disease occurs more frequently in young adults, women more than men, and is more common and severe in African Americans. The incidence of ocular involvement in patients with diagnosed systemic sarcoid is estimated to be 17%.[67] An anterior uveitis is present in 66% of the cases with ocular involvement. In some cases the ocular involvement is the only presentation. In a study of patients with iridocyclitis, Rothova and others[22] found a causally related systemic condition in 26% of patients, and sarcoid was the systemic disease in 7% of all patients with iridocyclitis.

Although sarcoid may affect any part of the eye, anterior uveitis is the most common finding.[23] *In younger patients with acute sarcoid, the uveitis is often unilateral and nongranulomatous,* whereas the systemic features are erythema nodosum and bilateral hilar adenopathy. These two features are called Lofgren's syndrome when associated with acute iritis. *In older patients, 35 to 50 years, the uveitis tends to be chronic, granulomatous, and bilateral.* Busacca or Koeppe nodules can be associated with the granulomatous presentation. The systemic features are pulmonary fibrosis, lupus pernio, and bone cysts.[1]

Other anterior segment ocular involvement in sarcoid includes keratitis sicca from invasion of the lacrimal gland, conjunctival granulomas, yellow fleshy nodules, and sarcoid plaques (lupus pernio), or lid granulomas (Fig. 18-13). A band keratopathy can occur in patients who also have hypercalcemia. If sarcoid occurs in children under 4 years, it presents with uveitis, arthritis, and a papillomacular skin rash with no pulmonary component.[24] This can be confused with the iridocyclitis of JRA. In these cases tests for ANA, RF, ACE, and serum lysozyme may be needed.

The diagnosis of sarcoid is made with compatible clinical and radiologic pictures and on granuloma tissue biopsy. Of patients with ocular sarcoid 90% have abnormal chest radiographs.[1] Lung biopsy by tracheobronchial fiberoptic technique is about 90% accurate in diagnosing sarcoid.[1] Biopsy of the lacrimal gland when enlarged and of a conjunctival granuloma can give histologic evidence supporting the diagnosis of sarcoidosis. The ACE is usually elevated in patients with active sarcoid. Other conditions that have an associated uveitis can also have elevated ACE, including tuberculosis, histoplasmosis, and ankylosing spondylitis. *However, a granulomatous uveitis in the presence of an elevated ACE is suggestive of sarcoid uveitis.* Elevated serum lysozyme and elevated serum ACE together have a very high predictive value for sarcoid.[24]

In addition, tears of patients with sarcoid-induced keratitis sicca have a normal or increased level of lysozyme, compared with low levels in keratitis sicca. A gallium citrate–enhanced computed tomography scan of the head, neck, and chest can be used to locate sites of inflammation. Even though the gallium scan may be positive despite a normal chest radiograph, the combination of elevated serum ACE and a positive gallium scan is highly sensitive and specific for the diagnosis

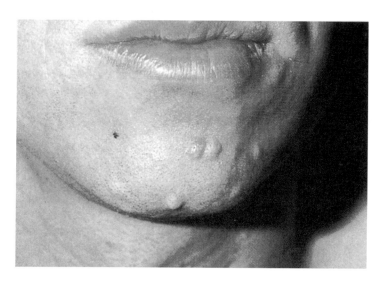

FIG. 18-12 Sarcoid nodules of the skin. *(From Lawrence CM and Cox NH: Physical signs in dermatology: color atlas and text, London, 1993, Wolfe Medical Publishers, Ltd.)*

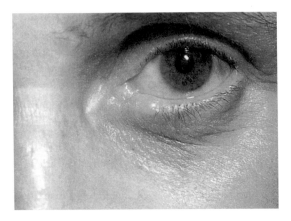

FIG. 18-13 Sarcoidosis with lid granulomas. Biopsy of these lid lesions can confirm the presence of sarcoid. *(From Lawrence CM and Cox NH: Physical signs in dermatology: color atlas and text, London, 1993, Wolfe Medical Publishers, Ltd.)*

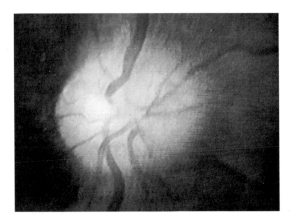

FIG. 18-14 Papilledema in a case of sarcoidosis.

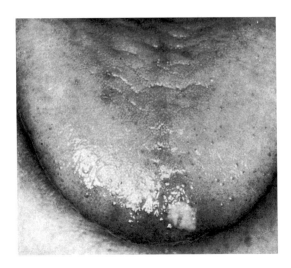

FIG. 18-15 Behçet's syndrome. Several painful ulcers on the tongue. These may be recurrent for years. *(From Cawson RA and others: Pathology: The mechanisms of disease, St. Louis, 1989, Mosby–Year Book.)*

of sarcoidsis.[61] Additionally, patients with active sarcoid often exhibit anergy. Skin testing is the most practical way of evaluating cellular immunity. A candida or trichophyton challenge in active sarcoid shows anergy.

Sarcoid involvement of the posterior pole has significant consequences which are discussed in Chapter 19 (Fig. 18-14).

Behçet's Syndrome

Behçet's disease is an idiopathic multisystem disease associated with HLA-B5[25] and characterized by recurrent attacks of uveitis, hypopyon, aphthous ulcers of the mouth (Fig. 18-15) and genitalia, and skin lesions including erythema nodosum, pustules, and ulceration. (Note: The oral ulcers are painful, which differentiates them from those of Reiter's syndrome.) The disease usually affects young men of Mediterranean countries and the Far East, especially Japan. Onset is between the ages of 20 and 40, with acute recurrent episodes becoming chronic after several attacks of iridocyclitis, hypopyon, and mucous membrane ulceration. Virtually all patients have the oral ulceration, and for many it is the first sign. Genital ulceration occurs in about 90% of patients, being more troublesome in men. The recurrent bilateral nongranulomatous

ocular inflammation is present in 70% of patients with Behçet's disease.[1] Other associated problems are thrombophlebitis, an asymmetric nondeforming arthritis typically of the large joints, and central nervous system involvement, including brainstem syndrome and meningoencephalitis with confusional states.

Although no specific laboratory tests or procedures aid in the diagnosis of Behçet's syndrome, there is some relationship with the HLA-B5 antigen.[11] The diagnosis is made by the presence of the major signs and associated problems listed above. Behçet's syndrome is a classic ocular inflammation associated with hypopyon.[2] Many of the patients with Behçet's syndrome exhibit a phenomenon in which a tuberculin-like skin reaction occurs after simple breaking of the skin with a hypodermic needle, as in blood drawing.[1]

The two basic ocular processes in Behçet syndrome are a panuveitis and perivasculitis. Patients often seek eye care because of the recurrent nongranulomatous anterior uveitis, with or without hypopyon. The vasculitis, which is bilateral, involves the retinal arteries and veins, causing retinal edema, necrosis, and atrophy. Secondary neovascularization may cause retinal detachment.[2] Posterior segment involvement can have a poor long-term visual prognosis if not discovered early in the disease process.

Corticosteroids often do not control the inflammation. The use of the immunosuppressive drug chlorambucil has been reported to be beneficial, but it may have serious oncogenic and cytotoxic systemic side effects.[5] A further discussion of posterior segment involvement is found in Chapter 19.

Vogt-Koyanagi-Harada (VKH) Syndrome

This syndrome is an idiopathic disorder that typically affects pigmented individuals and occurs more frequently in people of Asian, Latin American, and Native American descent. The following are the groups of signs generally considered to establish the diagnosis of VKH syndrome[1]:

1. Cutaneous signs: Alopecia, poliosis, and vitiligo
2. Neurologic signs: Headache; central nervous system involvement manifested by convulsions, cranial nerve palsies, and paresis; dysacusis; and in the acute phase cerebrospinal fluid lymphocytosis
3. Anterior uveitis: A bilateral *granulomatous* uveitis that may affect one eye first
4. Posterior uveitis: This may manifest as bilateral panuveitis with vitritis, multifocal choroiditis, disc edema, retinal edema, hemorrhages, and exudative retinal detachment

The prodromal stage occurs a few days before the ocular presentation and is characterized by headache, orbital pain, vitiligo, slight fever, and occasional photophobia and lacrimation. The ocular stage has the bilateral granulomatous anterior uveitis with sudden blurring of vision, dysacusis, and posterior uveitis. In the convalescent stage, the uveitis subsides but there is continuous dysacusis, poliosis, vitiligo, and alopecia. The fundus has depigmented spots and scarring.[35]

The uveitis is treated aggressively with topical, periocular, and systemic corticosteroids. Early treatment may shorten the duration and prevent progression of the disease. Untreated, the prognosis is poor because recurrence is high and may last for months or years.

Seronegative Spondyloarthropathies

The seronegative spondyloarthropathies are a group of diseases of unknown cause that have a high incidence of inflammatory eye disease. This group includes ankylosing spondylitis, Reiter's syndrome, arthritis associated with inflammatory bowel disease, and psoriatic arthritis (see Chapter 7). These conditions are distinguished from rheumatoid arthritis because they are seronegative for RF. The most common ocular presentation of the seronegative (RF-negative) spondyloarthropathies is a nongranulomatous, acute, recurrent iridocyclitis occurring in the young adult aged 16 to 40.[5] Although both eyes may be affected during the course of the disease, generally one eye at a time is affected.[4] An episode may have nongranulomatous KPs, considerable cells and flare in the anterior chamber such that a "plastic iritis" may be present, and possible posterior synechiae.

The seronegative *spondyloarthropathies* are closely associated with the histocompatability antigen *HLA-B27* and are characterized systemically by spondylitis, sacroilitis, and peripheral joint disease. Nussenblatt and Palestine[3] reported a study identifying the following classification of types of anterior uveitis: (a) idiopathic anterior uveitis, that is, not associated with any defined clinical syndrome, occurring in 52% of the study population; (b) HLA-B27 with ankylosing spondylitis, occurring in 8% of the study population; (c) HLA-B27 with Reiter's syndrome, occurring in 3% of the study population; (d) *36% of the population having an anterior uveitis associated with the HLA-B27 antigen and no systemic signs or symptoms.* The significant factor is that many uveitis patients have no systemic association, and a large percentage of uveitis patients with the HLA-B27 association at present have no associated systemic condition.

Ankylosing Spondylitis. This is a chronic inflammatory disease of the spinal articulations causing bony fusion (ankylosis) of the spinal articular and ligamentous structures. Ankylosing spondylitis is found in 0.1% to 0.2% of the population. Although this disease was once considered to be predominate among young adult males aged 20 to 40, recent studies suggest that it may be more evenly distributed among men and women. It may be milder in women because they are less likely to have progressive spinal disease.[15,27] The most characteristic sign of ankylosing spondylitis is low back pain or tenderness over the sacroiliac joints which improves with activity (morning stiffness). In the later stages there is restriction of motion from the ankylosis. Radiographic evidence of sacroilitis is diagnostic of the disease.

These patients are seronegative and may have an elevated ESR. The HLA-B27 antigen is associated with 90% of Caucasian and 50% of African-American patients diagnosed with ankylosing spondylitis.[5] Twenty-five percent of the patients with ankylosing spondylitis have at least one attack of iridocyclitis during the course of the disease.[19] The incidence of HLA-B27 in patients with acute iridocyclitis is about 45%.[1] The incidence of HLA-B27 in patients with ankylosing spondylitis and acute iridocyclitis is about 95%.[1] It is recommended that male patients with acute recurrent iridocyclitis have sacroiliac joint radiographs even when there are no symptoms of lower back pain, because in 50% of patients the radiographs may be positive before the patient is symptomatic.[2] The combination of acute iridocyclitis, lower back pain, positive radiographs, and HLA-B27 confirms the diagnosis of ankylosing spondylitis. A

rheumatology consultation is recommended every 2 years for HLA-B27–positive patients with iridocyclitis but no radiographic evidence of ankylosing spondylitis.

The acute iridocyclitis found in ankylosing spondylitis is of rapid onset with photophobia, pain, and blurry vision with nongranulomatous KPs and heavy flare and cells. There can be a fibrinous "plastic" iritis and hypopyon if the cellular presence is severe (Fig. 18-16). It is usually unilateral but may be alternating in recurrence. The uveitis has no correlation with the severity of the spondylitis. The episodes of uveitis in ankylosing spondylitis are less likely to cause a progressive visual impairment than those in Reiter's syndrome.[69]

Ankylosing spondylitis should be part of the differential diagnostic scheme for any unilateral, alternating, recurrent iridocyclitis in a young male. Sarcoid iridocyclitis is more granulomatous and often has mutton-fat KPs and Koeppe or Busacca iris nodules. The ACE and serum lysozyme are elevated in sarcoid. Do not overtest for HLA-B27 because it is not specific for ankylosing spondylitis.

These patients should be co-managed with a rheumatologist.

Reiter's Syndrome. Reiter's syndrome is an un-

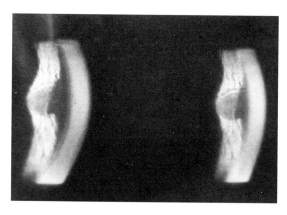

FIG. 18-16 Acute plasmoid iridocyclitis in a patient with ankylosing spondylitis. Note the high fibrin content on the aqueous around the pupil. *(Courtesy of Jane Stein.)*

common clinical condition that affects mainly men and is characterized by urethritis (cervicitis in women), followed by seronegative arthritis, conjunctivitis, and/or iridocyclitis. Although the conjunctivitis is seen more frequently, the recurrent, acute, nongranulomatous uveitis is the more serious ocular complication. The anterior uveitis occurs in about 20% of affected patients. Approximately 90% of patients have the HLA-B27 antigen.[28] The diagnosis can be made without the urethral and ocular findings if the arthritis is present with the other characteristics such as keratoderma blennorrhagicum, circinate balanitis, onycholysis, and *painless* ulcers of the mouth (as differentiated from the painful aphthous ulcers of Behçet's syndrome). The cause is probably linked to the HLA-B27 antigen and a genitourinary or gastrointestinal infection.

The first ocular sign can be a mucopurulent conjunctivitis that follows the urethritis. The urethritis usually precedes the arthritis by days or weeks and can be unresponsive to antibiotic treatment. Urethral cultures are used to determine if the urethritis is treatable, as it would be with an infectious cause such as gonococcal infection. The urethritis may even be overlooked by the patient because the discharge may be noticeable only in the morning before urination.[29] Because the conjunctivitis may appear early in the disease course and the patient is seen later, the history should determine if there has been a red eye and if there have been any episodes of arthritis, urethritis, or cervicitis.

The arthritis is acute in onset, migratory, asymmetric, and perhaps pauciarticular or polyarticular, involving the large joints and the weight-bearing joints of the lower extremities. There are three musculoskeletal manifestations: (1) A diffuse swelling of the fingers or toes, causing the descriptive term "sausage digits." This also occurs in psoriatic arthritis. (2) Swelling at the region of the Achilles tendon insertion or tenderness at the insertion of the plantar fascia causing heel pain. (3) Low back pain as seen in ankylosing spondylitis. Sacroiliac radiographic changes are present in 32% of patients.[30]

The iridocyclitis may follow the conjunctivitis or may be the only ocular manifestation. It is usually acute in onset and severe in presentation. Heavy cells (3+) and flare and tendency to form posterior synechiae are present. There may be spillover cells in the anterior vitreous. The cornea may have subepithelial infiltrates that affect the central cornea first and then the periphery, clearing in several weeks. Although the urethritis, ocular signs, skin lesions, and arthritis usually occur simultaneously in the initial episode, the recurrence is less acute and not necessarily in combination. The recurrences may be frequent enough to require long-term management.[16]

In the differential diagnostic scheme of Reiter's syndrome, the presence of keratoderma blennorrhagicum (scaling plaquelike skin lesions on the palms of the hands and the soles of the feet) and circinate balanitis (painless erythematous erosion of the glans penis) are characteristic. Tests of the uretheral discharge help to determine if a treatable infection is present. The ESR and white blood cell count can be elevated. The ocular presentation of an iridocyclitis of rapid onset with conjunctival injection, heavy cells, and flare with a tendency to form posterior synechiae can be characteristic of Reiter's syndrome.

Rheumatology and urology consultations are warranted in the care of any patients suspected of Reiter's syndrome.

Psoriatic Arthritis. This is a syndrome characterized by the presence of psoriasis and an associated inflammatory arthritis. The arthritic condition is seronegative, anodular, and asymmetric, involving the interphalangeal joints of the hands and feet and giving rise to sausage-shaped deformities of the fingers. The psoriasis, usually present before the arthritis, is characterized by erythematous macular lesions with silvery scales. It occurs on extensor surfaces, elbows, scalp, and chest and back. Nail changes including pitting are found in psoriatic arthritis. Psoriasis is found in about 1% to 3% of the population,[33] and 7% of these patients have psoriatic arthritis.[32] HLA-B27 is present in 60% of patients who have psoriatic spondylitis.[32]

The ocular presentations are conjunctivitis in

20% of patients, iridocyclitis in about 7%, and scleral disease in 2% of all patients with psoriatic arthritis.[31] As with other HLA-B27–related arthropathies, the iridocyclitis is acute, recurrent, and nongranulomatous. Dermatology and rheumatology consultations are appropriate in the management of patients with psoriatic arthritis.

Inflammatory Bowel Disease. Ulcerative colitis and Crohn's disease are chronic inflammatory conditions of the bowel, both of unknown cause (see Chapter 12). The inflammation in ulcerative colitis affects the colonic mucosa, usually at the rectum, and extends proximally for a variable distance. Crohn's disease or regional enteritis is a focal granuloma that can involve any part of the gastrointestinal tract from the mouth to the rectum; however, it usually involves the terminal ileum and the anorectal areas. The major characteristics of inflammatory bowel disease are diarrhea, which may be bloody, and abdominal pain. Sigmoidoscopy with mucosal biopsy can differentiate the two conditions. In ulcerative colitis, the mucosa is hyperemic, edematous, and granular. A normal mucosa in the presence of chronic diarrhea is more indicative of Crohn's disease. The involvement of the colon in ulcerative colitis is continuous from the rectum proximally, and in Crohn's disease it is segmental (focal) and often involves the right colon and terminal part of the ileum. The associated systemic features include low-grade fever, weight loss, arthritis, mucous membrane disease, erythema nodosum, liver disease, and ocular involvement. In general, these extracolonic features occur when the colitis is active. In both conditions, a majority of those affected are young adults at the time of onset, and a familial relationship seems most prevalent in the Jewish population.[34]

Ocular manifestations are found in 4% to 6% of patients with inflammatory bowel disease and exacerbate with the activity and treatment of the intestinal inflammation. An episcleritis, iritis, and peripheral keratopathy are found. An acute nongranulomatous recurrent iridocyclitis is the more frequent presentation, and it is related to the presence of spondylitis and HLA-B27. Fifty percent of patients with spondylitis and inflammatory bowel disease are HLA-B27 positive.[19] Thirty percent of these patients are likely to develop iridocyclitis. A differential diagnosis can be made with the iridocyclitis of ankylosing spondylitis because that of inflammatory bowel disease is frequently associated with exacerbations of the colitis.[5] When arthritis and Crohn's disease are present, the incidence of iritis is increased from 2% to 30%.[21] Ulcerative colitis is rarely associated with ocular complications, although 20% of these patients have ankylosing spondylitis.[21]

The differential diagnostic criteria for patients with iridocyclitis is the history of gastrointestinal symptoms of diarrhea, indigestion, abdominal pain, and bleeding. The acute iridocyclitis is milder and is not accompanied by as much pain and redness as in other spondyloarthropathies.

An internal medicine or gastroenterology consultation is warranted for co-management of these patients.

Syphilis

With the resurgence of venereal diseases,[68] it is likely that there will be an increased number of patients with syphilitic ocular disease. Syphilis is still a rare cause of uveitis, estimated to be the cause in only 1% of all uveitis.[36] *However, the disease must be considered in any case of recurrent ocular inflammation that is indolent, progressive, and resistant to conventional anti-inflammatory therapy.* Syphilis is caused by the spirochete *Treponema pallidum* and may be acquired or congenital (see Chapter 6).

Congenital syphilis can present with a chorioretinitis and a "salt and pepper" fundus, retinal pigment epithelium hypertrophy, interstitial keratitis, and a pale optic nerve.

Acquired syphilis has four stages:
1. Primary: This is characterized by the primary sign of infection, the chancre, which appears 21 days after inoculation. This painless, indurated ulcer is usually found on the genitalia but can be found on other mucous membranes, such as the anus and mouth. The chancre heals in 2 to 6 weeks, leaving no scar.[37] With adequate treatment of the primary lesion, second-

ary changes do not occur. Ocular involvement is rare other than an occasional chancre on the conjunctiva or eyelid.

2. Secondary: The hallmark of this stage, which occurs 6 weeks to 6 months after exposure, is the appearance of a maculopapular rash. The lesions are erythematous and symmetric and can involve any part of the body, although lesions of the palms and soles (see Fig. 18-17) of the feet are highly suggestive of secondary syphilis. Other complications such as malaise, fever, arthritis, periostitis, and uveitis may occur.[38] An iridocyclitis occurs in about 4% of patients with secondary syphilis. The inflammation is acute, may be granulomatous, and in 50% of the cases involves both eyes.[1] The patient may also have iris roseolae, papules, or nodules. The course of ocular syphilis is one of gradual worsening and progression from the iridocyclitis to frank involvement of the optic nerve.

3. Latent: This is a silent stage during which a patient may have relapses of secondary syphilis.

4. Tertiary: Three forms of the disease in this stage are cardiovascular syphilis, neurosyphilis, and benign gummas. Before the development of penicillin, 30% of patients developed tertiary syphilis, whereas today this stage is rare.[38]

Because the ocular presentation may cause the patient to seek eye care and in order to differentiate the condition from an unresponsive anterior uveitis, the optometrist should be familiar with the tests to confirm the diagnosis of syphilis. A complete description is found in Chapter 6. There are two basic types of tests, a nonspecific reagin antibody (a nontreponemal test) and a specific antitreponemal antibody.

The *rapid plasma reagin (RPR)* and the veneral disease research laboratory (VDRL) tests are tests for the nonspecific syphilis-related antibody reagin. These tests become reactive in primary syphilis as the titer rises and then become less reactive as the titer decreases in time, even in untreated patients. The titer also falls after treatment, and the rate of fall appears dependent on the duration of infection before treatment. These tests are most sensitive when titers are high during secondary syphilis. Because these are nonspecific tests for syphilis, biologic false-positive (BFP) tests may occur in nonsyphilitic disease, such as mononucleosis, pregnancy, acute infectious hepatitis, lupus erythematosus, rheumatoid arthritis, illicit drug use, pneumonia, and tuberculosis.[39]

The specific treponemal tests detect antibodies against *T. pallidum*. These tests are the FTA-ABS (fluorescent treponemal antibody absorption test) and the *MHA-TP* (microhemagglutination trepone-

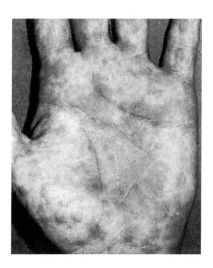

FIG. 18-17 Syphilis. Maculopapular rash of the palms is suggestive of syphilis. *(From Cawson RA and others:* Pathology: The mechanisms of disease, *St. Louis, 1989, Mosby–Year Book.)*

mal pallidum test). These are of greatest value in helping to distinguish between BFP tests and truly reactive reagin tests for syphilis in patients with clinical evidence of syphilis. BFP tests can occur in patients with SLE and other autoimmune diseases.[40] Because the treponemal tests are not titratable, become reactive in primary syphilis, and remain reactive for life, they are not used to monitor disease activity as the VDRL and RPR are.

A rationale for using these tests would be to use the RPR as a screening test. A nonreactive result is acceptable in patients with no signs or symptoms of syphilis. However, a positive result should be confirmed with an FTA-ABS or MHA-TP. Patients with signs and symptoms of syphilis or with unresponsive iridocyclitis should have the specific treponemal antibody tests.

The differential diagnosis of syphilitic uveitis with iritis as the presentation includes the HLA-B27 syndromes, sarcoid iridocyclitis, tuberculous iridocyclitis, and cytomegalovirus or other opportunistic infections in immunosuppressed individuals, such as herpes simplex or herpes zoster. Syphilitic uveitis has no pathognomonic features. The iridocyclitis may be unilateral or bilateral, acute or chronic, anterior or posterior.

Tuberculosis

Tuberculosis is a communicable chronic infection caused by *Mycobacterium tuberculosis*. Airborne transmission results in lung infection with possible spread to the lymph nodes and through the systemic circulation seeding of the bacilli in other areas of the body. The host develops a cell-mediated immune response to the bacilli. If the cell-mediated response is successful, multiplication of the bacilli decreases and dissemination ceases. These individuals are asymptomatic and noninfectious. The healed site is fibrotic and calcified, and these lesions show on chest radiography. If the cell-mediated response is not effective, the bacilli continue to multiply and spread through the lungs and into the bloodstream. These individuals are highly contagious.

Post-primary tuberculosis is due to reinfection or reactivation, usually found in elderly or debili-

tated patients and/or immunosuppressed patients. The dormant lesions of the primary infection break down, allowing dispersion of the tubercle bacilli and causing pulmonary and disseminated or miliary tuberculosis. The bacilli can affect any part of the body, and it is through this extrapulmonary involvement that an ocular infection may occur. Active ocular infection can occur as primary infection by direct introduction of the bacilli into the eye by hands or sputum with bacilli; however, active ocular infection is usually by hematogenous spread from a primary or secondary active site. The resultant granuloma has a propensity for the choroid but may involve the lids, conjunctiva, cornea, sclera, uvea, optic nerve, and orbit. Immune reaction to the tuberculoproteins is related to interstitial keratitis, phylectenular keratoconjunctivitis, episcleritis, and granulomatous uveitis.[41]

The most diagnostic test for tuberculosis is culture confirmation from sputum. Chest radiographs can also support the diagnosis. When clinical evidence of ocular tuberculosis exists, chest radiography and the PPD should be used. A positive response is indicative of past exposure, not necessarily active infection. The chest radiograph and PPD should be used for differential diagnosis with patients who have iridocyclitis that is unresponsive to conventional therapy or iridocyclitis and a clinical history of weight loss, night sweats, recurrent pulmonary infection, or past exposure to tuberculosis.[41]

The most common associated ocular involvement is uveitis. Anterior uveitis is usually granulomatous with mutton-fat KPs and possibly Koeppe and Busacca nodules on the iris. Because tuberculosis patients may already have a compromised immune system, systemic corticosteroids should be used with caution because of the additive immunosuppressive effect. The primary treatment should always be for the systemic disease. Isoniazid, rifampin, and ethambutol are three of the primary drugs used for systemic treatment. Consultation with an internist or pulmonary specialist should be made for the primary diagnosis and treatment of the systemic disease.

Fuchs' Heterochromic Iridocyclitis

Fuchs' heterochromic iridocyclitis is a unilateral, chronic, nongranulomatous iridocyclitis of insidious onset in quiet eyes of middle-aged adults.[42] The heterochromia is the classic sign, although it may be absent or difficult to detect. An affected brown eye becomes less brown, a blue eye more blue, a gray eye more greenish because the iritic stromal atrophy allows greater visibility of the underlying pigment epithelium through the thinned stroma.[3] The color differences are best seen in natural light before dilation. The patient is usually asymptomatic until the vision decreases due to cataract or the patient notices a color difference between the eyes. Occasionally the condition is found during a routine ocular examination of an asymptomatic patient.

The clinical picture is blurring of the iris stroma and loss of detail and denseness of the iris surface due to stromal atrophy, which can be seen with careful slit-lamp (Fig. 18-18) examination. There may be patchy loss of the posterior pigment layer detected with transillumination (Fig. 18-19). In the later stages patients have a moth-eaten appearance

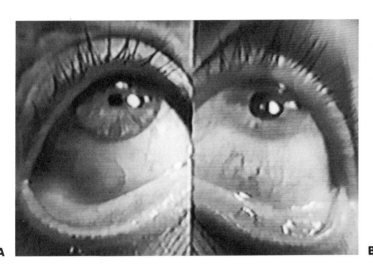

A **B**

FIG. 18-18 A, Normal right eye reveals small pupil, good iris detail, and dark blue color. **B,** Involved left eye reveals the classic characteristics of Fuch's heterochromic iridocyclitis: a mid-dilated pupil, loss of iris detail, and a pale blue color.

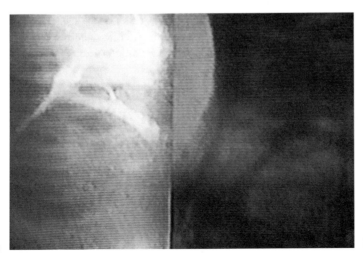

A **B**

FIG. 18-19 A, Atrophy of the iris stroma reveals a "moth-eaten" appearance. **B,** The same area of iris reveals transillumination of the area of atrophy.

of the pupillary border and may exhibit poor pupillary responses because of involvement of the iris sphincter. Low-grade cells and flare are usually present in the anterior chamber. The KPs are scattered uniformly over the corneal endothelium rather than in Arlt's triangle as usually found in acute inflammatory iridocyclitis. They have a characteristic small round or stellate appearance and are gray-white with thin fibrin filaments between the precipitates.[1]

Fuchs' heterochromic iridocyclitis has a chronic clinical course complicated by the development of cataracts and open-angle glaucoma. The disease process may be so quiet that the cataract changes produce the initial symptoms of a vision change.[42] Fifty to 100 percent of the patients develop a posterior subcapsular cataract secondary to the chronic inflammation causing a change in the permeability of the posterior lens capsule[21] (Fig. 18-20). Glaucoma, believed to be due to trabecular sclerosis, is the more serious consequence, occurring in about 20% of patients.[44] Initially, the pressure elevation is intermittent, then becomes chronic. The glaucoma becomes resistant to medical therapy and poorly responsive to laser trabeculoplasty and eventually requires filtering surgery.[43]

Observation is the best clinical approach in the treatment of Fuchs' heterochromic iridocyclitis. Topical corticosteroids may have some limited effect, but if there is no significant response, the steroids should be tapered and discontinued. Mydriatics are not required because posterior synechiae usually do not form.[2] Fuchs' patients may have aqueous flare indefinitely, as do those with other forms of anterior segment inflammation, especially after severe insults to the iris vasculature and the blood-aqueous barrier. Treatment with dilators and topical steroids is usually not necessary. Overtreatment only advances the cataract formation and the glaucoma.[2]

The differential diagnosis is usually made by the clinical picture of typical KPs, a well-dilated pupil, heterochromia, no synechiae, and mild cells and flare that do not respond to steroid therapy. In typical cases, no laboratory testing is recommended except to rule out other anterior segment inflammations. In atypical cases a PPD test, chest radiography, VDRL test, and FTA-ABS are recommended.

Lyme Disease

Lyme disease was recognized as a multisystem disease entity in the mid-1970s (see Chapter 6). The spirochete *Borrelia burgdorferi*, borne by the deer tick *(Ixodes dammini)*, has been established as the causative agent in humans. The most distinctive feature occurs in the first stage of the condition. A cutaneous rash, erythema chronicum migrans, occurs at the site of the tick bite, usually within the first 3 weeks following the bite. The rash begins as a red papule and develops into a large annular lesion with a red border and a clear center. Systemic features of fever, chills, and malaise often accompany the presentation of the rash.

Stage 2 is characterized by a disseminated infection with neurologic and cardiac involvement. The neurologic involvement is often manifested predominantly as meningoencephalitis and the cardiac involvement as a conduction defect. Stage 3 is a persistent infection with chronic neurologic, cardiac, and joint involvement.[50] After 1 to 16 weeks a relapsing monoarticular or oligoarticular arthritis occurs. The knees, shoulders, elbows, ankles, and wrists can be involved. The duration is variable, lasting from days to weeks.[51]

The ocular involvement includes conjunctivitis,

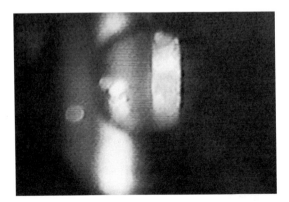

FIG. 18-20 Posterior subcapsular cataract in a patient with Fuch's heterochromic iridocyclitis.

episcleritis, uveitis, optic neuritis, panophthalmitis, and cranial nerve palsies. Most of these occur in stage 2 or 3 except for the conjunctivitis, which can occur in stage 1. Lyme uveitis is uncommon but important because of the nonspecific presentation and variable clinical picture. The anterior uveitis can be a mild iritis or a severe granulomatous reaction with granulomatous KPs and posterior synechiae. Most of the cases are bilateral in presentation.[50]

With classic presentation, the diagnosis of Lyme disease is straightforward—erythema migrans rash and typical systemic symptoms of flu and arthritis. Direct visualization and culture of the spirochete from patient specimens is difficult. A positive titer using the IgM ELISA technique is useful in diagnosis during the first stage. However, serologic cross-reactions with *Treponema pallidum* do occur. It may be necessary to use the FTA-ABS, the MHA-TP, and the VDRL for differentiation because the VDRL is negative in Lyme disease.

The differential diagnosis in Lyme disease can be diagnostically challenging because of the similarity of the ocular presentation of this and several other uveitic entities with a systemic cause. The clinical history is important, especially if the erythema migrans rash is absent. Serologic testing can be helpful but may be negative. From an ocular perspective, JRA and syphilis are of prime consideration.

Masquerade Syndromes

Iridocyclitis can be mimicked by many conditions that are not primarily inflammatory in nature. Because the signs and symptoms of these conditions suggest a primary inflammatory uveitis, they are referred to as "masquerade syndromes." Many clinicians use this descriptive term for any malignant process that simulates benign disease. The major groups of masquerade syndromes are intraocular foreign bodies, chronic retinal detachments, and intraocular tumors. The first two are relatively self explanatory. The following is a review of intraocular tumors that can be mistaken for primary uveitis.

Retinoblastoma. Retinoblastoma is the most common childhood intraocular malignancy.[45] It usually occurs in children under the age of 3 years and is accompanied by leukokoria, strabismus, and intraocular inflammation.[2] A pseudohypopyon occurs owing to the presence of malignant cells in the anterior chamber. Clinically the pseudohypopyon is not as mobile as an inflammatory hypopyon. Other anterior segment characteristics of retinoblastoma are nodules in the iris and free-floating cells in the aqueous.[6] Usually the retinoblastoma can be detected with ophthalmoscopy, ultrasonography, or computed tomography.

Any child under 4 years of age with uniocular inflammation should have both eyes examined by binocular indirect ophthalmoscopy. The differential diagnosis should also rule out trauma and tumor.

Juvenile Xanthogranuloma. Juvenile xanthogranuloma is a benign condition, usually involving the skin and the eye and occurring in infants and children under the age of 15.[2] The first sign may be a spontaneous hyphema (Fig. 18-21) and anterior segment inflammation. The skin lesions

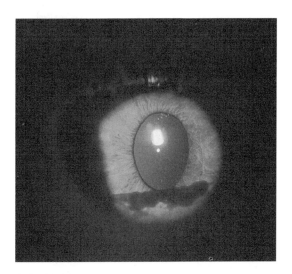

FIG. 18-21 Resolving hyphema in a case of juvenile xanthogranuloma. Note dark area of blood in the anterior chamber transversing the view of the inferior pupil and iris.

are usually red-brown or orange and are found on the head, neck, and proximal limbs. The ocular lesions commonly involve the iris and ciliary body and cause the recurrent spontaneous hyphema and subsequent secondary glaucoma.[52] The skin lesions tend to regress spontaneously without adverse effect, and the ocular consequences tend to recur, leading to progressive loss of vision with the glaucoma.[49] The condition responds to systemic corticosteroids and low-dose radiotherapy. It has been associated with neurofibromatosis and Niemann-Pick disease.[53,54]

Malignant Melanoma. Because uveal melanomas can produce media opacity, inflammation, and cataract, all adults with unexplained unilateral media opacity and inflammation require a thorough evaluation utilizing appropriate imaging studies. Melanomas can present as primary tumors or as

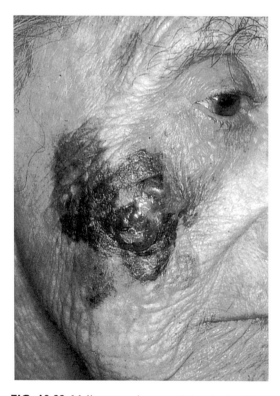

FIG. 18-22 Malignant melanoma of the cheek. *(From Habif TB:* Clinical dermatology, *St. Louis, 1990, Mosby–Year Book.)*

metastases to the eye (Figs. 18-22 and 18-23). As many as 50% of patients with metastases to the eye can present for ocular examination prior to the discovery of the primary malignancy.[47] Melanomas can cause glaucoma and inflammation by direct invasion of the trabecular meshwork. Large posterior necrotic tumors can cause a posterior and anterior inflammatory response or seed tumor cells to the anterior segment. Iris melanomas can produce cells and flare.[6] Ultrasonography is used to rule out the presence of posterior tumors when the media is too hazy for visualization and fluorescein angiography.

Reticulum Cell Sarcoma. Reticulum cell sarcoma is an uncommon intraocular lymphoma found most often in patients over 60 years of age. The name "reticulum cell" is a misnomer because the malignant cells have been shown to be malignant lymphoid cells, not reticulum cells. Thus the more appropriate name is intraocular lymphoma.[42] The neoplastic disease has two forms: the central nervous system (CNS) form and the visceral form. The CNS form involves the eye and CNS and the visceral form involves the visceral organs.

The condition often presents as an intermediate uveitis that can be unilateral but becomes bilateral. There is a painless loss of vision in an otherwise

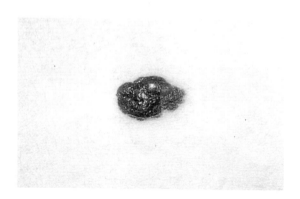

FIG. 18-23 Close-up of malignant melanoma of the skin. Note the irregular spreading pigmentation around the ulcerated black nodule. *(From Lawrence CM and Cox NH:* Physical signs in dermatology: color atlas and text, *London, 1993, Wolfe Medical Publishers, Ltd.)*

quiet eye. A common finding is cells that look like inflammatory cellular infiltrates in the vitreous cavity. These cells can be dense enough to obscure the fundus. Other ocular findings can be an anterior uveitis, chorioretinitis, and retinal infiltrates. Reticulum cell sarcoma should be suspected in elderly patients with neurologic findings and vitreal cells that do not respond to systemic or periocular corticosteroids.[48,55] The diagnosis is made with fine-needle aspiration biopsy. Patients with intraocular lymphoma should have cerebrospinal fluid cytology, brain magnetic resonance imaging, abdominal and chest computed tomography scans, blood studies, and bone marrow biopsies.[45]

References

1. Kanski JJ: *Uveitis: A colour manual of diagnosis and treatment,* London, 1987, Butterworth & Company.

2. Smith RE and Nozik RM: *Uveitis: A clinical approach to diagnosis and management,* Baltimore, 1983, Williams & Wilkins.

3. Nussenblatt RB and Palestine AG: *Uveitis fundamentals and clinical practice,* Chicago, 1989, Year Book Medical Publishers.

4. Rosenbaum JT: Characterization of uveitis associated with spondyloarthritis, *J Rheumotol* 16:792, 1989.

5. Godfrey WA: *Acute anterior uveitis.* In Tesman W and Jaeger EA (eds): *Clinical ophthalmology,* Philadelphia, 1992, JB Lippincott.

6. Giles CL: *Uveitis in childhood.* In Tasman W and Jaeger EA, editors: *Duane's clinical ophthalmology,* Philadelphia, 1981, JB Lippincott.

7. Muchnick B: Taking the mystery out of uveitis, *Rev Optometry.* Nov. 15, 1989:45.

8. Schlaegel TF Jr: *Essentials of uveitis,* Boston, 1969, Little, Brown & Co.

9. Hogan MJ, Kimura SJ, and Thygeson P: Signs and symptoms of uveitis, *Am J. Ophthalmol* 47:155, 1959.

10. Bloch-Michael E and Nussenblatt RB: International Uveitis Study Group recommendations for the evaluation of intraocular inflammatory disease, *Am J Ophthalmol* 103:234, 1987.

11. Sheppard JD and Nazik RA: *Practical diagnostic approach to uveitis.* In Tasman W and Jaeger EA (eds): *Duane's clinical ophthalmology,* Philadelphia, 1992, JB Lippincott.

12. Waltzman MB and King CD: Prostaglandin influences on intraocular pressure and pupillary size. *Am J Physiol* 212:329, 1967.

13. Parker JA and Nazik RA: *Laboratory tests in diagnosis of uveitis.* In Karsioglu WA, editor: *Laboratory diagnosis in opththalmology,* New York, 1987, Macmillan.

14. Rosenbaum JT and Wernick R: Selection and interpretation of laboratory tests for patients with uveitis, *Int Ophthalmol Clin* 30:238, 1990.

15. Calin A and Fries JF: Striking prevalence of ankylosing spondylitis in "healthy" W-27 positive males and females: a controlled study, *N Engl J Med* 293:835, 1975.

16. Fox R, Calin A, and Gerber R: The chronicity of symptoms and disability in Reiter's syndrome: an analysis of 131 consecutive patients, *Ann Intern Med* 91:190, 1979.

17. Kanski JJ: Screening for uveitis in juvenile chronic arthritis, *Br J Ophthalmol* 73:225, 1989.

18. Forre G and others: HLA antigens in juvenile rheumatoid arthritis, *Arthritis Rheum* 26:35, 1983.

19. Jabs DA: *Ocular manifestations of rheumatic disease.* In Tasman W and Jaeger EA (eds): *Clinical ophthalmology,* Philadelphia, 1992, JB Lippincott.

20. Glass and others: Early onset pauciarticular rheumatoid arthritis associated with HLA-DR S, iritis, and antinuclear antibody, *J Clin Invest* 66:246, 1980.

21. Pauesio CE and Nozik RA: Anterior and intermediate uveitis, *Int Ophthalmol Clin* 30, 245, 1990.

22. Rothova A and others: Uveitis and systemic disease, *Br J Ophthalmol* 76:137, 1992.

23. Klintuorin GK: *Sarcoidois.* In Gold DH and Weingeist TA, editors: *The eye in systemic disease,* Philadelphia, 1990, JB Lippincott.

24. Mayers M: Ocular sarcoidosis. *Int Opthalmol Clin* 30, 257, 1990.

25. Ohnos and others: Close association of HLA BW51 with Behçet's disease, *Arch Ophthalmol* 100:1455, 1982.

26. Arnett FC, Blas WB and Stevens MB: Juvenile onset chronic arthritis: clinical and roentgenographic features of a unique HLA-B27 subset, *Am J Med* 69:369, 1980.

27. Russel ML: Ankylosing spondylitis: the case of the underestimated female, *J Rheumatol* 12:1, 1985.

28. Morris R and others: HLA-27: a clue to the diagnosis and pathogenesis of Reiter's syndrome, *N Engl J Med* 290:554, 1974.

29. Stevens MB: *Differential diagnosis of multisystem disease.* In Harvey AM and others: *The principles and practice of medicine,* Norwalk, CT, 1984, Appleton & Lange.

30. Sharp JT: *Reiter's syndrome (reactive arthritis).* In McCarty DJ, editor: *Arthritis and allied conditions,* Philadelphia, 1985, Lea & Febiger.

31. Lambert JR and Wright V: Eye inflammation in psoriatic arthritis, *Ann Rheum Dis* 35:354, 1976.

32. Wright V: *Psoriatic arthritis.* In Kelly WN and others, editors: *Textbook of rheumatology,* Philadelphia, 1985, WB Saunders Co.

33. Rish DC: *Management of psoriasis.* In Gorall AH and May LA, editors: *Primary care medicine,* Philadelphia, 1981, JB Lippincott.

34. Bayless TM, Shuster MM, and Hendrix TR: *Diarrhea and constipation.* In Harvey AM and others, editors: *The principles and practice of medicine,* Norwalk, CT, 1988, Appleton & Lange.

35. Chan CC, Palenstine AG and Nussenblatt RB: *Sympathetic ophthalmia and Vogt-Koyanagi-Harada syndrome.* In Tasman W and Jaeger EA editors: *Clinical ophthalmology,* Philadelphia, 1989, JB Lippincott.

36. Henderly OE and others: Changing patterns of uveitis, *Am J Ophthalmol* 103:131, 1987.

37. Simons HB: *Management of syphillis and other venereal diseases.* In Gorall AH and May LA (eds): *Primary care medicine,* Philadelphia, 1981, JB Lippincott.

38. Quinn TC and Bender B: *Sexually transmitted diseases.* In Harvey AM and others (eds): *The principles and practice of medicine,* Norwalk, CT, 1988, Appleton & Lange.

39. Roberts SD: Optometric utilization of clinical laboratory tests. In Applanal DP and others: Problems in optometry, Philadelphia, 1990, JB Lippincott.

40. Thoburn R: *Antibiotics and infectious diseases.* In Smith JW, editor: *Manual of medical therapeutics,* Boston, 1962, Little, Brown & Co.

41. Deschenes J, Seamore C, Bok Cha S: *Tuberculosis and atypical mycobacteria.* In Tasman W and Jaeger EA editors: *Duane's clinical ophthalmology,* Philadelphia, 1991, JB Lippincott.

42. Godfrey WA: *Chronic iridocyclitis.* In Tesman W and Jaeger EA, editors: *Duane's clinical ophthalmology,* Philadelphia, 1987, JB Lippincott.

43. Leisegong TJ: Clinical features and prognosis in Fuch's uveitis syndrome, *Arch Ophthalmol* 100:1622, 1981.

44. Schuab IR: Fuch's heterochromic iridocyclitis, *Int Ophthalmol Clin* 30:252, 1990.

45. Char D: *Intraocular masquerade syndrome.* In Tasman W and Jaeger EA, editors: *Duane's clinical ophthalmology,* Philadelphia, 1992, JB Lippincott.

46. Burke PJ: *The lymphoid leukemias.* In Harvey AM and others, editors: *The principles and practice of medicine,* Norwalk, CT, 1988, Appleton & Lange.

47. Ferry AD and Font RL: Carcinoma metastic to the eye and orbit, *Arch Ophthalmol* 92:276, 1974.

48. Schlaegel TF: *Differential diagnosis (masquerade syndromes).* In Tasman W and Jaeger EA, editors: *Duane's clinical ophthalmology,* Philadelphia, 1982, JB Lippincott.

49. Jakodiec VA and Nelson D: *Lymphomatous, plasmacytic, histiocytic and hematopoietic tumors of the orbit.* In Tasman W and Jaeger EA, editors: *Duane's clinical ophthalmology,* Philadelphia, 1992, JB Lippincott.

50. Copeland RA: Lyme uveitis. *Int Ophthalmol Clin* 40:29, 1990.

51. Ziminiski CM: *Infectious arthritis.* In Harvey AM, and others, editors: *The principles and practice of medicine,* Norwalk, CT, 1988, Appleton & Lange.

52. Zimmerman LE: Ocular lesions of juvenile xanthogranuloma: neuroxanthoendothelioma, *Trans Am Acad Ophthalmol* 69:412, 1965.

53. Newell GB, Stone OJ, and Mullins JF: Juvenile xanthogranuloma and neurofibromatosis, *Arch Dermatol* 107:262, 1973.

54. Sibulkin D and Olichney J: Juvenile xanthogranuloma in a patient with Niemann-Pick disease, *Arch Dermatol* 108:830, 1973.

55. Lam S and Tessler HH: *Intermediate uveitis*. In Tasman W and Jaeger EA, editors: *Duane's clinical ophthalmology*, Philadelphia, 1992, JB Lippincott.

56. Craft JE, Grodzick RL, and Steere AC: Antibody response in Lyme disease: evaluation of diagnostic tests. *J Infect Dis* 149:78, 1984.

57. Tilkian SM, Conover MB and Tilkian AG: Clinical implications of laboratory tests. St. Louis, 1987, CV Mosby–Year Book.

58. Arnett FC: *Ankylosing spondylitis and related disorders*. In Harvey AM and others, editors: *The principles and practice of medicine*, Norwalk, CT, 1988, Appleton & Lange.

59. Heiss LI and Palmer DL: Anergy in patients with leukocytosis, *Am J Med* 56:323, 1974.

60. McGavin DD and others: Episcleritis and scleritis: a study of their clinical manifestations and association with rheumatoid arthritis, *Br J Ophthalmol* 60:192, 1976.

61. Nasal and others: Angiotensin converting enzyme and gallium scan in non-invasive evaluation of sarcoidosis, *Ann Intern Med* 90:328, 1979.

62. Schultz T, Miller WC, and Bedrossian C: Clinical applications of measurement of angiotensin converting enzyme, *JAMA* 242:439, 1979.

63. Gold DH, Morris DA, and Heinkind P: Ocular findings in systemic lupes erythematosus. *Br J Ophthalmol* 56:800, 1972.

64. Schaller JG and others: The association of antinuclear antibodies with chronic iridocyclitis of juvenile rheumatoid arthritis, *Arthritis Rheum* 17:409, 1974.

65. Zweiman B and Lisak RP: *Autoantibodies: autoimmunity and immune complexes*. In Henry JB (ed): *Clinical diagnosis and management by laboratory methods*, Philadelphia, 1984, WB Saunders Co.

66. Zizic TM: *Rheumatoid arthritis*. In Harvey AM and others: *The principles and practice of medicine*, Norwalk, CT, 1984, Appleton & Lange.

67. Johns CJ and others: Longitudinal study of chronic sarcoidosis with low dose maintenance corticosteroid therapy, *Ann NY Acad Sci* 465:702, 1986.

68. Centers for Disease Control: Continuing increase in infectious syphilis—United States. *Arch Dermatol* 124:509, 1988.

69. Biewerten DA and others: Acute anterior uveitis and HLA-27. *Lancet* 2:994, 1973.

19

The Posterior Segment in Systemic Disease

LEONARD V. MESSNER

KEY TERMS

Toxoplasmosis
Toxocariasis
Vitrectomy
Cytomegalovirus
Zidovudine (AZT)
Treponema Pallidum
Posterior Uveitis

Papillitis
Perineuritis
Acute Retinal Necrosis (ARN)
Gallium Scanning
Branch Retinal Vein
Occlusion (BRVO)

Central Retinal Vein
Occlusion (CRVO)
Central Retinal Artery
Occlusion (CRAO)
Branch Retinal Artery
Occlusion (BRAO)

INFLAMMATORY DISEASE OF THE RETINA AND CHOROID

A Review of Ocular Immunology

The eye is a structure that is unique with regard to immunology and inflammation. Of particular interest is the lack of lymphatic drainage, resulting in the direct drainage of ocular antigens into the bloodstream instead of into regional lymph nodes for processing.[35,171] The blood-retina and blood-aqueous barriers prohibit the direct communication of circulatory substances with the intraocular structures. However, in the event of intraocular inflammation, a breakdown of these barriers allows for the migration of leukocytes and proteins into surrounding intercellular spaces. Inflammation of the posterior segment often leads to the disruption of the retinal pigment epithelium, with the subsequent effusion of inflammatory elements into the sensory retina from the choroid.

The immunologic activity of the eye is in large part related to its ability to process endogenous antigens. Rahi and others[152] have classified uveitis according to specific antigenic substrates that include muscle (myositis), nerve and myelin (neuritis), melanocytes (melanocytopathy), retinal pig-

394

ment epithelium and outer segments (retinitis with choroidal vasculitis), and immune complex disease. This final category deals with the ability of the uvea to act as a filtering structure for circulating blood. In this way, the uvea functions as a sponge in which circulating immune complexes are permitted to lodge within the uveal tract with the subsequent precipitation of intraocular inflammation.

It is perhaps easiest to group uveitis into one of two categories: (1) endogenous intraocular inflammation and (2) uveitis caused by inflammation elsewhere within the body. the causative mechanisms of the latter include infection, immunologic disorders, and neoplasms. As mentioned above, the spongelike ability of the uvea to trap circulating antigen-antibody complexes makes it particularly susceptible to Type III hypersensitivity reactions caused by underlying systemic disease.

Toxoplasmosis

Toxoplasmosis is a zoonosis that is a frequent cause of retinochoroiditis in humans. The offending organism is the obligate intracellular protozoan *Toxoplasma gondii*. Exposure to *T. gondii* is relatively ubiquitous, with more than 60% of the general population in the United States and 75% of the world's population expressing some degree of seropositivity.[3,63-65,164] *T. gondii* was first discovered within a laboratory rodent in 1908, with the subsequent identification of intraocular tissue cysts by Janku in 1923.[102]

T. gondii is a coccidian of the subclass Sporozoa that has been shown to thrive within a variety of mammal and bird hosts. The most commonly established intermediate host is the cat.[118,134,151,178,182] Toxoplasma exists within humans in two forms: (1) tachyzoites (trophozoities), which represent actively motile organisms, and (2) brachyzoities (tissue cysts), which are the encysted form of *T. gondii*. The sporozoites containing oocysts are produced within the intestinal tract of the cat.[164,169,170] Oocysts are excreted within fecal material, where they can lie dormant in the soil or can be ingested by other animals, resulting in toxoplasmic infection.

Human acquisition of *T. gondii* is by one of several possible routes: (1) ingestion of contaminated, undercooked meat or dairy products (beef, lamb, pork, chicken, and eggs); (2) direct or indirect ingestion of cat feces or feces-contaminated products; (3) inhalation of fecal fragments; and (4) transplacental transmission of the parasite to a developing fetus from a recently infected mother.[63-64,127,161,178,182] Within a human host, mobile tachyzoites are free to migrate throughout the body, with a predilection for neural and retinal tissues. Because tachyzoites represent the most vulnerable form of *Toxoplasma,* they rapidly become self-encapsulated as tissue cysts in which the brachyzoites can lie dormant for many years.[169] In the event of reduced immune function (such as organ transplantation or acquired immunodeficiency syndrome [AIDS]) or in young patients with an immature immune system, the brachyzoites can erupt, liberating toxoplasma organisms and causing subsequent inflammatory precipitation.[34,154,160,167,187]

Historically, transplacental migration was thought to be the exclusive mode of infection by *T. gondii.* Definitive evidence now supports the premise of acquired infection in addition to congenital toxoplasmosis.[5,73,126] Acquired toxoplasmosis typically presents as a "silent" infection, with only a small percentage of affected individuals experiencing flulike symptoms. These constitutional symptoms are usually self-limiting unless the individual is immunosupressed, in which case they may be life threatening.

Congenital toxoplasmosis accounts for the majority of clinical cases. Transplacental migration to a developing fetus is possible among women who have become infected either just before or during pregnancy.[117,127,194] Systemic involvement can be quite serious, especially if acquired early in pregnancy. The characteristic triad of convulsions, cerebral calcification, and chorioretinitis is well described in the literature and constitutes the "3 Cs" of congenital toxoplasmosis. Immediate therapy is required for the survival of these individuals.

The hallmark of ocular toxoplasmosis is a focal, necrotizing retinitis that often progresses to involve the choroid. The inflammatory response is predominantly mononuclear, with a liberation of lymphocytes, macrophages, epithelioid cells, and plasma cells.[151] An intense overlying vitritis produces the characteristic "headlights in a fog" ophthalmoscopic appearance (Fig. 19-1). Retinitic lesions typically form contiguous with old, previously inactive lesions (Fig. 19-2) or may occur in an independent fashion. Although all retinal territories can be affected, there is a tendency for macular involvement, perhaps because of the increased blood supply to this region with end-arteriole termination. Vasculitis is common with ocular toxoplasmosis and contributes to the breakdown of the blood-retina barrier, leading to retinal thickening. The inflammatory response can produce a concomitant granulomatous or nongranulomatous anterior chamber response, but the presence of anterior uveitis in the absence of posterior segment inflammation is highly unlikely with toxoplasmosis.

The extent of vision loss with active retinochoroiditis depends on the location of the lesion and the amount of inflammatory response. The macula can be involved either directly or indirectly in the form of cystoid macular edema or choroidal neovascularization (Fig. 19-3). Lesions affecting the optic nerve or papillomacular bundle also result in profound vision loss, as can an intense vitritis. Other complications include serous retinal detachment, cataracts, glaucoma, posterior synechiae formation, and branch retinal artery or vein occlusion. Patients with peripheral retinitic lesions and minimal vitreous inflammation often remain asymptomatic and are discovered later during the course of routine ocular examination.

As the inflammatory process abates, a well-delineated and excavated chorioretinal scar forms in the area of previously active inflammation. Retinal gliosis is common, and fibrous membranes can sometimes be appreciated emanating from the lesion into the vitreous. The presence of a punched-out, well-delineated, focal chorioretinitic lesion is highly suggestive of previous toxoplasmotic uveitis.

Laboratory diagnosis for active retinochoroiditis is geared toward the detection of circulating antibodies against *Toxoplasma*. Absolute diagnosis predicated on sereopositivity is confounded by the high degree of exposure to *Toxoplasma* within the general population. On the other hand, individu-

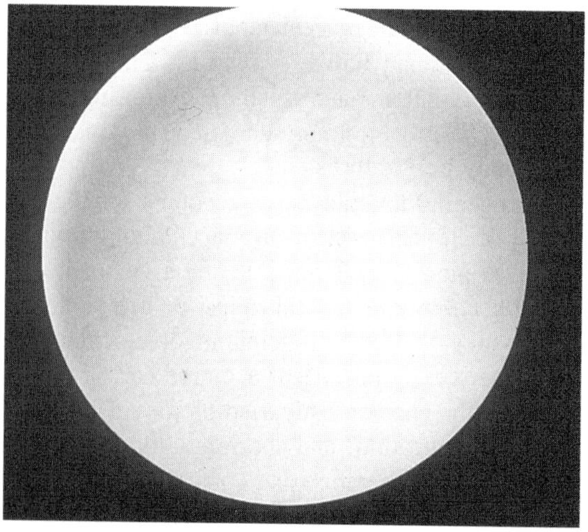

FIG. 19-1 A juxtapapillary retinitis with severe overlying vitritis in an 8-year-old boy who is seropositive for *Toxoplasma gondii.*

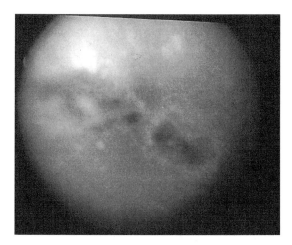

FIG. 19-2 Reactivation of *Toxoplasma* retinochoroiditis. Active retinitis can be appreciated as a fluffy white area that is contiguous with a pigmented, previously active chorioretinitic lesion. Inflammatory cells are evident in the vitreous overlying the area of active inflammation.

als afflicted with AIDS may not be capable of producing sufficient quantities of IgG or IgM, resulting in false negativity. In general, the presence of any reactive antibody titer accompanying active chorioretinitis should warrant a high index of suspicion for toxoplasmosis until proven otherwise.

Studies for *Toxoplasma* antibodies include the Sabin-Feldman dye test, indirect fluorescent antibody (IFA) test, enzyme-linked immunosorbant assay (ELISA) for *Toxoplasma,* indirect hemagglutination test for toxoplasmosis, complement fixation test, aqueous human antibody testing, and the *Toxoplasma* skin test. Of these, the IFA and ELISA are the most common tests routinely employed for diagnosis. The IFA uses killed tachy-

zoite antigens to detect circulating IgG and IgM antibodies directed against *Toxoplasma.* Titers of 1:8 or greater are generally considered to be positive for acute infection.[127,151] Although it is highly sensitive, false-positive results are possible in the presence of antinuclear antibodies (ANA) and rheumatoid factor.[151] The ELISA for *Toxoplasma* has recently gained favor owing to its high degree of sensitivity and limited cross-reaction with ANA and rheumatoid factor.[151]

The management of ocular toxoplasmosis is a two-pronged approach: (1) the eradication of the parasite along with (2) suppression of the inflammatory response. Treatment is most imperative for ocular lesions that threaten the macula or optic

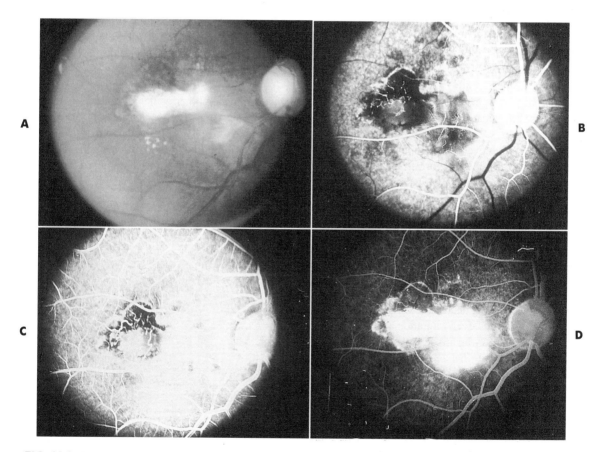

FIG. 19-3 A, An inactive, macular toxoplasmotic lesion with associated subretinal fibrosis and lipid. **B,** to **D,** Fluorescein angiography reveals a subfoveal choroidal neovascular membrane that progressively fills with fluorescein and shows profound leakage late in the angiogram.

nerve or produce a severe vitritis. Pyrimethamine (Daraprim) and sulfadiazine both inhibit the folic acid metabolism required for *Toxoplasma* survival and exhibit a synergistic effect when used together. The classic "triple therapy" treatment regimen combines pyrimethamine and sulfadiazine with corticosteroids and remains the most accepted treatment regimen for ocular toxoplasmosis.

The antibiotic clindamycin has proven to be of significant benefit, especially for the treatment of ocular toxoplasmosis.[179,180] Clindamycin can be used as alternative to or combined with pyrimethamine and sulfadiazine. Laser photocoagulation and cryotherapy are of limited therapeutic value for active retinochoroiditis. Topical steroids and cycloplegics are recommended to minimize the complications of anterior uveitis.

Toxocariasis

Toxocariasis is a parasitic infection attributed to the roundworm *Toxocara canis*. The development and reproductive cycles of *T. canis* are unique in that the ascarid is capable of full maturation with the laying of eggs within dogs but in humans develops only to the level of an immature larva. The disease process can be categorized as the constellation of systemic findings known as visceral larval migrans or as ocular toxocariasis.

Toxocariasis is most commonly a disease of dog handlers, breeders, and children, the later group being associated with geophagic tendencies. Human infection is the result of ingestion of ova-contaminated canine feces with subsequent deposition of the eggs within the intestinal tract, followed by the hatching and liberation of larvae. The nonocular visceral larval migration involves distant organ systems, which include the liver, lungs, and brain, producing hepatitis, pneumonitis, and encephalitis, respectively. The degree of systemic involvement depends upon the number of larva ingested and the immune status of the patient.

T. canis larvae enter the eye by way of the retinal circulation, inciting an inflammatory response in the form of a unilateral granulomatous retinochoroiditis. The posterior pole is the most common site of involvement, although peripheral lesions are not uncommon. The acute histologic presentation of ocular toxocariasis is an eosinophilic abscess that evolves to a well-delineated granuloma composed of macrophages, multinucleated giant cells, lymphocytes, plasma cells, and epithelioid cells.[70,131,168] In the acute phase, endophthalmitis is evident, often with an intense overlying vitritis that obscures underlying retinal detail. As the inflammatory response abates, a focal granulomatous retinochoroiditic lesion can be appreciated, often with associated fibrous membranes that emanate from the lesion and extend to insert at the optic disc or macula (Fig. 19-4). A progressive contraction of these membranes occurs with time which can result in profound traction on the retina, leading in some cases to traction and rhegmatogenous retinal detachment (Fig. 19-5). Occasionally, retinochoroidal anastomotic vessels can be appreciated in concordance with the inflammatory foci.

In addition to retinochoroidal involvement, *T. canis* can invade other ocular structures, including the optic nerve,[19,31,136,148] cornea,[12,93] conjunctiva, and lens.[108,168] Gass and others[69] have described the condition termed diffuse unilateral subacute neuroretinitis thought to be caused by *Toxo-*

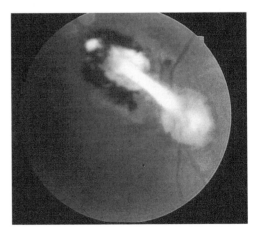

FIG. 19-4 A focal toxocaral granuloma with fibrous traction band extending into the optic nerve head. *(From Messner LV: Toxocariasis. In Onofrey BE, editor:* Clinical optometric pharmacology and therapeutics, *Philadelphia, 1991, JB Lippincott Co.)*

cara which results in optic atrophy and disseminated pigmentary hyperplasia.

Ocular toxocariasis should be considered in the differential diagnosis when one encounters fulminant endophthalmitis, especially in a young individual. The empirical laboratory study is the ELISA for *T. canis*. Owing to its high degree of specificity and sensitivity, the ELISA has virtually replaced all other immunoassays used in the diagnosis of toxocariasis with titers of 1:32 considered positive for visceral larva migrans and 1:8 positive for ocular toxocariasis. Analysis of vitreous and aqueous aspirate for hypereosinophilia or reactive ELISA titers may be required to confirm toxocariasis if the diagnosis remains elusive by conventional means.

The management of ocular toxocariasis depends upon the location, time frame, and extent of the inflammatory process. Patients with active endophthalmitis often show a favorable response when treated with anthelmintic agents such as thiabendazole and diethylcarbazine. The augmentation

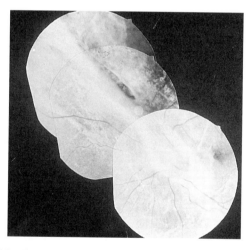

FIG. 19-5 Peripheral *Toxocara* inflammatory lesion with extensive transvitreal fibrosis communicating with the optic nerve. The optic disc and macula have been dragged toward the superonasal quadrant. Linear retinal breaks are evident adjacent to and below the fibrous vitreal membrane. *(From Messner LV:* Toxocariasis. *In Onofrey BE, editor:* Clinical optometric pharmacology and therapeutics, *Philadelphia, 1991, JB Lippincott Co.)*

of these agents with corticosteroids is advisable in many cases to further quell the inflammatory response.[49] Laser photocoagulation of toxocaral granulomas remains a controversial procedure because the "wounding" of encapsulated larvae often promotes an even more intense inflammatory response than was previously evident. It is generally accepted that photocoagulation should be attempted only if the larva is clearly visible and is located 3 mm or more from the foveola.[168] *Vitrectomy* with scleral buckling is useful in the event of traction or rhegmatogenous retinal detachment.

Cytomegalovirus

Cytomegalovirus (CMV) is a double-stranded DNA herpesvirus accounting for opportunistic infection among immunocompromised individuals. Multisystem involvement is associated with CMV infection that includes the eyes, lungs, kidneys, gastrointestinal tract, and reticuloendothelial system.[66,85,191] CMV retinitis was first reported by Foerster in 1959,[59] with only sporadic case reports until the advent of AIDS. Subsequently, the incidence of CMV retinitis has increased exponentially, making it now the most common cause of infectious posterior segment inflammation and the major cause of vision loss among AIDS patients.[85,142]

CMV retinitis is the most common opportunistic infection in AIDS patients, affecting more than 46% of these individuals.[84] Although CMV retinitis can present at any time during the course of AIDS, it is most commonly encountered during the latter stages of the disease process. CMV retinitis typically presents in a unilateral fashion, with over one half of all cases progressing to bilateral involvement.[96]

If untreated, CMV retinitis is a progressively blinding disorder. Cotton-wool spots seen in AIDS patients are commonly associated with noninfectious AIDS retinopathy (Fig. 19-6) as self-limited areas of nerve fiber infarction, or they may represent antecedent foci of CMV infection.[87,88,145] Retinitic lesions typically develop near the arcades and midperipheral retina, with progressive spreading to involve the peripheral fundus and posterior

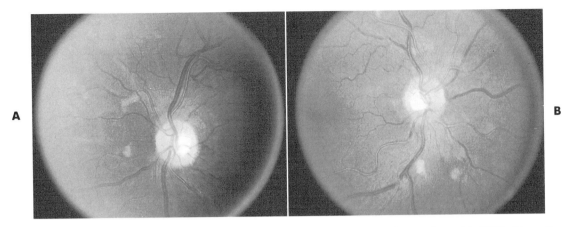

FIG. 19-6 Cotton-wool spots surrounding the left (**A**) and right (**B**) optic discs in a patient with AIDS. Nerve fiber layer infarcts represent the most common presentation of noninfectious retinal microangiopathy associated with AIDS.

pole. Patients in the early stage of retinitis evolution may be totally asymptomatic or may notice spots within the visual field due to vitreous involvement. The ophthalmoscopic features of early CMV retinitis include yellow-white granular dots that appear to coalesce, resulting in fluffy-white zones of inflammation (Fig. 19-7). Associated with this are areas of pigmentary mottling and dispersion due to disruption of the retinal pigment epithelium.[85] Intraretinal hemorrhage is usually evident along with sheathed and attenuated retinal vessels. The borders of these lesions are somewhat feathered and indistinct, with adjacent satelite lesions often observable that denote active areas of viral replication. The rubrics "pizza pie" and "brushfire" retinopathy are commonly used to describe the constellation of findings associated with CMV infection. Vitreous inflammation is typically minimal but may be severe in some cases.

The natural course of CMV retinitis is that of a progressive, necrotizing retinitis. The resultant thinned and atrophic retina is extremely susceptible to the formation of atrophic retinal holes, retinal tears, and ultimately rhegmatogenous retinal detachment.[28,61,85,163,181,188] Exudative retinal detachment has also been reported as a complication of CMV retinitis.[145]

The diagnosis of CMV retinitis is usually based on the clinical findings. Serodiagnosis is of limited use, and viral isolation in culture is extremely slow and often does not yield a positive result.[157] Chorioretinal tissue biopsy may be required if the absolute diagnosis remains elusive, with the presence of "owl's eye" inclusion bodies considered to corroborate CMV infection.

The medical management of CMV retinitis has resulted in the retention and stabilization of vision for many CMV victims owing to the development of newer antiviral agents. Ganciclovir and foscarnet are antivirals similar in structure to acyclovir, with pharmacokinetic actions directed toward the inhibition of CMV DNA polymerase.[37,77,84,96,98,120,149,158] At the present time, foscarnet is gaining in popularity because it has less marrow-suppressive activity than ganciclovir and is able to combat ganciclovir-resistant CMV.[98] The reduced neutropenia associated with foscarnet allows many patients to continue with *zidovudine (AZT)* therapy, which has resulted in a slightly longer life expectancy among these individuals.[42,119] In addition to periodic ophthalmoscopic evaluation, Bachman and associates[11] have recommended repeated visual field examinations to determine the efficacy of virostatic therapy in relation to retinal stability with CMV retinitis. The management of CMV-induced retinal detachment is complicated by the fragile and atrophic nature of the retina, making retinal reattachment surgery

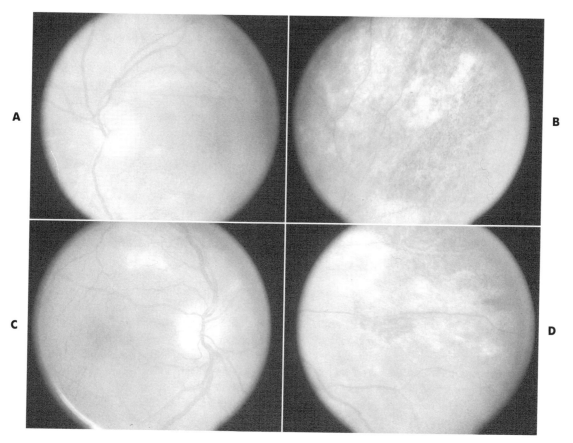

FIG. 19-7 CMV retinitis in a patient with AIDS. **A,** Localized areas of retinitis are seen above and below the left optic disc. **B,** The mid-peripheral eyegrounds of the left eye reveal confluent areas of necrotizing retinitis along with intraretinal hemorrhage and pigmentary mottling. **C,** In the right eye, patchy areas of retinitis are evident along the superotemporal arcade and superonasal to the optic disc. **D,** Confluent retinitis along with intraretinal hemorrhage, pigmentary disruption, and sheathed vessels can be observed nasal to the right optic nerve head. Note the presence of "satellite" lesions along the peripheral border of confluent retinitis, representing areas of active viral replication.

more difficult. Because of this, the relative risks versus potential benefits associated with surgery must be considered on an individual basis.

Syphilis

Syphilis is a multisystem disease caused by the spirochete *Treponema pallidum. T. pallidum* is transmitted by intimate sexual contact and enters the body via mucous membranes or through microabrasions of the skin. The disease presents in congenital and acquired forms, with ocular manifestations being common signatures of both.

Syphilis can be categorized according to a four-stage system. Primary syphilis is characterized by the presence of a painless, indurated chancre indicating the site of spirochete penetration. The chancre resolves spontaneously within 2 to 12 weeks, and the patient enters into a period of latency lasting 6 to 8 weeks before developing secondary syphilis. Secondary syphilis is generally associated with maculopapular skin eruptions along with constitutional symptoms. These findings typically persist for 2 to 6 weeks, at which time, if untreated, the patient enters a protracted period of latency.

During the latent stage, the patient is symptom-free while remaining seropositive for lues. The majority of patients who progress to latent syphilis remain at this stage of the disease; however, approximately 25% of these individuals eventually proceed to late or tertiary syphilis. The forms of tertiary syphilis include benign gummatous syphilis, cardiovascular syphilis, and neurosyphilis.

The ocular manifestations of syphilis are practically endless; however, patients should be viewed with a reasonably high index of suspicion for lues, particularly if they present with any of the following clinical findings: chronic or recurrent anterior or *posterior uveitis, papillitis, perineuritis,* optic atrophy, and abnormal or unexplained pupillary abnormalities.[16,122,130,162,174] The most common ocular presentation of syphilis is uveitis. Syphilitic uveitis is typically bilateral, can be granulomatous or nongranulomatous in nature, and can affect both the anterior and posterior segments. Historically, uveitis has been perceived as a strong marker for secondary syphilis, but an increasing number of patients with syphilitic uveitis are now showing cerebrospinal fluid abnormalities, implying that the incidence of uveitis associated with neurosyphilis may be higher than was originally thought.

Posterior luetic uveitis typically presents as a disseminated chorioretinitis with overlying vitritis. Vascular sheathing, as is seen with other inflammatory disorders, is also common with syphilis. Recent literature shows syphilitic chorioretinitis to present typically in one of two forms: a confluent necrotizing retinitis peripheral to the arcades[177] or a central chorioretinitis, often with profound vision loss.[43] Gass and others[68] have described large, solitary, placoid, pale-yellow lesions of the posterior pole as being pathognomonic of syphilitic chorioretinitis and have termed the entity acute syphilitic posterior placoid chorioretinitis.

With resolution of the inflammatory process, a diffuse pigmentary retinopathy is usually evident involving areas of previously active chorioretinitis (Fig. 19-8). Perivascular dispersion of pigment produces a "bone spicule–like" appearance which mimics that seen with retinitis pigmentosa and may obscure the correct diagnosis. Cases of sectoral or unilateral retinitis pigmentosa should be viewed with great skepticism, as most are in reality caused by syphilis or other inflammatory disorders.

Visual acuity can be reduced for a number of reasons, with the most common causes being intense vitreous inflammation, cystoid macular edema, and optic nerve involvement. Vision often improves dramatically after the patient is placed on antibiotic therapy.

An accurate diagnosis of syphilis is most easily obtained by serologic evaluation for circulating antibodies directed against *T. pallidum*. Nontreponemal tests such as the rapid plasma reagin (RPR) and the venereal disease research laboratory (VDRL) tests usually become positive during primary syphilis and reach maximal seroactivity during stage two. A significant number of these individuals become nonreactive during latent and tertiary syphilis.[78,174] In contrast, the treponema-specific studies, which include the fluorescent treponemal antibody absorbtion (FTA-ABS) and microhemagglutination for *T. pallidum* (MHA-TP), show reactivity with early syphilis and maintain some degree of positivity throughout the life of most syphilitic patients. Although more than 90% of individuals infected with *T. pallidum* show a positive FTA-ABS, seronegative syphilis, especially in combination with AIDS, has been reported, making the diagnosis elusive in some cases.[86,172]

Penicillin remains the drug of choice for the treatment of all forms of syphilis. It is generally accepted that syphilitic chorioretinitis should be treated in the same manner as tertiary syphilis, with the administration of 2.0 units of intravenous penicillin every 4 hours for 1 week. Although this therapeutic regimen is considered optimal therapy for most patients, there is, nevertheless, no acceptable agreement on a dosage and schedule for antibiotic therapy that absolutely ensures the total eradication of *T. pallidum*. For this reason, all victims of syphilis must be continually monitored for reactivation or exacerbation of the disease process.

The incidence of syphilis combined with AIDS is constantly increasing.[14,143,173] The luetic process among these individuals tends to be more ag-

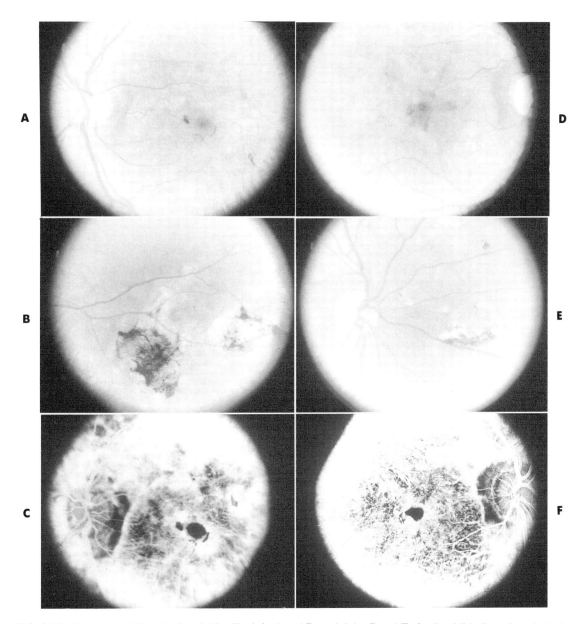

FIG. 19-8 Bilateral syphilitic chorioretinitis. The left (**A** and **B**) and right (**D** and **E**) fundi exhibit disseminated chorioretinitic lesions with chorioretinal scarring and pigmentary hyperplasia. Fluorescein angiography (**C** and **F**) shows extensive disruption of the retinal pigment epithelium, depicted as generalized, hyperfluorescent window defects.

gressive owing to the depressed immune status of HIV-infected individuals.[18,104,143] The reason for this is partly the commonality of the patient population at risk for both infectious diseases. Consequently, all patients with AIDS should be evaluated for syphilis and vice versa.

Tuberculosis

Once thought to be something of a "dead" disease, tuberculosis is being reported anew, predominantly among lower socioeconomic areas of both urban and rural United States.[115] *Mycobacterium tuberculosis* is transmitted through the inhalation of contaminated droplet secretions, inciting a granulomatous reaction within the lungs with subsequent hematogenous spread to extrapulmonary sites.

The most common ocular manifestation of tuberculosis is granulomatous anterior uveitis with posterior synechia formation.[2] Periphlebitis and disseminated choroiditis are common retinal and choroidal complications.[2,60] Peripheral periphlebitis with retinal neovascularization (Eale's disease) has been well documented with tuberculosis in the literature.[50,60]

Most cases of ocular tuberculosis are presumptive, given the difficulty of isolating *M. tuberculosis* within ocular tissues.[2] The purified protein derivative is considered positive for tuberculosis if 10 mm or more of induration and erythema are noted within a 24- to 72-hour time frame. Pulmonary radiographic findings include apical scarring, pleural thickening, and cavitary lesions (Ghon's complex). In patients with active systemic disease, acid-fast bacilli may be identified within the sputum, cerebrospinal fluid, pus, and urine.

Chemotherapy remains the accepted method of treatment for tuberculous uveitis, with isoniazid being the drug of choice. Corticosteroids and cycloplegics are indicated to quell the inflammatory response and prevent posterior synechia formation. Abrams and Schlaegel[2] have proposed an isoniazid therapeutic test for suspected tuberculous uveitis for individuals with positive skin tests and uveitis. If the uveitis abates within 3 weeks, during which time the patient is placed on a trial course

of isoniazid (300 mg/day), a firm diagnosis is established and the patient should undergo full-course antituberculosis therapy.

Herpes Virus Retinitis (Acute Retinal Necrosis)

Both herpes simplex and varicella-zoster are known be associated with *acute retinal necrosis (ARN)*.[39] Historically, ARN has been characterized as a self-limited necrotizing retinitis of otherwise healthy individuals with no significant predilection for gender, age, or race. Recent reports, however, have described several cases of ARN among AIDS patients,[32,39,86,97,146] implying a possible link between immunosuppression and ARN.

The clinical characteristics of ARN have been well delineated within the literature[58,81,186,193,196] and include diffuse uveitis, confluent peripheral areas of retinal whitening, vasculitis (arteritis), vitritis, and optic neuritis. The involved retina undergoes full-thickness necrosis, leaving it fragile and highly susceptible to retinal tear and subsequent rhegmatogenous retinal detachment. Retinal detachment occurs in 65% to 75% of affected eyes[189] and often results in profound vision loss. Retinal neovascularization from retinal ischemia has been reported as a rare complication of ARN.[189]

Bilateral ARN occurs in 36% of all cases, with involvement of the fellow eye usually occurring within 6 weeks of the initial presentation.[144]

Treatment of ARN during the early phase is best accomplished through the use of intravenous acyclovir,[23] yielding good resolution of active retinitis. The management of retinal detachment is complicated by the tenous nature of the necrotic retina and the high incidence of proliferative vitreoretinopathy associated with the syndrome.

Sarcoidosis

Sarcoidosis is a multisystem, granulomatous disease that involves the lungs, lymph nodes, spleen, skin, eyes, nervous system, and musculoskeletal system. In North America, sarcoidosis is found almost exclusively within the black population. The disease is most common between the ages of 20 and 40, with a gender skew toward women.[89,94] Ocular involvement occurs in 15% to 20% of all patients with sarcoidosis[94,99,101] and represents 3% to 7% of all cases of uveitis.[100]

No precise cause for sarcoidosis has been defined, although HLA positivity among some patients suggests the possibility of a genetic predisposition.[94] Whatever the cause, the hallmark of the disease is a T cell–mediated formation of granulomatous tissue.[38,90]

The most common anterior segment manifestation of sarcoidosis is iridocyclitis, which is often associated with large, greasy ("mutton fat") keratitic precipitates on the endothelial surface (Fig. 19-9). Chronic anterior uveitis may lead to posterior synechia formation, glaucoma, and cataracts. Nodules composed of granulomatous tissue may be observed and can involve the iris, conjunctiva, and cornea. Granulomatous infiltration of the lacrimal gland, orbit, and extraocular muscles may also occur.

Posterior segment involvement occurs in more than 28% of all cases of ocular sarcoidosis.[36,95,99,138] The disease is typified by a disseminated chorioretinitis with overlying vitritis. A profound periphlebitis is highly pathognomonic of sarcoidosis and has been termed "candle wax drippings" owing to the leukocytic infiltration of the vessel walls (Fig. 19-10). Cellular aggregates within the vitreous are common with sarcoidosis and can mimic the "snowballs" associated with pars planitis. Capillary closure can result from the inflammatory process, leading to retinal neovascularization and vitreous hemorrhage (Fig. 19-11).[176] The occurrence of neuroretinitis is exceedingly rare with sarcoidosis. Choroidal granulomas can be observed in some cases as elevated, cream-colored lesions of variable distinction (Fig. 19-12) and may precede the development of exudative retinal detachment.

Optic nerve involvement in the form of papilledema or direct granulomatous infiltration of the optic nerve is relatively rare in sarcoidosis, with the former caused by elevated intracranial pressure from intracranial granulomas.[94]

Absolute diagnosis of sarcoidosis is often arbitrary, with empirical certainty obtained only through autopsy.[10] Serologic studies for sarcoidosis are numerous, but none of those tests available is necessarily specific for the disease. Angiotensin-1-converting enzyme (ACE) and serum lysozyme are produced by epithelioid cells

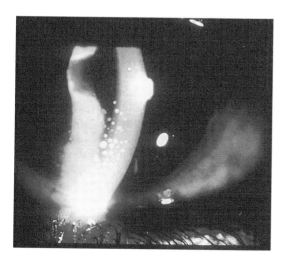

FIG. 19-9 "Mutton fat" keratitic precipitates with sarcoid uveitis.

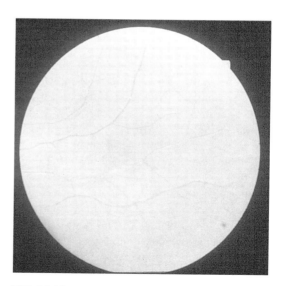

FIG. 19-10 Sheathed retinal venule in conjunction with sarcoidosis.

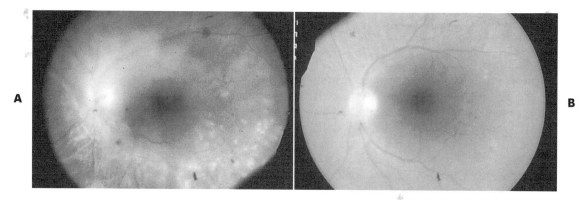

FIG. 19-11 A, Disseminated, white retinitic foci along with vitritis and vitreous hemorhage. **B,** The same patient after a 6-week treatment regimen of oral prednisone. Note the regression of the inflammatory process and vitreous hemorrhage.

and macrophages contained within granulomas, with their subsequent release triggered by helper T lymphocytes.[10] Elevated ACE levels in excess of 50 units/L are generally considered to be positive for sarcoidosis, especially if other clinical signs are manifest. Baarsma and colleagues[10] established a sensitivity of 84% and a specificity of 95% for sarcoidosis among individuals with elevated serum ACE levels. ACE is also found to be concentrated within the tears of patients with systemic and ocular sarcoidosis.[92] It is important to note that an increase in serum ACE is not exclusive for sarcoidosis and that other systemic illnesses produce these findings.[10,190] Serum lysozyme levels when taken alone are of limited predictive value for sarcoidosis but may be of diagnostic significance when associated with elevated ACE.[10] Both ACE and serum lysozyme production are inhibited by corticosteroids so that sarcoidosis may be masked by such treatment.

Radiologic evaluation is highly valuable in the investigation of sarcoidosis. Approximately 90% of affected individuals exhibit some evidence of abnormality on chest radiography at some time during the disease process.[9] Common radiographic findings include pulmonary infiltrates and bilateral hilar adenopathy. Radioactive gallium is readily taken up by activated macrophages of sarcoid granulomas and can be detected through *gallium scanning* of the head, neck, and thoracic regions.[109] Gallium scanning, however, is not nec-

essarily specific for sarcoidosis, as gallium uptake is also associated with other inflammatory and neoplastic disorders.[55,175] Karma and associates[109] have found significant gallium uptake over the orbits and parotid glands of many individuals with ocular sarcoid involvement.

Histologic confirmation of noncaseating granulomas is generally accepted as the most definitive test for sarcoidosis. Common biopsy sites include the conjunctiva, lacrimal, salivary, and parotid glands, peripheral and mediastinal lymph nodes, lungs, and liver. Skin testing for sarcoidosis (Kveim-Siltzbach test) is controversial and is rarely if ever performed.

Corticosteroids remain the mainstay of treatment for ocular and systemic sarcoidosis. Topical corticosteroids combined with cycloplegia are effective for anterior uveitis but are of negligible value in the management of posterior segment inflammation. Active retinal vasculitis and chorioretinitis typically require systemic treatment and generally respond favorably to oral prednisone. Sub-Tenon injection of methylprednisolone or triamcinolone may be indicated for patients who cannot tolerate systemic prednisone.

There is some debate as to the requirement of steroid therapy for posterior segment inflammation. General indications for treatment include significant vision loss from macular edema or severe vitritis, choroidal granulomas, optic nerve involvement, and retinal neovascularization. Conversely,

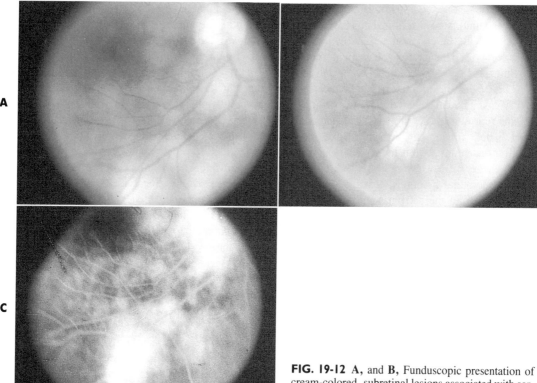

FIG. 19-12 A, and **B,** Funduscopic presentation of cream-colored, subretinal lesions associated with sarcoid choroiditis. **C,** Fluorescein angiography shows late staining of the choroidal granulomas.

if the vision remains good and no complicating factors occur, systemic treatment may not be necessary.

Given the chronic and recurrent nature of the disease process, long-term therapy is often required. Care must therefore be taken to recognize steroid-related systemic and ocular complications. Patients committed to oral steroids should be started on 40 to 80 mg of prednisone per day and maintained at this dosage level for several weeks, followed by a tapered withdrawal that is compatible with the resolution of the uveitis.

RETINAL VASCULAR DISEASE

Diabetic Retinopathy

Diabetes is the leading cause of new cases of blindness reported among individuals between the ages of 20 and 74 years in the United States.[110] Diabetic retinopathy represents the leading cause of

vision loss in patients under the age of 60 years.[139] The prevalence of diabetic retinopathy among diabetics increases proportionately to the duration of diabetes mellitus.[111-113] Although proliferative diabetic retinopathy is typically associated with the most severe form of vision reduction, diabetic macular edema is the most common cause of reduced vision among individuals with diabetic retinopathy.[129]

A number of systemic events have been described as "risk factors" in the exacerbation of diabetic retinopathy. Included among these are uncontrolled hypertension,[111-114] elevated hyperglycemia,[113,153] and diabetic nephropathy.[192] Rapid improvement of hyperglycemia and pregnancy can produce a worsening of the clinical presentation of diabetic retinopathy.[45]

Diabetic retinopathy can generally be categorized as microangiopathic nonproliferative retinopathy or proliferative retinopathy. Chronic tissue hypoxia associated with hyperglycemia leads to vasodilation of the retinal microvasculature.[76,116,165] This long-standing vasodilation results in pericyte degeneration, basement membrane thickening, and endothelial proliferation,[4,7,41,165] with the ultimate formation of microaneurysms[40,165] and capillary closure. Microaneurysms represent the earliest clinical manifestation of diabetic retinopathy and typically develop as focal outpouchings within the capillary bed of the outer sensory retina. Owing to the lack of normal tight endothelial junctions, leakage of blood and lipoprotein into the surrounding extracellular spaces produces the classic blot and dot forms of retinal hemorrhage along with circinate lipoproteinaceous exudate.

With increased capillary closure comes a hightened level of retinal ischemia. Historically, several angiogenic compounds have been postulated in the development of retinal neovascularization.[17,80,132] It is currently accepted that the angiogenic substance termed "retina-derived growth factor" is liberated from ischemic retinal tissue, allowing it to bind to adjacent areas of perfused retina and stimulating new vessel formation and direction.[165] These new vessels growing on the surface of the retina are fragile and prone to rupture, with subsequent vitreous hemorrhage. As fibrous tissue is laid down, a fibrovascular matrix is formed, leading to profound vitreoretinal traction and potentially traction or rhegmatogenous retinal detachment.

Clinically, diabetic retinopathy may be categorized as background, preproliferative, or proliferative. Background diabetic retinopathy is typified by the presence of intraretinal microangiopathy, which includes the presence of microaneurysms, hemorrhage, "hard" exudates, and retinal edema. As mentioned earlier, microaneurysms are the earliest clinical manifestation of diabetic retinopathy and represent focal outpouchings of the retinal microvasculature. The hemorrhagic component of background retinopathy originates within the deeper layers of the sensory retina and produces the characteristic dot and blot configuration due to the accumulation of blood within the outer plexiform layer. Hard exudates are composed of li-

poprotein that has extravasated from leaky vessels. A circinate quality is often appreciated in conjunction with the exudative response, with the epicenter of the ring defining the source of leakage (Fig. 19-13). If the macula is involved, an incomplete macular star is often observable as a result of the accumulation of lipid within Henle's layer. The presence of hard exudate is significant for vascular leakage at some point in time during the course of the disease process but does not necessarily imply active leakage. Retinal edema may be focal or diffuse in nature. Focal leakage typically originates from microaneurysms, whereas diffuse leakage usually occurs as a result of the breakdown of tight endothelial junctions of retinal vessels as well as at the level of the retinal pigment epithelium. The associated retinal thickening can be best appreciated through high magnification, through stereoscopic evaluation of the sensory retina (using the biomicroscope with a contact or other condensing lens), or with fluorescein angiography.

Preproliferative diabetic retinopathy is heralded by progressive capillary closure with resultant retinal ischemia. The ophthalmoscopic signature of preproliferative retinopathy is cotton-wool spots, which represent areas of focal nerve fiber layer infarction with axonal swelling. Intraretinal microvascular abnormalities, venous beading, and venous duplication ("omega loops") are also signs of retinal ischemia. The ocular fundus at this stage often exhibits a relative paucity of intraretinal hemorrhage owing to the destruction of the vascular source of leakage. This "featureless" retinal appearance can be documented as a generalized loss of vascular structure, with vessel sclerosis that is best quantified by fluorescein angiography (Fig. 19-14). Nonperfusion to the macula (macular ischemia) results in photoreceptor damage with irreversible vision loss (Fig. 19-15).

The hallmark of proliferative diabetic retinopathy is retinal neovascularization. Neovascular vessels at the optic disc and elsewhere throughout the retina have a fine and tortuous "angel hair pasta–like" quality with interdigitation into the vitreous (Fig. 19-16). As the vitreous contracts, these fragile vessels are extremely prone to rupture with subsequent bleeding into the vitreous. With time, fi-

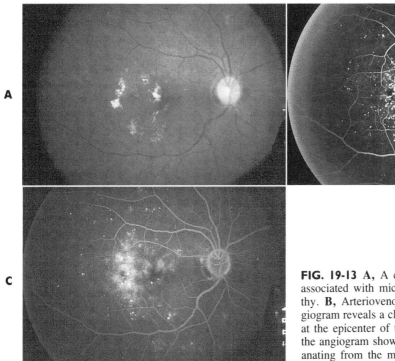

FIG. 19-13 A, A circinate, lipoproteinaceous ring associated with microangiopathic diabetic retinopathy. **B,** Arteriovenous phase of the fluorescein angiogram reveals a cluster of microaneurysms located at the epicenter of the lipid ring. **C,** Late phase of the angiogram shows focal, intraretinal leakage emanating from the microaneurysms, producing clinically significant macular edema.

brous tissue is also laid down along with the neovascular vessels, producing a fibrovascular complex that contracts, exerting a traction force on the underlying retina. This sequence of events commonly leads to traction or rhegmatogenous retinal detachment, with profound loss of vision if the macula is involved (Fig. 19-17).

Clinically significant macular edema is the most common cause of permanent vision loss among diabetics[129,139] and has been well described by the Early Treatment Diabetic Retinopathy Study.[51] Argon laser photocoagulation for focal leakage from microaneurysms as well as for diffuse leakage is warranted for clinically significant macular edema in order to preserve and in some cases improve visual function.[51,52,54,56,128,139] For patients with proliferative retinopathy, panretinal photocoagulation using argon green or argon blue-green laser has been shown to be effective in the prevention of vision loss due to vitreous hemorrhage.[44,195] Because of its minimal absorption

by hemoglobin, krypton red photocoagulation may be a beneficial alternative to argon if vitreous hemorrhage is present[106] and the fundus can be viewed. Vitrectomy for nonclearing vitreous hemorrhage[1,46-48,133,183,184] and tractional macular detachments[20,21,121,155,156] has restored vision for many individuals who have suffered devastating visual and ocular complications from diabetic retinopathy. Peripheral retinal cryopexy instead of vitrectomy has been reported as an adjunct to panretinal photocoagulation for patients with subtotal vitreous hemorrhage.[159]

Aspirin therapy has previously been reported to have no substantial effect on the course of diabetic retinopathy.[53] The effect of glycemic control on diabetic retinopathy has remained a topic of clinical debate. The Diabetes Control and Complications Trial is a multicenter study that is currently investigating the relationship between tight glycemic control and the progression diabetic complications, including nephropathy and retinopathy.

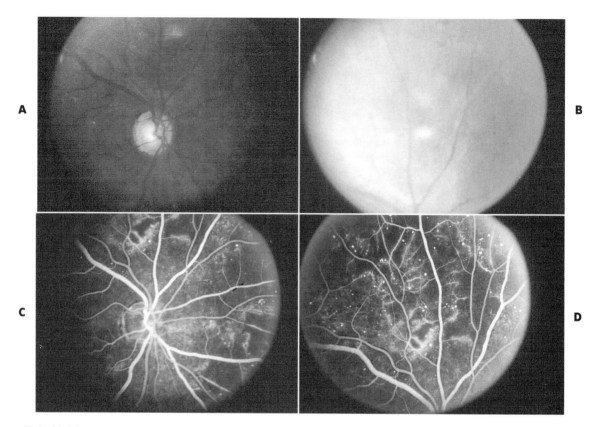

FIG. 19-14 Preproliferative diabetic retinopathy. **A,** and **B,** Infarction of the nerve fiber layer is evident in the form of cotton-wool spots located superior to the optic disc. Retinal ischemia may be inferred from the "featureless" quality of the retina which is observed as a generalized loss of microvascular circulation along with absence of nerve fiber layer striations. Fluorescein angiography reveals a patchy loss of retinal capillaries nasal **(C)** and superior **(D)** to the optic disc. Intraretinal microvascular disruption can be appreciated with leakage of fluorescein surrounding a hypofluorescent cotton-wool spot above the optic nerve head.

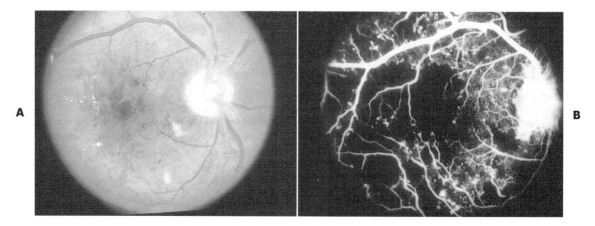

FIG. 19-15 Proliferative diabetic retinopathy with macular ischemia. **A,** Sclerotic, nonperfused vessels are evident above the macula. **B,** Fluorescein angiography shows profound nonperfusion to the macula and surrounding retina.

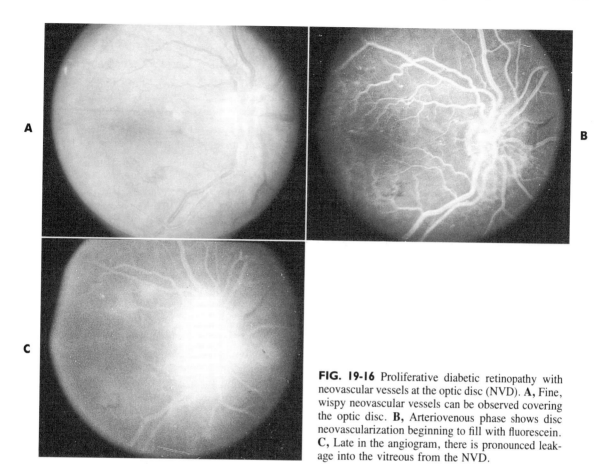

FIG. 19-16 Proliferative diabetic retinopathy with neovascular vessels at the optic disc (NVD). **A,** Fine, wispy neovascular vessels can be observed covering the optic disc. **B,** Arteriovenous phase shows disc neovascularization beginning to fill with fluorescein. **C,** Late in the angiogram, there is pronounced leakage into the vitreous from the NVD.

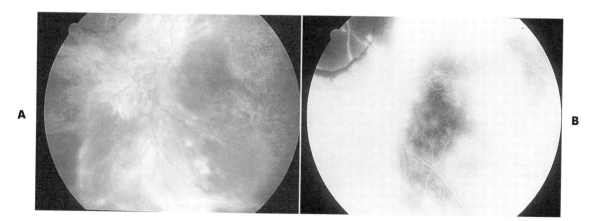

FIG. 19-17 Severe proliferative diabetic retinopathy with traction retinal detachment. **A,** Extensive fibrovascular proliferation is observable throughout the posterior pole. The underlying retinal vessels appear undulated owing to traction retinal detachment. **B,** There is leakage into the vitreous from retinal neovascularization along with stark retinal nonperfusion that is most evident in the upper right segment of the frame.

Venous Occlusive Disease

Vein occlusions are second only to diabetes in occurrence among common retinal vascular disorders.[141] Retinal vein occlusions are most common among elderly individuals who are hypertensive or who present with arteriolar sclerotic disease.

Branch retinal vein occlusion (BRVO) develops as a result of arteriolar sclerosis with secondary compression of the underlying retinal venule. The increased vascular turbulence at the arteriovenous crossing results in the formation of a thrombus, with ultimate lumen stenosis and occlusion. Risk factors associated with BRVO include hypertension,[22,75,105] diabetes,[22,103,105] male gender,[105] hyperopia,[105] and chronic open-angle glaucoma.[22,105]

The clinical presentation of BRVO is typically a wedge-shaped area of intraretinal hemorrhage with the apex of the hemorrhagic retinopathy pointing to the site of venous occlusion (Fig. 19-18). Additional retinal findings include edema, lipid exudate, and nerve fiber infarcts. The veins within the affected segment are often dilated and tortuous and exhibit a delayed filling pattern evident with fluorescein angiography. Collateral vessels frequently develop in an attempt to divert blood around the area of obstruction. The observation of collaterals bridging the horizontal raphae is particularly pathognomonic for BRVO. In addition to collaterals, recanalization of the thrombosed lumen has been reported by Bowers and associates.[24]

Macular edema has been reported in approximately 58% of patients with BRVO[75] and is the leading cause of vision loss among these individuals. Spontaneous visual improvement in eyes with macular edema has been reported in one third to one half of all cases.[57] If vision loss due to macular edema is 20/40 or worse and persists longer than 6 months and there is no evidence of macular ischemia compatible with the reduced acuity, grid photocoagulation to the area of vascular incompetence should be considered to improve visual function (Fig. 19-19). The Branch Vein Occlusion Study[26] has shown an improvement of two or more lines of vision in 63% of patients following argon laser grid photocoagulation for chronic macular edema versus 36% for untreated patients.

Some amount of capillary closure is to be expected with all presentations of BRVO. As a general rule, the larger the territory affected, the greater the degree of ischemia. BRVOs are defined as ischemic if the amount of nonperfusion as evidenced by fluorescein angiography is 5 disc diameters or more in size (Fig. 19-20). Nonperfused BRVOs are associated with a 36% risk for the development of retinal neovascularization, with approximately 60% of these progressing to vitreous hemorrhage.[25,57] The Branch Vein Occlusion Study showed a reduction in the incidence of vitreous hemorrhage from 61% in patients who were not treated compared with 29% of those who underwent scatter photocoagulation.[25] For this reason, scatter photocoagulation should be recommended for patients with retinal neovascularization secondary to ischemic BRVO in order to prevent vision loss from vitreous hemorrhage.

Tissue plasminogen activator (t-PA)[140] and other clot-lysing agents have been reported in the medical management of BRVO. Given the systemic and ocular complications associated with anticoagulation therapy, such management remains highly controversial. Because hypertension is the leading risk factor in association with BRVO, it seems logical to assume that adequate control of systemic hypertension may lessen an individual's chance of developing BRVO.

Central retinal vein occlusion (CRVO) is a com-

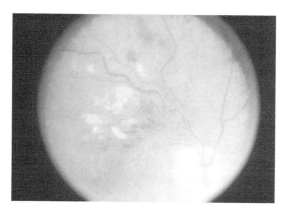

FIG. 19-18 Branch retinal vein occlusion.

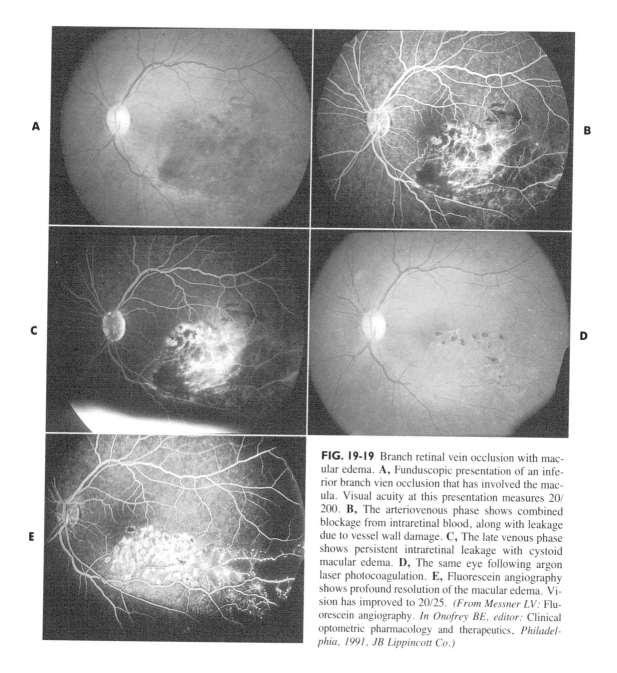

FIG. 19-19 Branch retinal vein occlusion with macular edema. **A,** Funduscopic presentation of an inferior branch vien occlusion that has involved the macula. Visual acuity at this presentation measures 20/200. **B,** The arteriovenous phase shows combined blockage from intraretinal blood, along with leakage due to vessel wall damage. **C,** The late venous phase shows persistent intraretinal leakage with cystoid macular edema. **D,** The same eye following argon laser photocoagulation. **E,** Fluorescein angiography shows profound resolution of the macular edema. Vision has improved to 20/25. *(From Messner LV:* Fluorescein angiography. *In Onofrey BE, editor:* Clinical optometric pharmacology and therapeutics, *Philadelphia, 1991, JB Lippincott Co.)*

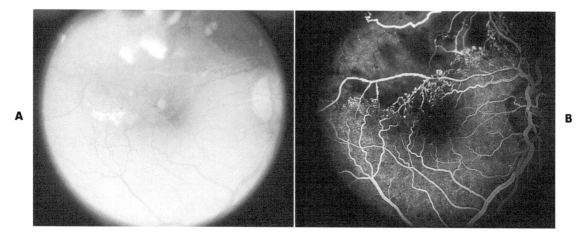

FIG. 19-20 A, Funduscopic presentation of an ischemic branch retinal vein occlusion. **B,** Note the extensive retinal nonperfusion within the territory of the vein occlusion as evidenced by fluorescein angiography.

mon retinal vascular disorder that usually occurs in patients over the age of 50 years.[74] Risk factors associated with CRVO are similar to those found with BRVO and include hypertension, arteriosclerotic heart disease, and diabetes mellitus.[74] The incidence of CRVO among young adults is quite low. Frucht and Yanko[167] reported that a significant history of systemic vascular disease was evident among younger patients who developed ischemic CRVO. Lupus anticoagulant and anticardiolipin antibodies have been implicated among younger individuals with retinal venous or arterial thrombosis who present with a lupus-like syndrome.[150]

The pathogenesis of CRVO has been linked to thrombosis of the central retinal vein in the area of the lamina cribrosa, leading to obstructed venous return from the sensory retina.[72] Most patients experience sudden and unprovoked vision loss and present with striate retinal hemorrhage in all quadrants, disc edema, retinal edema, and nerve fiber infarcts (Fig. 19-21). Hayreh's classification scheme reported in 1977,[79] using the terms "hemorrhagic" and "venous stasis retinopathy" to describe the fundus in CRVO, is rarely used any longer. At present, the common descriptors for CRVO classification are perfused (nonischemic) and nonperfused (ischemic).

Perfused CRVO presents with adequate retinal capillary circulation and demonstrates few if any cotton-wool spots upon ophthalmoscopic examination. Visual acuity can be severely reduced owing to macular edema or may be minimally affected. Collateral vessels at the optic disc are often pathognomonic of perfused CRVO and may develop as a result of venous thrombosis posterior to the lamina cribrosa.[79] In general, these individuals have a relatively favorable long-term prognosis, with many showing significant resolution of macular edema. Minturn and Brown[135] have reported that 5% to 20% of patients initially presenting with nonischemic CRVO eventually progress to the ischemic variant and that poor vision, severe macular edema, and progressive intraretinal bleeding may herald this transition.

Nonperfused CRVO can be categorically defined as having 10 disc diameters or more of retinal nonperfusion, as evidenced by fluorescein angiography (Fig. 19-22). The fundi of these individuals are typically noteworthy for the presence of many cotton-wool spots indicative of retinal ischemia. Rubeosis iridis is a common complication of ischemic CRVO and occurs in 40% to 60% of these patients,[33] with many cases progressing to neovascular glaucoma.[82] Barber and others[13] have reported electroretinographic abnormalities in

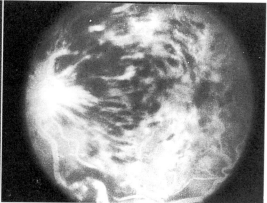

A

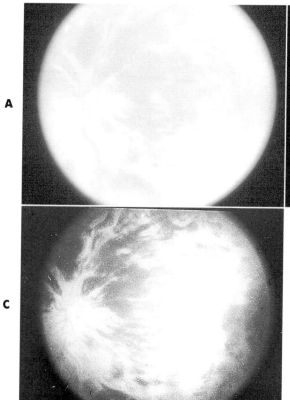

B

C

FIG. 19-21 **A,** Clinical presentation of a central retinal vein occlusion showing striate intraretinal hemorrhage in all four quadrants, retinal edema, disc edema, and a few cotton-wool spots inferotemporal to the optic disc. **B,** Arteriovenous phase of the fluorescein angiogram showing blockage from intraretinal hemorrhage along with leakage from the vessels of the optic disc and sensory retina. **C,** The late venous phase reveals extensive leakage from incompetent retinal vessels resulting in profound macular edema.

the form of reduced b/a ratios among patients with CRVO which progresses to iris neovascularization. Panretinal photocoagulation is generally recommended for patients with extensive retinal nonperfusion, whether or not iris neovascularization is evident, in order to reduce the risk of neovascular glaucoma. A multicenter study sponsored by the National Eye Institute, the Central Vein Occlusion Study, is currently underway to determine the value of photocoagulation therapy in the prevention of neovascular glaucoma in eyes with nonperfused CRVOs and also to evaluate the efficacy of grid photocoagulation for vision loss from macular edema.

Arterial Occlusive Disease

Retinal artery occlusion is a disease process found most commonly among the elderly. Associated systemic illnesses include hypertension,[29] diabe-

tes,[29] cardiac valvular disease,[6,29] carotid artery disease,[166] and giant cell arteritis.[71] Among younger individuals, migrainous vasospasm is the most common cause of retinal artery obstruction.[30,91] Retinal artery occlusions can be classified as *central retinal artery occlusion (CRAO)* or *branch retinal artery occlusion (BRAO)*.

The most common presenting symptom of CRAO is sudden and unprovoked vision loss that may be preceded by episodes of transient visual obscuration (amaurosis fugax). Visual acuity with acute CRAO ranges from hand motion to light perception and is accompanied by an afferent pupillary defect. Funduscopic examination reveals pallid edema corresponding to the infarcted retinal territories (Fig. 19-23). The fovea takes on the appearance of a "cherry-red spot" owing to the relative thinness of the retina in this area, allowing for visualization of the underlying choroidal circula-

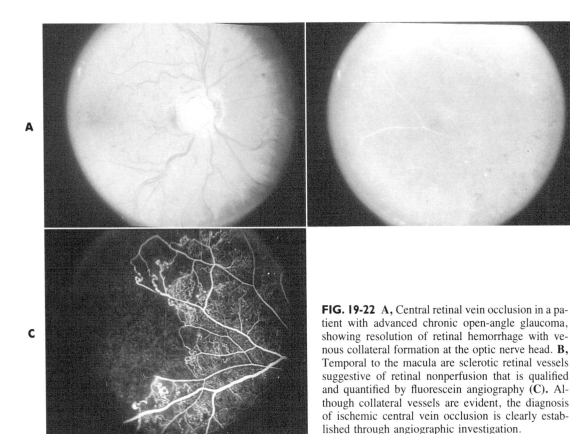

FIG. 19-22 A, Central retinal vein occlusion in a patient with advanced chronic open-angle glaucoma, showing resolution of retinal hemorrhage with venous collateral formation at the optic nerve head. **B,** Temporal to the macula are sclerotic retinal vessels suggestive of retinal nonperfusion that is qualified and quantified by fluorescein angiography **(C).** Although collateral vessels are evident, the diagnosis of ischemic central vein occlusion is clearly established through angiographic investigation.

tion. The retinal arterioles appear uniformly attenuated but may return to a more normal caliber following reperfusion. Fluorescein angiography, if performed, reveals a marked delay in retinal arteriole filling and arteriovenous transit time (Fig. 19-23). Residual perfusion to the retina may be evident along the distribution of cilioretinal arteries owing to their origination from the choroidal vasculature. Macular perfusion may be preserved along with some functional vision if there is cilioretinal supply to the macula.[107,123]

The presence of retinal emboli in the form of cholesterol (Hollenhorst plaques) or fibrinoplatelet aggregates may be observed within the arteriolar circulation. The source of these embolic fragments is usually the ipsilateral carotid artery which has undergone atheromatous degeneration.

The natural progression of CRAO produces a gradual clearing of the cloudy retinal swelling over a period of several weeks. The infarcted retina is replaced by supportive glial tissue, and the optic disc takes on a pale and atrophic quality. The incidence of retinal[124,125] and iris[71,83,147] neovascularization following CRAO is quite low, but it may develop, especially in the event of a chronic or incomplete CRAO.

Visual prognosis for CRAO is poor. This is in part due to the delay in seeking attention common among many individuals who have suffered central artery obstruction. Paracentesis, if performed within 24 hours of the occlusion, may be effective in dislodging embolic material, allowing for retinal reperfusion with return of visual function in some cases.[8] Digital massage, inhalation of carbogen, injectable vasodilators, and fibrinolytic agents seem to be of little therapeutic value.

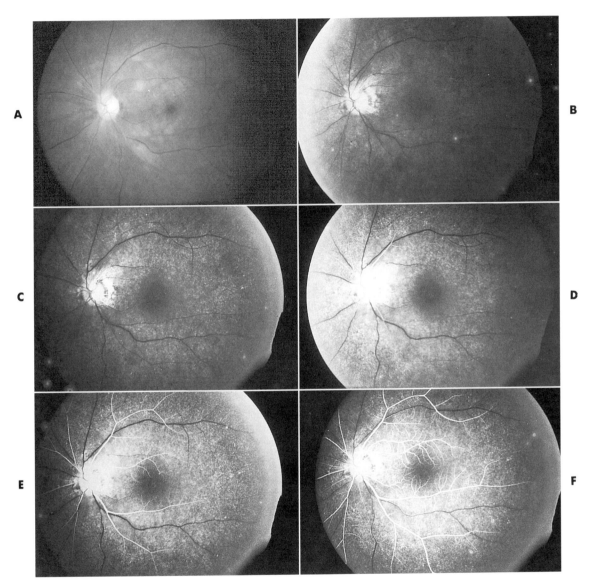

FIG. 19-23 A, Ophthalmoscopic presentation of pallid retinal edema along with arteriolar attenuation consistent with a central retinal artery occlusion. **B,** Ten seconds after the injection of fluorescein, there is patchy filling of the choriocapillaris along with the short posterior ciliary arteries supplying the optic nerve. The retinal arterioles have not yet begun to fluoresce. **C,** Several seconds later there is further expansion of the choroidal flush with no apparent filling of the retinal arterioles. **D,** Incomplete retinal arteriolar filling is first appreciated approximately 25 seconds into the transit. **E,** Several seconds later there is increased filling of the arteriolar segments. The retinal venules remain nonperfused. **F,** Several minutes after the injection of fluorescein, the arterioles have finally filled to completion and laminar venous flow is now evident.

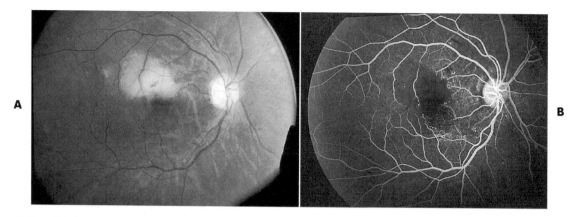

FIG. 19-24 A, Branch retinal artery obstruction in a patient with atheromatous degeneration of the ipsilateral internal carotid artery. A small fragment of cholesterol embolic material can be appreciated lodged within the proximal segment of the infarcted arteriole. **B,** Retinal nonperfusion is evident corresponding to territory of the occluded arteriole. Note the relative hypofluorescence of the occluded arteriole that may be observed as this vessel is superimposed over the perfused choroidal vasculature. *(From Messner LV,* Fluorescein angiography. *In Onofrey BE, editor:* Clinical optometric pharmacology and therapeutics, *Philadelphia, 1991, JB Lippincott Co.)*

Among elderly individuals who have suffered CRAO, the investigation of atherosclerotic disease elsewhere in the body is often of greatest clinical importance. Ipsilateral carotid stenosis or occlusion has been reported in approximately 45% of cases.[166] This is particularly important given the increased incidence of stroke among these patients[185] and the preliminary results of the North American Symptomatic Carotid Endarterectomy Trial, which indicate significant therapeutic value associated with endarterectomy for patients with high-grade stenosis.[137] Duplex evaluation of the carotid arteries is appropriate to verify carotid stenosis, with digital subtraction angiography or direct arteriography being recommended if surgery becomes an option.[15] Likewise, cardiovascular evaluation should be considered mandatory for individuals who have experienced transient ischemic attacks, retinal infarcts, or retinal emboli because 30% of these patients experience a myocardial infarction within 5 years, with an 18% death rate during the same interval.[185]

BRAO (Fig. 19-24) shares the same risk factors and causative mechanisms that have been discussed for CRAO. Visual acuity may be minimally affected or unaffected by the BRAO, depending the location of the infarcted vessel. Although no specific ocular treatment is recommended, patients who suffer BRAO face the same risks for stroke and cardiovascular disease as with CRAO and should be evaluated accordingly.

References

1. Aaberg TM and Abrams GW: Changing indications and techniques for vitrectomy in management of complications of diabetic retinopathy, *Ophthalmology* 94:775-779, 1987.

2. Abrams J and Schlaegel TF: The role of the isoniazid therapeutic test in tuberculous uveitis, *Am J Ophthalmol* 94:511-515, 1982.

3. Acers TE: Letter to the editor, *Arch Ophthalmol* 73:306-307, 1965.

4. Addison DJ, Garner A, and Ashton N: Degeneration of intramural pericytes in diabetic retinopathy, *Br Med J* 1:264-266, 1970.

5. Akstein RB, Wilson LA, and Teutsch SM: Acquired toxoplasmosis, *Ophthalmology* 89:1299-1302, 1982.

6. Appen RE, Wray SH, and Cogan DG: Central retinal artery occlusion, *Am J Ophthalmol* 79:374-381, 1975.

7. Ashton N: Vascular basement membrane changes in diabetic retinopathy, *Br J Ophthalmol* 58:344-366, 1974.

8. Augsburger JJ and Magargal LE: visual prognosis following treatment of acute central retinal artery obstruction, *Br J Ophthalmol* 64:913-917, 1980.

9. Austin MW and Clearkin LG: Radiological investigation in the management of uveitis, *Eye* 2:578-579, 1988.

10. Baarsma GS and others: The predictive value of serum angiotensin converting enzyme and lysozyme levels in the diagnosis of ocular sarcoidosis, *Am J Ophthalmol* 104:211-217, 1987.

11. Bachman DM and others: Visual field testing in the management of cytomegalovirus retinitis, *Ophthalmology* 99:1393-1399, 1992.

12. Baldone JA, Clark WB, and Jung RC: Nematode ophthalmitis: report of two cases, *Am J Ophthalmol* 57:763-766, 1964.

13. Barber C and others: The role of the electroretinogram in the management of central retinal vein occlusion, *Doc Ophthalmol Proc Ser* 40:149-159, 1984.

14. Becerra LI and others: Syphilitic uveitis in human immunodeficiency virus–infected and noninfected patients, *Ophthalmology* 96:1727-1730, 1989.

15. Becker WL and Burde RM: Carotid artery disease: a therapeutic enigma, *Arch Ophthalmol* 106:34-39, 1988.

16. Belin MW, Baltch AL, and Hay PB: Secondary syphilitic uveitis, *Am J Ophthalmol* 92:210-214, 1981.

17. BenEzra D: Neovasculogenic ability of prostaglandins, growth factors, and synthetic chemoattractants, *Am J Ophthalmol* 86:455-461, 1978.

18. Berry CD and others: Neurologic relapse after benzathine penicillin therapy for secondary syphilis in a patient with HIV infection, *N Engl J Med* 316:1587-1589, 1987.

19. Bird AC, Smith JL, and Curtin VT: Nematode optic neuritis, *Am J Ophthalmol* 69:72-77, 1970.

20. Blankenship GW: Stability of pars plana vitrectomy results for diabetic retinopathy complications: a comparison of five-year and six-month postvitrectomy findings, *Arch Ophthalmol* 99:1009-1012, 1981.

21. Blankenship GW and Machemar R: Long-term diabetic vitrectomy results, *Ophthalmology* 92:503-506, 1985.

22. Blankenship GW and Okun E: Retinal tributary vein occlusion: history and management by photocoagulation, *Arch Ophthalmol* 89:363-368, 1973.

23. Blumenkranz MS and others: Treatment of the acute retinal necrosis syndrome with intravenous acyclovir, *Ophthalmology* 93:296-300, 1986.

24. Bowers DK and others: Branch retina vein occlusion. A clinicopathologic case report, *Retina,* 7:252-259, 1987.

25. Branch Vein Occlusion Study Group: Argon laser scatter photocoagulation for prevention of neovascularization and vitreous hemorrhage in branch vein occlusion, *Arch Ophthalmol* 104:34-41, 1986.

26. Branch Vein Occlusion Study Group: Argon laser photocoagulation for macular edema in branch vein occlusion, *Am J Ophthalmol* 98:271-282, 1984.

27. Braunstein RA and Gass JDM: Branch artery obstruction caused by acute toxoplasmosis, *Arch Ophthalmol* 98:512-513, 1980.

28. Broughton WL, Cupples HP, and Parver LM: Bilateral retinal detachment following cytomegalovirus retinitis, *Arch Ophthalmol* 96:618-619, 1978.

29. Brown CG and Magargal LE: Central retinal artery obstruction and visual acuity, *Ophthalmology* 89:14-19, 1982.

30. Brown GC and others: Retinal arterial obstruction in children and young adults, *Ophthalmology* 88:18-25, 1981.

31. Brown GC and Tasman WS: Retinal artery obstruction in association with presumed *Toxocara* neuroretinitis, *Ann Ophthalmol* 13:1385-1387, 1981.

32. Chess J and Marcus DM: Zoster-related bilateral acute retinal necrosis syndrome as presenting sign in AIDS, *Ann Ophthalmol* 20:421-428, 1988.

33. Clarkson JG: *Central retinal vein occlusion.* In Ryan SJ and others, editors: *Retina, Vol 2, medical retina,* St. Louis, 1989, Mosby–Year Book.

34. Cohen SN: Toxoplasmosis in patients receiving immunosuppressive therapy, *JAMA* 211:657-660, 1970.

35. Corwin JM and Weiter JJ: Immunology of chorioretinal disorders, *Surv Ophthalmol* 25:287-305, 1981.

36. Crick RP, Hoyle C, and Smellie H: The eyes in sarcoidosis, Br J *Ophthalmol* 45:461-481, 1961.

37. Crumpacker CS: Mechanism of action of foscarnet against viral polymerases, *Am J Med* 92(suppl 2A):3-7, 1992.

38. Crystal RG and others: Pulmonary sarcoidosis: a disease characterized and perpetuated by activated lung T-lymphocytes, *Ann Intern Med* 94:73-94, 1981.

39. Culbertson WW: Infections of the retina in AIDS, *Int Ophthalmol Clin* 29:108-118, 1989.

40. Davis MD: *Vascular complications of diabetes.* In Kimura SJ and Caygill WM, editors: *Vascular complications of diabetes mellitus with special emphasis on microangiopathy of the eye,* St Louis, 1967, Mosby–Year Book.

41. DeOleveira F: Pericytes in diabetic retinopathy, *Br J Ophthalmol* 50:134-143, 1966.

42. deSmet MD and Nussenbatt RB: Ocular manifestations of AIDS, *JAMA* 266:3019-3022, 1991.

43. de Souza EC and others: Unusual central chorioretinitis as the first manifestation of early secondary syphilis, *Am J Ophthalmol* 105:271-276, 1988.

44. Diabetic, Retinopathy Study Research Group: Photocoagulation treatment of proliferative diabetic retinopathy (Diabetic Retinopathy Study report 2), *Ophthalmology* 85:82-106, 1978.

45. Diabetic Retinopathy Study Group, St. Thomas Hospital: Three year prospective study of visual function and retinopathy in diabetics with improved glycaemic control, *Eye* 1:744-749, 1987.

46. Diabetic Retinopathy Vitrectomy Study Research Group: Early vitrectomy for severe vitreous hemorrhage in diabetic retinopathy. Four-year results of a randomized trial (Diabetic Retinopathy Study report 5), *Arch Ophthalmol* 108:958-964, 1990.

47. Diabetic Retinopathy Vitrectomy Study Research Group: Early vitrectomy for severe proliferative diabetic retinopathy in eyes with useful vision. Results of a randomized trial (Diabetic Retinopathy Vitrectomy Study report 3), *Ophthalmology* 95:1307-1320, 1988.

48. Diabetic Retinopathy Vitrectomy Study Research Group: Early vitrectomy for severe vitreous hemorrhage in diabetic retinopathy. Two-year results of a randomized trial (Diabetic Retinopathy Vitrectomy Study report 2), *Arch Ophthalmol* 103:1644-1652, 1985.

49. Dinning WJ and others: Toxocariasis: A practical approach to management of ocular disease, *Eye* 2:580-582, 1988.

50. Duke-Elder S: *Disease of the retina.* In Duke-Elder, editor: *System of ophthalmology,* St. Louis, 1961, Mosby–Year Book.

51. Early Treatment Diabetic Retinopathy Study Research Group: Photocoagulation for diabetic macular edema (Early Treatment Diabetic Retinopathy Study report 1), *Arch Ophthalmol* 103:1796-1806, 1985.

52. Early Treatment Diabetic Retinopathy Study Research Group: Treatment techniques and clinical guidelines for photocoagulation of diabetic macular edema (Early Treatment Diabetic Retinopathy Study report 2), *Ophthalmology* 94:761-774, 1987.

53. Early Treatment Diabetic Retinopathy Study Research Group: Effects of aspirin treatment on diabetic retinopathy (Early Treatment Diabetic Retinopathy Study report 8), *Ophthalmology* 98:757-765, 1991.

54. Early Treatment Diabetic Retinopathy Study Research Group: Early photocoagulation for diabetic retinopathy (Early Treatment Diabetic Retinopathy Study report 9), *Ophthalmology* 98:766-785, 1991.

55. Edwards CL and Hayes RL: Tumor scanning with ^{67}Ga citrate, *J Nucl Med* 10:103-5, 1969.

56. Ferris FL and Patz A: Macular edema. A complication of diabetic retinopathy, *Surv Ophthalmol* 28:452-461, 1984.

57. Finkelstein D: Retinal branch vein occlusion. In Ryan SJ and others, editors: *Retina, vol 2, medical retina,* St. Louis, 1989, Mosby–Year Book.

58. Fisher JP and others: The acute retinal necrosis syndrome. Part 1: clinical manifestations, *Ophthalmology* 89:1309-1316, 1982.

59. Foerster HW: Pathology of granulomatous uveitis, *Surv Ophthalmol* 4:283-326, 1959.

60. Fountain JA and Werner RB: Tuberculous retinal vasculitis, *Retina* 4:48-50, 1984.

61. Freeman WR and others: Prevalence, pathophysiology, and treatment of rhegmatogenous retinal detachment in treated cytomegalovirus retinitis, *Am J Ophthalmol* 103:527-536, 1987.

62. Freeman WR and others: Demonstration of herpes group virus in acute retinal necrosis syndrome, *Am J Ophthalmol* 102:701-709, 1986.

63. Frenkel JK: Breaking the transmission chain of *Toxoplasma:* a program for the prevention of toxoplasmosis, *Bull NY Acad Med* 50:228-239, 1974.

64. Frenkel JK: Toxoplasmosis, *Pediatr Clin North Am* 32:917-932, 1985.

65. Frenkel JK: Toxoplasmosis: mechanism of infection, laboratory diagnosis and management, *Curr Top Pathol* 54:28-75, 1971.

66. Friedman AH and others: Cytomegalovirus retinitis: a manifestation of the acquired immune deficiency syndrome (AIDS), *Br J Ophthalmol* 67:372-380, 1983.

67. Frucht J, Yanko L: Central retinal vein occlusions in young adults, *Acta Ophthalmol* 62:780-786, 1984.

68. Gass JDM, Braunstein RA, and Chenoweth RG: Acute syphilitic posterior placoid chorioretinitis, *Ophthalmology* 97:1288-1297, 1990.

69. Gass JDM and others: Diffuse unilateral subacute neuroretinitis, *Ophthalmology* 85:521-545, 1978.

70. Ghafoor SYA and others: Experimental toxocariasis: a mouse model, *Br J Ophthalmol* 68:89-96, 1984.

71. Gold D: Retinal artery occlusion, *Trans Am Acad Ophthalmol Otolaryngol* 83:392-408, 1977.

72. Green WR and others: Central retinal vein occlusion: A prospective histopathologic study of 29 eyes in 28 cases, *Retina* 1:27-55, 1981.

73. Gump DW and Holden RA: Acquired chorioretinitis due to toxoplasmosis, *Ann Intern Med* 90:58-60, 1979.

74. Gutman FA: Evaluation of a patient with central retinal vein occlusion, *Ophthalmology* 90:481-483, 1983.

75. Gutman FA and Zegarra H: The natural course of temporal branch vein occlusion, *Trans Am Acad Ophthalmol Otolaryngol* 78:178-192, 1974.

76. Guyton AC and others: Evidence for tissue oxygen demand as the major factor causing autoregulation, *Circ Res* 14(Suppl 1):1-60; 15:1-68, 1964.

77. Hardy WD: Foscarnet treatment of acyclovir-resistant herpes simplex virus infection in patients with acquired immunodeficiency syndrome: preliminary results of a controlled, randomized, regimen-comparative trial, *Am J Med* 92(suppl 2A):30-35, 1992.

78. Hart G: Syphilis tests in diagnostic and therapeutic decision making, *Ann Intern Med* 104:368-376, 1986.

79. Hayreh SS: Central retinal vein occlusion: Differential diagnosis and management, *Trans Am Acad Ophthalmol Otolaryngol* 83:379-391, 1977.

80. Hayreh SS: Ocular neovascularization, *Int Ophthalmol* 2:27-32, 1980.

81. Hayreh MMS and others: Acute retinal necrosis. ARVO abstracts, *Invest Ophthalmol Vis Sci* 19(suppl):48, 1980.

82. Hayreh SS and others: Ocular neovascularization with retinal vascular occlusion. III. Incidence of ocular neovascularization with retinal vein occlusion, *Ophthalmology* 90:488-506, 1983.

83. Hayreh SS and Podhaysky P: Ocular neovascularization with retinal vascular occlusion. II. Occurrence in central and branch retinal artery occlusion, *Arch Ophthalmol* 100:1585-1596, 1982.

84. Heinmann MH: Long-term intravitreal ganciclovir therapy for cytomegalovirus retinopathy, *Arch Ophthalmol* 107:1767-1772, 1989.

85. Hennis HL, Scott AA, and Apple DJ: Cytomegalovirus retinitis, *Surv Ophthalmol* 34:193-203, 1989.

86. Hicks CB, Benson PM, Lupton GP, et al: Seronegative secondary syphilis in a patient with the human immunodeficiency virus (HIV) with Kaposi sarcoma, *Ann Intern Med* 107:492-495, 1987.

87. Holland GN and others: Ocular disorders associated with a new severe acquired cellular immundeficiency syndrome, *Am J Ophthalmol* 93:393-402, 1982.

88. Holland GN and others: Acquired immune deficiency syndrome: ocular manifestations, *Ophthalmology* 90:859-873, 1983.

89. Hoover DL, Khan JA, and Giangiacomo J: Pediatric ocular sarcoidosis, *Surv Ophthalmol* 30:215-228, 1986.

90. Hunninghake GW and Crystal RG: Pulmonary sarcoidosis: a disease mediated by excess helper T-lymphocyte activity at sites of disease activity, *N Engl J Med* 305:429-434, 1981.

91. Hupp SL, Kline LB, and Corbett JJ: Visual disturbances of migraine, *Surv Ophthalmol* 33:221-236, 1989.

92. Immonen I and others: Concentration of angiotensin-converting enzyme in tears of patients with sarcoidosis, *ATA Ophthalmol* 65:27-29, 1987.

93. Irvine AR: Nematodiasis: *clinical description and pathology*, In Kimura, editor: *Retinal diseases symposium on differential diagnostic problem of posterior uveitis*, Philadelphia, 1966, Lea & Febiger.

94. Jabs DA: *Sarcoidosis*. In Ryan SJ and others, editors: *Retina, vol 2, medical retina*, St. Louis, 1989, Mosby–Year Book.

95. Jabs DA and Johns CJ: Ocular involvement in chronic sarcoidosis, *Am J Ophthalmol* 102:297-301, 1986.

96. Jabs DA, Enger C, and Bartlett JG: Cytomegalovirus retinitis and acquired immunodeficiency syndrome, *Arch Ophthalmol* 107:75-80, 1989.

97. Jabs DA and others: Presumed varicella zoster retinitis in immunocompromised patients, *Retina* 7:9-13, 1987.

98. Jacobson MA: Maintenance therapy for cytomegalovirus retinitis in patients with acquired immunodeficiency syndrome: foscarnet, *Am J Med* 92(suppl 2A):26-29, 1992.

99. James DG: Ocular sarcoidosis, *Ann NY Acad Sci* 465:551-563, 1986.

100. James DG, Neville E, and Langley DA: Ocular sarcoidosis, *Trans Ophthalmol Soc UK* 96:133, 1976.

101. James DG and others: A worldwide review of sarcoidosis, *Ann NY Acad Sci* 278:321-334, 1976.

102. Janku J: Pathogenesis and pathologic anatomy of coloboma of the macula lutea in an eye of normal dimensions and in a microphthalmic eye with parasites in the retina, Casop Lek Cesk 62:1021, 1052, 1081, 1111, 1138, 1923.

103. Joffe L and others: Macular branch vein occlusion, *Ophthalmology* 87:91-98, 1980.

104. Johns DR, Tierney M, and Felsenstein D: Alteration in the natural history of neurosyphilis by concurrent infection with the human immunodeficiency virus, *N Engl J Med* 316:1569-1572, 1987.

105. Johnston RL and others: Risk factors of branch retinal vein occlusion, *Arch Ophthalmol* 103:1831-1832, 1985.

106. Johnson RN, Irvine AR and Wood IS: Histopathology of krypton red laser panretinal photocoagulation, a clinicopathologic correlation, *Arch Ophthalmol* 105:235-238, 1987.

107. Justice J and Lehmann RP: Cilioretinal arteries: a study based on review of stereo fundus photographs and fluorescein angiographic findings, *Arch Ophthalmol* 94:1355-1358, 1976.

108. Karel I and others: Larval migrans lentis, *Ophthalmologica* 174:14-19, 1977.

109. Karma A, Poukkula AA, and Ruokonen AO: Assessment of activity of ocular sarcoidosis by gallium scanning, *Br J Ophthalmol* 71:361-367, 1987.

110. Klein R and Klein BEK: Vision disorders in diabetes. In National Diabetes Data Group. Diabetes in America: diabetes data compiled 1984. Bethesda, MD, 1985 US Department of Health and Human Services. XII-1-XII-36 (DHHS publ. no. (NIH) 85-1486).

111. Klein R and others: The Wisconsin Epidemiologic Study of Diabetic Retinopathy. II. Prevalence and risk of diabetic retinopathy when age at diagnosis is less than 30 years, *Arch Ophthalmol* 102:520-526, 1984.

112. Klein R and others: The Wisconsin Epidemiologic Study of Diabetic Retinopathy. III. Prevalence of diabetic retinopathy when age at diagnosis is 30 or more years, *Arch Ophthalmol* 102:527-532, 1984.

113. Klein R, Moss SE and Klein BEK: New management concepts for timely diagnosis of diabetic retinopathy treatable by photocoagulation, *Diabetes Care* 10:633-638, 1987.

114. Knowler WC, Bennett PH and Ballantine EJ: Increased incidence of retinopathy in diabetics with elevated blood pressure: a six year follow-up study of Pima Indians, *N Engl J Med* 302:645-650, 1980.

115. Knox DL: *Syphilis and tuberculosis.* In Ryan SJ and others, editors: *Retina,* vol 2, *medical retina,* St. Louis, 1989, Mosby–Year Book.

116. Kohner EM: Dynamic changes in the microcirculation of diabetics as related to diabetic microangiopathy, *Acta Med Scand* 578(Suppl):41-47, 1975.

117. Koppe JG, Kloosterman GJ, and deRoerer-Bonnet H: Toxoplasmosis and pregnancy with long-term follow-up of the children, *Eur J Obstet Gynecol Reprod Biol* 43:101-110, 1974.

118. Krick JA and Remington JS: Toxoplasmosis in the adult—an overview, *N Engl J Med* 298:550-553, 1978.

119. Le Hoang P and others: Foscarnet in the treatment of cytomegalovirus retinitis in acquired immune deficiency syndrome, *Ophthalmology* 96:865-874, 1989.

120. Lietman PS: Clinical pharmacology: foscarnet, *Am J Med* 92(suppl 2A):8-11, 1992.

121. Liggett PE and others: Intraoperative argon endophotocoagulation for recurrent vitreous hemorrhage after vitrectomy for diabetic retinopathy, *Am J Ophthalmol* 103:146-149, 1987.

122. Lim SH, Heng LK, and Puvanendran K: Secondary syphilis presenting with optic perineuritis and uveitis, *Ann Acad Med* 19:413-415, 1990.

123. Lorentzen SE: Incidence of cilioretinal arteries, *Acta Ophthalmol* 48:518-524, 1970.

124. Manschot WA and Lee WR: Development of retinal neovascularisation in vascular occlusive disease, *Trans Ophthalmol Soc UK* 104:880-886, 1985.

125. Manschot WA and Lee WR: Retinal neovascularisation arising from hyalinised blood vessels, *Graefes Arch Clin Exp Ophthalmol* 222:63-70, 1984.

126. Masur H and others: Outbreak of toxoplasmosis in a family and documentation of acquired retinochoroiditis, *Am J Med* 64:396-402, 1978.

127. McCabe RE and Remington JS: *Toxoplasma gondii.* In Mandell GL, Douglas RG Jr, and Bennett JE, editors: *Principles and practice of infectious disease,* ed 2, New York, 1985, John Wiley & Sons.

128. McDonald HR and Schatz H: Grid photocoagulation for diffuse macular edema, *Retina* 5:65-72, 1985.

129. McMeel JW, Trempe CL and Franks EB: Diabetic maculopathy, *Trans Am Acad Ophthalmol Otolaryngol* 83:476-485, 1977.

130. McPhee SJ: Secondary syphilis: uncommon manifestations of a common disease, *West J Med* 140:35-42, 1984.

131. Messner LV: *Toxocariasis.* In Onofrey BE, editor: *Clinical optometric pharmacology and therapeutics,* Philadelphia, 1991, JB Lippincott Co.

132. Michaelson IC: The mode of development of the vascular system of the retina, with some observations on its significance for certain retinal disease, *Trans Ophthalmol Soc UK* 68:137-180, 1948.

133. Michels RG, Rice TA and Rice EF: Vitrectomy for diabetic vitreous hemorrhage, *Am J Ophthalmol* 95:12-21, 1983.

134. Miller NL, Frenkel JK, and Dubey JP: Oral infections with *Toxoplasma* cysts and oocysts in felines, other mammals, and in birds, *J Parasitol* 58:928-937, 1972.

135. Minturn J and Brown GC: Progression of nonischemic central retinal vein obstruction to the ischemic variant, *Ophthalmology* 93:1158-1162, 1986.

136. Molk R: Treatment of toxocaral optic neuritis, *J Clin Neuro-ophthalmol* 2:109-112, 1982.

137. North American Symptomatic Carotid Endarterectomy Trial Collaborators: Beneficial effect of carotid endarterectomy in symptomatic patients with high-grade carotid stenosis, *N Engl J Med* 325:445-453, 1991.

138. Obenauf CD and others: Sarcoidosis and its ophthalmic manifestations, *Am J Ophthalmol* 86:648-655, 1978.

139. Olk RJ: Modified grid argon (blue-green) laser photocoagulation for diffuse diabetic macular edema, *Ophthalmology* 93:938-950, 1986.

140. Oncel M, Peyman GA and Khoobehi B: Tissue plasminogen activator in the treatment of experimental retinal vein occlusion, *Retina* 9:1-7, 1989.

141. Orth DH and Patz A: Retinal branch vein occlusion, *Surv Ophthalmol* 22:357-376, 1978.

142. Palestine AG and others: Ophthalmic involvement in acquired immunodeficiency syndrome, *Ophthalmology* 91:1092-1099, 1984.

143. Passo MS and Rosenbaum JT: Ocular syphilis in patients with human immundeficiency virus infection, *Am J Ophthalmol* 106:1-6, 1988.

144. Pepose JS: Acute retinal necrosis syndrome. In Ryan SJ and others, editors: *Retina, vol 2, medical retina,* St. Louis, 1989, Mosby–Year Book.

145. Pepose JS: Cytomegalovirus infections of the retina. In Ryan SJ and others, editors: *Retina, vol 2, medical retina,* St. Louis, 1989, The CV Mosby Co.

146. Pepose JS and others: Acquired immune deficiency syndrome. Pathogenic mechanisms of ocular disease, Ophthalmology 92:472-484, 1985.

147. Perraut LE and Zimmerman LE: The occurrence of glaucoma following occlusion of the central retinal artery: a clinicopathologic report of six new cases with a review of the literature, *Arch Ophthalmol* 61:845-865, 1959.

148. Phillips CI and Mackenzie AD: Toxocaral larval papillitis, *Br Med J* 1:154-155, 1973.

149. Polis MA: Design of a randomized controlled trial of foscarnet in patients with cytomegalovirus retinitis associated with acquired immunodeficiency syndrome, *Am J Med* 92(suppl 2A):22-25, 1992.

150. Pulido JS, et al: Antiphospholipid antibodies associated with retinal vascular disease, *Retina* 7:215-218, 1987.

151. Quinlan P and Jabs DA: *Ocular toxoplasmosis.* In Ryan SJ and others, editors: *Retina, Vol 2, medical retina,* St. Louis, 1989, Mosby–Year Book.

152. Rahi AH and others: *What is endogenous uveitis?* In Silverstein AM and O'Connor GR, editors: *Immunology and immunopathology of the eye,* New York, 1979, Masson Publishing.

153. Rand LI and others: Multiple factors in the prediction of risk of proliferative diabetic retinopathy, *N Engl J Med* 313:1433-1438, 1985.

154. Reynolds ES, Walls KW and Pfeiffer RI: Generalized toxoplasmosis following renal transplantation: report of a case, *Arch Intern Med* 118:401-405, 1966.

155. Rice TA and Michels RG: Long-term anatomic and functional results of vitrectomy for diabetic retinopathy, *Am J Ophthalmol* 90:297-303, 1980.

156. Rice TA, Michels RG, and Rice EF: Vitrectomy for diabetic traction retinal detachment involving the macula, *Am J Ophthalmol* 95:22-33, 1983.

157. Richman DD and others: Rapid viral diagnosis, *J Infect Dis* 149:298-310, 1984.

158. Rosecan LR and others: Antiviral therapy for cytomegalovirus retinitis in AIDS with dihydroxy propoxymethyl guanine, *Am J Ophthalmol* 101:405-418, 1986.

159. Ross WH and Gottner MJ: Peripheral retinal cryopexy for subtotal vitreous hemorrhage, *Am J Ophthalmol* 105:377-382, 1988.

160. Ruskin J and Remington JS: Toxoplasmosis in the compromised host, *Ann Intern Med* 84:193-199, 1976.

161. Sacks JJ, Roberto RR and Brooks NF: Toxoplasmosis infection associated with raw goat's milk, *JAMA* 248:1728-1732, 1982.

162. Schlaegel TF and Kao SF: A review of 28 presumptive cases of syphilitic uveitis, *Am J Ophthalmol* 93:412-414, 1982.

163. Schuman JS and Friedman AH: Retinal manifestations of the acquired immune deficiency syndrome (AIDS): cytomegalovirus,

Candida albicans, cryptococcus, toxoplasmosis and *Pneumocystis carinii, Trans Ophthalmol Soc UK* 103:177-190, 1983.

164. Scott EH: New concepts in toxoplasmosis, *Surv Ophthalmol* 18:255-274, 1974.

165. Sebag J and McMeel JW: Diabetic retinopathy. Pathogenesis and the role of retina-derived growth factor in angiogenesis, *Surv Ophthalmol* 30:377-384, 1986.

166. Shah HG, Brown GC, and Goldberg RE: Digital subtraction carotid angiography and retinal artery obstruction, *Ophthalmology* 92:68-72, 1985.

167. Shepp DH and others: *Toxoplasma gondii* reactivation identified by detection of parasitemia in tissue culture, *Ann Intern Med* 103:218-221, 1985.

168. Shields JA: Ocular toxocariasis: a review, *Surv Ophthalmol* 28:361-381, 1984.

169. Shimada K, O'Connor GR and Yoneda C: Cyst formation by *Toxoplasma gondii* (RH strain) in vitro, *Arch Ophthalmol* 92:496-500, 1974.

170. Shoukrey N and Tabbara KF: *Eye related parasitic diseases.* In Tabbara KF and Hyndiuk RA, editors: *Infections of the eye,* Boston, 1986, Little, Brown & Co.

171. Silverstein AM, Welter S, and Zimmerman LB: A progressive immunization reaction in the actively sensitized rabbit eye, *J Immunol* 86:312-323, 1961.

172. Smith JL: Seronegative ocular and neurosyphilis, *J Clin Neuro-ophthalmol* 8:157-159, 1988.

173. Smith JL: Syphilis/lyme/AIDS, *J Clin Neuro-ophthalmol* 7:196-197, 1987.

174. Spoor TC and others: Ocular syphilis: acute and chronic, *J Clin Neuro-ophthalmol* 3:197-203, 1983.

175. Staab EV and McCartney WH: Role of gallium 67 in inflammatory disease, *Semin Nucl Med* 8:219-234, 1978.

176. Steahly LP: Sarcoidosis and peripheral neovascularization, *Ann Ophthalmol* 20:426-430, 1988.

177. Stoumbos VD and Klein ML: Syphilitic retinitis in a patient with acquired immundeficiency syndrome-related complex, *Am J Ophthalmol* 103:103-104, 1987.

178. Swartzberg JE and Remington JS: Transmission of *Toxoplasma, Am J Dis Child* 129:777-779, 1975.

179. Tabbara KF and O'Connor GR: Treatment of ocular toxoplasmosis with clindamycin and sulfadiazine, *Ophthalmology* 87:129-134, 1980.

180. Tabbara KF, Nozik RA and O'Connor GR: Clindamycin effects on experimental ocular toxoplasmosis in the rabbit, *Arch Ophthalmol* 92:244-247, 1974.

181. Teich SA, Orellana J, and Friedman AH: Prevalence, pathophysiology, and treatment of rhegmatogenous retinal detachment in treated cytomegalovirus retinitis (letter), *Am J Ophthalmol* 104:312-314, 1987.

182. Teutsch SM and others: Epidemic toxoplasmosis associated with infected cats, *N Engl J Med* 300:695-699, 1979.

183. Thompson JF and others: Results and prognostic factors in vitrectomy for diabetic vitreous hemorrhage, *Arch Ophthalmol* 105:191-195, 1987.

184. Thompson JF and others: Results of vitrectomy for proliferative diabetic retinopathy, *Ophthalmology* 93:1571-1573, 1986.

185. Trobe JD: Carotid endarterectomy. Who needs it? *Ophthalmology* 94:725-730, 1987.

186. Urayama A and others: Unilateral acute uveitis with periarteritis and detachment, *Jpn J Clin Ophthalmol* 25:607-619, 1971.

187. Vietzke WM and others: Toxoplasmosis complicating malignancy: experience at the National Cancer Institute, *Cancer* 21:816-827, 1968.

188. Visser OHE and Bos PJM: Kaposi's sarcoma of the conjunctiva and CMV-related retinitis in AIDS, *Doc Ophthalmol* 64:77-85, 1986.

189. Wang CL and others: Retinal neovascularization associated with acute retinal necrosis, *Retina* 3:249-252, 1983.

190. Weinreb RN and Tessler H: Laboratory diagnosis of ophthalmic sarcoidosis, *Surv Ophthalmol* 28:653-664, 1984.

191. Weller TH: The cytomegalovirus: ubiquitious agents with protean clinical manifestations, *N Engl J Med* 285:203-214, 267-274, 1971.

192. West KM, Erdreich LJ, and Stober JA: A detailed study of risk factors for retinopathy and nephropathy in diabetes, *Diabetes* 29:501-508, 1980.

193. Willerson D Jr, Aaberg TM, and Reeser FH: Necrotizing vaso-occlusive retinitis, *Am J Ophthalmol* 84:209-219, 1977.

194. Wilson CB, Remington JS, Stagno S, et al: Development of adverse sequelae in children born with subclinical congenital *Toxoplasma* infection, *Pediatrics* 66:767-774, 1980.

195. Wilson DJ and Green R: Argon laser panretinal photocoagulation for diabetic retinopathy, *Arch Ophthalmol* 105:239-242, 1987.

196. Young NJA and Bird AC: Bilateral acute retinal necrosis, *Br J Ophthalmol* 62:581-590, 1978.

APPENDIX A

Injection Techniques Specifically Tailored for the Optometrist

JANICE L. GLASS

*I*njectable drugs can be administered in several ways; the two routes that are emphasized here are the subcutaneous (SQ) route and the intramuscular (IM) route. The time for an injectable medication to take effect can vary from seconds to longer than 30 minutes by the purposeful choice of the drug, dosage, and route of administration. Although this control is a distinct advantage of the parenteral technique, injections are the most hazardous way to administer a drug. Exercising caution and maintaining proper technique prevent infection and avoid damage to the patient's nerves, blood vessels, tissues, and bones.

Note: Injections are potentially dangerous techniques that should be attempted by the optometrist only after receiving advanced training and appropriate certification.

THE SUBCUTANEOUS ROUTE

Use. The SQ route is used to deliver a dose of epinephrine to mitigate an allergic reaction; epinephrine is effective in this instance when given by the SQ route. Owing to its high potency, epi-

nephrine given IM could cause life-threatening arrhythmias and hypertension.

Contraindications. To prevent damage to subcutaneous tissue, drugs that are irritating, oil-based, or concentrated are given by the IM route. Mistakenly giving one of these solutions by the SQ route could cause tissue extravasation, necrosis, abscess, or tissue ischemia.

Subcutaneous Sites. An injection into SQ tissue is usually best done at a site where there are no blood vessels, bones, or nerve endings near the surface. Frequently used sites are the flabby tissue above the elbow of the upper arm, the fat pad of the lower abdomen, the thighs, and the hips (Figs. A1, A2, A3, and A4).

Subcutaneous Needle. Choose a 25- to 27-gauge, ⅝-inch needle with a 3-ml syringe or a tuberculin syringe. The volume range for SQ injections is 0.1 ml to 1.0 ml.

Onset and Duration of Action. Onset is in minutes (as in the case of epinephrine) to hours (as in some types of insulin and heparin). The duration of action is hours to weeks.

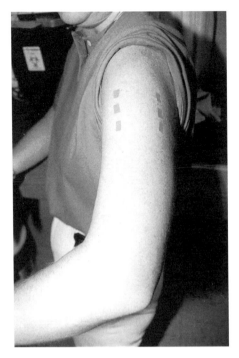

FIG. A1 SQ sites of arm.

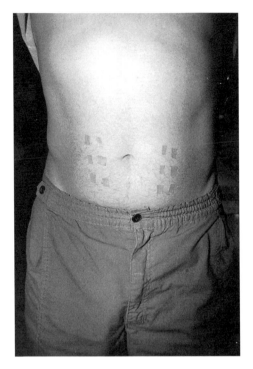

FIG. A2 SQ sites of abdomen.

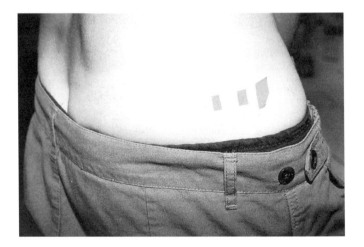

FIG. A3 SQ sites of hip.

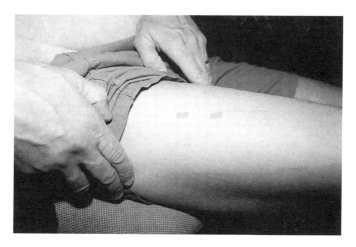

FIG. A4 SQ sites of thigh.

Administration by Subcutaneous Injection

STEP 1: Obtain equipment and medication. Assemble syringe and needle according to manfacturer's instruction if necessary. Today, most are preassembled and sterilized.

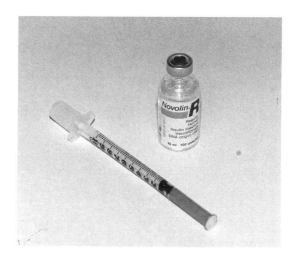

STEP 2: Withdraw the drug by inverting the vial and pulling back on the plunger to the desired dose at eye level. Withdraw needle from vial and depress plunger to remove air from barrel.

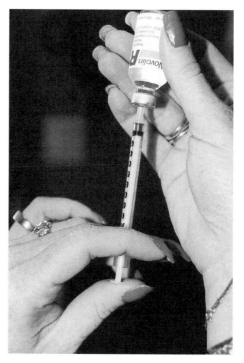

STEP 3: Select the site. Pinch at least a 1-inch fat fold. Select whatever angle permits the needle to reach the tissue between the muscle and the fat.

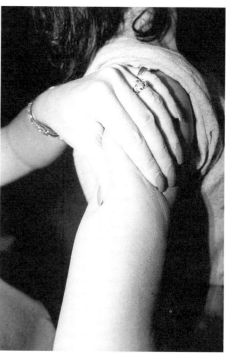

STEP 4: Cleanse the skin area in a circular, outward motion with an alcohol swab and let air dry.

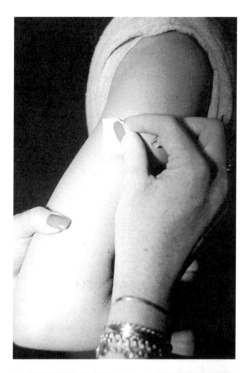

STEP 5: Insert the needle quickly with a dartlike motion (it is not necessary to aspirate) at a 45- to 90-degree angle.

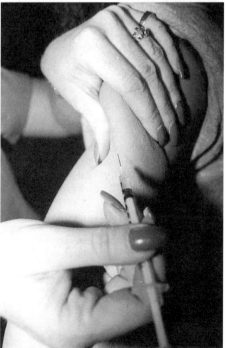

STEP 6: Inject the drug slowly and withdraw the needle. If there is bleeding, apply gentle pressure with a dry, sterile sponge. Do not massage the site.

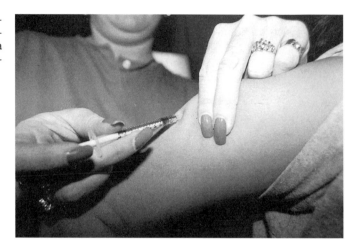

THE INTRAMUSCULAR ROUTE

The IM route is used when one is delivering a larger volume of drug than with the SQ route, when giving an irritating drug, or when a more rapid onset is needed. Absorption into the bloodstream is faster than with the SQ route owing to the greater blood supply to the muscles.

Complications from IM injections include necrosis, skin sloughing, abscesses, nerve injury, and persistent pain. To safely administer an IM injection, the site chosen should not be near large blood vessels and large nerves.

Intramuscular Sites

The ventrogluteal (gluteus medius and minimus) site has dense muscles and no major blood vessels or nerves.

The dorsogluteal (gluteus maximus) site is the most dangerous. An injection too close to the buttocks crease could puncture the superior gluteal artery and damage the sciatic nerve permanently. However, this is a common site of injection. To locate the proper area, picture a cross superimposed on the right gluteus maximus with the intersection of the horizontal and vertical lines located in the center of the right cheek. The only safe area for an IM injection in the dorsogluteal site is in the superior lateral box formed by the cross.

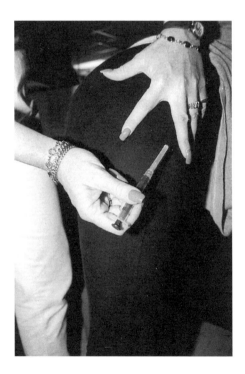

The vastus lateralis (outer mid-thigh) site has no major arteries or blood vessels. It is easily located but can be painful owing to the large number of nerve endings in the muscle. It is often used in children.

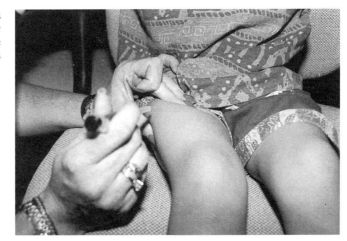

The deltoid site is easily accessible but is a small muscle; therefore no more than 2 ml of medication can be given in one injection. You may give up to 2 ml of medication in each arm if necessary.

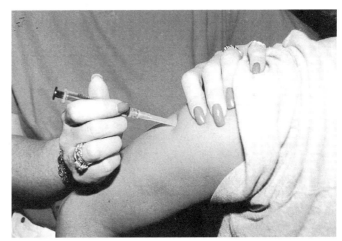

The Needle. Choose a 22- to 25-gauge, 1.5-inch needle for the deltoid. Choose a 20- to 23-gauge, 1.5- to 3-inch needle for the dorsogluteal, ventrogluteal, and vastus lateralis sites. For children, use the vastus lateralis site with a 23- to 26-gauge, 1.5-inch needle.

Onset and Duration of Action. Onset is less than 1 hour, and the duration is hours to weeks.

Administration by Intramuscular Route

STEP 1: Obtain equipment and medication.

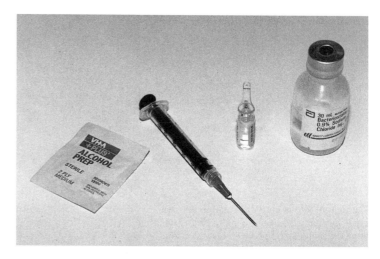

STEP 2: Withdraw the drug by inverting the vial and injecting a small amount of air into the vial. Pull back on the plunger to the desired dose at eye level.

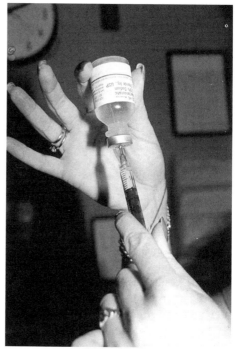

STEP 3: If breaking an ampule, first flick the solution into the bottom.

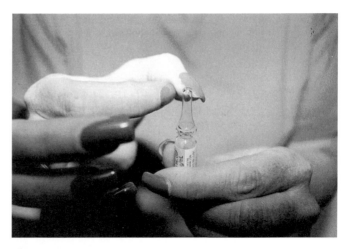

STEP 4: Using an alcohol swab or 2 × 2-inch gauze pad, break the ampule at the neck and withdraw the medication.

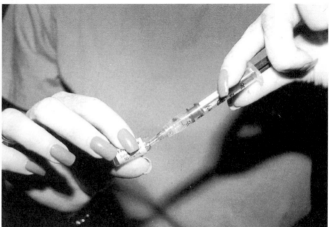

STEP 5: Select the site. Cleanse the site in a circular outward motion with an alcohol swab; let dry.

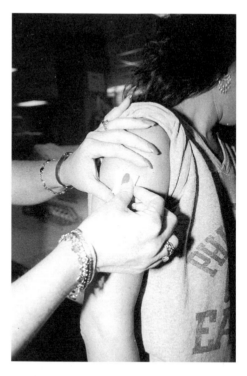

STEP 6: With your nondominant hand, stretch the skin taut with your thumb and index finger.

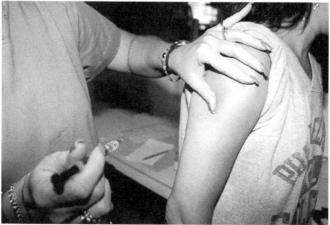

STEP 7: With your dominant hand, insert the needle quickly at a 90-degree angle with a dartlike motion.

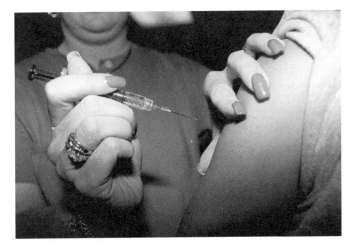

STEP 8: Aspirate the plunger by pulling back on its handle. If blood is present, withdraw the syringe and start again because you have entered a blood vessel.

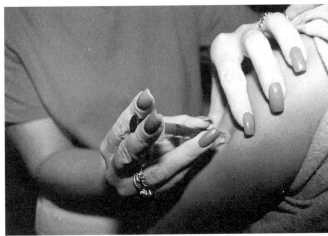

STEP 9: If no blood is present, inject the medication. Then slowly withdraw the needle at the same angle you inserted it.

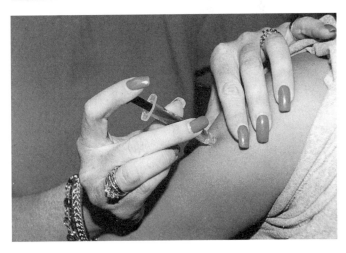

STEP 10: Apply pressure with a sterile sponge. Massaging the site is not necessary.

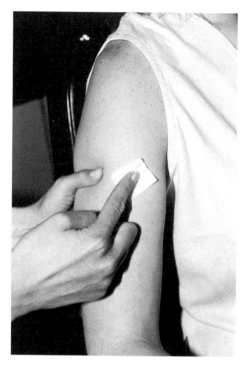

STEP 11: Dispose of all needles in a proper container.

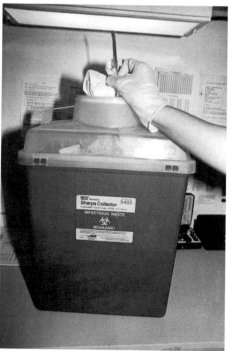

Bibliography

Hahn K: Brush up on your injection technique, *Nursing 90,* 20:54, 1990.

Newton M, Newton D, and Fudin J: Mastering the big three injection routes, Nursing *92,* 22:34, 1992.

Wolfe L, Weitzel MH, and Fuerst EV: *Fundamentals of nursing,* ed 6, Philadelphia, 1979, JB Lippincott Co.

Video Recording Techniques for the Optometric Examination

BRUCE G. MUCHNICK

Video documentation of ocular pathology imaged through a biomicroscope has the advantage of high-resolution, real-time motion picture recording combined with the low cost and easy storage of videotapes. Unfortunately, most video slit-lamp apparatuses are prohibitively expensive, and the camera usually can be used only for the filming of biomicroscopic views and not for home use.

Described below is an easy and inexpensive technique for video recording slit-lamp images with any biomicroscope and any home video camera. The technique does not rely on special video cameras and does not require any camera-to-biomicroscope attachment. Disadvantages of this technique include the inability to reduce magnification power below $30\times$ in order to film low-power views, the need to use one hand to hold the camera and the other hand to manipulate the slit-lamp (making hands-on procedures difficult to videotape), and the need to view through the camera monitor and not the slit-lamp ocular.

In spite of these disadvantages, this technique provides an inexpensive way to film sharp and colorful videos of most internal and external ocular structures and pathology. (Note: Before videotaping, written permission to film should be obtained from the patient.)

DESCRIPTION OF METHOD

Prepare Camera

STEP 1: Load videotape. If video camera has a screw mount, screw in a skylight or ultraviolet filter in front of camera lens to prevent the slit-lamp ocular from scratching the camera lens.

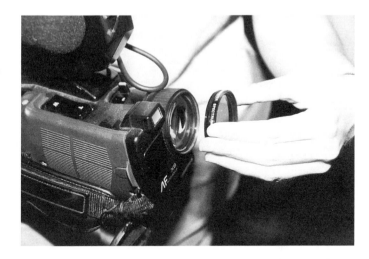

STEP 2: Set video camera focus system to manual focus if possible. (Automatic focusing units may turn the camera lens as it touches the slit-lamp ocular, causing scratching of the lens.)

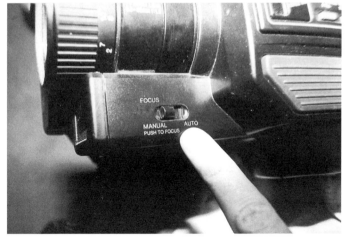

STEP 3: Set zoom lens of camera on lowest power (widest field).

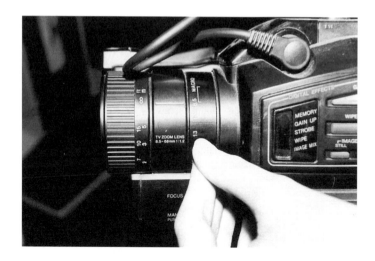

Prepare Biomicroscope

STEP 4: Position patient comfortably into slit-lamp chin and head-rest. Set illumination system on moderate brightness with slit-beam wide open (full field illumination).

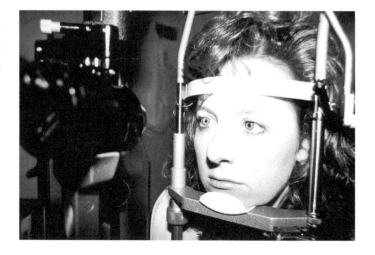

STEP 5: Magnification should be on lowest setting. Fold back rubber eyeguard around slit-lamp ocular. With joystick focus on area of eye to be filmed.

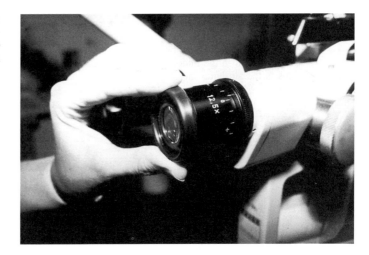

Videotaping

STEP 6: Once area to be filmed is centered in the slit-lamp eyepiece, position the video camera lens in direct alignment with the visual axis of the slit-lamp ocular. Lightly touch the camera lens (or skylight filter) against the slit-lamp eyepiece (or rubber guard).

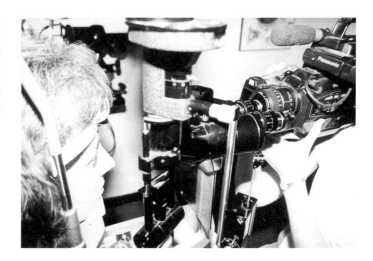

STEP 7: Look into the camera monitor (viewfinder). Move camera around slightly until you see a small, white, overexposed, and blurry patch of light in the middle of a black field (this is the slit-lamp image of the patient's eye).

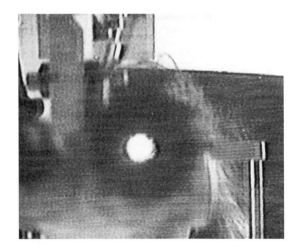

STEP 8: Zoom into that image using the camera's telephoto lens system. As you zoom in, the blurry image becomes larger until it fills the camera monitor.

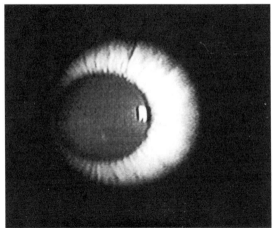

STEP 9: Focus the image in the camera monitor with the slit-lamp joystick. Total magnification is the power of the slit-lamp multiplied by the camera telephoto power.

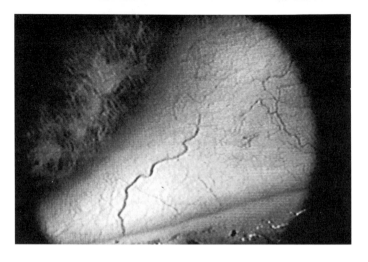

STEP 10: Press record button and begin videotaping the slit-lamp image. Increased power is obtained by zooming to higher powers with the video camera or by increasing power on the slit lamp. Higher magnification necessitates higher illumination.

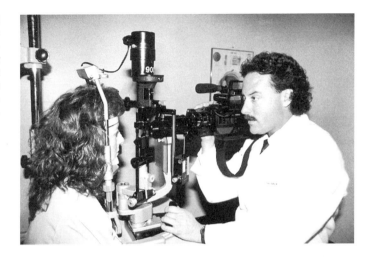

STEP 11: Once the camera is held steady with one hand, the examiner's other hand is free to hold open the patient's lid or hold a biomicroscope lens.

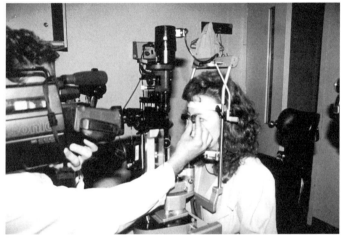

Index